ELECTRON SPIN RESONANCE

A Comprehensive Treatise
on Experimental Techniques

BOOKS EDITED BY THE AUTHOR

The author has edited the English language editions of the following Russian books:

Electron Paramagnetic Resonance, S. A. Al'tshuler and B. M. Kozyrev, translated by Scripta Technica, Academic Press, New York, 1964.

Diamagnetism and the Chemical Bond, Ya. G. Dorfman, translated by Scripta Technica, Academic Press, New York, 1965.

Spectroscopic Analysis of Gaseous Mixtures, O. P. Bochkova and E. Ya. Schreyder, translated by Scripta Technica, Academic Press, New York, 1965.

The Theory of Nuclear Magnetic Resonance, I. V. Aleksandrov, translated by Scripta Technica, Edward Arnold, London, 1966.

The Chemical Bond in Semiconductors and Solids, N. N. Sirota, Ed., translated by Consultants Bureau, Plenum Press, New York, in press.

Figures 4–9, 4–10, 4–11, 4–15, 8–11, and 8–15 are reprinted from *Principles of Radar*, by Reintjes and Coate, by permission of The M.I.T. Press.

Figure 14–27 is reprinted from the article "Junction-Diode Amplifiers," by A. Uhlir, Jr., by permission of *Scientific American*.

CHEMISTRY

Printed in the United States of America

Electron Spin Resonance

A Comprehensive Treatise on Experimental Techniques

CHARLES P. POOLE, Jr.

DEPARTMENT OF PHYSICS
UNIVERSITY OF SOUTH CAROLINA
COLUMBIA, SOUTH CAROLINA

1967

INTERSCIENCE PUBLISHERS

a division of John Wiley & Sons

New York · London · Sydney

TO MY MOTHER AND FATHER

Preface

The field of electron spin resonance (ESR) was founded about twenty years ago. It has experienced a continuous growth since then, and is now expanding more rapidly than ever before. During the first ten years of its existence, the experimental techniques and the theoretical superstructure were developed to the point where extensive summaries of the field became necessary, and books on this subject made their appearance. Several of these books included excellent summaries of the experimental techniques in one or more introductory chapters. However, the main purpose of each volume was the presentation of the theory and experimental results. Those who wished to build entire spectrometers or elaborate auxiliary equipment found it necessary to consult the literature for the required information. In addition, expositions of the mechanics of recording spectra and obtaining data therefrom took a secondary place to the explication of data interpretation. During the past ten years the literature has continued to proliferate. The existing experimental techniques are being continuously refined, and occasionally new ones are introduced. As a result, the research worker who is interested in instrumentation has been forced to rely upon the journal literature.

This book was written in the belief that an overall summary and bibliography of ESR experimental techniques has been long overdue. It is an attempt to present a balanced treatment of both the theoretical and the practical aspects of the instrumentation. Although the presentation is in no sense historical, nevertheless some space has been reserved for the early apparatus which was built by the pioneers, and used to carry out the definitive experiments in ESR. Much of the discussion is devoted to the exposition of general principles which underlie ESR instrumentation, such as electromagnetic theory and the mechanism of magnetic field modulation. The *MIT Radiation Laboratory Series* (*RLS*) is extensively paraphrased. Recent developments such as enhancement techniques, helices, and acoustic spin resonance are covered. Thus this book is an attempt to present the general background material, the basic principles, and the main applications of ESR experimental techniques. It endeavors to show the reader how to design, build, and use an ESR spectrometer.

At the present time, scientists from many diverse disciplines such as physics, chemistry, biology, and medicine carry out ESR research. They approach the subject with a variety of backgrounds in mathematics, electronics, ship experience, etc. Therefore, to properly achieve the above objectives, it has been necessary to write for several disparate audiences. Some sections are of a theoretical nature, and will be of greatest interest to physicists. Other sections are of a more descriptive nature, and are written for those who are more interested in the qualitative results of the theory, or in the design details of a specific component. Numerous cross references and a minimum of presuppositions in each chapter should enable the reader to garner much information from the latter chapters without a prior reading of the earlier ones. The last paragraph of Sec. 1-A discusses the interrelationship between the subject matter in the various chapters. In terms of relative mathematical sophistication the chapters might be classified in difficult (Chaps. 2–5, 8, 10, 14, and 20), average (12, 13, 18, and 19), and easy (1, 6, 7, 9, 11, 15–17, and 21) groups.

This volume is intended mainly as a general reference book. However, the use of ESR spectrometers has become so widespread that many university departments will be interested in including some instrumentation instruction in their curriculum. A biennial special topics course in ESR instrumentation will greatly benefit those university departments which have active programs in the field. For this purpose one might wish to cover the first four introductory chapters and various sections in Chaps. 6–12. Extra time might be spent on the subject matter in Chap. 14 since this brings into focus much of the material covered earlier. Chapters 18–20 might be discussed next, and the course concluded with selected topics from Chaps. 13 and 15–17. The material in Chap. 5 constitutes good supplementary reading for the better students. The author taught such a course from this volume during the fall semester of 1965 at the University of South Carolina. Those professors who now teach a general introduction to magnetic resonance might consider the inclusion in the courses of material from Chaps. 1, 8, 10, 14, and 18–21, with an emphasis on Chaps. 14 and 20.

The principal references for each subject are arranged alphabetically by author at the end of the appropriate chapter. The literature is covered through most of 1965. *Physics Abstracts* was found to be an excellent source of references. Since this is an experimental techniques book, the following abbreviations were used for the principal instrumentation journals:

ETP   *Experimentelle Technik der Physik*

JSI   *Journal of Scientific Instruments*

PTE   *Pribory i Tekhnika Eksperimenta* [English trans.: *Instruments and Experimental Techniques*] This journal resembles the *Journal of the Chemical Society* in its inconvenient lack of volume numbers.

RSI   *Review of Scientific Instruments*

All the references are given in the standard form. The references to *Paramagnetic Resonance (1963)* refer to the *Proceedings of the 1962 Jerusalem Conference* edited by W. Low. When the page number is known in the English translation of a foreign language journal, such as *PTE*, it is often inserted in parentheses between original page and the year.

Parts of Chaps. 1, 18, and 20 originally appeared in an unpublished report, "The Dance of the Nucleons," written at the University of Maryland in 1957.

This book concerns electron spin resonance or ESR. This branch of science has several equivalent names. In the older literature, the field was often referred to as paramagnetic resonance, and some authors still use this name. A large number of contemporary scientists refer to the field as electron paramagnetic resonance or EPR. Several other names have appeared on occasion. The present author has adopted the name ESR more or less out of personal taste. *De gustibus non est disputandum.*

Many treatises on electromagnetic theory make use of the Meter-Kilometer-Second or MKS system of units, while most of the published ESR literature is written in the centimeter-gram-second or cgs system. We have adopted the MKS system for the introductory Chaps. 2–5 and also for much of Chaps. 8, 9, and 14 since these treat electromagnetic theory. We would have preferred to write the entire book using MKS units, but it seemed too much at variance with the generally accepted notation. Accordingly, cgs units appear throughout much of the remainder of the book. It is believed that very little confusion will result from this arrangement. Some of the principal units merely require powers of ten for their conversion (e.g., webers/meter^2 $\longleftrightarrow$ gauss, joule $\longleftrightarrow$ erg, meter $\longleftrightarrow$ centimeter, kilogram $\longleftrightarrow$ gram, and the Bohr magneton units joule meter^2/weber $\longleftrightarrow$ erg/gauss). Appendix A presents the principal equations in each system of units, and lists the main conversion factors. In other ways we have followed a uniform system of nomenclature throughout the book in conformity with the list of symbols found on p. xxi. Chapter 13 constitutes an exception because therein we present block diagrams of typical spectrometers in their original form. This serves to introduce the reader to the divergent notation that he will encounter throughout the literature. The unit of length, inch (1 in. = 2.54 cm) appears occasionally in the text.

In the preparation of this volume I have benefited greatly from the encouragement and criticism of my colleagues and students. Especial appreciation is due to O. F. Griffith III for reading the entire manuscript and to D. A. Giardino and T. C. Sayetta for reading close to half of the text in manuscript form. Their critiques were very valuable. The following read particular chapters and offered helpful comments: W. E. Barr, R. L. Childers, C. W. Darden III, R. D. Edge, W. R. Ferris, R. G. Fellers, F. H. Giles, Jr., T. J. Hardwick, J. S. Hyde, J. F. Itzel, W. K. Jackson, Jr., E. R. Jones, Jr., R. P. Kohin, S. Kumar, E. C. Lerner, E. E. Mercer, D. E. O'Reilly, G. S. Painter, O. F. Schuette, J. C. Schug, J. E. Sees, J. R. Singer, M. P. Stombler, E. F. Strother, J. Taylor, H. H. Tobin, and T. G. Weismann. Miss Elizabeth Obear kindly checked the accuracy of the long lists of references.

I wish to thank many colleagues and the following corporations, journals, and publishing houses for granting their permission to reproduce a number of their figures: Academic Press, American Chemical Society, American Institute of Physics, *Arch. Sci.*, Bell Telephone Laboratories, Cambridge University Press, Central Scientific Co.,

Cornell University Press, Eastman Kodak, Faraday Society, Institute of Electronics and Electrical Engineers, Institute of Physics, Instruments Publishing Co., McGraw-Hill, National Research Council of Canada, Pergamon Press, Physical Society, Physical Society of Japan, Radio Corp. of America. Reinhold Publishing Corp., Royal Society of London, Societé Française de Physique, Springer-Verlag, Taylor and Francis, Ltd., Technology Press MIT, Van Nostrand, Varian Assoc., VEB Deutscher Verlag, der Wissenschaften, Verlag Birkhäuser, and Z. *Naturforschung.*

In addition, thanks are due to the Gulf Research and Development Company for the drafting on some of the figures. Reprints sent to me by numerous colleagues were of inestimable value in the preparation of this volume. Please continue to send me reprints of your current work.

I wish to express my appreciation to my wife, Kathleen, for her diligent typing of the first draft of the manuscript, and to my daughter Elizabeth whose birth during this period did not unduly delay the proceedings. I wish to thank the members of the secretarial staff here at the Physics Department of USC, Miss Patricia Acton, Mrs. Teresa Horton, Mrs. Jean Josey, and Mrs. Jean Padgett for their painstaking typing of the second draft and its revisions. Their patience with my cacography is certainly appreciated.

CHARLES P. POOLE, JR.

Columbia, South Carolina

Contents

Greek Symbols

α	Attenuation constant
α_ϵ	Attenuation constant due to dielectric losses
α_M	Mass absorption coefficient
α_R	Attenuation constant due to conductor losses
β	Bohr magneton; cavity coupling coefficient; current sensitivity of a crystal detector; feedback ratio; phase constant
β_N	Nuclear magneton
Γ	Reflection coefficient
γ	Gyromagnetic ratio; propagation constant ($\alpha + j\beta$)
Δ	Weiss constant; hyperfine structure anomaly
δ	Deviation ratio (in FM); skin depth
ϵ	Dielectric constant; extinction coefficient
ϵcd	Optical density
ϵ'	Real part of dielectric constant
ϵ''	Imaginary part of dielectric constant
ϵ_0	Dielecrric constant of free space
$\hat{\theta}$	Unit vector in θ direction
θ_i	Temperature of ith spin system (used only in Sec. 18-A)
θ_p	Brewster or polarizing angle
Λ	Shape constant of absorption curve
Λ'	Shape constant of absorption derivative
λ	Spin orbit coupling constant; wavelength
λ_c	Cutoff wavelength
λ_g	Guide wavelength
μ	Amplification factor of vacuum tube; magnetic moment
μ_c	Electric moment
μ	Permeability
μ_0	Permeability of free space
ν	Frequency
Π_i	Formation of a product
π	3.14159
ρ	Charge density; electron density; mass density; resistivity

σ	Electrical conductivity
$\tau_{1/2}$	Time to scan between half power points
τ_0	Response time
$\hat{\varphi}$	Unit vector in φ direction
Φ	Scalar potential
ϕ	Magnetic flux
χ	Magnetic susceptibility
χ'	Real part of magnetic susceptibility
χ''	Imaginary part of magnetic susceptibility
χ_e	Electric susceptibility
χ_0	Static magnetic susceptibility
ψ	Wave function
Ω	Ohm
ω	Angular frequency $(2\pi f, 2\pi \nu)$
ω_0	Resonant frequency

Roman Symbols

A	Area; incident wave amplitude; acetonitrile
A, A_i	Hyperfine coupling constant
A_N	Hyperfine coupling constant of nitrogen
A_p	Hyperfine coupling constant of proton
A	Vector potential
α	Attenuation
AM	Amplitude modulation
ATR	Anti-transmit-receive (tubes); attenuated total reflectance
af	Audio frequency
AFC	Automatic frequency control
At	Ampere turn
B	Reflected wave amplitude; susceptance; noise bandwidth
B	Magnetic induction or magnetic flux density
bcc	Body centered cubic
BeV	Billion electron volt
C	Coulomb
C	Capacitance
c	Concentration; velocity of light *in vacuo*; curie
cgs	Centimeter-gram-second (system of units)
CRO	(Cathode ray) oscilloscope
cw	Continuous wave
D	Detectability; multiplicity factor; zero field splitting for axial symmetry
D	Electric displacement (electric flux density)
dc	Direct current; zero frequency (analogical use)
DME	Dimethoxyethane
DMF	Dimethylformamide
DMSO	Dimethylsulfoxide
dN	Noise power
DPPH	α,α'-Diphenyl-β-picryl hydrazyl
E	Zero field splitting for lower than axial symmetry

E_i	Crystal field energy
E_m	Maximum value of electric field **E**
E	Electric field
ENDOR	Electron nuclear double resonance
ESR	Electron spin resonance
e	Charge of electron
emf	Electromotive force
EPR	Electron paramagnetic resonance
eV	Electron volt
F	Force; noise figure
F_{amp}	Amplifier noise figure
F_K	Klystron noise figure
FM	Frequency modulation
f	Frequency
f_c	Cutoff frequency
f_{mod}	Modulation frequency
fcc	Face centered cubic
G	Gauss
G	Conductance; gain
Gc	Gigacycle (10^3 Mc $= 1$ Gc)
GeV	Gigaelectron volt (10^9 eV)
g	Spectroscopic splitting factor or g factor
H	Henry
H	Magnetic field strength
H_1	rf magnetic field
H_m	Maximum value of magnetic field H
H_t	Magnetic field tangential to surface
$\mathcal{3C}_N$	Nuclear spin energy (Hamiltonian)
$\mathcal{3C}_Q$	Quadrupole energy (Hamiltonian)
$\mathcal{3C}_{CF}$	Crystal field energy (Hamiltonian)
$\mathcal{3C}_{elect}$	Electronic energy (Hamiltonian)
$\mathcal{3C}_{hfs}$	Hyperfine structure energy (Hamiltonian)
$\mathcal{3C}_{LS}$	Spin orbit energy (Hamiltonian)
$\mathcal{3C}_{SS}$	Spin-spin energy (Hamiltonian)
$\mathcal{3C}_{Zee}$	Zeeman energy (Hamiltonian)
h	Planck's constant
$\hbar$	$h/2\pi$
hfs	Hyperfine structure
I	Electric current; nuclear spin

Im	Imaginary part of
ir	Infrared
J	Exchange integral
J_m	mth order Bessel function
J	Electron current density; total angular momentum $(\mathbf{J} = \mathbf{L} + \mathbf{S})$
JSI	*Journal of Scientific Instruments*
j	$(-1)^{1/2}$
K	A constant [e.g., eq. (1-G-31)]; voltage gain scans feedback
k	Boltzmann's constant
kc	Kilocycles $\sec^{-1}$
keV	Kiloelectron volt
kK	Kilokaiser (1000 cm^{-1})
L	Conversion loss; inductance; insertion loss; load (subscript)
L	Orbital angular momentum
LET	Linear energy transfer
LO	Local oscillator
l	Length
lf	Low frequency
M	Figure of merit of a crystal detector; magnetization
M_I, m_i	Projection of nuclear spin I along magnetic field direction
Mc	Megacycle $\sec^{-1}$
MeV	Million electron volt
MKS	Meter-Kilometer-Second (system of units)
m	Meter
m	Mass (of electron); modulation index
mmf	Magnetomotive force
N	Noise power (also dN); number of spins
N_{hfs}	Number of hyperfine components
NBS	National Bureau of Standards
NMR	Nuclear magnetic resonance
Np/m	Nepers per meter
n	Index of refraction; transformer turns ratio
n_i	Number of hyperfine components; population of ith energy level
P	Polarization; power
P_B	Bucking power

P_c	Power in cavity
P_w	Power in waveguide
P	Poynting vector
$\mathcal{P}$	Parity operator
PMR	Paramagnetic resonance
PTE	*Pribory i Tekhniki Exsperimenta*
ppm	Parts per million
Q	A constant in eqs. (1-G-28) and (1-G-31); electric charge; quality factor
Q_L	Loaded Q
Q_x	"Sample" Q
Q	Quadrupole moment (electric)
q	Electric charge
q_i	Excess charge density
R	Resistance
R_c	Cavity resistance
R_{dc}	dc resistance (video resistance)
R_g	Generator resistance
R_s	Surface resistivity
$\mathcal{R}$	Reluctance
RBE	Relative biological effectiveness
rd	Rutherford
Re	Real part of
RSI	*Review of Scientific Instruments*
r	Normalized resistance R/Z_0; radius; reflected (subscript); ripple factor
$\hat{\mathbf{r}}$	Unit vector in r direction
rf	radio frequency
rms	Root mean square
S	Area of surface; signal power; stabilization factor; slowing factor
S	Spin angular momentum
SCE	Saturated calomel electrode
T	Temperature
T_1	Spin-lattice (longitudinal) relaxation time
T_2	Spin-spin (transverse) relaxation time
T_d	Detector temperature
T_s	Sample temperature
T_x	Exchange relaxation time; $T_x{}^{ij}$

TE	Transverse electric
TEM	Transverse electromagnetic
TM	Transverse magnetic
TMAI	Tetramethylammoniumiodide
TNBAP	Tetra-n-butylammoniumperchlorate
TNPAP	Tetra-n-propylammoniumperchlorate
TR	Transmit-receive (microwave tube)
t	Noise temperature; time; transmitted (subscript)
U	Energy; energy density
U_E	Energy stored in electric fields
U_H	Energy stored in magnetic fields
uhf	Ultra high frequency
uv	Ultraviolet
V	Crystal field potential; potential due to electric (multipole) moment; voltage
V_c	Resonant cavity volume
V_e	Potential due to electric (multipole) moment
V_w	Volume of waveguide $\frac{1}{2}\ g$ long
$\mathbf{V}$	Vector
VSWR	Voltage standing wave ratio
v	Velocity
v_g	Group velocity
v_p	Phase velocity
Wb	Weber
WWV	NBS radio station
X	Reactance
x	Normalized reactance X/Z_0
$\hat{x}$	Unit vector in x direction
Y	Admittance; ESR amplitude or line shape; signal-to-noise ratio
$Y_l{}^m$	Spherical harmonic
Y_0	Characteristic admittance
YIG	Yttrium iron garnet
$\hat{y}$	Unit vector in y direction
Z	Impedance

CHAPTER 1

Introduction

A. Historical Background

In 1934, Cleeton and Williams constructed a primitive microwave spectrometer and detected the inversion of the ammonia molecule. Two years later Gorter (1936) attempted to detect nuclear magnetic resonance in solids by observing an increase in temperature, and he showed remarkable insight by attributing the negative result of his experiment to a long spin-lattice relaxation time ($T_1 > 10^{-2}$ sec). Both groups were severely hampered in their studies by the limitations of the available experimental equipment. During the 1930's the state of the art had not developed sufficiently to provide the components that are required for constructing magnetic resonance or microwave spectrometers. As a result these fields remained inactive until the middle of the next decade.

During World War II a great deal of research was carried out in the development of radar. The technical problems which were solved by those engaged in this work included (*1*) the development of high power microwave generators called magnetrons to produce the radar signal, (*2*) the design of highly directional antennae to transmit the signal and receive the echo, (*3*) the construction of sensitive (crystal) detectors to detect the echo, (*4*) the development of electronic methods for distinguishing the echo from the transmitted signal and for determining the distance of the target by the time delay of the echo after the transmitted pulse, (*5*) the perfection of narrow band amplifiers, lock-in detectors and other noise-reducing circuits to increase the sensitivity of the radar system, and (*6*) the design of data display systems such as special oscilloscope arrangements. The wartime effort included fundamental studies of new fields of science such as microwave engineering and semiconductor devices in addition to the design of hardware.

At the close of the war, microwave and electronic technology had advanced to the point where electron spin resonance and microwave spectrometers could be constructed with the required sensitivity and resolution. Bleaney and Penrose (1946) and Good (1946) carried out more detailed microwave absorption studies on the ammonia molecule while Zavoisky (1945) and Cummerow and Halliday (1946) detected electron spin resonance absorption in solids, and Griffiths (1946) observed ferromagnetic resonance. At the same time, Bloch (1946), Bloch, Hansen, and Packard (1946), Purcell (1946), Purcell, Bloembergen, and Pound (1946), and Purcell, Torrey, and Pound (1946) founded the field of nuclear magnetic resonance. During the past twenty years these fields of research have grown tremendously, and their publications to date are numbered in the thousands.

At the close of the war some of the principal scientists who directed and carried out the radar research at the Radiation Laboratory of the Massachusetts Institute of Technology collected and recorded the results of the concentrated radar research in twenty-eight volumes called the *Radiation Laboratory Series* (*RLS*). These are listed at the end of Chap. 4. Almost twenty years later these volumes still constitute the principal source for solving microwave engineering problems, and they are widely used by workers in the fields of electron spin resonance and microwave spectroscopy. The basic problem in radar is the generation of very high power microwave pulses, and the detection of a very, very weak microwave echo signal. The fundamental problem in electron spin resonance, on the other hand, is the production of continuous (CW) intermediate power microwaves and the detection of a very small change in this power level. Despite this basic difference, most of the components which enter into the construction of a modern ESR spectrometer have their origin in the *Radiation Laboratory Series*.

During the past two decades a large number of spectrometers have been constructed at various universities and research laboratories, and described in the literature. In addition, several commercial models are on the market. Various types of auxiliary equipment have been designed for variable temperature investigations, high pressure work, irradiation studies, sample pretreatments, etc. Nuclear magnetic resonance, optical absorption (pumping), and acoustic (ultrasonic) absorption experiments were combined with electron spin resonance to open up the field of double resonance.

TABLE

Summary of the Various

Branch	Frequency, cps	Wavelength	Typical energy unit	
			Name[a]	Value in joules
Static	0–60		Joule	1
			Calorie	4.186
Low or audio frequency	10^3–10^5	3–300 km	Kc	6.62377×10^{-31}
Radio frequency	10^6–10^8	300–3 m	Joule	1
			Cm^{-1}	1.98574×10^{-23}
Microwaves	10^9–10^{11}	30 cm to 3 mm	Mc	6.62377×10^{-28}
Infrared	10^{12} to 3×10^{14}	300–1μ	Cm^{-1}	1.98574×10^{-23}
			kk	1.98574×10^{-20}
			Kcal/m	4.186×10^3
			Joule	1
Visible, ultraviolet	4×10^{14} to 3×10^{15}	0.8–0.1μ	Erg	1×10^{-7}
			eV	1.60207×10^{-19}
			Mc	6.62377×10^{-28}
X-rays	10^{16}–10^{19}	30–0.03 mμ	eV	1.60207×10^{-19}
			KeV	1.60207×10^{-16}
γ-rays	10^{19}–10^{22}	3×10^{-9} to 3×10^{-12} cm	MeV	1.60207×10^{-13}
Low energy, nuclear	10^{19}–10^{23}	3×10^{-9} to 3×10^{-13} cm	MeV	1.60207×10^{-13}
High energy, nuclear	10^{23}–10^{26}	3×10^{-13} to 3×10^{-17} cm	BeV	1.60207×10^{-10}
			GeV	1.60207×10^{-7}
High energy cosmic rays	$>10^{25}$		BeV	1.60207×10^{-10}
			GeV	1.60207×10^{-7}

[a] A kilokayser (kk) is 1000 cm.$^{-1}$

[b] NQR denotes nuclear quadrupole resonance, NMR signifies nuclear magnetic resonance, and ESR means electron spin resonance.

[c] TWO means travelling wave oscillator.

Sophisticated techniques have been devised for determining relaxation times. Several new microwave devices such as isolators (gyrators), circulators, and helices have been incorporated into ESR spectrometers. In other words, the information contained in the *Radiation Laboratory Series* was supplemented by recent advances in microwave engineering, and combined with other experimental techniques to produce the modern sophisticated electron spin resonance spectrometers.

The state of the art in the field of ESR instrumentation has reached maturity during the past few years, and so it is fitting to gather together in one volume the information that is required to design, build, modify, and use an ESR spectrometer. For some time there has been a need for such a volume because the required information is scattered throughout twenty-seven Radiation Laboratory volumes and hundreds of journal articles. This book will present the basic principles and main applications of ESR instrumentation, and will supply references to additional sources of information. It is believed that future advances in ESR technology will build upon existing systems, and that the basic principles of the field will not change radically during the next decade. In the future there will no doubt be refinements in instrumentation to produce a spectrometer which provides a spectrum on chart paper labeled with an accurate ordinate scale in absolute intensity units, and an abscissa scale in precise magnetic field units. In addition, a computer will automatically calculate the spin concentration, line width and shape, relaxation times, etc. Optical spectroscopy and high resolution NMR still lead ESR in these refinements.

The first five chapters of the book present the background which will help the reader to better understand the remainder, and to read the literature. The next seven chapters describe the principal parts of an ESR spectrometer, and they are followed by Chap. 13 which describes some existing spectrometers and tabulates the characteristics of many others. Chapter 14 discusses sensitivity and synthesizes some of the material presented in the earlier chapters. The next three chapters discuss auxiliary equipment and are followed by two chapters which explain specialized techniques that are frequently used in ESR. Chapter 20 presents an analysis of line shapes. The book concludes with a brief summary of spectrometer operation. Most of the sections can be read without a mastery of Chaps. 2 to 5, but nonetheless, the results that are obtained in these chapters are used throughout the book. An attempt has been made to keep most of the chapters self-contained.

B. Spectroscopy

The general field of spectroscopy is subdivided into several regions depending on the energy involved in a typical quantum jump. A summary of the various branches of spectroscopy is presented in Table 1-1. Historically they developed as separate fields of research; each employed particular experimental techniques, and these instrumentation differences just happened to coincide with different physical phenomena such as the progressively increasing energies associated with rotational, vibrational, and electronic spectra.

Electron spin resonance (ESR) is frequently considered to be in the microwave branch of spectroscopy, and nuclear magnetic resonance (NMR) is usually classified in radiofrequency spectroscopy, but these are merely instrumental characterizations based, for example, on the last two columns of Table 1-1. In terms of the observed phenomena, ESR studies the interaction between electronic magnetic moments and magnetic fields. Occasionally, electron spin resonance studies are carried out with NMR instrumentation using magnetic fields of several gauss rather than several thousand gauss. The splitting of energy levels by a magnetic field is customarily referred to as the Zeeman effect, and so we may say that ESR is the study of direct transitions between electronic Zeeman levels while NMR is the study of direct transitions between nuclear Zeeman levels. In concrete terms it may be said that ESR and NMR study the energy required to reorient electronic and nuclear magnetic moments, respectively, in a magnetic field.

Straight microwave spectroscopy uses apparatus similar to that employed in ESR, but in contrast to ESR, it measures molecular rotational transitions directly, and when it employs a magnetic field, it is usually for the purpose of producing only a small additional splitting of the rotational energy levels. In fact, in this branch of spectroscopy it is much more customary to produce Stark effect splittings by means of an applied electric field. In ESR, on the other hand, a strong magnetic field is an integral part of the experimental arrangement.

C. Electric Mom

The previous section mentioned that ES between an electronic magnetic moment Classically, this is similar to the more familia an electric moment and an electric field, so the lat first.

The potential V_e due to a monopole or point charg r is given by

$$V_e = e/4\pi\epsilon r$$

where ϵ is the dielectric constant of the medium.

The electric field intensity E is radial, with the value

$$E = -\partial V_e/\partial r = e/4\pi\epsilon r^2$$

A dipole consists of two charges e and $-e$ separated by a distance l. As shown on Fig. 1-1, the potential due to this dipole at the point P is

$$V_{e_1} = \frac{e}{4\pi\epsilon}\left[\frac{1}{r - \frac{1}{2}l\cos\theta} - \frac{1}{r + \frac{1}{2}l\cos\theta}\right] \tag{3}$$

$$= \frac{\mu_e\cos\theta}{4\pi\epsilon r^2} \tag{4}$$

where $r \gg l$ and μ_e is the electric dipole moment defined by

$$\mu_e = el \tag{5}$$

The electric field intensities in the r, θ, and φ spherical coordinate directions are

$$E_r = -\frac{\partial V}{\partial r} = \frac{\mu_e\cos\theta}{2\pi\epsilon r^3} \tag{6}$$

$$E_\theta = -\frac{1}{r}\frac{\partial V}{\partial\theta} = \frac{\mu_e\sin\theta}{4\pi\epsilon r^3} \tag{7}$$

$$E_\varphi = -\frac{1}{r\sin\theta}\frac{\partial V}{\partial\varphi} = 0 \tag{8}$$

1–1

Branches of Spectroscopy

Phenomenon[b]	Typical radiation generator	Typical detector
	Battery	Ammeter Voltmeter
Dielectric absorption	Mechanical	Ammeter Voltmeter
NQR, NMR, Dielectric absorption	Tuned circuit Crystal	Antenna
Molecular rotations, ESR	Klystron Magneton TWO[c]	Antenna Crystal Bolometer
Molecular vibrations	Heat source	Bolometer PbS cell
Electronic transitions	Incandescent lamp	Photocell Photographic film
Electronic transitions	Discharge tube	Photocell
Inner shell electronic transitions	Heavy element bombardment	Geiger counter Photomultiplier
Nuclear energy level transitions	Naturally radioactive nuclei	Scintillation detector
Strange particle creation	Accelerator (e.g., synchrotron)	Bubble chamber Spark chamber
Extraterrestrial	Star, magnetic field in galaxy	Extensive shower detector

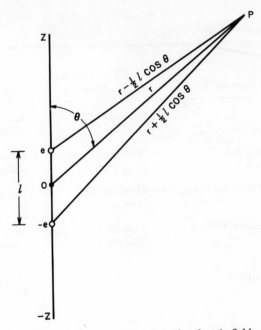

Fig. 1–1.   Coordinate system for calculating the electric field strength at the point P due to an electric dipole.

In vector notation the electric field $\mathbf{E}$ of a dipole is often written

$$\mathbf{E} = \frac{1}{4\pi\epsilon r^3}\left[3\frac{(\mathbf{\mu}_e \cdot \mathbf{r})\mathbf{r}}{r^2} - \mathbf{\mu}_e\right] \tag{9}$$

The first term of this expression is

$$(\mathbf{\mu}_e \cdot \mathbf{r})\mathbf{r} = \mu_e\hat{\mathbf{r}}\,r^2\cos\theta \tag{10}$$

where $\hat{\mathbf{r}}$ and $\hat{\theta}$ are dimensionless unit vectors. The second term in (9) gives

$$\mathbf{\mu}_e = \mu_e\hat{z} = \mu_e\,(\hat{\mathbf{r}}\cos\theta - \hat{\vartheta}\sin\theta) \tag{11}$$

so that

$$\mathbf{E} = \frac{\mu_e}{4\pi\epsilon r^3}\,(\hat{\vartheta}\sin\theta + 2\hat{\mathbf{r}}\cos\theta) \tag{12}$$

$$= \hat{\vartheta}E_\theta + \hat{\mathbf{r}}E_r \tag{13}$$

in agreement with eqs. (6) and (7).

An axial electric quadrupole moment may be constructed by placing two oppositely directed dipoles with the moments $\mu_e = el_1$, a distance l_2 apart as shown in Fig. 1-2. As before, the potential at the point P is

$$V_{e_2} = \frac{el_1 \cos \theta}{4\pi\epsilon} \left[\frac{1}{(r - \frac{1}{2} l_2 \cos \theta)^2} - \frac{1}{(r + \frac{1}{2} l_2 \cos \theta)^2} \right]$$

$$= \frac{\mu_{e_2} \cos^2 \theta}{4\pi\epsilon r^3} \tag{14}$$

where the quadrupole moment μ_{e_2} (often denoted eQ) is defined by

$$\mu_{e_2} = eQ = 2el_1l_2 \tag{15}$$

The electric field intensities arising from the quadrupole moment may be computed easily from eqs. (6)–(8)

$$E_r = \frac{3 \mu_{e_2} \cos^2 \theta}{4\pi\epsilon r^4} \tag{16}$$

$$E_\theta = \frac{2 \mu_{e_2} \sin \theta \cos \theta}{4\pi\epsilon r^4} \tag{17}$$

$$E_\varphi = 0 \tag{18}$$

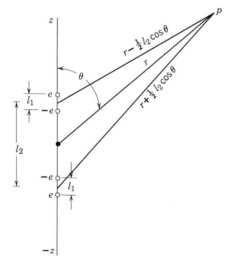

Fig. 1-2. Coordinate system for calculating the electric field strength at the point P due to an axial electric quadrupole.

The potentials due to the monopole V_e, the dipole V_{e_1} and the quadrupole V_{e_2} may be written as follows:

$$V_e = \frac{e}{4\pi\epsilon}\left(\frac{1}{r}\right) \tag{19}$$

$$V_{e_1} = -\frac{\mu_e}{4\pi\epsilon}\frac{\partial}{\partial z}\left(\frac{1}{r}\right) \tag{20}$$

$$V_{e_2} = \frac{\mu_{e_2}}{8\pi\epsilon}\frac{\partial^2}{\partial z^2}\left(\frac{1}{r}\right) \tag{21}$$

where

$$\frac{\partial}{\partial z}\left(\frac{1}{r}\right) = -\frac{1}{r^2}\frac{\partial r}{\partial z} = -\frac{\cos\theta}{r^2} \tag{22}$$

If successive axial dipoles are constructed in the above manner, the potential of the lth will be given by

$$V_{e_l} = (-1)^l\frac{\mu_{e_l}}{4\pi\epsilon l!}\frac{\partial^l}{\partial z^l}\left(\frac{1}{r}\right) \tag{23}$$

For the octopole moment, $l = 3$, and for the hexadecapole moment, $l = 4$ [see Stratton (1941)].

D. Magnetic Moments

If magnetic monopoles existed they would be analogs of electric charges, and one could write the potential V_m for such a monopole m as

$$V_m = \frac{\mu}{4\pi}\frac{m}{r} \tag{1}$$

where μ (or μ-bar) is the permeability of the medium.   Indeed, in analogy to the electric case one may write the potential V_l for the lth axial magnetic moment μ_l as

$$V_l = (-1)^l\frac{\mu}{4\pi l!}\mu_l\frac{\partial^l}{\partial z^l}\left(\frac{1}{r}\right) \tag{2}$$

Thus the magnetic potential V_l may be derived from the corresponding electric potential V_{e_l} by replacing the dielectric constant ϵ with the reciprocal of the permeability μ and by replacing the electric moment μ_{e_l} with the magnetic moment μ_l.

No isolated magnetic monopoles have ever been found in nature. A constant electric current I flowing in a planar loop of wire possesses a magnetic dipole moment given by

$$\mathbf{\mu}_1 = \mathbf{\mu} = IA\mathbf{\hat{n}} \tag{3}$$

where A is the area enclosed by the loop and $\mathbf{\hat{n}}$ is the unit vector perpendicular to the plane of the loop. This magnetic dipole moment formula is valid for distances from the wire that are much greater than the longest loop "diameter," since close to the wire there are additional multipole terms in the "near field" expression for the magnetic field. Such a loop of wire may be excited by an rf field, and in this case it constitutes a magnetic dipole antenna such as the one discussed in RLS-12, p. 95.

The preceding treatment discussed magnetic multipoles in terms of their analogy with electric multipoles. This analogy does not reveal an essential aspect of magnetic moments, which is their relationship to angular momentum. For example, the magnetic dipole moment μ is proportional to the angular momentum $\mathbf{J}\hbar$, and the constant of proportionality is

$$\mathbf{\mu} = (ge/2m)\,(\mathbf{J}\hbar) \tag{4}$$

$$= g\beta\mathbf{J} \tag{5}$$

where g is the g factor (spectroscopic splitting factor), β is the Bohr magneton, e is the electric charge of an electron, $\hbar$ is Planck's constant divided by 2π, and m is the electronic mass.

The unit of electron magnetic moments is the Bohr magneton β and that of nuclear magnetic moments is the nuclear magneton β_N. These two constants have the ratio

$$\frac{\beta}{\beta_N} = \frac{e\hbar/2m}{e\hbar/2m_p} = \frac{9.2838 \times 10^{-24}\ \mathrm{Jm^2/Wb}}{5.0538 \times 10^{-27}\ \mathrm{Jm^2/Wb}} = \frac{9.2838 \times 10^{-21}\ \mathrm{erg/G}}{5.0538 \times 10^{-24}\ \mathrm{erg/G}}$$

$$= 1838 \tag{6}$$

which is the ratio of the rest mass m_p, of the proton to the rest mass m of the electron.   Thus ESR energies are generally about 2000 times as big as NMR energies.

In NMR one usually expresses the magnitude of a particular nuclear magnetic moment by its gyromagnetic ratio γ.   The gyromagnetic ratio is related to the g factor by the expression

$$\gamma = g\beta/\hbar \tag{7}$$

$$= 8.809 \times 10^{10}g \text{ rad m}^2/\text{Wb} \tag{8a}$$

$$= 8.809 \times 10^6 g \text{ rad/G} \tag{8b}$$

where g is dimensionless, and γ has the units ($2\pi \times$ cps/magnetic field strength).

E. High Order Multipole Moments

The generalized lth order electric multipole moment μ_{e_l} has $2l + 1$ components, and following Blatt and Weisskopf (1952) it is defined in terms of the normalized spherical harmonic function $Y_{lm}(\theta,\varphi)$

$$\mu_{e_l} = \int r^l Y_{lm}^*(\theta,\varphi) \rho(r,\theta,\varphi) d\tau \tag{1}$$

where $\rho(r, \theta, \varphi)$ is the charge density.   This is a classical formula, and has the quantum mechanical analog.

$$\mu_{e_l} = e \sum_{i=1}^{N} \int r_i{}^l Y_{lm}^*(\theta,\varphi)|\psi(r_1,r_2,\cdots r_N)|^2 d\tau \tag{2}$$

The generalized lth order magnetic multipole moment μ_l also has $2l + 1$ components, and following Blatt and Weisskopf (1952) is defined in terms of the gradient of the magnetization (magnetic moment density) $M(r)$.   In other words

$$\rho(r,\theta,\varphi) \xrightarrow{\text{becomes}} -\nabla \cdot \mathbf{M}(r) \tag{3}$$

in eq. (1).

The parity operator $\mathcal{P}$ is an operator which inverts the coordinates

$$\mathcal{P}\, \psi(x,y,z) = \psi(-x,-y,-z) \tag{4}$$

and functions of even and odd parity are defined by

$$\mathcal{P}\, \psi(x,y,z) = +\, \psi(x,y,z) \quad \text{even}$$
$$= -\, \psi(x,y,z) \quad \text{odd} \tag{5}$$

Nuclear ground states have definite parities so that

$$\mathcal{P}|\psi(x,y,z)|^2 = |\psi(x,y,z)|^2 \tag{6}$$

and the parity of a spherical harmonic function $Y_{lm}(\theta,\varphi)$ is given by $(-1)^l$

$$\mathcal{P}\, Y_{lm}(\theta,\varphi) = (-1)^l\, Y_{lm}(\theta,\varphi) \tag{7}$$

The integral of an odd function times an even function over all space vanishes, as may be seen by considering the functions

$$x^2\, e^{-z^2} \qquad \text{even function} \tag{8}$$

$$\frac{1}{x(1-y^2)} \qquad \text{odd function} \tag{9}$$

integrated over all space. The result is

$$\int_{-\infty}^{\infty} x\,dx \int_{-\infty}^{\infty} \frac{dy}{1-y^2} \int_{-\infty}^{\infty} e^{-z^2}dz$$

$$= (0) \times \left(2\int_{0}^{\infty} \frac{dy}{1-y^2}\right) \times \left(2\int_{0}^{\infty} e^{-z^2}dz\right) = 0 \tag{10}$$

where the odd function vanishes and the even functions "double" when the limits of integration are changed from $(-\infty \to \infty)$ to $(0 \to \infty)$. As a result of this parity rule the electric multipole moments vanish for odd values of l. In particular, this means that nuclei in their ground or stationary states do not have electric dipole moments.

The lower order electric multipoles are defined for $m = 0$ as follows:

(1) Electric monopole:

$$\mu_{e_0} = \frac{1}{(4\pi)^{1/2}} \int \rho(x,y,z)d\tau \tag{11}$$

(2) Electric dipole:

$$\mu_{e_1} = \left(\frac{3}{4\pi}\right)^{1/2} \int z\rho(x,y,z)d\tau \tag{12}$$

(3) Electric quadrupole:

$$\mu_{e_2} = \left(\frac{5}{16\pi}\right)^{1/2} \int (3z^2 - r^2)\rho(x,y,z)d\tau \tag{13}$$

(4) Electric octopole:

$$\mu_{e_3} = \left(\frac{7}{16\pi}\right)^{1/2} \int (5z^3 - 3r^2z)\rho(x,y,z)d\tau \tag{14}$$

(5) Electric hexadecapole moment:

$$\mu_{e_4} = \frac{3}{16(\pi)^{1/2}} \int (35z^4 - 30z^2r^2 + 3r^4)\rho(x,y,z)d\tau \tag{15}$$

and analogous formulae may be written down for magnetic multipoles.

F. Orbital and Spin Moments

The magnetic moment of an electron spin μ_S is given by

$$\mu_S = 2\beta\mathbf{S} \tag{1}$$

while the magnetic moment associated with orbital momentum μ_L is

$$\mu_L = \beta\mathbf{L} \tag{2}$$

where the Bohr magneton β defined by*

$$\beta = e\hbar/2m \tag{3}$$

is a convenient unit of magnetic moment, **S** is the spin angular momentum operator, and **L** is the angular momentum operator. One may write eqs. (1) and (2) in terms of the g factor

$$\mathbf{\mu}_S = g\beta\mathbf{S} \tag{4}$$

$$\mathbf{\mu}_L = g\beta\mathbf{L} \tag{5}$$

where $g = 2$ and 1 for the spin and orbital motion, respectively. The g factor is the ratio of the magnetic moment to the angular momentum expressed in dimensionless units by means of the Bohr magneton.

If an electron has both spin and orbital motion, then the total angular momentum **J** is obtained by the vector addition

$$\mathbf{J} = \mathbf{L} + \mathbf{S} \tag{6}$$

where **J** has the possible magnitudes $|L - S|$, $|L - S + 1|$, . . . , $|L + S|$. For example, a single S electron has $S = \frac{1}{2}$, $L = 0$, and $J = \frac{1}{2}$ while a single D electron has $S = \frac{1}{2}$, $L = 2$, and $J = 5/2$ or $3/2$.

As a result of eqs. (1) and (2) the vector addition of the orbital and spin components to the magnetic moment gives a value

$$\mathbf{\mu} = g\beta\mathbf{J} \tag{7}$$

for the overall magnetic moment, where the Landé g factor has the form

$$g = \frac{3}{2} + \frac{S(S + 1) - L(L + 1)}{2J\,(J + 1)} \tag{8}$$

which is usually derived in texts on modern physics [e.g., see French (1958)]. Of course, for pure spin or orbital motion these expressions reduce to eqs. (1) and (2), respectively.

---

* This is an MKS formula. In the cgs system, we have $\beta = e\hbar/2mc$.

In solids the electronic orbital motion interacts strongly with the crystalline electric fields and becomes decoupled from the spin, a process called "quenching." The more complete the quenching, the closer the g factor approaches the free electron value. For example, $g = 2.0037$ in the free radical α, α'-diphenyl-β-picryl hydrazyl, which is very close to the free-electron value of 2.0023. It equals 1.98 in many chromium compounds, and it sometimes exceeds 6 for Co^{+2}. Thus the amount of quenching varies with the spin system.

The g factor is very often anisotropic and varies with the direction (x', y', z') in a single crystal. In the general case the g factor may be a symmetric tensor g' with six components g'_{ij}

$$g' = \begin{bmatrix} g'_{x'x'} & g'_{x'y'} & g'_{x'z'} \\ g'_{y'x'} & g'_{y'y'} & g'_{y'z'} \\ g'_{z'x'} & g'_{z'y'} & g'_{z'z'} \end{bmatrix} \tag{9}$$

where

$$g'_{ij} = g'_{ji} \tag{10}$$

It is always possible to find the principal axes (x, y, z) where the g tensor is diagonal

$$g = \begin{bmatrix} g_{xx} & 0 & 0 \\ 0 & g_{yy} & 0 \\ 0 & 0 & g_{zz} \end{bmatrix} = \begin{bmatrix} g_x & 0 & 0 \\ 0 & g_y & 0 \\ 0 & 0 & g_z \end{bmatrix} \tag{11}$$

and in this case one subscript is often omitted for convenience. The similarity transformation, A, that is used to convert g' to g by the relation

$$g = Ag'A^{-1} \tag{12}$$

where A^{-1} is the inverse of A, leaves the trace of the g tensor invariant, so one may write

$$g_{xx} + g_{yy} + g_{zz} = g'_{x'x'} + g'_{y'y'} + g'_{z'z'} \tag{13}$$

It is very common for the **g** tensor to have axial symmetry, in which case

$$g_\parallel = g_{zz} \tag{14}$$

$$g_\perp = g_{xx} = g_{yy} \tag{15}$$

where the z axis is taken as the symmetry axis. For an arbitrary orientation of a crystal in a magnetic field one obtains a resonance characterized by the g factor

$$g = (g_{xx}{}^2 \cos^2 \theta_x + g_{yy}{}^2 \cos^2 \theta_y + g_{zz}{}^2 \cos^2 \theta_z)^{1/2} \tag{16}$$

where, for example, θ_x is the angle between the x axis and the magnetic field direction and $\cos \theta_x$ is called the direction cosine of x. The three direction cosines obey the relation

$$\cos^2 \theta_x + \cos^2 \theta_y + \cos^2 \theta_z = 1 \tag{17}$$

so one of them may be easily eliminated from eq. (16). For axial symmetry eq. (16) has the form

$$g = [g_\perp{}^2 (\cos^2 \theta_x + \cos^2 \theta_y) + g_\parallel{}^2 \cos^2 \theta_z]^{1/2} \tag{18}$$

and the use of eq. (17) simplifies this to

$$g = (g_\perp{}^2 \sin^2 \theta + g_\parallel{}^2 \cos^2 \theta)^{1/2} \tag{19}$$

where the subscript z is dropped since θ is understood to be the angle between the symmetry axis (along $g_\parallel$) and the magnetic field direction.

Electron spin resonance measurements from randomly oriented radicals produce ESR spectra whose line shapes are powder patterns of eqs. (16) or (19), and these are discussed in Chap. 20.

The sign of the g factor may be obtained with circularly polarized microwaves [Eshbach and Strandberg (1952), Kastler (1954); Charru (1956); Portis and Teaney (1958); Portis (1959); Teaney, Blumberg, and Portis (1960)]. In most ESR experiments only the magnitude of g is determined.

G. The Spin Hamiltonian

The interaction energy of a paramagnetic atom in a constant magnetic field $\mathbf{H}_0$ is given by the spin Hamiltonian $\mathcal{H}$ [Abragam and Pryce (1951); Bleaney and Stevens (1953)].

$$\mathcal{H} = \mathcal{H}_{elect} + \mathcal{H}_{cf} + \mathcal{H}_{LS} + \mathcal{H}_{SS} + \mathcal{H}_{Zee} + \mathcal{H}_{hfs} + \mathcal{H}_Q + \mathcal{H}_N$$

and the various terms have the following typical forms and magnitudes

$$\mathcal{H}_{elect} = \text{electronic energy} \approx 10^4 - 10^5 \text{ cm}^{-1} \text{ (optical region)} \tag{1}$$

$$\mathcal{H}_{cf} = \text{crystal field energy} \approx 10^3 - 10^4 \text{ cm}^{-1} \text{ (infrared or optical region)} \tag{2}$$

$$\mathcal{H}_{LS} = \text{spin orbit interaction} = \lambda L \cdot S \approx 10^2 \text{ cm}^{-1} \tag{3}$$

$$\mathcal{H}_{SS} = \text{spin-spin interaction} = D(S_z^2 - \tfrac{1}{3}S(S+1)) \tag{4}$$
$$= 0\text{-}1 \text{ cm}^{-1}$$

$$\mathcal{H}_{Zee} = \text{Zeeman energy} = \beta \mathcal{H} \cdot (L + 2S) = \beta(g_x \mathcal{H}_x S_x \tag{5}$$
$$+ g_y \mathcal{H}_y S_y + g_z \mathcal{H}_z S_z) = 0\text{-}1 \text{ cm}^{-1}$$

$$\mathcal{H}_{hfs} = \text{hyperfine structure} = (A_x S_x I_x + A_y S_y I_y \tag{6}$$
$$+ A_z S_z I_z) = 0\text{-}10^{-2} \text{ cm}^{-1}$$

$$\mathcal{H}_Q = \text{quadrupole energy} = \{3eQ/[4I(2I - 1)]\} \tag{7}$$
$$\times (\partial^2 V/\partial z^2)[I_z^2 - \tfrac{1}{3}I(I+1)] = 0\text{-}10^{-2} \text{ cm}^{-1}$$

$$\mathcal{H}_N = \text{nuclear spin energy} = \gamma \beta_N H \cdot I = 0\text{-}10^{-3} \text{ cm}^{-1} \tag{8}$$

Several of the symbols in these eight equations are defined as follows:

λ = spin orbit coupling constant

$\left. \begin{array}{c} S_z \\ L_z \end{array} \right\}$ = z component (along $\mathcal{H}$) of the spin and orbital angular moments, respectively

D = zero field splitting constant

β = Bohr magneton

g_z = z component of g factor

A_z = z component of hyperfine coupling constant A

I_z = z component of nuclear spin I

e = electronic charge

Q = nuclear electric quadrupole moment
V = crystalline electric field potential
γ = nuclear gyromagnetic ratio
β_N = nuclear magneton

The energy $\mathcal{H}_{elect}$ is the electronic energy of the paramagnetic ion in the free state, and the energy $\mathcal{H}_{cf}$ is the interaction energy of the free ion's electronic structure with the crystalline electric field. This term helps to determine the g factor, as may be exemplified by Polder's values [Polder (1942); Ingram (1955), p. 142] for Cu^{+2} in a tetragonal crystalline electric field

$$g_{\parallel} = 2 - [8\lambda/(E_3 - E_1)] \tag{9}$$

$$g_{\perp} = 2 - [2\lambda/(E_4 - E_1)] \tag{10}$$

where λ is the spin orbit coupling constant and E_1, E_2, E_3, and E_4 are the four levels into which the crystal field splits the $3d^9$, ^2D Cu^{+2} ground electronic level. For Cu^{+2}, $\lambda = -852$ cm^{-1}, and the energy denominators are over ten times this value, so the g factors for Cu^{+2} vary from 2.15 to 2.4. Formulae similar in form to these relations may be obtained for other transition metal ions in lattice sites of various symmetries.

The crystal field splitting between the ground orbital level E_1 and the next excited orbital level E_2 helps to determine the spin lattice relaxation time T_1 (in seconds) produced by the direct and Raman processes, and for $S = \frac{1}{2}$, Kronig (1939) gave the relations

$$T_1 = \frac{10^4 (E_2 - E_1)^4}{\lambda^2 H^4 T} \qquad \text{direct process} \tag{11}$$

$$T_1 = \frac{10^4 (E_2 - E_1)^6}{\lambda^2 H^2 T^7} \qquad \text{Raman process} \tag{12}$$

where E_1, E_2, and λ are in cm^{-1}, H is in gauss, and T is the absolute temperature. A direct process corresponds to a transition between two spin states with the emission or absorption of a phonon, while a Raman process entails the absorption of one phonon and the emission of another. (A phonon is a quantized lattice vibration.)

The spin orbit interaction $\lambda L \cdot S$ further splits the optical energy levels, influences the g factor in the manner shown in eqs. (9) and (10), and affects the spin lattice relaxation time T_1 in accordance with eqs. (11) and (12). The variation of the spin orbit coupling constant λ is given in Fig. 1-3 for the neutral atoms in several transition series. The quantity ζ is related to λ by

$$\zeta = \pm 2S\lambda \tag{13}$$

where S is the spin. The negative sign refers to a more than half filled shell, and the positive sign refers to a half filled or a less than

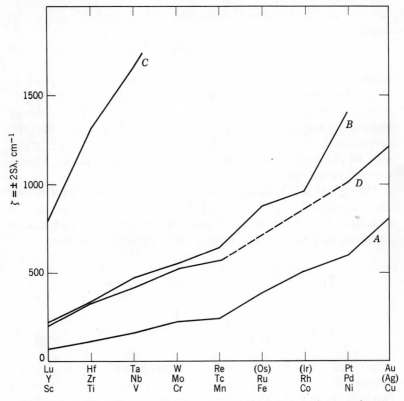

Fig. 1-3.   The spin-orbit coupling constant ζ for d electrons in neutral atoms. (A) First series; (B) second series; (C) third series; (D) third series sealed down by a factor of 4.   [Griffith (1961)].

half filled shell.   Some authors call ζ the spin orbit coupling constant, while others refer to λ by the same name.

The spin-spin interaction is sometimes the same order of magnitude as the Zeeman energy, and in this case it leads to a very complicated system of energy levels which is strongly dependent on the orientation of the crystal in the magnetic field.   Ruby (Cr^{+3}/Al_2O_3) is a satisfactory maser material because the spin-spin term $(D = 0.193$ cm$^{-1})$ is energetically comparable to the Zeeman energy, and the magnetic field strength and direction may be adjusted to give convenient maser operating conditions, as the energy level scheme in Fig. 1-4 indicates.   A strong exchange interaction or rapid re-orientation effects, such as one finds in liquids, can average out the influence of the spin-spin interaction, and render the resonant line narrow and isotropic.

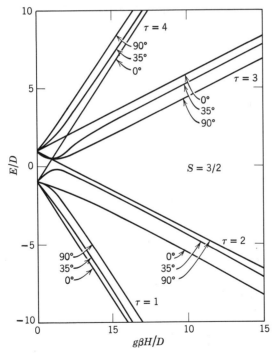

Fig. 1–4. Angular dependence of the energy levels (ordinate) of Cr^{+3} as a function of the normalized magnetic field strength (abscissa). The four energy levels are labeled with their τ values. [Davis and Strandberg (1957)].

The Zeeman term given in eq. (5) and its axially symmetric form were described in the previous section.   Electron spin resonance may be described as the measurement of the Zeeman energy $\mathcal{3C}_{\text{Zee}}$, and in essence ESR does nothing more than study the manner in which the other Hamiltonian terms perturb or are perturbed by the Zeeman energy.

When the crystalline electric field has a symmetry lower than axial there is sometimes a lower symmetry spin-spin interaction of the form $E(S_x{}^2 - S_y{}^2)$, and ordinarily $|D| > |E|$.

The interaction of nuclear spins with an unpaired electron produces hyperfine structure (hfs).   When the electronic spin of a transition metal interacts with its own nuclear spin, the hfs is described by the Hamiltonian term given by eq. (6),

$$\mathcal{3C}_{\text{hfs}} = A I \cdot S \tag{14}$$

which for axial symmetry has the form

$$\mathcal{3C}_{\text{hfs}} = A_\perp (S_x I_y + S_y I_y) + A_\parallel S_z I_z \tag{15}$$

In some systems, such as aromatic molecules, the unpaired electron circulates among several atoms, and the resulting hyperfine structure is the result of a Hamiltonian term of the form

$$\mathcal{3C}_{\text{hfs}} = \sum A_i m_i \tag{16}$$

where the projection m_i of the ith nuclear spin on the magnetic field direction may take on the following $2I_i + 1$ values: $I_i, I_i - 1$, $I_i - 2, \ldots, 1 - I_i, -I$. The hyperfine coupling constant varies with the nuclear species, and it is a measure of the strength of the interaction between the nuclear and electronic spins.

When several $I = \frac{1}{2}$ nuclei are equally coupled (i.e., have same A_i), they produce an intensity ratio that follows the binomial coefficient distribution, as shown in Fig. 1-5.   The figure indicates that spectral lines are well resolved when their separation exceeds their width, and when this is not true they tend to merge together or coalesce into one line.   This figure is useful for comparing with experimentally determined spectra [see also the more detailed spectra calculated by Lebedev, Chernikova, Tikhomirova, and Voevodskii (1963)]. As shown in Tables 1–2 and 1–3, the intensity ratio of 1–3–3–1 is obtained with the methyl radical CH_3 ($I = \frac{1}{2}$) while the ratio of 1–2–3–2–1 is obtained with two equally coupled nitrogen nuclei ($I = 1$) such as the ones found in DPPH. A system contain-

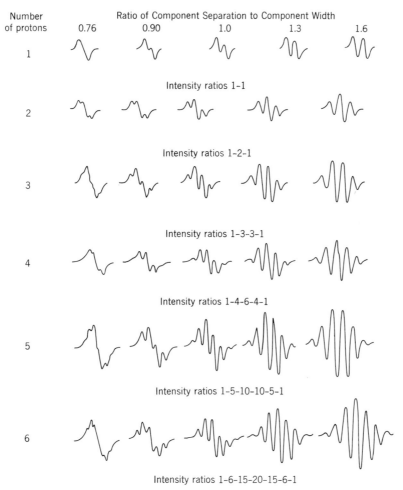

Fig. 1–5. Theoretical hyperfine structure curves for a Gaussian line shape [Poole (1958); Poole and Anderson (1959)].

TABLE 1–2

Determination of Hyperfine Structure Intensity Ratios for Three Equally
Coupled $I = 1/2$ Nuclei (e.g., Protons)

Spin configuration			m_1	m_2	m_3	$M = m_1 + m_2 + m_3$	Intensity ratio
↑	↑	↑	1/2	1/2	1/2	3/2	1
↑	↑	↓	1/2	1/2	−1/2		
↑	↓	↑	1/2	−1/2	1/2	1/2	3
↓	↑	↑	−1/2	1/2	1/2		
↑	↓	↓	1/2	−1/2	−1/2		
↓	↑	↓	−1/2	1/2	−1/2	−1/2	3
↓	↓	↑	−1/2	−1/2	1/2		
↓	↓	↓	−1/2	−1/2	−1/2	−3/2	1

TABLE 1–3

Determination of Hyperfine Structure Intensity Ratios for Two Equally Coupled
$I = 1$ Nuclei (e.g., Nitrogen) Such As the Ones Found in DPPH

Spin configurations		m_1	m_2	$M = m_1 + m_2$	Intensity ratio
↑	↑	1	1	2	1
↑	→	1	0		
→	↑	0	1	1	2
↑	↓	1	−1		
→	→	0	0	0	3
↓	↑	−1	1		
→	↓	0	−1		
↓	→	−1	0	−1	2
↓	↓	−1	−1	−2	1

ing three equally coupled protons (A_p) and two equally coupled
nitrogens (A_N) possesses an hfs Hamiltonian with the form

$$\mathcal{H}_{hfs} = A_p(m_1 + m_2 + m_3) + A_N(m_4 + m_5) \qquad (17)$$

where m_1, m_2, and m_3 assume the values $\pm\frac{1}{2}$ and m_4 and m_5 may
equal 0 or ± 1. If the coupling constant $A_p \gg A_N$, the spectrum

will consist of four widely separated groups of lines with the relative intensity ratio 1–3–3–1 each of which is split into a 1–2–3–2–1 quintet while when $A_p \ll A_N$, the main split is into a widely spaced 1–2–3–2–1 quintet with each of these components further split into a 1–3–3–1 quartet as shown on Fig. 1-6. One may easily compute that when $A_p = A_N$ in eq. (17), the resulting spectrum has eight lines with the intensity ratio 1–5–12–18–18–12–5–1 as shown on Fig. 1-6c.

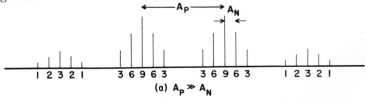

(a) $A_P \gg A_N$

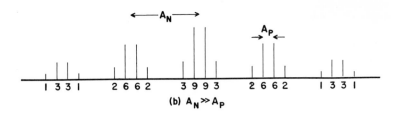

(b) $A_N \gg A_P$

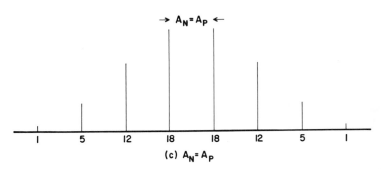

(c) $A_N = A_P$

Fig. 1–6. Hyperfine structure patterns for three equally coupled $I = 1/2$ nuclei with coupling constant A_p and two equally coupled $I = 1$ nuclei with coupling constant A_N.

If there are n nuclei with $I = \frac{1}{2}$ contributing to the hfs, then there will be 2^n different hyperfine components if all of the coupling constants differ and no degeneracy occurs. For example, five protons give the result from Fig. 1-5:

$$1 + 5 + 10 + 10 + 5 + 1 = 32 = 2^5 \tag{18}$$

If there are n nuclei with the nuclear spin I then there will be $(2I + 1)^n$ hyperfine components. For several nuclei with the individual values I_i and n_i the total number of hyperfine components N_{hfs} will be

$$N_{\mathrm{hfs}} = \Pi_i (2I_i + 1)^{n_i} \tag{19}$$

where the symbol Π_i denotes the formation of a product. For example, the system depicted in Fig. 1-6 has

$$I_{\mathrm{p}} = \tfrac{1}{2} \quad n_{\mathrm{p}} = 3$$

$$I_{\mathrm{N}} = 1 \quad n_{\mathrm{N}} = 2 \tag{20}$$

with the results that

$$N_{\mathrm{hfs}} = [2(\tfrac{1}{2}) + 1]^3 (2 + 1)^2 = 72 \tag{21}$$

This may be checked by adding the intensities shown on Fig. 1-6c:

$$1 + 5 + 12 + 18 + 18 + 12 + 5 + 1 = 72 \tag{22}$$

When some nuclei are equivalent to others, the resulting degeneracy has the effect of decreasing the number and increasing the amplitude of the components in the hyperfine pattern without affecting the overall integrated intensity.

Usually, all of the hyperfine components have the same line width and shape, but sometimes relaxation mechanisms cause deviations from this rule as explained in Sec. 20-L.

The quadrupolar interaction $\mathcal{3C}_Q$ has the form

$$[I_z^2 - \tfrac{1}{3}I(I + 1)] = [m_I^2 - \tfrac{1}{3}I(I + 1)] \tag{26}$$

where $m_I = I_z$ is the z component of the nuclear spin I. The hyperfine structure Hamiltonian alone produces a symmetric pattern and the quadrupole Hamiltonian produces energy level shifts which, in accordance with the selection rule $\Delta m_I = 0$, do not disturb the observed spectrum to first order. For example, when $I = 5/2$,

$$m_I{}^2 - \frac{1}{3} I(I + 1) = \begin{cases} \dfrac{10}{3} & m_I = \pm \dfrac{5}{2} \\[2mm] -\dfrac{2}{3} & m_I = \pm \dfrac{3}{2} \\[2mm] -\dfrac{8}{3} & m_I = \pm \dfrac{1}{2} \end{cases} \qquad (27)$$

and the levels for a given m_I are shifted equally, as shown in Fig. 1-7. If $\mathcal{3C}_Q$ becomes appreciable relative to $\mathcal{3C}_{zee}$, then second order quadrupole effects become important, and the observed hyperfine pattern becomes unsymmetrical.

Hydrogen atoms in the gaseous state have a hyperfine splitting of about 1420 Mc or 507 G [Wittke and Dicke (1956)] which is one of the largest ever observed. This splitting constant varies slightly for hydrogen atoms trapped in solid matrices [Livingston, Zeldes, and Taylor (1955)]. Jen, Foner, Cochran, and Bowers (1956) found that in solid matrices deuterium atoms gave hyperfine intervals of 76.7 and 78.7 G with the overall triplet splitting of 155.4 G. The ratio of the H^1 splitting of 508.7 G to the D overall splitting in the solid state equals the ratio μ_H/μ_D of the nuclear magnetic moments of hydrogen and deuterium. In aromatic hydrocarbons the hyperfine splitting A_i due to one proton of a C—H group is about 28 G times the electron density ρ_i at the carbon atom, so an aromatic hydrocarbon radical ion usually has an overall hyperfine splitting of 28 G. The electron density ρ_i is the fraction of the time that the unpaired electron spends on the ith carbon, and the above relation is usually expressed quantitatively as [McConnell (1956)]

$$A_i = Q\rho_i \qquad (28)$$

$$= 28\rho_i \quad \text{gauss} \qquad (29)$$

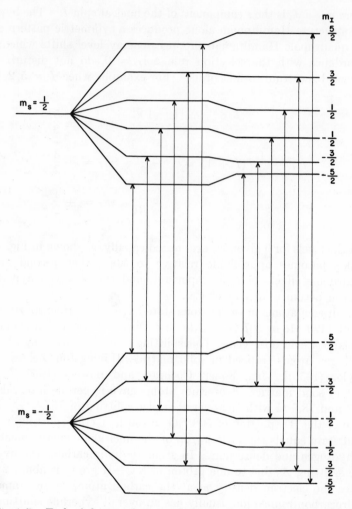

Fig. 1–7.   Each of the two electron spin energy levels on the left is split into six equally spaced levels shown in the center by the hyperfine interaction for $I = 5/2$. To first order the nuclear quadrupole interaction splits these levels unequally as indicated on the right, but the six allowed transitions denoted by the arrows remain equal in energy.

for aromatic hydrocarbons, where

$$\sum \rho_i = 1 \tag{30}$$

A more precise formula is [Colpa and Bolton (1963)]:

$$A_i = (Q + Kq_i)\partial_i \qquad (31)$$

where q_i is the excess charge density on the ith carbon and the constants Q and K have the values 17 and 31.2 [see also Sayetta and Memory (1963)]. Charge densities may also be negative.

The nuclear spin energy $\gamma\beta_N\mathcal{3C}\cdot I$ is very small and can usually be neglected.

The optical spectra of solids containing transition metals arise from the crystal field energy splittings perturbed by the spin orbit coupling. It is also possible to observe directly the spin-spin coupling energy $\mathcal{3C}_{SS}$ or the nuclear quadrupole interaction $\mathcal{3C}_Q$ in the absence of a magnetic field by employing the proper microwave frequency. Sometimes the application of an electric field is employed to assist in the location and identification of such zero field levels. The subject of pure nuclear quadrupole resonance has an extensive literature, and several pertinent books and review articles are listed at the end of the chapter [Cohn and Reif (1957); Das and Hahn (1958); Grechishkin (1959); Grivet and Bassompierre (1961)].

H. Information Gained from Electron Spin Resonance

The principal information gained from electron spin resonance spectra is an evaluation of the various terms in the spin Hamiltonian as discussed in the preceding section. Usually $\mathcal{3C}_{zee}$ and $\mathcal{3C}_{hfs}$ are evaluated directly from ESR data, while the crystal field and spin orbit energies are independently evaluated from optical spectra, and are then correlated with ESR data. The experimentally determined ESR data for transition metal ions are tabulated in three review articles [Bowers and Owen (1953); Orton (1959); Low and Offenbacher (1965)], and two books [Pake (1962); Al'tshuler and Kozyrev (1964)]. The bibliography at the end of the book lists sources of data for other systems, [e.g., Bagguley and Owen (1957)].

To be most informative an ESR spectrum of a particular paramagnetic system will be recorded at several temperatures, several frequencies, and several microwave powers. Sometimes one may employ the ESR spectrum to identify an unknown transition metal ion or lattice defect, or it may distinguish between several valence states of the same ion.   The ESR spectrum frequently identifies the lattice site and symmetry of the paramagnetic species, particularly if single crystal data are available.   Considerable information can be obtained about the nuclei in the immediate neighborhood of the absorbing spin, and sometimes relaxation time data detect long range effects.   Diffusion constants, correlation times, and the type of hydration can be determined from the ESR spectra of solutions. Chemical bonds in molecules and crystals sometimes may be characterized by ESR studies.   The effective masses of atoms in semiconductors may be deduced.   The concentrations of paramagnetic species may be determined.   ESR studies furnish detailed information on ferromagnetic, antiferromagnetic, and ferrimagnetic materials.

The preceding is just a brief enumeration of some of the types of information that are furnished by electron spin resonance investigations.   There are a number of books, proceedings of conferences and review articles which devote considerable space to this topic, and these are listed in the Selected Bibliography at the end of the book.

I. Systems Studied by Electron Spin Resonance

A large number of systems have been studied by electron spin resonance, and this section will enumerate the principal ones.   There is some overlap in these categories.

*Biological Systems:** (1) hemoglobin (Fe); (2) nucleic acids; (3) enzymes; (4) chloroplasts when irradiated; (5) riboflavin (before and after uv irradiation).

Chemical Systems: (1) polymers; (2) catalysts; (3) rubber; (4) free radicals.

Conduction Electrons: (1) solutions of alkali metals in liquid ammonia; (2) alkali and alkaline earth metals (fine powders); (3) alloys (e.g., small amount of paramagnetic metal alloyed; with another metal); (4) nonresonant absorption of microwaves by superconductors.

Free Radicals: (1) stable solid free radicals (a single exchange narrowed resonance); (2) stable free radicals in solution (hfs obtained); (3) free radicals produced by irradiation (usually at low temperature, sometimes single crystals); (4) condensed discharges

---

* The presence of water produces large dielectric losses.

(free radicals produced in gas and condensed on solid at low temperature); (5) biological systems; (6) biradicals; (7) electrochemical generation of ion-radicals (polarography); (8) triplet states; (9) paramagnetic molecules (e.g., NO, NO_2, ClO_2).

Irradiated Substances: (1) ionic crystals (e.g., alkali halides), (F centers and other centers); (2) solid organic compounds; (3) liquid organic compounds; (4) organic single crystals; (5) polymers; (6) semiconductors (e.g., Ge and Si); (7) photoconductors (e.g., dyes).

Naturally Occurring Substances: (1) mineral with transition elements [e.g., ruby (Cr/Al_2O_3), dolomite $Mn/(Ca, Mg)(CO_3)$]; (2) minerals with defects (e.g., quartz); (3) hemoglobin (Fe); (4) petroleum; (5) coal; (6) rubber.

Semiconductors: (1) cyclotron resonance (e.g., Ge, Si, InSb); (2) doped semiconductors (e.g., Si with As, Sb, P); (3) irradiated semiconductors; (4) graphite.

*Transition Elements:** (1) single crystals (1% in diamagnetic crystal, anisotropic g factors, and hfs constants evaluated); (2) relaxation time studies (mostly liquid He temperature, low power); (3) chelates, sandwich compounds; (4) alloys.

Experimental data and theoretical discussions of these systems may be found in the books, proceedings of conferences, and review articles listed in the Selected Bibliography at the end of the book.

J. Comparison of Electron Spin Resonance Results with Information Obtained from Magnetic Susceptibility Measurements

An electron spin resonance measurement consists of the simultaneous determination of the microwave frequency ν and the magnetic field strength H. These data are used to calculate the g factor from the relation

$$g = (h/\beta) (\nu/H) \tag{1}$$

where the constant of proportionality is the ratio of Planck's constant to the Bohr magneton. A magnetic susceptibility measurement carried out with a paramagnetic sample entails the determination of the force exerted on a sample in a magnetic field as a function

* Most of the work has been with the first transition series (Ti to Cu).

of the absolute temperature T. The data are used to calculate the susceptibility χ, the Weiss constant Δ, and the g factor by means of the Curie-Weiss Law

$$\chi = \frac{Ng^2\beta^2 S(S+1)}{3k(T+\Delta)} \tag{2}$$

where S is the spin, k is Boltzmann's constant, and N is the number of spins in the sample. This is the spin-only formula used for a quenched orbital angular momentum. In the absence of quenching one replaces $\mathbf{S}$ by $\mathbf{J}$ where

$$\mathbf{J} = \mathbf{L} + \mathbf{S} \tag{3}$$

Thus both ESR and magnetic susceptibility methods provide the g factor. The ESR technique singles out each ion and electronic state and resolves the corresponding spectra, while the magnetic susceptibility technique measures an average of the susceptibilities of all the paramagnetic states in the sample. Electron spin resonance provides additional information concerning hyperfine interactions with nuclear spins. Both methods furnish information on zero field splittings, with the ESR results being more specific. The Weiss constant Δ determined by magnetic susceptibility measurements may be employed to evaluate the exchange integral (exchange energy) J between two paramagnetic ions by the approximation

$$\Delta = \tfrac{2}{3} zS(S+1)J/k \tag{4}$$

One should not confuse this use of J with the total angular momentum. This same approximation may be employed with the Curie temperature T_C (or Néel temperature T_N) which separates paramagnetic and ferromagnetic or antiferromagnetic behavior

$$T_C = \tfrac{2}{3} zS(S+1)J/k \tag{5}$$

where z is the number of paramagnetic nearest neighbor ions exchange-coupled to each paramagnetic ion. It must be emphasized that the last two equations are only rough approximations since usually $T_C \neq \Delta$, and often Δ exceeds T_C by a factor of 2 to 4 [Nagamiya, Yosida, and Kubo (1955)].

The hyperfine structure, quadrupole moment and zero field splitting affect the susceptibility and contribute to the specific heat of paramagnetic salts at extremely low temperatures [Bleaney (1950)].

References

A. Abragam and M. H. L. Pryce, *Proc. Roy. Soc.*, **A205**, 135 (1951).

S. A. Al'tshuler and B. M. Kozyrev, *Electron Paramagnetic Resonance*, translated by Scripta Technica, English language edition edited by C. P. Poole, Jr., Academic, N. Y., 1964.

D. M. S. Bagguley and J. Owen, *Rept. Progr. Phys.* **20**, 304 (1957).

J. M. Blatt and V. F. Weisskopf, *Theoretical Nuclear Physics*, Wiley, N. Y., 1952.

B. Bleaney, *Phys. Rev.*, **78**, 214 (1950).

B. Bleaney and R. P. Penrose, *Nature*, **157**, 339 (1946).

B. Bleaney and K. W. H. Stevens, *Rept. Progr. Phys.*, **16**, 108 (1953).

F. Bloch, *Phys. Rev.*, **70**, 460 (1946).

F. Bloch, W. W Hansen, and M. Packard, *Phys. Rev.*, **69**, 127 (1946).

K. D. Bowers and J. Owen, *Rept. Progr. Phys.*, **18**, 304 (1955).

A. Charru, *C. R. Acad. Sci.*, **243**, 652 (1956).

C. E. Cleeton and N. H. Williams, *Phys. Rev.*, **45**, 234 (1934).

M. H. Cohn and F. Reif, *Solid State Phys.*, **5**, 322 (1957).

J. P. Colpa and J. R. Bolton, *Mol. Phys.*, **6**, 273 (1963).

R. L. Cummerow and D. Halliday, *Phys. Rev.*, **70**, 433 (1946).

T. P. Das and E. L. Hahn, *Nuclear Quadrupole Resonance Spectroscopy*, Solid State Physics Suppl. I, Academic, N. Y., 1958.

C. F. Davis and M. W. P. Strandberg, *Phys. Rev.*, **105**, 447 (1957).

J. R. Eshbach and M. W. P. Strandberg, *RSI*, **23**, 623 (1952).

A. P. French, *Principles of Modern Physics*, Wiley, N. Y., 1958.

W. E. Good, *Phys. Rev.*, **69**, 539 (1946).

C. J. Gorter, *Physica*, **3**, 995 (1936).

V. S. Grechishkin, *Usp. Fiz. Nauk.*, **69**, 189 (699) (1959).

J. S. Griffith, *The Theory of Transition Metal Ions*, Cambridge University Press, Cambridge, England, 1961, p. 113.

J. H. E. Griffiths, *Nature*, **158**, 670 (1946).

P. Grivet and A. Bassompierre, *Acad. Roy. Belg. Classe Sci. Mem. Collection in 8°*, **33**, 219 (1961).

D. J. E. Ingram, *Spectroscopy at Radio and Microwave Frequencies*, Butterworths, London, 1955.

C. K. Jen, S. N. Foner, E. L. Cochran, and V. A. Bowers, *Phys. Rev.*, **104**, 846 (1956).

A. Kastler, *C. R. Acad. Sci.*, **238**, 669 (1954).

R. deL. Kronig, *Physica*, **6**, 33 (1939).

Ya. S. Lebedev, D. M. Chernikova, N. N. Tikhomirova, and V. V. Voevodskii, *Atlas of Electron Spin Resonance Spectra*, Consultants Bureau, N. Y., 1963.

R. Livingston, H. Zeldes, and E. H. Taylor, *Discussions Faraday Soc.*, **19**, 166 (1955).

W. Low and E. L. Offenbacher, *Solid State Phys.*, **17**, 135 (1965).

H. M. McConnell, *J. Chem. Phys.*, **24**, 632, 764 (1956).

T. Nagamiya, Y. Yosida, and R. Kubo, *Advan. Phys.*, **4**, 1 (1955).

J. W. Orton, *Rept. Progr. Phys.*, **22**, 204 (1959).

G. E. Pake, *Paramagnetic Resonance*, Benjamin, N. Y., 1962.

D. Polder, *Physica*, **9**, 709 (1942).

C. P. Poole, Jr., Thesis, Department of Physics, University of Maryland, 1958.

C. P. Poole and R. S. Anderson, *J. Chem. Phys.*, **31**, 346 (1959).

A. M. Portis, *J. Phys. Chem. Solids*, **8**, 326 (1959).

A. M. Portis and D. T. Teaney, *J. Appl. Phys.*, **29**, 1962 (1958).

E. M. Purcell, *Phys. Rev.*, **69**, 681 (1946).

E. M. Purcell, N. Bloembergen, and R. V. Pound, *Phys. Rev.*, **70**, 986, 988 (1946).

E. M. Purcell, H. C. Torrey, and R. V. Pound, *Phys. Rev.*, **69**, 37 (1946).

RLS-12.

T. C. Sayetta and J. D. Memory, *J. Chem. Phys.*, **40**, 2748 (1964).

J. A. Stratton, *Electromagnetic Theory*, McGraw-Hill, N. Y., 1941.

D. T. Teaney, W. E. Blumberg, and A. M. Portis, *Phys. Rev.*, **119**, 1851 (1960).

J. P. Wittke and R. H. Dicke, *Phys. Rev.*, **103**, 620 (1956).

E. Zavoisky, *J. Phys. USSR*, **9**, 211 (1945).

CHAPTER 2

Transmission Lines

A. Introduction

Electron spin resonance spectrometers employ waveguide "transmission lines," and a knowledge of transmission line theory is a necessary prerequisite for understanding the principles that will be presented later when waveguides are discussed. Transmission lines may be analyzed either in terms of current and voltage or in terms of electric and magnetic fields. As a result they constitute an intermediate case between low frequency circuitry, and high frequency electromagnetic theory. The present chapter merely serves as an introduction to transmission line theory. For a more complete treatment the reader is referred to other texts such as the one by Ramo, Whinnery, and Van Duzer (1965).

B. The Lossless Transmission Line

A transmission line is made up of two conductors separated by a dielectric, and in a typical case it connects a voltage (or current) generator to a load. The transmission line has a distributed inductance per unit length L and a distributed capacitance per unit length C as shown on Fig. 2-1. Across the length increment dz the current changes from I to $I + (\partial I/\partial z)dz$ and the voltage changes from V to $V + (\partial V/\partial z)dz$. The voltage change is the negative of the inductance $L\,dz$ times the rate of change of the current, and the current change is the negative of the capacity $C\,dz$ times the time rate of change of the voltage. In other words

$$\partial V/\partial z = -L(\partial I/\partial t) \tag{1}$$

and

$$\partial I/\partial z = -C(\partial V/\partial t) \tag{2}$$

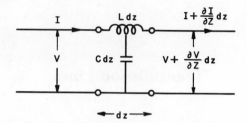

Fig. 2–1. Schematic representation of inductance Ldz and capacitance Cdz associated with an increment dz along a lossless transmission line. The effect of these reactances on the voltage V and current C is shown.

These two equations may be combined by differentiating the first with respect to z and the second with respect to t, giving the wave equation,

$$\partial^2 V/\partial z^2 = LC(\partial^2 V/\partial t^2) \tag{3}$$

since

$$(\partial/\partial z)\,(\partial/\partial t) = (\partial/\partial t)\,(\partial/\partial z) \tag{4}$$

The analogous current wave equation arises when eq. (1) is differentiated with respect to t and eq. (2) with respect to z, and has the form

$$\partial^2 I/\partial z^2 = LC(\partial^2 I/\partial t^2) \tag{5}$$

Equations (3) and (5) are of the same form, so only one will be discussed. The voltage wave equation may be written

$$\partial^2 V/\partial z^2 = (1/v^2)\,(\partial^2 V/\partial t^2) \tag{6}$$

where the velocity v is given by

$$v = 1/(LC)^{1/2} \tag{7}$$

This equation has a solution of the form

$$V = V_1(t - z/v) + V_2\,(t + z/v) \tag{8}$$

If this solution is put into eq. (1), I may be obtained by a partial integration with respect to t, and if it is put into eq. (2), I may be evaluated by a partial integration with respect to z. A comparison of the two results shows that the current I has the form

$$I = (1/Z_0) \left[V_1(t - z/v) - V_2(t + z/v) \right] \tag{9}$$

plus an additive constant, where the transmission line characteristic impedance Z_0 is

$$Z_0 = (L/C)^{1/2} \tag{10}$$

The function $V_1 (t - z/v)$ corresponds to a wave traveling in the positive z direction and the function $V_2(t + z/v)$ corresponds to a wave traveling in the negative z direction.

If there is a discontinuity in the transmission line it may be represented by the circuit shown in Fig. 2-2. The line contains a forward traveling wave V_1 and I_1 and a backward traveling wave V_2 and I_2. The current and voltage must both be continuous across the discontinuity, and must satisfy the requirements

$$V_L = V_1 + V_2 \tag{11}$$

and

$$I_L = I_1 + I_2 \tag{12}$$

From eq. (9) one may write

$$I_L = V_1/Z_0 - V_2/Z_0 \tag{13}$$

and since $V_L = I_L Z_L$, this becomes

$$V_L/Z_L = V_1/Z_0 - V_2/Z_0 \tag{14}$$

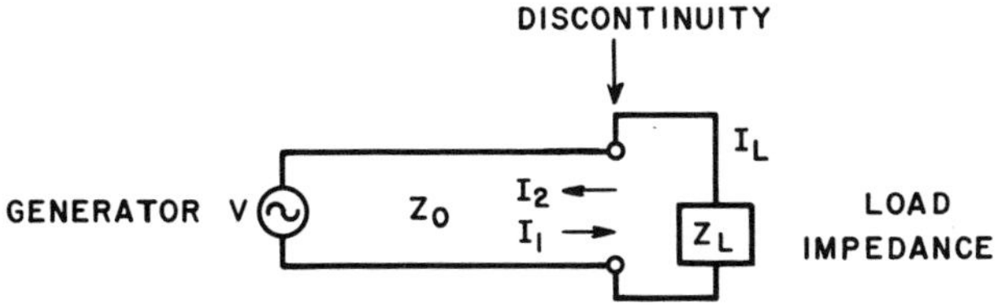

Fig. 2-2. Transmission line of characteristic impedance Z_0 with a discontinuity followed by a load impedance Z_L.

Employing eqs. (11) and (14) one may compute the voltage reflection coefficient Γ and voltage transmission coefficient T

$$\Gamma = V_2/V_1 = (Z_L - Z_0)/(Z_L + Z_0) \tag{15}$$

and

$$T = V_L/V_1 = 2Z_L/(Z_L + Z_0) \tag{16}$$

Along a uniform transmission line the voltage goes through maxima and minima when one moves from points where V_1 and V_2 add, to positions where they subtract. Thus there are places of maximum voltage

$$V_{\max} = |V_1| + |V_2| \tag{17}$$

and points of minimum voltage

$$V_{\min} = |V_1| - |V_2| \tag{18}$$

The voltage standing wave ratio VSWR is defined by

$$\mathrm{VSWR} = V_{\max}/V_{\min} = (1 + |\Gamma|)/(1 - |\Gamma|) \tag{19}$$

which may be rearranged to

$$|\Gamma| = (\mathrm{VSWR} - 1)/(\mathrm{VSWR} + 1) \tag{20}$$

The current along the line reaches a maximum

$$I_{\max} = (|V_1| + |V_2|)/Z_0 \tag{21}$$

where the voltage reaches a minimum, and vice versa

$$I_{\min} = (|V_1| - |V_2|)/Z_0 \tag{22}$$

and as a result the impedance Z passes through maxima and minima given by

$$Z_{\max} = (\mathrm{VSWR})Z_0 \tag{23}$$

$$Z_{\min} = Z_0/(\mathrm{VSWR}) \tag{24}$$

If a transmission line is "matched" or terminated by its characteristic impedance Z_0, then there is no reflected wave V_2, and the

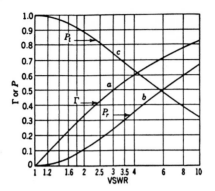

Fig. 2-3. Relation between VSWR and (a) reflection coefficient Γ, (b) relative reflected power P_r, and (c) relative transmitted power P_t (*RLS*-10, p. 17).

voltage standing wave ratio is one. Thus the amount by which the VSWR exceeds unity is a measure of the amount of mismatch. A transmission line of infinite length is equivalent to one terminated by its characteristic impedance.

Some microwave engineers make use of the power standing wave ratio PSWR which is related to the voltage standing wave ratio by

$$PSWR = (VSWR)^2 \tag{25}$$

The relationship between the reflection coefficient Γ, the relative reflected power P_r, and the relative transmitted power P_t are shown in Fig. 2-3 (see *RLS*-8, p. 64) where

$$P_r = |\Gamma|^2 \tag{26}$$

$$P_t = 1 - |\Gamma|^2 \tag{27}$$

and of course

$$P_t + P_r = \text{incident power} \tag{28}$$

C. The Smith Chart

Transmission line calculations are greatly simplified by the use of the Smith or hemisphere chart [Smith (1939), (1944)] which is discussed in most books on microwaves [e.g., Ramo, Whinnery, and Van Duzer (1965)], and is shown on Fig. 2-4. This section will present a brief description of the chart.

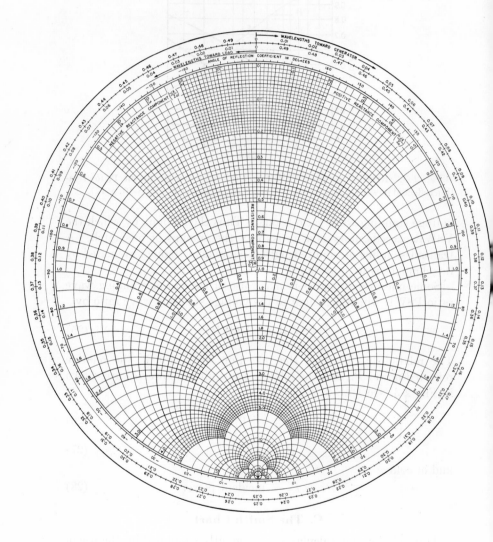

Fig. 2–4. The Smith chart. The circles of constant resistance and constant reactance are shown, while the circles of constant reflection coefficient are omitted [Smith (1944)].

Let the impedance Z at any point along the line be normalized to the characteristic impedance Z_0 and decomposed into its real and imaginary parts R and X, respectively,

$$Z/Z_0 = R/Z_0 + j(X/Z_0) \tag{1}$$

This expression is usually written

$$z = r + jx \tag{2}$$

where $z = Z/Z_0$, etc. Constant resistance (r) circles are arranged in the pattern shown on Fig. 2-5a, and constant reactance (x) circles form the configuration shown on Fig. 2-5b. It should be noted that the family of constant resistance circles is orthogonal to the family of constant reactance circles. Figure 2-5c presents circles of constant VSWR. The numbers around the perimeter of Figs. 2-5a, b, and c give the number of (guide) wavelengths toward the load.

The actual Smith chart is shown on Fig. 2-4. Its use may be illustrated by drawing the VSWR = 2 and VSWR = 5 circles on Fig. 2-4 and graphically picking off the per unit reactance r and susceptance x values for several positions along the transmission line, as shown on Table 2-1. Thus the Smith chart may be used to

TABLE 2-1

Values of per Unit Reactance r and per Unit Susceptance x as a Function of Wavelength along the Transmission Line

VSWR	Wavelength toward generator	Wavelength toward load	Reactance r	Susceptance x
2	0	0.500	0.5	0.0
2	0.125	0.375	0.8	0.6
2	0.152	0.348	1.0	0.7
2	0.250	0.250	2.0	0.0
2	0.348	0.152	1.0	0.7
2	0.375	0.125	0.8	0.6
2	0.5000	0	0.5	0.0
5	0	0.500	0.2	0.0
5	0.125	0.375	0.39	0.92
5	0.250	0.250	5.0	0.0
5	0.375	0.125	0.39	0.92
5	0.500	0	0.2	0.0

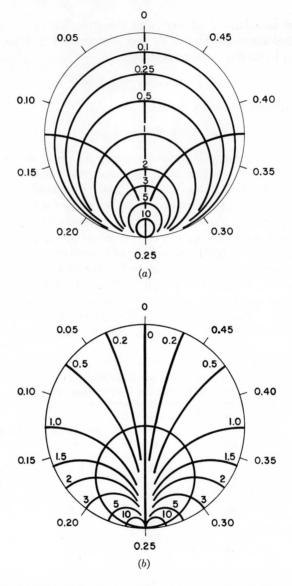

Fig. 2–5. (a) Loci of constant resistance circles on the Smith chart. Their centers lie on the lower half of the vertical diameter. (b) Loci of constant reactance circles on Smith chart. Their centers lie on the horizontal line which is tangent to the lowest point on the chart (i.e., where $\lambda = 0.25$).

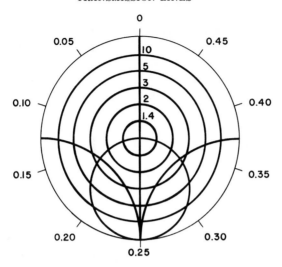

Fig. 2–5.   (c) Loci of concentric constant VSWR circles on the Smith chart.

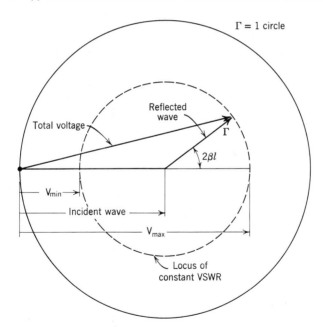

Fig. 2–6.   Vector diagram to illustrate the reflection coefficient representation
of the Smith chart [Ginzton (1957)].

ascertain the value of the impedance along the transmission line, and since $V = ZI$ this shows how the current and voltage vary. The vector relationship between the total voltage and the voltage in the incident and reflected wave is illustrated on Fig. 2-6. The Smith chart is useful as an aid in analyzing and solving waveguide transmission problems such as the effect that slide screw tuners, resonant cavities, crystals, etc. have on the configuration of the electromagnetic waves in waveguides. Its use will be illustrated several times later in the book.

The standing wave configuration in a waveguide is easily measured by means of a slotted line equipped with a crystal detector as described in RLS-11. The crystal current supplies the ratio V_{max}/V_{min} and thereby furnishes the VSWR.

Wilmshurst, Gambling, and Ingram (1962) analyzed the performance of various types of ESR spectrometers in terms of their operating points on a Smith chart.

D. Transmission Lines with Losses

The effect of losses on the transmission line may be represented by adding a series resistance per unit length R and a shunt conductance per unit length G to the transmission line equations (2-B-1) and (2-B-2). The resulting expressions are

$$\partial V/\partial z = - L(\partial I/\partial t) - RI \tag{1}$$

$$\partial I/\partial z = - C(\partial V/\partial t) - GV \tag{2}$$

and for a sinusoidal time dependence $e^{j\omega t}$ of both the current and the voltage eqs. (1) and (2) become

$$\partial V/\partial z = - (R + j\omega L)I \tag{3}$$

and

$$\partial I/\partial z = - (G + j\omega C)V \tag{4}$$

One may eliminate either I or V from these equations by a differentiation with respect to z followed by a substitution, with the result that

$$\partial^2 V/\partial z^2 = \gamma^2 V \tag{5}$$

and

$$\partial^2 I/\partial z^2 = \gamma^2 I \tag{6}$$

where the propagation constant γ is defined in terms of the attenuation constant α and the phase constant β

$$\gamma = \alpha + j\beta = [(R + j\omega L)\,(G + j\omega C)]^{1/2} \tag{7}$$

The solution to eq. (5) is

$$V = V_1 e^{-\gamma z} + V_2 e^{\gamma z} \tag{8}$$

and substitution of this solution in eq. (3) gives for the current

$$I = (1/Z_0)\,(V_1 e^{-\gamma z} - V_2 e^{\gamma z}) \tag{9}$$

where the characteristic impedance Z_0 is

$$Z_0 = [(R + j\omega L)/(G + j\omega C)]^{1/2} \tag{10}$$

Thus a lossy transmission line supports a forward traveling wave $V_1 e^{-\alpha z - j\beta z}$ and a backward traveling wave $V_2 e^{-\alpha z + j\beta z}$ each of which decreases exponentially with the attenuation constant α. Table 2–2 summarizes the properties of lossy transmission lines, and compares them to lossless transmission lines.

Most transmission lines encountered in practical cases have low losses so that

$$R \ll \omega L \tag{11}$$

and

$$G \ll \omega C \tag{12}$$

Therefore

$$\alpha + j\beta = [(R + j\omega L)\,(G + j\omega C)]^{1/2} \tag{13}$$

$$\approx j\omega (LC)^{1/2}\,[1 - RG/\omega^2 LC - j(R/\omega L + G/\omega C)]^{1/2} \tag{14}$$

$$\approx j\omega (LC)^{1/2}\,[1 - \tfrac{1}{2}j(R/\omega L + G/\omega C)] \tag{15}$$

TABLE 2–2

Summary of Transmission Line Equations (from *RLS-9*, pp. 32–33)

No.	Quantity	General line	Ideal line	Approximation, low-loss line
1	Propagation constant $\gamma = \alpha + j\beta$	$[(R + j\omega L)(G + j\omega C)]^{1/2}$	$j\omega(LC)^{1/2}$	See α and β below
2	Phase constant β	$\mathrm{Im}\ \gamma$	$\omega(LC)^{1/2} = \omega/v_p = 2\pi/\lambda$	$\beta'[1 + \frac{1}{2}(\alpha_c/\beta' - \alpha_d/\beta')^2]$
3	Attenuation constant α	$\mathrm{Re}\ \gamma = (-1/2)(dP/Pdl)$	0	$\alpha_c + \alpha_d = R/2Z_0' + G/2Y_0'$
4	Characteristic impedance Z_0	$\left(\dfrac{R + j\omega L}{G + j\omega C}\right)^{1/2}$	$(L/C)^{1/2}$	$Z_0\left[1 + \frac{1}{2}\left(\dfrac{\alpha_c}{\beta'} - \dfrac{\alpha_d}{\beta'}\right)\left(\dfrac{\alpha_c}{\beta'} + \dfrac{3\alpha_d}{\beta'}\right)\right]$ $- jZ_0'\left(\dfrac{\alpha_c}{\beta'} - \dfrac{\alpha_d}{\beta'}\right)$
5	Input impedance Z_{-l}	$Z_0\dfrac{Z_r + Z_0 \tanh \gamma l}{Z_0 + Z_r \tanh \gamma l}$	$Z_0\dfrac{Z_r + jZ_0 \tan \beta l}{Z_0 + jZ_r \tan \beta l}$	$\dots$
6	Impedance of short-circuited line	$Z_0 \tanh \gamma l$	$jZ_0 \tan \beta l$	$Z_0\dfrac{\alpha l + j \tan \beta l}{1 + j\alpha l \tan \beta l}$
7	Impedance of open-circuited line	$Z_0 \coth \gamma l$	$-jZ_0 \cot \beta l$	$Z_0\dfrac{1 + j\alpha l \tan \beta l}{\alpha l + j \tan \beta l}$
8	Impedance of a line an odd number of quarter wavelengths long	$Z_0\dfrac{Z_r + Z_0 \coth \alpha l}{Z_0 + Z_r \coth \alpha l}$	Z_0^2/Z_r	$Z_0\dfrac{Z_0 + Z_r\alpha l}{Z_r + Z_0\alpha l}$
9	Impedance of a line an integral number of half wave-lengths long	$Z_0\dfrac{Z_r + Z_0 \tanh \alpha l}{Z_0 + Z_r \tanh \alpha l}$	Z_r	$Z_0\dfrac{Z_r + Z_0\alpha l}{Z_0 + Z_r\alpha l}$
10	Voltage V_{-l} along line	$V_i(1 + \Gamma_0 e^{-2\gamma l})$	$V_i(1 + \Gamma_0 e^{-2j\beta l})$	$\dots$
11	Current I_{-l} along line	$I_i(1 - \Gamma_0 e^{-2\gamma l})$	$I_i(1 - \Gamma_0 e^{-2j\beta l})$	$\dots$
12	Voltage reflection coefficient	$\dfrac{Z_r - Z_0}{Z_r + Z_0}$	$\dfrac{Z_r - Z_0}{Z_r + Z_0}$	$\dots$

R, L, G, C = distributed resistance, inductance, conductance, capacitance per unit length.

$\beta' = (L/C)^{1/2}$ = phase constant, neglecting losses.

$Z_0' = (L/C)^{1/2}$ = characteristic impedance, neglecting loss; $Y'_0 = 1/Z'_0$.

λ = wavelength measured along line.

v_p = phase velocity of line, equals velocity of light in dielectric of line for an ideal line.

Γ_0 = reflection coefficient at $z = 0$.

l = distance along line, from load end.

Subscript r denotes receiving end (load) quantities at $z = 0$.

Subscript $-l$ denotes input end, quantities at $z = -l$.

Subscript i denotes incident wave quantities.

α_c results from conductor losses.

α_d results from dielectric losses.

since $RG \ll \omega^2 LC$.   This gives for the attenuation constant

$$2\alpha = R/Z_0 + GZ_0 \text{ Np/m} \tag{16a}$$

$$= 8.686 \ (R/Z_0 + GZ_0) \text{ dB/m} \tag{16b}$$

in the units Np/m and dB/m.   In addition,

$$\beta = \omega \ (LC)^{1/2} \tag{17}$$

and as before in the lossless case

$$Z_0 = (L/C)^{1/2} \tag{18}$$

Another way of looking at lossy transmission lines is to consider that a traveling wave propagating along a transmission line has the current and voltage values

$$V = V_1 e^{-\alpha z} e^{j(\omega t - \beta z)} \tag{19}$$

and

$$I = I_1 e^{-\alpha z} e^{j(\omega t - \beta z)} \tag{20}$$

so that the average power P is

$$P = \tfrac{1}{2} |V_1 I_1| e^{-2\alpha z} \tag{21}$$

where the factor of a half arises from averaging the time dependence. The average power attenuation is the fractional rate of decrease of the power with distance

$$2\alpha = - \ (1/P) \ (\partial P / \partial z) \tag{22}$$

and

$$\alpha = \frac{1}{2} \left(\frac{\text{power lost per unit length}}{\text{power transmitted}} \right) \tag{23}$$

E. Miscellaneous Transmission Line Characteristics

When a transmission line is terminated in a short circuit the voltage will be zero and the current will be a maximum both at the short, and also at multiples of half wavelengths before the short.   Intermediate between these points the voltage will be a maximum and the current zero. The current and voltage are 90° out of time phase, and the ratio of the maximum current to the maximum voltage on the line equals the characteristic impedance. Since $V_{min} = I_{min} = 0$, the voltage standing wave ratio is infinite.

When an open circuit terminates a transmission line the roles of the voltage and current are interchanged, with the voltage reaching a maximum and the current vanishing at the open circuit, etc. The phase relations and characteristic impedance remain in the same. A transmission line terminated by a purely inductive or capacitive load is equivalent to one of slightly different length (within $\lambda/4$) which is terminated by either an open or a short circuit. Thus short circuit, open circuit, and inductive and capacitive terminations all produce infinite standing wave ratios, and they may be converted into each other by adding or subtracting a length of line equal to or less than a quarter of a wavelength.

An infinitely long transmission line has only a forward traveling wave, with no reflected wave. Such a line is electrically equivalent to a transmission line of finite length terminated in a resistance equal to the characteristic impedance, and it is said to be matched. When such a transmission line is actuated by a generator which is also "matched" to the line, then the VSWR becomes unity, and there is no reflected wave. If the transmission line is lossless, all of the energy supplied by the generator will be dissipated by the terminating load or impedance.

If the transmission line is terminated in a resistance other than the characteristic impedance, then some of the incident microwave power is dissipated in the load, and some is reflected. When the load impedance Z is complex

$$Z_L = R_L + jX_L \qquad (1)$$

then R_L dissipates some power and X_L changes the phase relations between V_1, V_2, I_1, and I_2.

If a transmission line possesses a discontinuity where its characteristic impedance changes abruptly from the value Z_0 to Z_0' there will arise an impedance mismatch, and standing waves will be set up (VSWR > 1). It is possible to "match" these two transmission lines and effectively nullify the disturbance from the discontinuity by the use of a quarter wave transformer which is an intervening quarter wavelength long section of transmission line whose characteristic impedance Z_0'' is the geometric mean of the other two

$$Z_0'' = (Z_0 Z_0')^{1/2} \tag{2}$$

Because of the requirement that such a transformer be a quarter of a wavelength (or an odd number of quarter wavelengths) long its matching properties are very frequency sensitive. The thin film applied to camera lenses to reduce reflections is an example of a quarter wave transformer designed to match the impedance of air to that of the lens glass at the center of the optical (visible) region of the electromagnetic spectrum.

References

E. L. Ginzton, *Microwave Measurements*, McGraw-Hill, N. Y., 1957, p. 233.

S. Ramo, J. R. Whinnery, and T. Van Duzer, *Fields and Waves in Communication Electronics*, Wiley, N. Y., 1965.

RLS-8.

RLS-10.

RLS-11.

P. H. Smith, *Electronics*, **12**, 29 (Jan. 1939); **17**, 130 (Jan. 1944).

T. H. Wilmshurst, W. A. Gambling, and D. J. E. Ingram, *J. Electron. Control*, **13**, 339 (1962).

CHAPTER 3

Electromagnetic Theory

A. Maxwell's Equations

Maxwell's equations are required for an understanding of microwave propagation in waveguides, energy storage in resonant cavities, and other topics which are essential to electron spin resonance spectrometers.

Maxwell's equations relate six basic electromagnetic quantities: (*1*) the electric field vector **E** with the units volts/meter; (*2*) the electric displacement or electric flux density vector **D** with the units coulombs/meter^2; (*3*) the magnetic field or field strength vector **H** with the units amperes per meter; (*4*) the magnetic induction or magnetic flux density vector **B** with the units webers/meter^2 = kilogram/coulomb second = 10^4 gauss; (*5*) the electric charge density ρ with the units coulombs/meter^3; and (*6*) the electric current density vector **J** with the units amperes/meter.[2]

The MKS (meter-kilogram-second) units are employed in the first five chapters of this book, and those who prefer cgs (centimeter-gram-second) units should consult Appendix A for the conversion factors between the two systems and some of the important equations rewritten in cgs units. The electron spin resonance literature frequently refers to the magnetic field **H** in units of gauss, and we will occasionally adapt this hybrid terminology.

In vector notation Maxwell's equations have the form

$$\nabla \cdot \mathbf{D} = \rho \qquad (1)$$

$$\nabla \cdot \mathbf{B} = 0 \qquad (2)$$

$$\nabla \times \mathbf{E} = - \partial \mathbf{B}/\partial t \qquad (3)$$

$$\nabla \times \mathbf{H} = \mathbf{J} + \partial \mathbf{D}/\partial t \qquad (4)$$

where eqs. (1) and (2) contain the divergence operator $\nabla \cdot$ and eqs. (3) and (4) contain the curl operator $\nabla \times$. When the rf fields vary sinusoidally in time at the angular frequency $2\pi f = \omega$ we may write

$$\partial \mathbf{B}/\partial t = j\omega \mathbf{B} \tag{5}$$

$$\partial \mathbf{D}/\partial t = j\omega \mathbf{D} \tag{6}$$

where $j = (-1)^{1/2}$. Equations (3) and (4) each have three components corresponding to the x, y, and z Cartesian coordinate directions, and so in scalar notation when the rf fields vary sinusoidally in time they have the form

$$\frac{\partial D_x}{\partial x} + \frac{\partial D_y}{\partial y} + \frac{\partial D_z}{\partial z} = \rho \tag{7}$$

$$\frac{\partial B_x}{\partial x} + \frac{\partial B_y}{\partial y} + \frac{\partial B_z}{\partial z} = 0 \tag{8}$$

$$\frac{\partial E_z}{\partial y} - \frac{\partial E_y}{\partial z} = -j\omega B_x \tag{9}$$

$$\frac{\partial E_x}{\partial z} - \frac{\partial E_z}{\partial x} = -j\omega B_y \tag{10}$$

$$\frac{\partial E_y}{\partial x} - \frac{\partial E_x}{\partial y} = -j\omega B_z \tag{11}$$

$$\frac{\partial H_z}{\partial y} - \frac{\partial H_y}{\partial z} = J_x + j\omega D_x \tag{12}$$

$$\frac{\partial H_x}{\partial z} - \frac{\partial H_z}{\partial x} = J_y + j\omega D_y \tag{13}$$

$$\frac{\partial H_y}{\partial x} - \frac{\partial H_x}{\partial y} = J_z + j\omega D_z \tag{14}$$

where the subscripts x, y, and z denote the components of the vectors.

Since these equations are in cartesian coordinates they are convenient for use with rectangular waveguides.   When one is interested in cylindrical waveguides and cylindrical resonant cavities, then Maxwell's equations (1) and (4) are usually written in the form,

$$\frac{1}{r} \frac{\partial}{\partial r} (rD_r) + \frac{1}{r} \frac{\partial D_\varphi}{\partial \varphi} + \frac{\partial D_z}{\partial z} = \rho \tag{15}$$

$$\frac{1}{r} \frac{\partial H_z}{\partial \varphi} - \frac{\partial H_\varphi}{\partial z} = J_r + \frac{\partial D_r}{\partial t} \tag{16}$$

$$\frac{\partial H_r}{\partial z} - \frac{\partial H_z}{\partial r} = J_\varphi + \frac{\partial D_\varphi}{\partial t} \tag{17}$$

$$\frac{1}{r} \frac{\partial}{\partial r} (rH_\varphi) - \frac{1}{r} \frac{\partial H_r}{\partial \varphi} = J_z + \frac{\partial D_z}{\partial t} \tag{18}$$

where the subscripts r, φ, and z denote vector components in the cylindrical coordinate system shown in Fig. 3-1.   Maxwell's other two equations may be easily written down in cylindrical coordinates by using eqs. (15)–(18) as models.

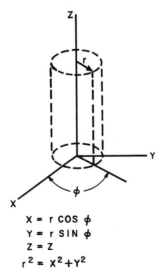

$$X = r \cos \phi$$
$$Y = r \sin \phi$$
$$Z = Z$$
$$r^2 = X^2 + Y^2$$

Fig. 3–1.   Cylindrical coordinate system.

For completeness we repeat eqs. (15)–(18) in spherical (polar) coordinates r, θ, and φ:

$$\frac{1}{r^2} \frac{\partial}{\partial r} (r^2 D_r) + \frac{1}{r \sin \theta} \frac{\partial}{\partial \theta} (D_\theta \sin \theta) + \frac{1}{r \sin \theta} \frac{\partial D_\theta}{\partial \varphi} = \rho \quad (19)$$

$$\frac{1}{r \sin \theta} \left[\frac{\partial}{\partial \theta} (H_\varphi \sin \theta) - \frac{\partial H_\theta}{\partial \varphi} \right] = J_r + \frac{\partial D_r}{\partial t} \quad (20)$$

$$\frac{1}{r} \left[\frac{1}{\sin \theta} \frac{\partial H_r}{\partial \varphi} - \frac{\partial}{\partial r} (r H_\varphi) \right] = J_\theta + \frac{\partial D_\theta}{\partial t} \quad (21)$$

$$\frac{1}{r} \left[\frac{\partial}{\partial r} (r H_\theta) - \frac{\partial H_r}{\partial \theta} \right] = J_\varphi + \frac{\partial D_\varphi}{\partial t} \quad (22)$$

where the corresponding coordinate system is given in Fig. 3-2. If Maxwell's equations are desired in other coordinate systems the reader should consult Stratton (1941), Margenau and Murphy (1943), or Ramo, Whinnery, and Van Duzer (1965) for details on the proper form of the vector operators.

B. Auxiliary Equations

The force **F** on a charge q moving with a velocity **v** in a region with an electric field **E** and magnetic induction **B** is given in vector notation by

$$\mathbf{F} = q[\mathbf{E} + \mathbf{v} \times \mathbf{B}] \quad (1)$$

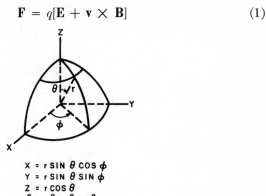

$$X = r \, SIN \, \theta \, COS \, \phi$$
$$Y = r \, SIN \, \theta \, SIN \, \phi$$
$$Z = r \, COS \, \theta$$
$$r^2 = X^2 + Y^2 + Z^2$$

Fig. 3-2.   Spherical polar coordinate system.

and the x component of the force F_x is

$$F_x = q[E_x + v_y B_z - v_z B_y] \qquad (2)$$

The y and z components may be obtained by permuting the indices. From Newton's law, $F = \text{mass} \times \text{acceleration}$, one may obtain the equation of motion.

The torque on a magnetic moment $\mathbf{\mu}$ possessing angular momentum $\hbar \mathbf{S}$ in a magnetic field of induction $\mathbf{B}$ is given by $\mathbf{\mu} \times \mathbf{B}$, and the equation of motion is

$$d(\hbar \mathbf{S})/dt = \mathbf{\mu} \times \mathbf{B} \qquad (3)$$

or

$$d\mathbf{\mu}/dt = \gamma \mathbf{\mu} \times \mathbf{B} \qquad (4)$$

and for a sinusoidally varying motion

$$j\omega\mathbf{\mu} = \gamma \mathbf{\mu} \times \mathbf{B} \qquad (5)$$

where the gyromagnetic ratio γ is the ratio of the magnetic moment to the angular momentum. This relation is the classical basis for both nuclear magnetic resonance and electron spin resonance, and will be discussed in detail later. The conduction current density obeys Ohm's law

$$\mathbf{J} = \sigma \mathbf{E} \quad \text{A/m}^2 \qquad (6)$$

where σ is the conductivity in mhos/meter.

The convection current density $\mathbf{J}$ resulting from a charge density ρ moving with velocity $\mathbf{v}$ is given by

$$\mathbf{J} = \rho \mathbf{v} \quad \text{A/m}^2 \qquad (7)$$

The permeability μ and the magnetic susceptibility χ are defined by

$$\mathbf{B} = \mu\mathbf{H} = \mu_0(\mathbf{H} + \mathbf{M}) = \mu_0\mathbf{H}(1 + \chi) \qquad (8)$$

where $\mathbf{M}$ is the magnetization or magnetic moment per unit volume. The symbol for permeability μ should not be confused with the magnetic moment vector $\mathbf{\mu}$ of eqs. (3)–(5). For free space $\mu_0 = 4\pi \times 10^{-7}$ H/m and for ferromagnetic ion alloys the relative permeability

μ/μ_0 varies from several hundred to several thousand. For non-ferromagnetic materials (diamagnetic, paramagnetic, or anti-ferromagnetic) the relative permeability is very close to the free space value. The susceptibility χ is negative for diamagnetic materials and positive for paramagnetic materials.

The dielectric constant ϵ is defined by

$$\mathbf{D} = \epsilon\mathbf{E} = \epsilon_0(\mathbf{E} + \mathbf{P}) = \epsilon_0\mathbf{E}(1 + \chi_e) \qquad (9)$$

where the electric susceptibility χ_e and the polarization or electric moment per unit volume $\mathbf{P}$ are analogous to χ and $\mathbf{M}$ of the magnetic case. In general, μ, ϵ, χ, and χ_e are all second rank tensors, and may vary with direction throughout the material. In the case of eq. (8) this means that

$$\begin{bmatrix} B_x \\ B_y \\ B_z \end{bmatrix} = \begin{bmatrix} \mu_{xx} & \mu_{xy} & \mu_{xz} \\ \mu_{yx} & \mu_{yy} & \mu_{yz} \\ \mu_{zx} & \mu_{zy} & \mu_{zz} \end{bmatrix} \begin{bmatrix} H_x \\ H_y \\ H_z \end{bmatrix} \qquad (10)$$

and for the x component of B

$$B_x = \mu_{xx}H_x + \mu_{xy}H_y + \mu_{xz}H_z \qquad (11)$$

In general it is always possible to find a coordinate system in which the x, y, and z axes are the principal axes and the permeability tensor is diagonal

$$\begin{bmatrix} B_x \\ B_y \\ B_z \end{bmatrix} = \begin{bmatrix} \mu_{xx} & 0 & 0 \\ 0 & \mu_{yy} & 0 \\ 0 & 0 & \mu_{zz} \end{bmatrix} \begin{bmatrix} H_x \\ H_y \\ H_z \end{bmatrix} \qquad (12)$$

so B and H do not mix components

$$B_x = \mu_{xx}H_x \qquad (13)$$

$$B_y = \mu_{yy}H_y \qquad (14)$$

$$B_z = \mu_{zz}H_z \qquad (15)$$

In terms of the susceptibility

$$\begin{bmatrix} B_x \\ B_y \\ B_z \end{bmatrix} = \mu_0 \begin{bmatrix} H_x \\ H_y \\ H_z \end{bmatrix} + \mu_0 \begin{bmatrix} \chi_{xx} & \chi_{xy} & \chi_{xz} \\ \chi_{yx} & \chi_{yy} & \chi_{yz} \\ \chi_{zx} & \chi_{zy} & \chi_{zz} \end{bmatrix} \begin{bmatrix} H_x \\ H_y \\ H_z \end{bmatrix} \qquad (16)$$

and for the x component

$$B_x = \mu_0(1 + \chi_{xx})H_x + \mu_0\chi_{xy}H_y + \mu_0\chi_{xz}H_z \qquad (17)$$

The tensor formulation is of more than academic interest since g factors are often anisotropic, which means that the corresponding rf magnetic susceptibilities are anisotropic and eqs. (4) and (5) must be generalized to include the gyromagnetic ratio tensor

$$\begin{bmatrix} \gamma_{xx} & \gamma_{xy} & \gamma_{xz} \\ \gamma_{yx} & \gamma_{yy} & \gamma_{yz} \\ \gamma_{zx} & \gamma_{zy} & \gamma_{zz} \end{bmatrix} \qquad (18)$$

instead of merely the scalar gyromagnetic ratio γ. The g factor tensor discussed in Sec. 1-F equals the gyromagnetic ratio tensor times $\hbar/\beta$ in agreement with eq. (1-D-7). The electric quantities ϵ and χ_e may also be tensors and should then be treated similarly, but their tensor properties will not concern us here. Throughout the remainder of the book the term susceptibility will normally mean magnetic susceptibility.

The continuity equation relates the spatial variation of the current density **J** (called the divergence of J) and time variation of the charge density ρ

$$\nabla \cdot \mathbf{J} + \partial\rho/\partial t = 0 \qquad (19)$$

$$\partial J_x/\partial x + \partial J_y/\partial y + \partial J_z/Jz + \partial\rho/\partial t = 0 \qquad (20)$$

For certain types of problems it is mathematically convenient to introduce the "fictitious" magnetic charge density ρ_M and magnetic current density J_M in eqs. (3-A-2) and (3-A-3) (*RLS*-12, Chap. 3)

$$\nabla \cdot \mathbf{B} = \rho_M \qquad (21)$$

$$\nabla \times \mathbf{E} = -\partial\mathbf{B}/\partial t - \mathbf{J}_M \tag{22}$$

$$\nabla \cdot \mathbf{J}_M + \partial\rho_M/\partial t = 0 \tag{23}$$

but such an approach will not be useful for the types of problems which will concern us in magnetic resonance.

C. The Integral Form of Maxwell's Equations

Two mathematical theorems may be employed to convert eqs. (3-A-1)–(3-A-4) to their integral form. Stokes' theorem states that the surface integral of the curl $\nabla \times \mathbf{V}$ of the vector $\mathbf{V}$ over any surface S equals the line integral of $\mathbf{V}$ along the boundary l of the surface

$$\iint_S \nabla \times \mathbf{V} \cdot d\mathbf{S} = \int_l \mathbf{V} \cdot d\mathbf{l} \tag{1}$$

The divergence theorem (Gauss' theorem) states that the volume integral of the gradient $\nabla \cdot \mathbf{V}$ of the vector over a volume τ equals the surface integral of $\mathbf{V}$ over the surface S which forms the boundary of τ

$$\iiint_\tau \nabla \cdot \mathbf{V} \, d\tau = \iint_S \mathbf{V} \cdot d\mathbf{S} \tag{2}$$

Stokes' theorem and the divergence theorem allow us to write four integral forms of Maxwell's equations; and each of these constitutes a well known and basic law of electromagnetism.

(1) Gauss' law states that at any time the electric flux flowing out of a closed surface equals the charge Q contained within

$$\iint_S \mathbf{D} \cdot d\mathbf{S} = \iiint_\tau \rho \, d\tau = Q \tag{3}$$

For a point charge q at the center of a spherical surface a distance r away, $d\mathbf{S} = r^2 \sin^2 \theta d\theta d\varphi$ in spherical coordinates and D is independent of angle, so

$$D = q/4\pi r^2 \tag{4}$$

which is well known from electrostatics.

(*2*) The magnetic induction flowing out of a closed surface at a given time is zero

$$\iint_S \mathbf{B} \cdot d\mathbf{S} = 0 \tag{5}$$

(*3*) Faraday's law states that the electromotive force (emf) or line integral of $\mathbf{E}$ about a closed path equals the negative of the rate of change of magnetic induction $\mathbf{B}$ through the path

$$\text{emf} = \int_l \mathbf{E} \cdot d\mathbf{l} = -\partial/\partial t \iint_S \mathbf{B} \cdot d\mathbf{S} \tag{6}$$

(*4*) Ampère's law states that the magnetomotive force mmf around a closed path l equals the current flowing through the path

$$\int_l \mathbf{H} \cdot d\mathbf{l} = \iint_S \mathbf{J} \cdot d\mathbf{S} + \partial/\partial t \iint_S \mathbf{D} \cdot d\mathbf{S} \tag{7}$$

$$\text{mmf} = I + \partial/\partial t \iint_S \mathbf{D} \cdot d\mathbf{S} \tag{8}$$

where I is the total current through the surface S bounded by the path l, and the last term on the right is the Maxwell displacement current.

D. Electromagnetic Energy Storage and Power Flow

It is well known from electrostatics that the energy U stored in a capacitance of C farads charged to a potential of V volts and a charge of Q coulombs is given by

$$U = \tfrac{1}{2}CV^2 = \tfrac{1}{2}Q^2/C \tag{1}$$

In like manner the energy stored in an inductance of L henrys carrying a constant current of I amperes is

$$U = \tfrac{1}{2}LI^2 \tag{2}$$

The power P dissipated in a resistance R is

$$P = IV = IR^2 = V^2/R \tag{3}$$

where a watt is a joule per second. Thus an inductance and a capacitance store energy without dissipating it, while a resistance dissipates energy without storing it.

The energy storage in a condenser may be considered as stored in the electric field E set up by the voltage and charge, and it is given by,

$$U = \tfrac{1}{2} \int \epsilon E^2 \, d\tau \quad \text{joules} \tag{4}$$

where the volume integration is carried out over the space in and around the condenser, and ϵ is the dielectric constant. In like manner the energy density $\Delta U/\Delta\tau$ associated with any electromagnetic field is,

$$\Delta U/\Delta\tau = \tfrac{1}{2}\epsilon E^2 \tag{5}$$

In general this energy density will be a function of time and position.

A similar treatment applies to inductances. The energy stored in an inductance is stored in the magnetic field, and may be expressed in the form,

$$U = \tfrac{1}{2} \int \mu H^2 \, d\tau \tag{6}$$

and the magnetic energy density $\Delta U/\Delta\tau$ is

$$\Delta U/\Delta\tau = \tfrac{1}{2}\mu H^2 \tag{7}$$

Under static conditions the inductance stores only magnetic energy and the capacitance stores only electric energy, so the energies of eqs. (4) and (6) are the total energies for these systems.

When electromagnetic standing waves are present in a region of space with dielectric constant ϵ and permeability μ the energy density at a given position in the space is given by

$$U = \tfrac{1}{2}\epsilon E^2 + \tfrac{1}{2}\mu H^2 \tag{8}$$

When the standing wave ratio is infinite the electric and magnetic fields are in both space quadrature and time quadrature. The first part of this statement means that the electric field is zero where the magnetic field is a maximum, and vice versa. The second part means that the instant in time when the electric fields reach their maximum values E_M the magnetic fields are everywhere zero, and vice versa. Thus the total energy keeps passing back and forth between the electric and magnetic fields, and it may be evaluated when one or the other is a maximum. Therefore

$$U = \tfrac{1}{2} \int \epsilon E_M{}^2 \, d\tau = \tfrac{1}{2} \int \mu H_M{}^2 \, d\tau \tag{9}$$

There is no energy propagation, but only energy storage. This is analogous to an LC tuned circuit where the energy goes back and forth between the capacitor and inductor, and may be evaluated at either maximum value,

$$U = \tfrac{1}{2} L I_M{}^2 = \tfrac{1}{2} C V_M{}^2 \tag{10}$$

The opposite situation occurs when the standing wave ratio is unity. In this case the $\mathbf{E}$ and $\mathbf{H}$ vectors are in phase and energy is propagated in accordance with Poynting's vector $\mathbf{P}$

$$\mathbf{P} = \tfrac{1}{2}\mathbf{E} \times \mathbf{H} \tag{11}$$

or more precisely

$$\mathbf{P} = \tfrac{1}{2}\mathrm{Re}\,(\mathbf{E} \times \mathbf{H}^*) \tag{12}$$

The total energy passing a surface in time t is

$$U = \int_0^t dt \int_S \mathbf{P} \times d\mathbf{S} \tag{13}$$

Poynting's vector $\mathbf{P}$ may be illustrated by a uniform plane wave moving at the velocity $\mathbf{v}$. This wave has the $\mathbf{E}$ vector perpendicular to the $\mathbf{H}$ vector, and both are perpendicular to the direction of propagation z with the following relations satisfied,

$$P = \tfrac{1}{2}\mathbf{E} \times \mathbf{H} \tag{14}$$

$$Z = |E|/|H| = (\mu/\epsilon)^{1/2} \tag{15}$$

$$v = 1/(\mu\epsilon)^{1/2} \tag{16}$$

and at each point

$$\tfrac{1}{2}\epsilon E^2 = \tfrac{1}{2}\mu H^2 \tag{17}$$

If one lets $E = E_x$ then H becomes H_y, but in a more general case E and H may have both x and y components, while remaining normal to each other.   In the former case,

$$E_x/H_y = -E_y/H_x = (\mu/\epsilon)^{1/2} = Z \tag{18}$$

If in addition to a forward wave there is also a backward traveling wave with components E' and H', then

$$E_x'/H_y' = -E_y'/H_x' = -(\mu/\epsilon)^{1/2} = -Z \tag{19}$$

and eqs. (14), (15), and (17) are valid for the total $\mathbf{E}$ and $\mathbf{H}$ vectors.

E. Electromagnetic Potentials

In solving electromagnetic problems it is frequently convenient to introduce two new variables called the vector potential $\mathbf{A}$ and the scalar potential ϕ.   These are defined by the relations

$$\mathbf{B} = \nabla \times \mathbf{A} \tag{1}$$

and

$$\mathbf{E} = -\nabla\phi - \partial\mathbf{A}/\partial t \tag{2}$$

with the Lorentz condition (Lorentz gauge)

$$\nabla \cdot \mathbf{A} + \mu\epsilon(\partial\phi/\partial t) = 0 \tag{3}$$

By using the vector identity

$$\nabla \times \nabla \times \mathbf{A} = \nabla(\nabla \cdot \mathbf{A}) - \nabla^2\mathbf{A} \tag{4}$$

one may easily derive the two wave equations

$$\nabla^2\mathbf{A} - \mu\epsilon(\partial^2\mathbf{A}/\partial t^2) = -\mu\mathbf{J} \tag{5}$$

$$\nabla^2\phi - \mu\epsilon(\partial^2\phi/\partial t^2) = -\rho/\epsilon \tag{6}$$

which have their analogs in the electric field and magnetic field wave equations

$$\nabla^2 \mathbf{E} - \mu\epsilon(\partial^2 \mathbf{E}/\partial t^2) = (1/\epsilon \nabla\rho + \mu(\partial \mathbf{J}/\partial t) \tag{7}$$

$$\nabla^2 \mathbf{H} - \mu\epsilon(\partial^2 \mathbf{H}/\partial t^2) = -\nabla \times \mathbf{J} \tag{8}$$

An elementary application of potential theory is to consider the electrostatic potential arising from a point charge q

$$\mathbf{D} = \epsilon\mathbf{E} = -\epsilon\nabla\phi \tag{9}$$

and eq. (3-C-4) is easily integrated to give

$$\phi = -q/4\pi\epsilon r \tag{10}$$

Another simple example is that in which φ is independent of time, so that eq. (6) reduces to Poisson's equation.

$$\nabla^2\phi = -\rho/\epsilon \tag{11}$$

If in addition there are no charges present then $\rho = 0$ and Laplace's equation results

$$\nabla^2\phi = 0 \tag{12}$$

F. Boundary and Continuity Conditions

In practice the solution of Maxwell's equations depends upon the value of the field vectors on boundaries and across interfaces. These boundary and continuity conditions are easily derived from the integral form of Maxwell's equations, and the reader is referred to any text on electromagnetic theory for their derivation. These conditions refer to the discontinuous change that occurs in the values of H, B, D, and E when passing from the first medium with the constituent parameters ϵ, μ, and σ to a second medium characterized by ϵ'', μ'', and σ''. The conditions are:

(1) The tangential component of the electric field intensity $E_\parallel$ (i.e., E parallel to the interface) is continuous across the boundary

$$E_\parallel = E_\parallel'' \tag{1}$$

and if the first medium is a conductor ($\sigma \sim \infty$) then

$$E_\parallel'' \sim 0 \tag{2}$$

(*2*) The tangential component of the magnetic field $H_\parallel$ is continuous across the boundary except when a surface current sheet J exists on the boundary. In the absence of J

$$H_\parallel = H_\parallel'' \tag{3}$$

For a perfect conductor ($\sigma \sim \infty$ and $H \sim 0$) there is a surface current density J along the boundary and

$$H_\parallel'' = J \tag{4}$$

(*3*) There is a discontinuity in the normal component of the electric displacement $D_\perp$ (i.e., the component perpendicular to the interface) equal to the surface charge ρ_S on the boundary

$$D_\perp - D_\perp'' = \rho_S \tag{5}$$

and when no such surface charge exists

$$D_\perp = D_\perp'' \tag{6}$$

(*4*) The normal component of the magnetic induction $B_\perp$ is continuous across the boundary

$$B_\perp = B_\perp'' \tag{7}$$

This relation is important in magnet design.

G. Incidence of Plane Waves on Dielectrics

The present section considers the oblique reflection of a plane wave at the planar interface between two dielectric regions. This case is somewhat more complicated than the reflection at a conductor surface because, in general, there will be both a transmitted and a reflected wave, as shown on Fig. 3-3. As in the conductor case, the angle of incidence θ equals the angle of reflection θ'

$$\theta = \theta' \tag{1}$$

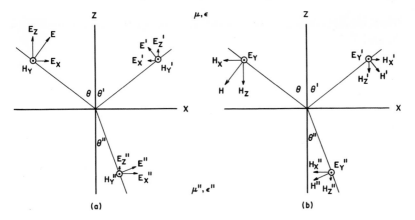

Fig. 3-3. The incidence of a plane wave on a dielectric interface: (a) with the E vector in the plane of incidence and H directed up from the paper, and (b) with the H vector in the plane of incidence and E directed up from the paper. The angle of incidence is θ, the angle of reflection θ', and the angle of refraction θ''.

and the angle of incidence θ is related to the angle of refraction θ'' by Snell's law

$$\sin \theta'' / \sin \theta = (\mu \epsilon / \mu'' \epsilon'')^{1/2} \tag{2}$$

where μ and ϵ refer to the first medium and μ'' and ϵ'' apply to the second medium. For most materials $\mu = \mu''$ so that Snell's law has the more familiar form

$$\sin \theta'' / \sin \theta = (\epsilon / \epsilon'')^{1/2} = n/n'' \tag{3}$$

where n is the index of refraction.

In the preceding section it was noted that across the dielectric boundary the tangential components of E and H are continuous and the normal components of D and B are continuous. One may use the first two of these boundary conditions and Fig. 3-3 to write down and analyze the electromagnetic waves.

When the electric field is polarized in the plane of incidence in accordance with Fig. 3-3a the boundary conditions give at the interface

$$E_x + E_x' = E_x'' \tag{4}$$

$$H_y + H_y' = H_y'' \tag{5}$$

The last equation may be written in terms of the wave impedances Z_z and Z_z''

$$E_x/Z_z - E_x'/Z_z = E_x''/Z_z'' \tag{6}$$

where

$$Z_z = E_x/H_y = -E_x'/H_y' \tag{7a}$$

$$Z_z'' = E_x''/H_y'' \tag{7b}$$

The reflection and transmission coefficients Γ and T, respectively, may now be written down

$$\Gamma = E_x'/E_x = (Z_z'' - Z_z)/(Z_z'' + Z_z) \tag{8}$$

$$T = E_x''/E_x = 2Z_z''/(Z_z'' + Z_z) \tag{9}$$

More explicitly, the wave impedances are

$$Z_z'' = (\mu''/\epsilon'')^{1/2} \cos \theta'' = (\mu/\epsilon'')^{1/2} [1 - (\mu\epsilon/\mu''\epsilon'') \sin^2 \theta]^{1/2} \tag{10}$$

and

$$Z_z = (\mu/\epsilon)^{1/2} \cos \theta \tag{11}$$

As a result the propagation constants in the first and second media are

$$\beta_x = k \sin \theta \tag{12}$$

$$\beta_z = k \cos \theta \tag{13}$$

$$\beta_x'' = k'' \sin \theta'' \tag{14}$$

$$\beta_z'' = k'' \cos \theta'' \tag{15}$$

where

$$k = 2\pi/\lambda = \omega(\mu\epsilon)^{1/2} \tag{16}$$

and

$$k'' = 2\pi/\lambda'' = \omega(\mu''\epsilon'')^{1/2} \tag{17}$$

The preceding expressions enable the electromagnetic wave configurations in the two media to be written down. When the **E** vector is polarized in the plane of incidence one has for the first medium

$$E_x = E \cos \theta \, [\exp (-j\beta_z z) + \Gamma \exp (j\beta_z z)] \exp (-j\beta_x x) \quad (18)$$

$$E_z = -(\mu/\epsilon)^{1/2} \sin \theta \, H_y \quad (19)$$

$$H_y = \frac{E}{(\mu/\epsilon)^{1/2}} \, [\exp (-j\beta_z z) - \Gamma \exp (j\beta_z z)] \exp (-j\beta_x x) \quad (20)$$

$$Z_z{}'' = (\mu''/\epsilon'')^{1/2} \, [1 - (\mu\epsilon/\mu''\epsilon'') \sin^2 \theta]^{1/2} \quad (10)$$

By a similar analysis one may show that when the **H** vector is polarized in the plane of incidence

$$E_y = E \, [\exp (-j\beta_z z) + \Gamma \exp (j\beta_z z)] \exp (-j\beta_x x) \quad (21)$$

$$H_x = -\frac{E}{(\mu/\epsilon)^{1/2}} \cos \theta \, [\exp (-j\beta_z z)$$

$$- \Gamma \exp (j\beta_z z)] \exp (-j\beta_x x) \quad (22)$$

$$H_z = \frac{1}{(\mu/\epsilon)^{1/2}} \sin \theta \, E_y \quad (23)$$

$$Z_z{}'' = (\mu''/\epsilon'')^{1/2} \, [1 - (\mu\epsilon/\mu''\epsilon'') \sin^2 \theta]^{-1/2} \quad (24)$$

It should be noted that eqs. (18)–(23) reduce to the wave configurations for reflection in the case of a perfect conductor when $\Gamma = -1$. This will be discussed in Sec. 4-A.

As in the conductor case, an incident plane wave of arbitrary polarization may be considered as a superposition of the two polarizations discussed above, and each component may be handled separately.

The reflection coefficient Γ for the dielectric interface has the form

$$\Gamma = (Z_z{}'' - Z_z)/(Z_z{}'' + Z_z) \quad (8)$$

When the wave impedance of the second medium is zero or infinity then

$$|\Gamma| = 1 \qquad (25)$$

and there is complete reflection. It may be objected that since the transmission coefficient

$$T = 2Z_z''/(Z_z'' + Z_z) \qquad (9)$$

becomes 2 when $|Z_z''| \gg |Z_z|$ one has an inconsistency in the previous section. To resolve this apparent inconsistency, consider the simple case of normal incidence with the plane wave of amplitude E_x and $H_y = E_x/Z$ incident on the dielectric interface. The reflected wave E_x' is

$$E_x' = \Gamma E_x \qquad (26)$$

and the transmitted wave E_x'' is

$$E_x'' = T E_x \qquad (27)$$

The power carried away by the reflected and transmitted waves P' and P'', respectively, is

$$P' = \tfrac{1}{2} E_x' H_y' = (E_x')^2/2Z_z = \Gamma^2 E_x^2/2Z_z \qquad (28)$$

and

$$P'' = \tfrac{1}{2} E_x'' H_y'' = (E_x'')^2/2Z_z'' = T^2 E_x^2/2Z_z'' \qquad (29)$$

Consider the ratio of the transmitted power P'' to the reflected power P in the limit $Z_z'' \gg Z_z$

$$\lim_{Z_z''/Z_z \to \infty} (P''/P) = (T^2/\Gamma^2)(Z_z/Z_z'') = 0 \qquad (30)$$

even though $T^2 = 4\Gamma^2$. The conservation of power may be demonstrated from the ratio of the reflected power to the incident power

$$\lim_{Z_z''/Z_z \to \infty} (P'/P) = \Gamma^2 = 1 \qquad (31)$$

Another instance in which total reflection occurs is when the wave impedance of the first medium Z_z is real, and that of the second medium Z_z'' is purely imaginary. In this case $Z_z'' = jX_z''$ and

$$| \Gamma | = \left| \frac{jX_z'' - Z_z}{jX_z'' + Z_z} \right| = \left[\frac{X_z''^2 + Z_z^2}{X_z''^2 + Z_z^2} \right]^{1/2} = 1 \qquad (32)$$

This is analogous to terminating a transmission line with a reactive load which does not dissipate power, but instead reflects it all.

A special case of total reflection occurs for

$$\sin \theta_c = (\mu'' \epsilon'' / \mu \epsilon)^{1/2} \qquad (33)$$

when either the **E** or **H** vector is polarized in the plane of incidence, since in this case the load impedance Z_z'' from eq. (10) vanishes and that from eq. (24) becomes infinite. Usually $\mu = \mu''$ and the critical angle θ_c is given by

$$\sin \theta_c = (\epsilon'' / \epsilon)^{1/2} = n'' / n \qquad (34)$$

The critical angle for θ exists only when $\epsilon'' < \epsilon$, and so this case of total reflection occurs only when the plane wave passes from a medium of high dielectric constant to one of low dielectric constant. In this case total reflection occurs when the angle of incidence exceeds the critical angle. When total reflection occurs electromagnetic energy does penetrate several wavelengths into the second medium, but its amplitude is rapidly attenuated with distance. This energy is used in the recently developed "attenuated total reflectance" (ATR) technique of infrared spectroscopy.

When total reflection occurs the phase relation between the incident and reflected waves is different for the two types of polarizations. As a result, when a wave of arbitrary polarization is totally reflected it will, in general, become elliptically polarized.

The preceding discussion concerned cases of total reflection and the absence of a propagating transmitted wave. When the electric field is polarized in the plane of incidence there is a particular angle called the polarizing angle or Brewster angle θ_z for which the wave impedances in the two media are identical,

$$Z_z = Z_z'' \qquad (35)$$

and this occurs when

$$(\mu/\epsilon)^{1/2} \cos \theta_P = (\mu''/\epsilon'')^{1/2} [1 - (\mu\epsilon/\mu''\epsilon'') \sin^2 \theta_P]^{1/2} \qquad (36)$$

from eqs. (10) and (11). When $\mu = \mu''$ a rearrangement gives

$$\tan \theta_P = (\epsilon''/\epsilon)^{1/2} = n''/n \qquad (37)$$

which may be satisfied for either $\epsilon'' > \epsilon$ or $\epsilon'' < \epsilon$. The plane wave polarized with E in the plane of incidence is completely transmitted at the Brewster angle. No such Brewster angle exists for polarization of H in the plane of incidence. Plane-polarized electromagnetic radiation may be obtained by letting an unpolarized beam of radiation be incident at the Brewster angle. All of the reflected radiation will then be plane polarized with the **H** vector in the plane of incidence.

H. Imperfect Dielectrics

Maxwell's fourth equation

$$\nabla \times \mathbf{H} = \mathbf{J} + \partial \mathbf{D}/\partial t \qquad (1)$$

for a temporal dependence $e^{j\omega t}$ has the form

$$\nabla \times \mathbf{H} = j\omega(\epsilon - j\sigma/\omega) \mathbf{E} \qquad (2)$$

where use was made of Ohm's law $J = \sigma E$. It is more customary to consider the relative dielectric constant ϵ/ϵ_0 as made up of a real part ϵ' and an imaginary part ϵ'' defined by

$$\epsilon/\epsilon_0 = \epsilon' - j\epsilon'' \qquad (3)$$

Care should be exercised not to confuse these quantities with the ϵ and ϵ'' used earlier in the chapter. Physically, ϵ''/ϵ' is the dimensionless ratio of the conduction current J to the displacement current $\partial D/\partial t$ in the dielectric, and it is sometimes referred to as the loss tangent or tan δ

$$\tan \delta = \epsilon''/\epsilon' = 36\pi\sigma/\omega\epsilon' \times 10^9 \qquad (4)$$

where σ is in mhos/meter. Values of tan δ and ϵ'/ϵ_0 are listed in Table 3-1 for a number of typical dielectric materials.

TABLE 3–1

Dielectric Constant ϵ'/ϵ_0 and Loss Tangent tan δ for Several Solids at Room Temperature[a]

Material	10^8 cps		10^{10} cps	
	ϵ'/ϵ_0	tan δ	ϵ'/ϵ_0	tan δ
Alumina, Al_2O_3	{ 9.34 11.54 }	—	—	—
Bakelite (BM-16981, not pre- formed or pretreated)	4.7	10^{-2}	4.5	1.2 $\times$ 10^{-2}
Lucite HM-119 (polyacrylate)	2.58	6.7 $\times$ 10^{-3}	2.57	4.9 $\times$ 10^{-3}
Plexiglass	—	—	2.59	6.7 $\times$ 10^{-3}
Polyamide resin (Nylon 66)	3.16	2.1 $\times$ 10^{-2}	—	—
Polyisobutylene	2.23	3 $\times$ 10^{-4}	—	—
Polytetrafluoroethylene (Teflon)	2.1	<2 $\times$ 10^{-4}	2.08	3.7 $\times$ 10^{-4}
Pyrex glass (Corning 7740)	4.52	4.5 $\times$ 10^{-3}	4.52	8.5 $\times$ 10^{-3}
Rubber; natural (vulcanized)	2.42	1.8 $\times$ 10^{-2}	—	—
Silica, fused	3.78	3 $\times$ 10^{-5}	3.78	1.7 $\times$ 10^{-4}
Styrofoam (polystyrene)	—	—	1.03	1.5 $\times$ 10^{-4}

[a] Data obtained from *American Institute of Physics Handbook*, 1963, Sec. 5.

When an electromagnetic wave propagates in the z direction through a dielectric medium the z dependence may be of the form

$$E = E_0 \exp (j\omega t - j\beta z - \alpha z) \tag{5}$$

where for simplicity only the positively traveling wave will be considered. In the absence of losses ($\epsilon'' = 0$ and $\alpha = 0$) the wave is undiminished in amplitude as it proceeds in the z direction with the velocity **v**

$$v = 1/(\mu\epsilon)^{1/2} \tag{6}$$

the propagation constant β

$$\beta = \omega(\mu\epsilon)^{1/2} = 2\pi/\lambda \tag{7}$$

and the characteristic impedance Z_0

$$Z_0 = (\mu/\epsilon)^{1/2} \tag{8}$$

When losses are present ϵ is complex and

$$\mathbf{v} = \mathrm{Re}\ 1/(\mu\epsilon)^{1/2} \tag{9}$$

$$\alpha = -\omega\ \mathrm{Im}\ (\mu\epsilon)^{1/2} \tag{10}$$

and

$$\beta = \omega\ \mathrm{Re}\ (\mu\epsilon)^{1/2} \tag{11}$$

In addition, the impedance Z has both a real part and an imaginary part. More explicitly

$$(\mu\epsilon)^{1/2} = (\mu\epsilon_0)^{1/2}\ (\epsilon' - [j\sigma/\omega\epsilon_0])^{1/2} \tag{12}$$

For a good conductor $\sigma \gg \omega\epsilon'\epsilon_0$ so that

$$\gamma = \omega\ (\mu\epsilon)^{1/2} = (1 - j)/\delta \tag{13}$$

and

$$\alpha = \beta = 1/\delta \tag{14}$$

where δ is the skin depth which will be explained in the next section. Further discussion of eq. (14) will be postponed until then.   For a low loss dielectric

$$\sigma/\omega\epsilon_0 \ll \epsilon' \tag{15}$$

and the square root in eq. (12) may be approximated by a binomial expansion

$$(\mu\epsilon)^{1/2} = (\mu\epsilon_0\epsilon')^{1/2}\ [1 - j\sigma/2\omega_0\epsilon_0\epsilon' + \tfrac{1}{8}\ (\sigma/\omega_0\epsilon_0\epsilon')^2] \tag{16}$$

As a result

$$\alpha = \pi\sigma/\lambda\omega\epsilon_0\epsilon' = (\pi/\lambda)\ \tan\delta \tag{17}$$

$$\beta = (2\pi/\lambda)\ [1 + \tfrac{1}{8}\ (\sigma/\omega\epsilon_0\epsilon')^2] \tag{18}$$

and

$$Z_0 = (\mu/\epsilon_0\epsilon')^{1/2}\ [1 - \tfrac{3}{8}\ (\sigma/\omega\epsilon_0\epsilon')^2 + j(\sigma/2\omega\epsilon_0\epsilon')] \tag{19}$$

One should bear in mind that

$$\epsilon = \epsilon_0 \, (\epsilon' - j\epsilon'')$$

$$\epsilon'' = \sigma/\omega\epsilon_0 \tag{20}$$

I. The Skin Effect

In a good conductor the conductivity σ is very high, and there are no free charges present. If any free charges were generated in a good conductor they would move to the surface with a time constant ϵ/σ which is extremely small. The conduction current J obeys Ohm's law $J = \sigma E$, and the displacement current $\partial D/\partial t$ is negligible compared with the conduction current J when $\omega\epsilon \ll \sigma$.

If we assume that the displacement current may be neglected, then the following equations hold within the conductor.

$$\nabla^2 \mathbf{H} = \sigma\mu(\partial \mathbf{H}/\partial t) = j\omega\sigma\mu\mathbf{H} \tag{1}$$

$$\nabla^2 \mathbf{E} = \sigma\mu(\partial \mathbf{E}/\partial t) = j\omega\sigma\mu\mathbf{E} \tag{2}$$

$$\nabla^2 \mathbf{J} = \sigma\mu(\partial \mathbf{J}/\partial t) = j\omega\sigma\mu\mathbf{J} \tag{3}$$

where a sinusoidal time variation is assumed. In the case of a plane conductor with no spatial variation in the current flow on the surface eq. (3) may be written

$$\partial^2 \mathbf{J}/\partial z^2 = j\omega\sigma\mu\mathbf{J} \tag{4}$$

where the z direction is perpendicular to the conductor surface. This equation has the solution

$$J = J_0 \exp{[-(1+j)(z/\delta)]} \tag{5}$$

where J_0 is the current density on the surface where $z = 0$, and the skin depth δ

$$\delta = (2/\omega\mu\sigma)^{1/2} \quad \text{meters} \tag{6}$$

is the depth at which the current decays to $1/e = 0.369$ of its value at the surface. The imaginary part of the exponential (5) indicates

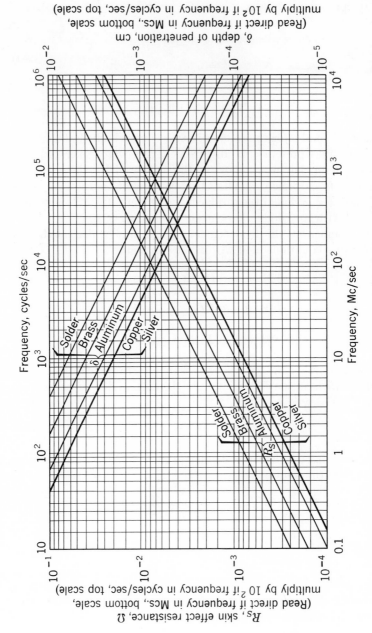

Fig. 3-4. Skin effect quantities for plane conductors [Ramo, Whinnery, and Van Duzer (1965), p. 252].

that there is also a phase change with depth. Numerical values of the skin depth for several important conductors may be obtained from Fig. 3-4. Included on this figure are values of the skin effect resistance R_S.

$$R_S = 1/\sigma\delta \tag{7}$$

which is the "surface" resistance of the conductor. From this figure we see that at the typical modulation frequency of 100 kc, the skin depth for copper is 0.2 mm, at the typical NMR frequency of 10 Mc, $\delta = 0.02$ mm for copper, and at the typical ESR frequency of 10^{10} cps the corresponding value is 6.6×10^{-4} mm. Thus microwaves only require conductors with a very thin metallic layer of high conductivity, and the electromagnetic energy is essentially confined to the surface. Fig. 3-5 shows the attenuation resulting from a thin layer of one metal on the surface of a second (see *RLS*-9, p. 128).

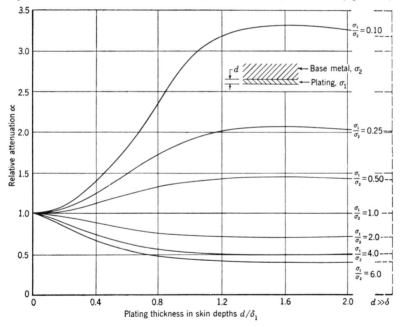

Fig. 3-5. Attenuation in plated conductors. The relative attenuation α is the ratio of the attenuation of the combination to the attenuation of the base metal (*RLS*-9, p. 128).

This is important because microwave cavities are frequently plated in this manner. The skin depth of 6.5 mm at 100 cps exceeds the 1.3-mm wall thickness of RG-52/U X band waveguide. Thus, low frequency audio modulation coils may be effectively located outside a cavity constructed from such a waveguide.

The derivation of eq. (4) assumes that the skin depth is much smaller than any curvature on the conductor surface. It should be emphasized that the current density J does actually penetrate below the skin depth, but its magnitude decreases exponentially with depth so that almost none is found below several skin depths.

References

American Institute of Physics Handbook, 2nd Ed., McGraw-Hill, N.Y., 1963, Sec. 5.

H. Margenau and G. M. Murphy, *The Mathematics of Physics and Chemistry*, Vol. 1, 2nd Ed., Van Nostrand, N.Y., 1956.

S. Ramo, J. R. Whinnery, and T. Van Duzer, *Fields and Waves in Communication Electronics*, Wiley, N.Y., 1965.

RLS-9.

J. A. Stratton, *Electromagnetic Theory*, McGraw-Hill, N.Y., 1941.

CHAPTER 4

Guided Electromagnetic Waves

A. Reflection of Plane Waves from Conductors

The reflection of a plane wave $E \exp [j(\omega t - \beta z)]$ vibrating in the x direction and normally incident on a perfect conductor is analogous to a transmission line terminated in a short circuit because the transverse **E** vector must be zero at the conductor. To satisfy this boundary condition the reflected electromagnetic wave sets up standing waves corresponding to $-E \exp [j(\omega t + \beta z)]$ so that

$$E_x = E\{\exp [j(\omega t - \beta z)] - \exp [j(\omega t + \beta z)]\} \tag{1}$$

$$= -2jE \sin \beta z e^{j\omega t} \tag{2}$$

as shown on Fig. 4-1. The **H** vector H_y vibrates at right angles to and in space quadrature with the **E** vector

$$H_y = (2E/Z_0) \cos \beta z e^{j\omega t} \tag{3}$$

where Z_0 is the characteristic impedance of the medium. The reflected wave carries away the same amount of energy that the incident wave brings to the conductor, so Poynting's vector at the surface averages to zero.

Another way to look at the problem is to consider the reflection coefficient Γ

$$\Gamma = (Z_L - Z_0)/(Z_L + Z_0) \tag{4}$$

where Z_L is the characteristic impedance of the conductor. One of Maxwell's equations is

$$\nabla \times \mathbf{H} = \mathbf{J} + \partial \mathbf{D}/\partial t \tag{5}$$

$$= (\sigma + j\omega\epsilon)\mathbf{E} \tag{6}$$

$$= j\omega[\epsilon - j(\sigma/\omega)]\mathbf{E} \tag{7}$$

77

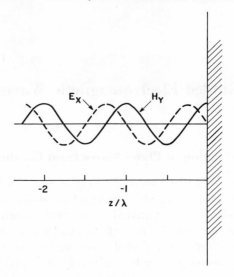

Fig. 4–1. Standing waves of E_x and H_y for plane wave normally incident on a conductor.

so the ratio of the conductivity to the angular frequency σ/ω constitutes an effective imaginary term in the dielectric constant. For the conductor as a termination and $\sigma/\omega \gg \epsilon$

$$Z_L = [\mu/(\epsilon - j\sigma/\omega)]^{1/2} = (1 + j)\,(\omega\mu/2\sigma)^{1/2} = (1 + j)R_s \quad (8)$$

where R_s is the surface resistivity which becomes very small when $\sigma/\omega \gg \epsilon$. Recall that for free space

$$Z_0 = (\mu_0/\epsilon_0)^{1/2} = 120\pi\ \Omega \tag{9}$$

and μ_0 in a conductor is usually equal to the permeability of free space, so that

$$Z_L \ll Z_0 \tag{10}$$

for the conductor. As a result

$$\Gamma \approx -1 \tag{11}$$

For copper

$$R_s = (\omega\mu/2\sigma)^{1/2} = 2.61 \times 10^{-7}\ (f)^{1/2}\ \Omega \tag{12}$$

where f is in cycles per second. Since for green light at a wavelength of 600 mμ $f = 5 \times 10^{14}$ cps, it follows that even at optical frequencies R_s for copper is less than 10 Ω, and eqs. (10) and (11) are still valid approximations.

When a plane wave $E \exp [-jk(x \sin \theta + z \cos \theta)]$ is incident on a plane conductor at an arbitrary angle of incidence the analysis is somewhat more complicated. There are two cases to consider: (1) the electric vector $\mathbf{E}$ in the plane of incidence, and (2) the magnetic vector $\mathbf{H}$ in the plane of incidence as illustrated on Fig. 4-2. The mathematical treatment for these cases is found in most texts on electromagnetic theory such as Stratton's (1941) and Jackson's (1962) and only a qualitative discussion will be given here.

The first general characteristic of reflection at oblique incidence is that for both polarizations the angle of incidence θ equals the angle of reflection θ'. When the $\mathbf{E}$ vector is polarized in the plane of incidence it remains in that plane after reflection, as shown in Fig. 4-2a. The $\mathbf{H}$ vector remains pointing in the same direction so that both $\mathbf{E}$ and $\mathbf{H}$ are still perpendicular to the direction of propagation. The electromagnetic field above the conductor has the form of a standing wave with respect to the z direction, and the form of a traveling wave in the x direction. From the boundary condition, the component of

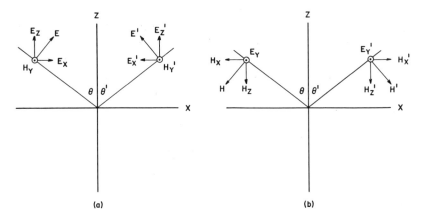

(a)   (b)

Fig. 4-2. The reflection of a plane wave at a conductor surface (a) with the $\mathbf{E}$ vector in the plane of incidence and $\mathbf{H}$ directed out of the paper, and (b) with the $\mathbf{H}$ vector in the plane of incidence and $\mathbf{E}$ directed out of the paper. The angle of incidence is θ and the angle of reflection is $\theta' = \theta$.

E in the x direction E_x vanishes at the conductor surface and at points nd above the surface, where the distance nd is

$$nd = \frac{n\pi}{\omega(\mu\epsilon)^{1/2}\cos\theta} = \frac{n\lambda}{2\cos\theta} \tag{13}$$

When the **H** vector is polarized in the plane of incidence it remains in this plane after reflection, as shown on Fig. 4-2b. The **E** vector remains pointing out of the paper, and again traveling waves are set up in the x direction and standing waves in the z direction, with eq. (13) satisfied for the vector **E**.

Whenever $\theta \neq 90°$ the phase velocities v_p in the x and z directions are

$$v_{px} = \omega/\beta_x = v/\sin\theta \tag{14}$$

and

$$v_{pz} = \omega/\beta_z = v/\cos\theta \tag{15}$$

where β_x and β_z are the real parts of the propagation constant in the x and z directions, respectively. It may seem paradoxical that this exceeds the velocity of light v

$$c = v = 1/(\mu\epsilon)^{1/2} \tag{16}$$

normal to the wavefront since it is generally believed that the velocity of light cannot be exceeded. However, a careful analysis will show that the electromagnetic energy flow **E** × **H** is normal to the wavefront and moves at the velocity v, so the phase velocity v_p is merely the velocity of points on the wavefront, and is not associated with the rate of propagation of electromagnetic energy. The nature of phase velocities will be clarified at the end of this chapter.

The wave impedance Z_z associated with oblique incidence between two media is the ratio of the **E** to the **H** vectors tangential to the boundary. For the **E** vector polarized in the plane of incidence one has

$$Z_z = E_x/H_y = -E_x'/H_y' = (\mu/\epsilon)^{1/2}\cos\theta \tag{17}$$

and for **H** in the plane of incidence

$$Z_z = -E_y/H_x = E_y'/H_x' = (\mu/\epsilon)^{1/2}\sec\theta \tag{18}$$

where the primed components denote the waves after reflection. Thus one polarization increases the wave impedance and one decreases it from the intrinsic impedance of the medium.   The wave impedance concept will be useful for the analysis of waveguides.

The electromagnetic wave configuration resulting from the plane wave

$$E \exp\left[-jk(x \sin\theta + z \cos\theta)\right] = E \exp\left[-j(\beta_x x + \beta_z z)\right] \quad (19)$$

$$H = E/(\mu/\epsilon)^{1/2} \quad (20)$$

with the propagation constants

$$\beta_x = k \sin\theta \quad (21)$$

$$\beta_z = k \cos\theta \quad (22)$$

$$k = 2\pi/\lambda = \omega(\mu\epsilon)^{1/2} \quad (23)$$

incident on a conductor surface becomes the superposition of the incident and reflected waves.   For the **E** field polarized in the plane of incidence it has the form

$$E_x = -2jE \cos\theta \sin\beta_z z \exp\left(-j\beta_x x\right) \quad (24)$$

$$E_z = -(\mu/\epsilon)^{1/2} \sin\theta \, H_y \quad (25)$$

$$H_y = [2E/(\mu/\epsilon)^{1/2}] \cos\beta_z z \exp\left(-j\beta_x x\right) \quad (26)$$

When the **H** vector is polarized in the plane of incidence the corresponding field configurations are

$$E_y = -2jE \sin\beta_z z \exp\left(-j\beta_x x\right) \quad (27)$$

$$H_x = -[2E/(\mu/\epsilon)^{1/2}] \cos\theta \cos\beta_z z \exp\left(-j\beta_x x\right) \quad (28)$$

$$H_z = [1/(\mu/\epsilon)^{1/2}] \sin\theta \, E_y \quad (29)$$

These wave configurations are useful for the analysis of waveguide propagation because the electromagnetic waves in waveguides may be considered as undergoing multiple reflections while they propagate.

When the incident wave is polarized in a direction other than the two discussed here it may be considered as a superposition of these two cases, and each component may be handled separately.

B. The Electromagnetic Field of Guided Waves

Two of Maxwell's equations have the form:

$$\nabla \times \mathbf{E} = -\partial \mathbf{B}/\partial t \tag{1}$$

and

$$\nabla \times \mathbf{H} = \mathbf{J} + \partial \mathbf{D}/\partial t \tag{2}$$

and in the interior of the microwave transmission line $\mathbf{J} = 0$. An electromagnetic wave propagated in the z direction has the propagation factor $\exp(j\omega t - \gamma z)$ where the propagation constant γ is defined by

$$\gamma = \alpha + j\beta \tag{3}$$

All of the time and z dependence is contained in the propagation factor, which considerably simplifies the curl eqs. (1) and (2). As a result they become

$$\partial E_z/\partial y + \gamma E_y = -j\omega\mu H_x \tag{4}$$

$$-\gamma E_x - \partial E_z/\partial x = -j\omega\mu H_y \tag{5}$$

$$\partial E_y/\partial x - \partial E_x/\partial y = -j\omega\mu H_z \tag{6}$$

$$\partial H_z/\partial y + \gamma H_y = j\omega\epsilon E_x \tag{7}$$

$$-\gamma H_x - \partial H_z/\partial x = j\omega\epsilon E_y \tag{8}$$

$$\partial H_y/\partial x - \partial H_x/\partial y = j\omega\epsilon E_z \tag{9}$$

There are three general types of wave configurations that may propagate along microwave transmission lines, namely, transverse electromagnetic (TEM) waves, transverse electric (TE) waves, and transverse magnetic (TM) waves. They have the following properties

$$H_z = E_z = 0 \qquad\qquad TEM \quad (10)$$

$$E_z = 0, \quad H_z \neq 0 \qquad\qquad TE \quad (11)$$

$$H_z = 0, \quad E_z \neq 0 \qquad\qquad TM \quad (12)$$

Some authors use the symbol H for TE waves and E for TM waves. A TEM mode is usually found in coaxial cables, while rectangular and cylindrical waveguides are unable to propagate TEM modes.

Maxwell's curl equations (1) and (2) are considerably simplified for transverse electromagnetic waves, and in this case eqs. (5), (7), (4), and (8), respectively, have the form

$$\gamma E_x = j\omega\mu H_y \tag{13}$$

$$j\omega\epsilon E_x = \gamma H_y \tag{14}$$

$$\gamma E_y = -j\omega\mu H_x \tag{15}$$

$$j\omega\epsilon E_y = -\gamma H_x \tag{16}$$

These four equations lead to the relation

$$\gamma^2 = \omega^2\mu\epsilon \tag{17}$$

with the velocity of propagation v

$$v = 1/(\mu/\epsilon)^{1/2} \tag{18}$$

and as a result the six Maxwell curl relations (4)–(9) simplify to

$$E_x = -j(\mu/\epsilon)^{1/2}H_y \tag{19}$$

$$E_y = j(\mu/\epsilon)^{1/2}H_x \tag{20}$$

$$\partial E_x/\partial y = \partial E_y/\partial x \tag{21}$$

$$\partial H_x/\partial y = \partial H_y/\partial x \tag{22}$$

For a Cartesian coordinate solution to these equations, let

$$E_x + jE_y = E_0 e^{j\theta} = E_0(\cos \theta + j \sin \theta) \tag{23}$$

$$H_x + jH_y = H_0 e^{j\theta'} = H_0 (\cos \theta' + j \sin \theta') \tag{24}$$

subject to the condition that

$$E_0 = (\mu/\epsilon)^{1/2} H_0 \tag{25}$$

and it follows from eqs. (19) and (20) that

$$\cos \theta = -\sin \theta' \tag{26}$$

$$\sin \theta = \cos \theta' \tag{27}$$

$$\cot \theta = -\tan \theta' \tag{28}$$

with the solution

$$\theta = \theta' + \pi/2 \tag{29}$$

Thus without loss of generality one may select **E** in the y direction, and the four eqs. (19)–(21) reduce to

$$E = (\mu/\epsilon)^{1/2} H \tag{30}$$

where

$$E = E_y \exp (j\omega t - \gamma z) \tag{31}$$

$$H = H_x \exp (j\omega t - \gamma z) \tag{32}$$

which constitutes a plane wave. This wave configuration or mode will propagate between lossless parallel plane conductors with the **E** vector perpendicular to the conductor surfaces. Of course, both vectors will be perpendicular to the direction of propagation, and the Poynting vector will move at the velocity of light $1/(\mu\epsilon)^{1/2}$, since it is a *TEM* mode. If the finite conductivity of the conducting planes is taken into account, a small electric field E_z will develop along the direction of propagation associated with the finite electric current that flows in the z direction on the guide walls. Aside from this weak axial electric field, the wave configuration remains nearly the same as in the lossless case.

A TEM mode in cylindrical coordinates is discussed in the next section on coaxial lines. It is not possible for TEM modes to propagate along hollow tubes such as rectangular, cylindrical, or elliptical waveguides. Both transverse electric and transverse magnetic waves are able to propagate between parallel planes, but they do not find much application in ESR, and so will not be discussed here. They are similar to the corresponding TE and TM waveguide modes, and may be derived therefrom by letting either the x or y waveguide dimension become much larger than the other dimension.

It is not possible for microwaves to propagate along a guiding system with both a longitudinal magnetic field component H_z and a longitudinal electric field component E_z in addition to the transverse **E** and **H** components. However it is possible to propagate wave configurations with either an H_z component (TE mode) or an E_z (TM mode) in addition to the transverse **E** and **H** components. The general boundary conditions on the three mode types (TEM, TE, and TM) are: (1) the magnetic field lines must form continuous closed loops which surround either a conduction current J or a displacement current $\partial D/\partial t$; (2) the electric field lines may form continuous closed loops which surround a changing magnetic field $\partial B/\partial t$; or (3) the electric field lines may end normally on a charge induced on the conductor surface. This last condition cannot be satisfied by a TEM mode.

C. Coaxial Lines

The usual mode found in coaxial lines is transverse electro–magnetic (TEM_{01}). The electric field E_r consists of radial lines of force extending from the inner conductor to the outer conductor, and the magnetic field H_φ consists of concentric circles which surround the inner conductor. The electric field E_r begins and ends on charges induced on the inner and outer conductors, and the magnetic field circles H_φ surround the conduction current J_z in the center conductor (J_z also flows in the outer conductor) to satisfy boundary conditions (1) and (3) mentioned at the end of the last section.

Since this is a TEM mode it travels at light velocity v

$$v = 1/(\mu/\epsilon)^{1/2} \qquad (1)$$

and the guide wavelength λ_g equals the free space wavelength λ. Because the guide wavelength is independent of the waveguide dimensions the cutoff wavelength λ_c is infinite, and there is no lower limit on the frequency which will propagate in this mode. The capacitance per unit length, inductance per unit length, and conductance per unit length are related to the natural logarithm of the ratio of the inner conductor radius r_i to the outer conductor radius r_0 as shown in Table 4-1.

Of more practical importance is the characteristic impedance Z_0 which is

$$Z_0 = (1/2\pi)(\mu/\epsilon)^{1/2} \ln (r_0/r_i) \ \Omega \qquad (2)$$

and for air or vacuum as the dielectric between the two conductors this simplifies to

$$Z_0 = 60 \ln (r_0/r_i) \ \Omega \qquad (3)$$

as shown graphically on Fig. 4-3.   The resistance per unit length R is

$$R = (R_s/2\pi) \ (1/r_0 + 1/r_i) \qquad (4)$$

where R_s is the surface resistivity. The attenuation due to the conductor losses α_R is

$$\alpha_R = R/2Z_0 \ \mathrm{Np/m} \qquad (5)$$

$$= 4.343 \ R/Z_0 \ \mathrm{dB/m} \qquad (5a)$$

Typical characteristic impedances for commercially available coaxial lines lie in the range 30 to 100 Ω, as shown in Table 4.2.   For a typical coaxial cable $r_i = 5 \times 10^{-4}$ m and $Z_0 = 50 \ \Omega$, giving

$$R \approx 320 R_s \qquad (6)$$

and

$$\alpha_R \approx 28 R_s \ \mathrm{dB/m} \qquad (7)$$

For copper

$$R_s = 2.61 \times 10^{-4} f^{1/2} \ \Omega \tag{8}$$

so that

$$\alpha_R \approx 7 \times 10^{-3} f^{1/2} \ \text{dB/m} \tag{9}$$

where the frequency f is in megacycles. For a typical X band frequency $f = 10^4$ Mc

$$\alpha_R \approx 0.7 \ \text{dB/m} \tag{10}$$

and a coaxial cable 4 m long will attenuate the microwave power by about 50%. The calculation for α_R is mainly illustrative because the actual values of α_R for coaxial cables shown in Fig. 4-4 exceed the calculated values due to the effect of dielectric losses, and increased conduction losses arising from braiding of the outer conductor. In practical cases, tabulated values from engineering handbooks should be employed in determining attenuation constants. A comparison of extrapolated attenuation constants from Fig. 4-4 with the attenuation of RG-52/U waveguide shown in Table 7-3 indicates that typical coaxial cables attenuate X band microwaves 10 times as effectively as the waveguide.

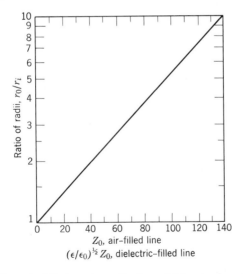

Fig. 4–3. Characteristic impedance Z_0 of coaxial line in ohms (RLS-9, p. 183).

TABLE 4–1
Transmission Line Formulae[a]
[Ramo, Whinnery, and Van Duzer (1965), p. 444].

	Coaxial line	Parallel wire line	Shielded parallel wire line[b]	Parallel bar line / Formulae for $a \ll b$
			$p = s/d$ $q = s/D$	
Capacitance C, F/m	$\dfrac{2\pi\epsilon}{\ln(r_0/r_i)}$	$\dfrac{\pi\epsilon}{\cosh^{-1}(s/d)}$	—	$\epsilon\, b/a$
External inductance L, H/m	$\mu/2\pi \ln(r_0/r_i)$	$\mu/\pi \cosh^{-1}(s/d)$	—	$\mu(b/a)$
Conductance G, mhos/m	$\dfrac{2\pi\sigma}{\ln(r_0/r_i)} = \dfrac{2\pi\omega\epsilon_0\epsilon''}{\ln(r_0/r_i)}$	$\dfrac{\pi\sigma}{\cosh^{-1}(s/d)} = \dfrac{\pi\omega\epsilon_0\epsilon''}{\cosh^{-1}(s/d)}$	—	$\sigma\, b/a = \omega\epsilon_0\epsilon'\, a/b$
Resistance R, Ω/m	$\dfrac{R_s}{2\pi}\left(\dfrac{1}{r_0}+\dfrac{1}{r_i}\right)$	$\dfrac{2R_s}{\pi d}\left[\dfrac{s/d}{\sqrt{(s/d)^2-1}}\right]$	$\dfrac{2R_{s2}}{\pi d}\left[1+\dfrac{1+2p^2}{4p^4}(1-4q^2)\right]$ $+\dfrac{8R_{s3}}{\pi D}q^2\left[1+q^2-\dfrac{1+4p^2}{8p^4}\right]$	$\dfrac{2R_s}{b}$
Internal inductance L_i, H/m (for high frequency)	\multicolumn{4}{c}{$\dfrac{R}{\omega}$}			

Characteristic impedance at high frequency Z_0, Ω	$\dfrac{\eta}{2\pi}\ln\left(\dfrac{r_0}{r_i}\right)$	$\dfrac{\eta}{\pi}\cosh^{-1}\left(\dfrac{s}{d}\right)$	$\dfrac{\eta_1}{\pi}\left\{\ln\left[2p\left(\dfrac{1-q^2}{1+q^2}\right)\right] - \dfrac{1+\frac{4p^2}{16p^4}(1-q^2)}{}(1-4q^2)\right\}$	$\eta(a/b)$
Z_0 for air dielectric	$60\ln\left(\dfrac{r_0}{r_i}\right)$	$120\cosh^{-1}(s/d)$ $\cong 120\ln(2s/d)$ if $s/d \gg 1$	$120\left\{\ln\left[2p\left(\dfrac{1-q^2}{1+q^2}\right)\right] - \dfrac{1+\frac{4p^2}{16p^4}(1-q^2)}{}(1-4q^2)\right\}$	$120\pi(a/b)$
Attenuation due to conductor α_c	$\dfrac{R}{2Z_0}$		
Attenuation due to dielectric α_d	$\dfrac{GZ_0}{2} = \dfrac{\sigma\eta}{2} = \dfrac{\pi\sqrt{\epsilon'\mu'}}{\lambda_0}\left(\dfrac{\epsilon''}{\epsilon'}\right)$		
Total attenuation dB/m	$8.686\,(\alpha_c + \alpha_d)$		
Phase constant for low loss lines β	$\omega\sqrt{\mu\epsilon} = 2\pi/\lambda$		

[a] All units above are mks.

$\epsilon = \epsilon_0(\epsilon' - j\epsilon'') = $ dielectric constant, F/m
$\mu = \mu'\mu_0 = $ permeability, H/m $\left.\right\}$ for the dielectric
$\eta = (\mu/\epsilon)^{1/2}$ Ω

$\epsilon'' = $ loss factor of dielectric $= \sigma/\omega\epsilon_0$
$R_s = $ skin effect surface resistivity of conductor, Ω
$\lambda = $ wavelength in dielectric $= \lambda_0/\sqrt{\epsilon'\mu'}$

[b] Formulae for shielded pair obtained from Green, Leibe, and Curtis, *Bell System Tech. Syst.*, **15**, 248 (1936).

TABLE 4-2

List of Standard Radio Frequency Cables[a]

[*American Institute of Physics Handbook* (1963), pp. 5-53 to 5-56]

Class of cables	JAN type	Inner conductor	Dielectric material[b]	Nominal diam of dielectric, in.	Shielding braid	Protective covering	Nominal over-all diam, in.	Weight, lb/ft	Approx. impedance, Ω[c]	Nominal capacitance, μμf/ft	Max operating voltage, rms	Remarks
General purpose	RG-5A/U RG-5B/U	16 Awg silvered copper	A	0.181	Silver-coated copper, double braid	Noncontaminating synthetic resin	0.332	0.087	50.0	28.5	3,000	Small-sized microwave cable
	RG-8/U RG-8A/U[d]	7/21 Awg copper	A	0.285	Copper, single braid	Synthetic resin	0.405	0.106	50.0	29.5	4,000	Medium-sized flexible cable
	RG-9A/U RG-9B/U[d]	7/21 Awg silvered copper	A	0.280	Silver-coated copper, double braid	Noncontaminating synthetic resin	0.420	0.150	50.0	30.0	4,000	Special medium-sized flexible cable
	RG-10/U RG-10A/U[d]	7/21 Awg copper	A	0.285	Copper, single braid	Noncontaminating synthetic resin and armor	0.475 max	0.146	50.0	29.5	4,000	Same as RG-8/U and RG-8A/U but with armor
	RG-14/U RG-14A/U[d]	10 Awg copper	A	0.370	Copper, double braid	Noncontaminating synthetic resin	0.545	0.216	50.0	29.5	5,500	Medium-sized power-transmission cable
	RG-17/U RG-17A/U[d]	0.188-in. copper	A	0.680	Copper, single braid	Noncontaminating synthetic resin	0.870	0.460	50.0	29.5	11,000	Large-sized, low-attenuation, high-power-transmission cable
	RG-18/U RG-18A/U[d]	0.188-in. copper	A	0.680	Copper, single braid	Noncontaminating synthetic resin and armor	0.945 max	0.585	50.0	29.5	11,000	Same as RG-17/U and RG-17A/U but with armor
	RG-19/U RG-19A/U[d]	0.250-in. copper	A	0.910	Copper, single braid	Noncontaminating synthetic resin	1.120	0.740	50.0	29.5	14,000	Very large, low-attenuation, high-power-transmission cable
	RG-20/U RG-20A/U[d]	0.250-in. copper	A	0.910	Copper, single braid	Noncontaminating synthetic resin and armor	1.195 max	0.925	50.0	29.5	14,000	Same as RG-19/U and RG-19A/U but with armor
	RG-55/U	20 Awg copper	A	0.116	Tinned copper, double braid	Polyethylene	0.206 max	0.034	50.0	28.5	1,900	Small-sized flexible cable

RG-58A/U RG-58C/U^d	19/0.0068 in. tinned copper	A	0.116	Tinned copper, single braid	Synthetic resin	0.195	0.025	50.0	28.5	1,900	Small-sized flexible cable
RG-74/U RG-74A/U^d	10 Awg copper	A	0.370	Copper, double braid	Noncontaminating synthetic resin and armor	0.615 max	0.310	50.0	29.5	5,500	Same as RG-14/U and RG-14A/U but with armor
RG-59/U RG-59A/U^d	22 Awg copper covered steel	A	0.146	Copper, single braid	Synthetic resin	0.242	0.032	70.0	21.0	2,300	General-purpose small-sized video cable
RG-11/U RG-11A/U^d	7/26 Awg tinned copper	A	0.285	Copper, single braid	Synthetic resin	0.405	0.096	70.0	20.5	4,000	Medium-sized flexible video and communication cable
RG-35/U RG-35A/U^d	9 Awg copper	A	0.680	Copper, single braid	Noncontaminating synthetic resin and armor	0.945 max	0.525	70.0	21.5	10,000	Large-sized high-power low-attenuation video and communication cable
RG-6/U RG-6A/U^d	21 Awg copper-covered steel	A	0.185	Inner: silver-coated copper; outer: copper	Noncontaminating synthetic resin	0.332	0.082	70.0	20.0	2,700	Small-sized video and communication cable
RG-13/U RG-13A/U^d	7/26 Awg tinned copper	A	0.280	Copper, double braid	Synthetic resin	0.420	0.126	70.0	20.5	4,000	Medium-sized flexible video and communication cable
RG-12/U RG-12A/U^d	7/26 Awg tinned copper	A	0.285	Copper, single braid	Noncontaminating synthetic resin	0.475 max	0.141	75.0	20.5	4,000	Similar to RG-11/U but with armor
RG-34/U RG-84A/U^d	9 Awg copper	A	0.680	Copper, single braid	Noncontaminating synthetic resin	1.000	1.325	71.0	21.5	10,000	Same as RG-35/U except lead sheath instead of armor for subterranean installations
RG-85/U RG-85A/U^d	9 Awg copper	A	0.680	Copper, single braid	Noncontaminating synthetic resin	1.565 max	2.910	71.0	21.5	10,000	Same as RG-84/U with special armor for subterranean installations
High-temperature RG-87A/U	7/20 Awg silvered copper	F (solid)	0.280	Silver-coated copper, double braid	Teflon-tape moisture seal, two braids fiber glass, silicone-varnish impregnated	0.425	—	50.0	29.5	4,000	Semiflexible cable, operating at temp. −55 to 250°C
RG-115/U	7/21 Awg silvered copper	F (tape)	0.250	Silver-coated copper, double braid	Teflon-tape moisture seal, two braids fiber glass, silicone-varnish impregnated	0.370	—	50.0	29.5	4,000	Semiflexible cable, operating at temp. −55 to 250°C

(continued)

TABLE 4-2 (*continued*)

Class of cables	JAN type	Inner conductor	Dielectric material[b]	Nominal diam of dielectric, in.	Shielding braid	Protective covering	Nominal over-all diam, in.	Weight, lb/ft	Approx. impedance, Ω^c	Nominal capacitance, $\mu\mu f/ft$	Max operating voltage, rms	Remarks
	RG-116/U	7/20 Awg silvered copper	F (solid)	0.280	Silver-coated copper, double braid	Teflon-tape moisture seal, two braids fiber glass, silicone-varnish impregnated and armor	0.475	—	50.0	29.5	4,000	Same as RG-87A/U but with armor
	RG-117/U	0.188-in. copper	F (solid)	0.620	Copper, single braid	Teflon-tape moisture seal, two braids fiber glass, silicone-varnish impregnated	0.730	—	50.0	29.0	22,000	Semiflexible cable, operating at temp. −55 to 250°C
	RG-118/U	0.188-in. copper	F (solid)	0.620	Copper, single braid	Teflon-tape moisture seal, two braids fiber glass, silicone-varnish impregnated and armor	0.780	0.610	50.0	29.0	22,000	Same as RG-117/U but with armor
	RG-119/U	0.102-in. copper	F (solid)	0.328	Copper, double braid	Teflon-tape moisture seal, two braids fiber glass, silicone-varnish impregnated	0.465	—	50.0	29.0	12,000	Semiflexible cable, operating at temp. −55 to 250°C
	RG-120/U	0.102-in. copper	F (solid)	0.328	Copper, double braid	Teflon-tape moisture seal, two braids fiber glass, silicone-varnish impregnated and armor	0.515	—	50.0	29.0	12,000	Same as RG-119/U but with armor
	RG-81/U	0.062-in copper	G	0.321	Copper tube		0.375	0.172	50.0	37.0	3,000	Small, semirigid cable, operating at temp. to 250°C
	RG-82/U	0.125-in. copper	G	0.650	Copper tube		0.750	0.698	50.0	36.0	4,000	Large semirigid cable, operating at temp. to 250°C

Pulse	RG-25/U	19/0.0117-in. tinned copper	D	0.308	Tinned copper, double braid	Synthetic rubber	0.565	0.205	50.0	50.0	8,000 peak	Special cable for twist application
	RG-26/U	19/0.0117-in. tinned copper	D	0.308	Tinned copper, single braid	Synthetic rubber and armor	0.525 max	0.189	50.0	50.0	8,000 peak	Medium-sized cable
	RG-27/U	19/0.0185-in. tinned copper	D	0.455	Tinned copper, single braid	Synthetic resin and armor	0.675 max	0.304	50.0	50.0	15,000 peak	Large-sized cable
	RG-28/U	19/0.0185-in. tinned copper	D	0.455	Inner: tinned copper; outer: galvanized steel	Synthetic rubber	0.805	0.370	50.0	50.0	15,000 peak	Large-sized cable
	RG-64/U	190/.0117-in. tinned copper	D	0.308	Tinned copper, double braid	Synthetic rubber	0.495	0.205	50.0	50.0	8,000 peak	Medium-sized cable
	RG-78/U RG-78A/U[d]	19/0.0117-in. tinned copper	E	0.288	Tinned copper, single braid	Polyethylene	0.385 max	—	50.0	50.0	8,000 peak	High-voltage cable
	RG-88/U RG-88A/U[d]	19/0.0117-in. tinned copper	E	0.288	Tinned copper, four braids	Polyethylene	0.490 max	—	50.0	50.0	8,000	Replaces RG-77/U in aircraft applications
Special characteristics	RG-22A/U RG-22B/U[d]	Each conductor 7/0.0152-in. copper	A	0.285	Tinned copper, double braid	Noncontaminating synthetic resin	0.420	0.151	95.0	16.0	1,000	Small-sized balanced twin-conductor cable
	RG-57/U RG-57A/U[d]	Each conductor 7/21 Awg copper	A	0.472	Tinned copper, single braid	Synthetic resin	0.625	0.225	95.0	17.0	3,000	Large-sized twin-conductor cable
	RG-111/U RG-111A/U[d]	Each conductor 7/0.0152-in. copper	A	0.285	Tinned copper, double braid	Noncontaminating synthetic resin and armor	0.490 max	0.146	95.0	16.0	1,000	Same as RG-22/U and RG-22A/U but with armor
	RG-21/U RG-21A/U[d]	16 Awg resistance wire	A	0.185	Silver-coated copper, double braid	Noncontaminating synthetic resin	0.332	0.087	50.0	29.0	2,700	Special high-attenuation cable with small temp. coefficient of attenuation
	RG-62/U RG-62A/U[d]	22 Awg copper-covered steel	A	0.146	Copper, single braid	Synthetic resin	0.242	0.0382	93.0	13.5	750	Small-sized, low-capacitance air-spaced cable
	RG-62B/U	7/32 Awg copper-covered steel	A	0.146	Copper, single braid	Noncontaminating synthetic resin	0.242	0.0283	93.0	13.5	750	Same as RG-62/U and RG-62A/U except inner conductor is stranded

(continued)

TABLE 4-2 (continued)

Class of cables	JAN type	Inner conductor	Dielectric material[b]	Nominal diam of dielectric, in.	Shielding braid	Protective covering	Nominal over-all diam, in.	Weight, lb/ft	Approx. impedance, Ω[c]	Nominal capacitance, μμf/ft	Max operating voltage, rms	Remarks
	RG-71/U	22 Awg copper-covered steel	A	0.146	Tinned copper, double braid	Polyethylene	0.250 max	0.0457	93.0	13.5	750	Small-sized low-capacitance air-spaced cable
	RG-63/U RG-63B/U	22 Awg copper-covered steel	A	0.285	Copper, single braid	Synthetic resin	0.405	0.0832	125.0	10.0	1,000	Medium-sized low-capacitance air-spaced cable
	RG-79/U RG-79B/U[d]	22 Awg copper-covered steel	A	0.285	Copper, single braid	Synthetic resin and armor	0.475 max	0.136	125.0	10.0	1,000	Same as RG-63/U and RG-63B/U but with armor
	RG-65/U RG-65A/U[d]	No. 32 formex, F, 0.128-in. diam meter (helix)	A	0.285	Copper, single braid	Synthetic resin	0.405	0.096	950.0	44.0	1,000	High-impedance video cable, high delay line

a The detail requirements for the cable types listed herein are covered by Specification JAN-C-17A. Power rating and attenuation characteristics of these cables will be available in the Armed Services Index of R. F. Transmission Lines and Fittings.

b Dielectric materials: (A) stabilized polyethylene; (D) layer of synthetic rubber between two layers of conducting rubber; (E) layer of conducting rubber plus two layers of synthetic rubber; (F) polytetrafluoroethylene (Teflon); (G) magnesium oxide.

c See individual specifications for nominal impedances and allowable tolerances.

d This cable is mechanically and electrically the same as the one listed with it but has the improved, noncontaminating, low-temperature synthetic resin jacket. This cable is preferred for all Signal Corps procurements.

e In pulse cable, the nominal diameter of dielectric is the diameter over the outer layer of conducting or synthetic rubber.

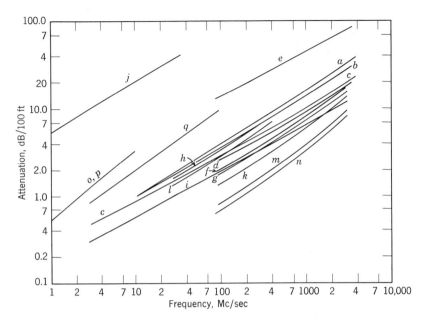

Fig. 4–4. Attenuation of standard rf cables vs. frequency. Cable RG-U number: (a) 55 and 58; (b) 59; (c) 62 and 71; (d) 5 and 6; (e) 21; (f) 8, 9, and 10; (g) 11, 12, and 13; (h) 22; (i) 63 and 79; (j) 65; (k) 14 and 74; (l) 57; (m) 17 and 18; (n) 19 and 20; (o) 25, 25A, 26, 26A, 64, 64A, 77, and 78; (p) 27 and 28; (q) 41 (30. 4 m = 100 ft) (RLS-17, p. 26; see also RLS-9, p. 268).

For comparative purposes Table 4-1 gives the electrical characteristics of a coaxial cable, of a parallel wire transmission line with and without a shield, and of a parallel bar transmission line. Parallel wire transmission lines tend to have higher characteristic impedances than coaxial lines, and they are balanced while the coaxial line is not. As an example of the application of each: (1) a shielded parallel wire line is often used to connect the output of a push–pull field modulation amplifier to the magnetic field modulation coils since one needs only to reverse the cable connector to reverse the phase of the modulation, and the entire system is balanced, while (2) a coaxial line often carries the signal from the output of the crystal to the preamplifier, since both the crystal and the preamplifier are electrically unbalanced. Table 4-2 lists the characteristics of some common coaxial cables.

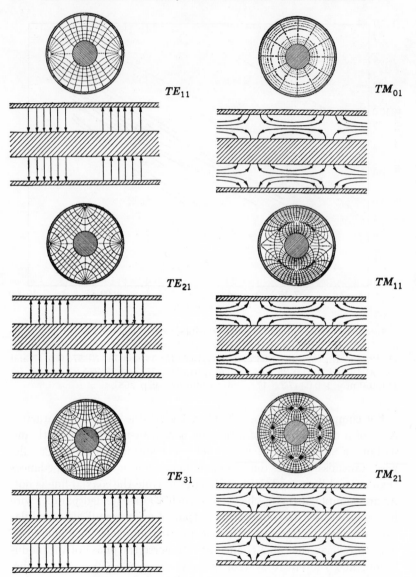

Fig. 4–5.   Transverse electric and tranverse magnetic modes in a coaxial transmission line.   (—) Electric field E; (. . .) magnetic field H (RLS-10, Sec. 2.4).

In conclusion, it should be mentioned that higher order waves of TE and TM type can propagate along coaxial lines, and the formulae in Table 4-1 do not apply to such modes (see RLS-8, p. 41; RLS-9, Chap. 2). For most coaxial line applications the wave length exceeds the average diameter (or circumference), and so these higher order modes are beyond cutoff, and cannot propagate. In these applications they only become important in the neighborhood of discontinuities. The wave configurations of several higher order coaxial modes are shown in Fig. 4-5.

D. Rectangular Waveguides

It was mentioned above that hollow waveguides cannot support TEM modes, so the rectangular waveguide shown on Fig. 4-6 will transmit only TE and TM modes. The generalized TE mode wave configuration may be obtained by setting $E_z = 0$ in eqs. (4-B-4) to (4-B-9) and the generalized TM mode results when $H_z = 0$ in these equations.   Each mode type will be discussed in turn.

Transverse Electric Modes: The magnetic field component H_z of the TE wave configuration satisfies the Laplace wave equation

$$\nabla^2 H_z = \mu\epsilon(\partial^2 H_z/\partial t^2) \tag{1}$$

and for the harmonic time dependence $e^{j\omega t}$

$$\nabla^2 H_z = -k^2 H_z \tag{2}$$

where

$$k^2 = \omega^2\mu\epsilon \tag{3}$$

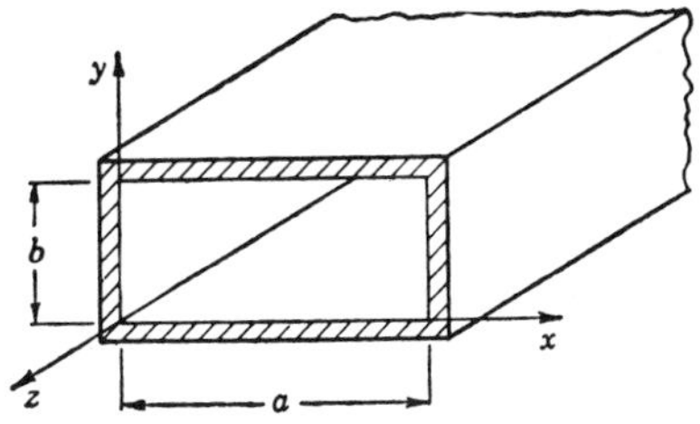

Fig. 4–6.   Rectangular waveguide coordinates (RLS-9, p. 38).

The entire z dependence of the H_z vector is contained in the propagation factor $e^{-\gamma z}$ so that

$$\partial^2 H_z / \partial z^2 = \gamma^2 H_z \tag{4}$$

and

$$\partial^2 H_z / \partial x^2 + \partial^2 H_z / \partial y^2 = -(k^2 + \gamma^2) H_z \tag{5}$$

It is now convenient to rewrite eqs. (4-B-4) and (4-B-5) with $E_z = 0$

$$E_y = -j(k/\gamma)\ (\mu/\epsilon)^{1/2} H_x \tag{6}$$

$$E_x = j(k/\gamma)\ (\mu/\epsilon)^{1/2} H_y \tag{7}$$

Equations (4-B-7) and (4-B-8) may now be solved for H_x and H_y

$$H_x = (\gamma/k_c{}^2)\ (\partial H_z / \partial x) \tag{8}$$

$$H_y = (\gamma/k_c{}^2)\ (\partial H_z / \partial y) \tag{9}$$

where

$$\gamma = \alpha + j\beta = (k_c{}^2 - k^2)^{1/2} \tag{10}$$

If we neglect the conductor attenuation for the present (i.e., $\alpha \ll \beta$), then

$$k_c = 2\pi/\lambda_c = (k^2 + \gamma^2)^{1/2} = 2\pi f_c(\mu\epsilon)^{1/2} \tag{11}$$

and

$$\gamma = j\beta = 2\pi j/\lambda_g = (k_c{}^2 - k^2)^{1/2} = j\omega(\mu\epsilon)^{1/2}\ [1 - (f_c/f)^2]^{1/2} \tag{10a}$$

for a perfect dielectric with zero loss tangent.

The boundary condition that the normal derivative of H_z

$$\partial H_z / \partial n = 0 \tag{12}$$

must vanish at the walls limits the possible functional dependence of the wave vector H_z. The solution of eqs. (6)–(9) with this boundary condition is

$$H_x = (\gamma k_x/k_c{}^2)\ H_0 \sin k_x\, x \cos k_y y \tag{13}$$

$$H_y = (\gamma k_y/k_c{}^2) H_0 \cos k_x \sin k_y y \tag{14}$$

$$H_z = H_0 \cos k_x x \cos k_y y \tag{15}$$

$$E_x = Z_{TE} H_y \tag{16}$$

$$E_y = -Z_{TE} H_x \tag{17}$$

where the characteristic impedance Z_{TE} for a TE mode is

$$Z_{TE} = (\mu/\epsilon)^{1/2} [1 - (f_c/f)^2]^{-1/2} \tag{18}$$

Several mode configurations are sketched on Fig. 4-7. The cutoff frequency f_c is defined by eq. (11), and it is the lower limit of the frequencies that will propagate for a given mode. The boundary conditions on k_x and k_y are

$$k_x = m\pi/a; \quad k_y = n\pi/b \tag{19}$$

where m and n are integers. Therefore

$$k_c = 2\pi/\lambda_c = [(m\pi/a)^2 + (n\pi/b)^2]^{1/2} = (k_x{}^2 + k_y{}^2)^{1/2} \tag{20}$$

where λ_c is the cutoff wavelength. One may write

$$1/\lambda^2 = 1/\lambda_g{}^2 + 1/\lambda_c{}^2 \tag{21}$$

where λ is the free space wavelength $= [f(\mu\epsilon)^{1/2}]^{-1}$ in the dielectric, and λ_g is the guide wavelength or wavelength in the direction of propagation z

$$\gamma = \alpha + (2\pi/\lambda_g)j \tag{22}$$

Thus for propagation to occur, it is necessary for the free space wavelength to be less than the cutoff wavelength. When this is not the case then the guide wavelength λ_g becomes imaginary and contributes to the attenuation constant α in eq. (22).

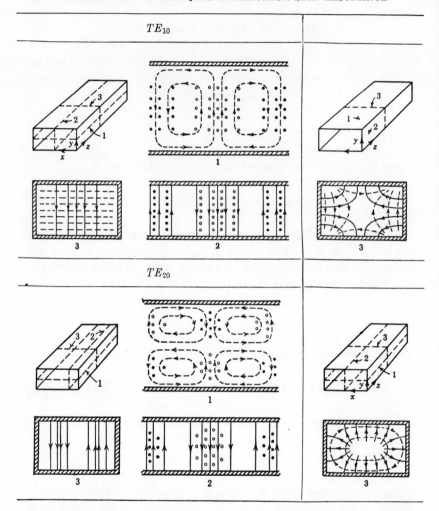

Fig. 4–7. Summary of wave types for rectangular guides. The symbol (●) denotes a vector directed up out of the paper and (○) one into the paper. Dotted lines refer to **H** and solid lines to **E** [Ramo, Whinnery, and Van Duzer (1965)].

TE_{11}

TE_{21}

TM_{11}

TM_{21}

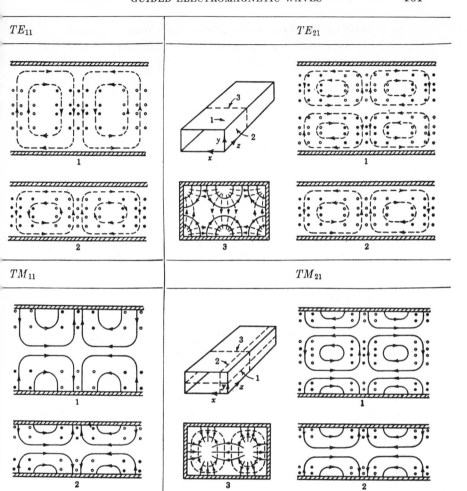

As a result of the ohmic losses in the conducting waveguide walls the microwave power is attenuated by the factor $\exp(-\alpha_R z)$. The attenuation constant α_R for the TE_{mn} mode is given by

$$\alpha_R = \frac{1}{2} \frac{\text{power dissipated in walls per meter}}{\text{power transmitted}} \qquad (23)$$

$$= \frac{R_s}{2} \frac{\oint (|H_x|^2 + |H_y|^2 + |H_z|^2)dl}{\int \text{Re } (\mathbf{E} \times \mathbf{H}^*)dA} \qquad (24)$$

$$= \frac{2R_s}{b(\mu/\epsilon)^{1/2}[1 - (f_c/f)^2]^{1/2}} \left[(1 + b/a)\,(f_c/f)^2 \right.$$
$$\left. + \left(1 - \left(\frac{f_c}{f}\right)^2\right)\left(\frac{b/a(b/a\,m^2 + n^2)}{b^2 m^2/a^2 + n^2}\right) \right] \quad \text{Np/m} \qquad (25)$$

which has the simpler form for the TE_{m0} mode [Ramo, Whinnery, and Van Duzer (1965), p. 422]

$$\alpha_R = \frac{R_s}{b(\mu/\epsilon)^{1/2}[1 - (f_c/f)^2]^{1/2}} \left[1 + \frac{2b}{a}\left(\frac{f_c}{f}\right)^2 \right] \quad \text{Np/m} \qquad (26)$$

The frequency dependence of the attenuation constant α_R for several modes is shown on Fig. 4-8. One may convert eqs. (23)–(26) to the units dB/m by multiplying the righthand side by 8.686. The transverse electric modes TE_{mn} are labeled by their m,n values, and the mode configurations of four of them are shown on Fig. 4-7.

The TE_{10} Mode: The dominant mode is the one with the lowest cutoff frequency, and from eq. (20) it is apparent that for rectangular waveguides the TE_{10} mode is dominant. The field configurations are obtained from eqs. (13)–(19) by letting $m = 1$ and $n = 0$, and renormalizing as follows

$$H_x = + H_0 \sin(\pi x/a) \qquad (27)$$

$$H_z = H_0(\lambda_g/2a) \cos(\pi x/a) \qquad (28)$$

$$E_y = - Z_{TE}H_0 \sin(\pi x/a) \qquad (29)$$

$$H_y = E_x = E_z = 0 \qquad (30)$$

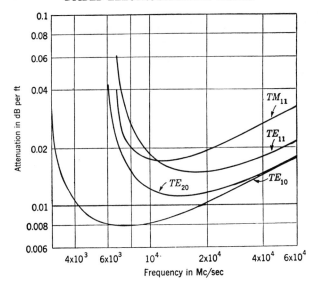

Fig. 4–8.   Ohmic attenuation α_R in rectangular copper waveguide for several modes: $a = 2$ in. $= 5.08$ cm; $b = 1$ in. $= 2.54$ cm (1 ft $= 304.8$ cm) (*RLS*-8, p. 48).

These equations are normalized differently in Sec. 8-H.   The cutoff wavelength λ_c, characteristic impedance Z_{TE}, group velocity v_g, and phase velocity v_p of this mode are given by

$$\lambda_c = 2a \tag{31}$$

$$Z_0 = \frac{(\mu/\epsilon)^{1/2}}{[1 - (\lambda/2a)^2]^{1/2}} \tag{32}$$

$$v_g = \frac{1}{(\mu\epsilon)^{1/2}} [1 - (\lambda/2a)^2]^{1/2} \tag{33}$$

$$v_p = \frac{1}{(\mu\epsilon)^{1/2}} [1 - (\lambda/2a)^2]^{-1/2} \tag{34}$$

The attenuation α_R due to the ohmic losses in the guide walls was given by eq. (26), and that due to dielectric losses α_ϵ is

$$\alpha_\epsilon = \frac{\omega (\mu\epsilon)^{1/2} (\epsilon''/\epsilon')}{2[1 - (\lambda/2a)^2]^{1/2}} \quad \text{Np/m} \tag{35}$$

$$= \frac{4.343 \, \omega (\mu\epsilon)^{1/2} (\epsilon''/\epsilon')}{[1 - (\lambda/2a)^2]^{1/2}} \quad \text{dB/m} \tag{36}$$

Three-dimensional sketches of several TE electromagnetic mode configurations are shown in Figs. 4-9 and 4-10, and the current distribution in the waveguide walls is shown in Fig. 4-11 for the TE_{10} mode. The top and bottom faces of the waveguide have the charge density ϵE_y since the electric field E_y V/m begins on the charge ϵE_y and ends on the charge $-\epsilon E_y$ C/m. The electric current density J A/m equals the tangential magnetic field component H_t at the walls. The magnetic field loops surround the displacement current $\partial D/\partial t$ A/m which completes the circuit from the top to the bottom of the waveguide. The guide wavelength and characteristic impedance of this mode are independent of the guide dimension b, but as b increases at a constant power level both the attenuation constant and the electric field strength decrease. For small b the electric field $\mathbf{E}$ can become so strong at the very high microwave power levels used in radar installations that arcing across the waveguide is likely to occur, but in ESR spectrometers this is almost never a problem. For most ESR applications one uses standard commercially available

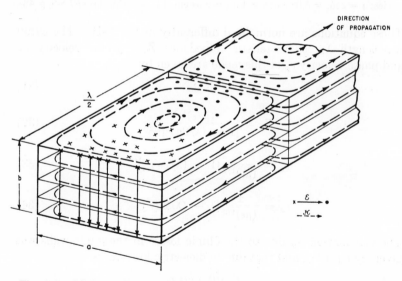

Fig. 4–9. Mode configuration for rectangular TE_{10} mode. The symbol ($\bullet$) denotes a vector directed up from the waveguide, ($\times$) refers to one aimed down into the waveguide, and (λ) corresponds to the guide wavelength [Reintjes and Coate (1952), p. 573].

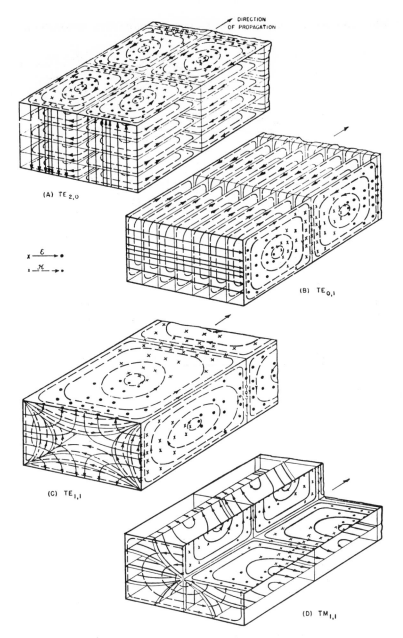

Fig. 4–10. Configurations of higher order modes in rectangular waveguides [Reintjes and Coate (1952), p. 589]; notation as in Fig. 4–9.

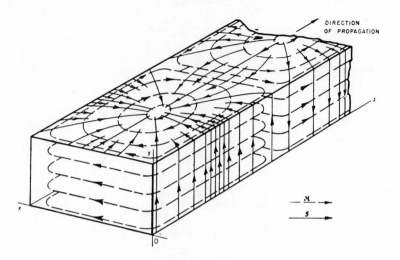

Fig. 4–11.   Current distribution (—) in waveguide walls for the rectangular TE_{10} mode [Reintjes and Coate (1952), p. 576].

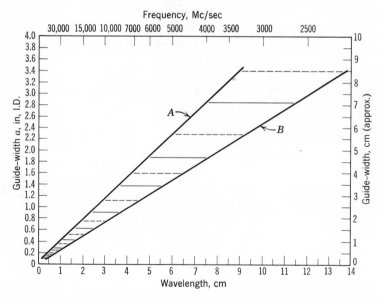

Fig. 4–12.   Preferred dimensions of rectangular waveguides suitable for various wavelength ranges: (A) limit dictated by higher order modes; (B) limit dictated by proximity to cutoff [Southworth (1950), p. 82].

rectangular waveguides operating in the TE_{10} mode, and the recommended frequency ranges of these waveguides are shown in Fig. 4-12.

Transverse Magnetic Modes: The electric vector E_z of a TM wave configuration satisfies Laplace's equation

$$\nabla^2 E_z = \mu\epsilon(\partial^2 E_z/\partial t^2) \tag{37}$$

The solution of this equation is obtained in a manner analogous to the solution of eq. (1) with the aid of the boundary condition that the electric field vector parallel to the boundary vanishes. The mathematical manipulations will be left as an exercise for the reader, and only the conclusions will be presented. The electromagnetic wave configurations for the TM modes are

$$E_x = -(\gamma k_x/k_c^2)\, E_0 \cos k_x x \, \sin k_y y \tag{38}$$

$$E_y = -(\gamma k_y/k_c^2)\, E_0 \sin k_x x \, \cos k_y y \tag{39}$$

$$E_z = E_0 \sin k_x x \, \sin k_y y \tag{40}$$

$$H_x = -E_y/Z_{TM} \tag{41}$$

$$H_y = E_x/Z_{TM} \tag{42}$$

$$H_z = 0 \tag{43}$$

The TM_{11} mode is sketched on Fig. 4-10.

The characteristic impedance Z_{TM} of a TM mode is given by

$$Z_{TM} = (\mu/\epsilon)^{1/2}\,[1 - (f_c/f)^2]^{1/2} \tag{44}$$

and the attenuation constant α_R arising from ohmic losses in the waveguide walls is [Ramo, Whinnery, and Van Duzer (1965), p. 423]

$$\alpha_R = \frac{2R_s}{b\,(\mu/\epsilon)^{1/2}\,[1 - (f_c/f)^2]^{1/2}}\left[\frac{m^2\,(b/a)^3 + n^2}{m^2\,(b/a)^2 + n^2}\right] \quad \text{Np/m} \tag{45}$$

The frequency dependence of eq. (45) for the TM_{11} mode is shown on Fig. 4-8. The remaining expressions (3), (10), (11), and (19)–(23) are valid for both TE and TM modes. It should be noted that by comparing eq. (18) to eq. (44) the characteristic impedance of the transverse electric wave exceeds that in the unbounded dielectric $(\mu/\epsilon)^{1/2}$, while that of a transverse magnetic wave is less than $(\mu/\epsilon)^{1/2}$. There exist TE_{mn} waves with either m or n equal to zero (but not both), while for TM modes both m and n must be positive integers.

In a dielectric filled waveguide the cutoff wavelength λ_c and k_c are still defined in terms of the waveguide dimensions by eq. (20) so that the cutoff frequency f_c is inversely proportional to the dielectric constant ϵ in accordance with eq. (11)

$$f_c \lambda_c (\mu\epsilon)^{1/2} = 1 \tag{46}$$

As a result the characteristic impedances $Z_{TE}{}^{\epsilon}$ and $Z_{TM}{}^{\epsilon}$ for TE and TM modes, respectively, in a dielectric filled waveguide are

$$Z_{TE}{}^{\epsilon} = (\epsilon_0/\epsilon)^{1/2} \left[1 - (\epsilon_0/\epsilon)(\lambda/\lambda_c)^2\right]^{-1/2} \tag{47}$$

$$Z_{TM}{}^{\epsilon} = (\epsilon_0/\epsilon)^{1/2} \left[1 - (\epsilon_0/\epsilon)(\lambda/\lambda_o)^2\right]^{1/2} \tag{48}$$

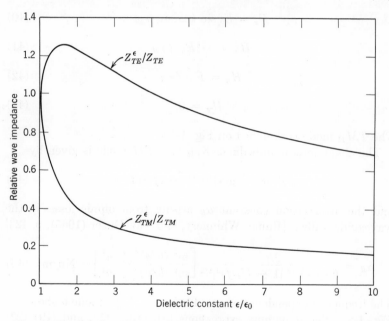

Fig. 4–13. Relative characteristic (wave) impedance as a function of the dielectric constant ϵ/ϵ_0 for TE modes ($Z_{TE}{}^{\epsilon}/Z_{TE}$) and TM modes ($Z_{TM}{}^{\epsilon}/Z_{TM}$) (*RLS*-8, p. 371).

where $\mu = \mu_0$ in the dielectric. Fig. 4-13 is a graph of the relative characteristic impedances $Z_{TE}{}^\epsilon/Z_{TE}$ and $Z_{TM}{}^\epsilon/Z_{TM}$ versus the relative dielectric constant ϵ/ϵ_0 for $(\lambda/\lambda_c)^2 = 0.8$. Further details are given in RLS-8, p. 369ff.

Sometimes space limitations such as those that exist in Dewars require the use of a waveguide with as small a cross section as possible. The cross section may be decreased by filling the waveguide with a dielectric material such as Teflon and scaling the dimensions in the ratio $(\epsilon/\epsilon_0)^{1/2}$ where ϵ_0 is the dielectric constant of air (or vacuum) and ϵ is the dielectric constant of Teflon.

The characteristics of standard rectangular waveguides are given in Table 7-3.

E. Cylindrical Waveguides

The electromagnetic wave configurations for the allowed TE (or TM) modes in cylindrical waveguides are obtained by solving the Laplace equation for H_z (or E_z) in cylindrical coordinates

$$\nabla^2 H_z = \frac{1}{r}\frac{\partial}{\partial r}\left(r\frac{\partial H_z}{\partial r}\right) + \frac{\partial^2 H_z}{\partial z^2} + \frac{1}{r^2}\frac{\partial^2 H_z}{\partial \varphi^2} = \mu\epsilon\frac{\partial^2 H_z}{\partial t^2} \tag{1}$$

The same equation holds for the other field components. As in the rectangular waveguide case one assumes the time and z dependence $\exp(j\omega t - \gamma z)$ where z is the direction of propagation. This gives

$$\frac{1}{r}\frac{\partial}{\partial r}\left(r\frac{\partial H_z}{\partial r}\right) + \frac{1}{r^2}\frac{\partial^2 H_z}{\partial \varphi^2} + k_c^2 H_z = 0 \tag{2}$$

where

$$k^2 = (2\pi/\lambda)^2 = \omega^2\mu\epsilon \tag{3}$$

$$k_c = 2\pi/\lambda_c = (k^2 + \gamma^2)^{1/2} = 2\pi f_c(\mu\epsilon)^{1/2} \tag{4}$$

The φ dependence for TE modes is of the form

$$A \sin m\varphi + B \cos m\varphi \tag{5}$$

and so for the z component of the magnetic field one obtains the expression

$$\frac{1}{r}\frac{\partial}{\partial r}\left(r\frac{\partial H_z}{\partial r}\right) + \left(k_c^2 - \frac{m^2}{r^2}\right)H_z = 0 \tag{6}$$

which is Bessel's equation.   For TM modes the corresponding equation holds for E_z

$$\frac{1}{r}\frac{\partial}{\partial r}\left(r\frac{\partial E_z}{\partial r}\right) + \left(k_c^2 - \frac{m^2}{r^2}\right)E_z = 0 \tag{7}$$

The solution of Bessel's equation is the mth order Bessel function $J_m(k_c r)$ and the electromagnetic field distributions are in terms of the Bessel function $J_m(k_c r)$ and its derivative $J_m'(k_c r)$

$$\frac{dJ_m(k_c r)}{d(k_c r)} = J_m'\ (k_c r) \tag{8}$$

Several miscellaneous relations that are important for cylindrical waveguide modes above cutoff $(f > f_c)$ are

$$\beta_z = (k_c^2 - k^2)^{1/2} = j\omega(\mu\epsilon)^{1/2}\,[1 - (f_c/f)^2]^{1/2} \tag{9}$$

$$\gamma = \alpha + j\beta \tag{10}$$

$$1/\lambda^2 = 1/\lambda_g^2 + 1/\lambda_c^2 \tag{11}$$

$$\lambda f = 1/(\mu\epsilon)^{1/2} = v \tag{12}$$

$$\lambda_g = 2\pi/\beta_z \tag{13}$$

$$\lambda_c = 2\pi/k_c = 1/[f_c(\mu\epsilon)^{1/2}] \tag{14}$$

where $(\mu\epsilon)^{1/2}$ is assumed to be real.

For transverse electric modes the electromagnetic wave configurations are

$$H_r = -\frac{\gamma}{k_c}H_0J_m'(k_c r)\begin{cases}\cos m\ \varphi \\ \sin m\ \varphi\end{cases} \tag{15}$$

$$H_\varphi = \frac{m\gamma}{k_c^2 r} H_0 J_m(k_0 r) \begin{cases} \sin m\,\varphi \\ -\cos m\,\varphi \end{cases} \tag{16}$$

$$H_z = H_0 J_m(k_c r) \begin{cases} \cos m\,\varphi \\ \sin m\,\varphi \end{cases} \tag{17}$$

$$E_r = Z_{TE} H_\varphi \tag{18}$$

$$E_\varphi = -Z_{TE} H_r \tag{19}$$

$$E_z = 0 \tag{20}$$

where the factor exp $(j\omega t - \gamma z)$ is understood in these expressions. Several TE mode configurations are sketched on Figs. 4-14 and 4-15. For the TE modes the characteristic impedance is

$$Z_{TE} = \frac{(\mu/\epsilon)^{1/2}}{[1 - (f_c/f)^2]^{1/2}} \tag{21}$$

The boundary condition on the radial component of the magnetic field is $H_r = 0$ at the conductor surface $r = a$, or

$$J_m'(k_c a) = 0 \tag{22}$$

There are an infinite number of solutions of this equation, and a typical solution is the nth order root $(k_c a)'_{mn}$. These roots are listed in Table 8-1 of Chap. 8 because their principal application in ESR is in the design of resonant cavities. From eq. (14) it follows that

$$\lambda_c = 2\pi a/(k_c a)'_{mn} = 1/[f_c(\mu\epsilon)^{1/2}] \tag{23}$$

and the attenuation constant α_R arising from ohmic losses in the guide walls is in Np/m (RLS-10, p. 70)

$$\alpha_R = \frac{R_s}{a(\mu/\epsilon)^{1/2}[1 - (f_c/f)^2]^{1/2}} \left[\left(\frac{f_c}{f}\right)^2 + \frac{m^2}{(k_c a)'_{mn}{}^2 - m^2} \right] \tag{24}$$

Wave Type	TM_{01}	TM_{02}
Field distributions in cross-sectional plane, at plane of maximum transverse fields	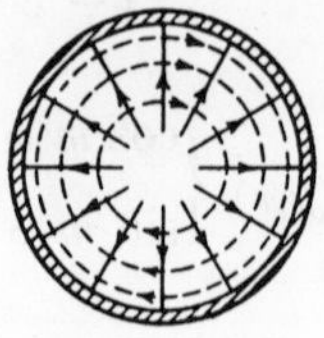	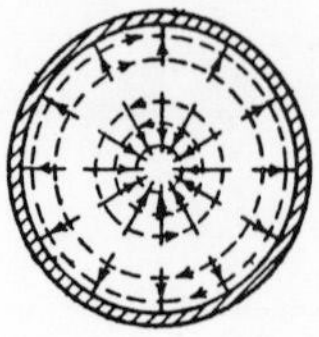
Field distributions along guide	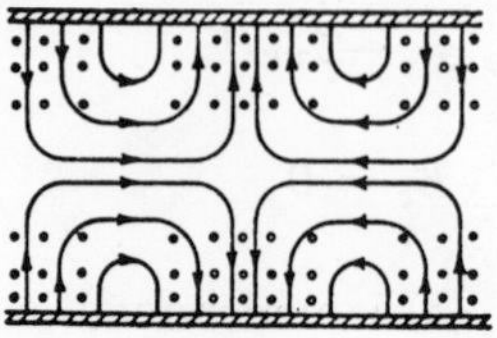	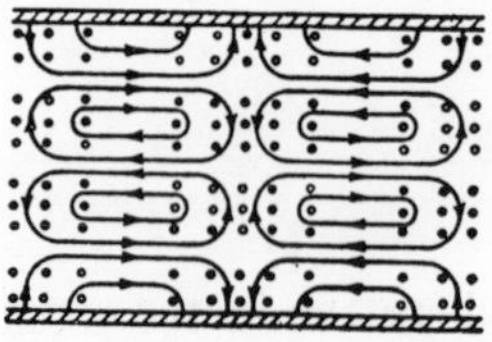
Field components present	E_z, E_r, H_ϕ	E_z, E_r, H_ϕ
p_{nl} or p'_{nl}	2.405	5.52
$(k_c)_{nl}$	$\dfrac{2.405}{a}$	$\dfrac{5.52}{a}$
$(\lambda_c)_{nl}$	$2.61a$	$1.14a$
$(f_c)_{nl}$	$\dfrac{0.383}{a\sqrt{\mu\,\epsilon}}$	$\dfrac{0.877}{a\sqrt{\mu\,\epsilon}}$
Attenuation due to imperfect conductors	$\dfrac{R_s}{a\eta}\dfrac{1}{\sqrt{1-(f_c/f)^2}}$	$\dfrac{R_s}{a\eta}\dfrac{1}{\sqrt{1-(f_c/f)^2}}$

Fig. 4–14.   Summary of wave types for cylindrical waveguides.   The notation follows Fig. 4-7 and $\eta = (\mu/\epsilon)^{1/2}$ [Ramo, Whinnery, and Van Duzer (1965), Table 8.04].

For transverse magnetic modes the electromagnetic wave configurations are

$$E_r = -\ \frac{\gamma}{k_c}\,E_0 J_m{}'(k_c r)\begin{cases}\cos m\ \varphi\\ \sin m\ \varphi\end{cases} \tag{25}$$

$$E_\varphi = -\ \frac{m\gamma}{k_c{}^2 r}\,E_0 J_m(k_c r)\begin{cases}\sin m\ \varphi\\ -\cos m\ \varphi\end{cases} \tag{26}$$

TM_{11}	TE_{01}	TE_{11}
Distributions Below Along This Plane		Distributions Below Along This Plane
$E_z, E_r, E_\phi, H_r, H_\phi$	H_z, H_r, E_ϕ	$H_z, H_r, H_\phi, E_r, E_\phi$
3.83	3.83	1.84
$\dfrac{3.83}{a}$	$\dfrac{3.83}{a}$	$\dfrac{1.84}{a}$
$1.64a$	$1.64a$	$3.41a$
$\dfrac{0.609}{a\sqrt{\mu\,\epsilon}}$	$\dfrac{0.609}{a\sqrt{\mu\,\epsilon}}$	$\dfrac{0.293}{a\sqrt{\mu\,\epsilon}}$
$\dfrac{R_s}{a\eta}\dfrac{1}{\sqrt{1-(f_c/f)^2}}$	$\dfrac{R_s}{a\eta}\dfrac{(f_c/f)^2}{\sqrt{1-(f_c/f)^2}}$	$\dfrac{R_s}{a\eta}\dfrac{1}{\sqrt{1-(f_c/f)^2}}\left[\left(\dfrac{f_c}{f}\right)^2+0.420\right]$

$$E_z = E_0 J_m(k_c r)\begin{cases}\cos m\,\varphi \\ \sin m\,\varphi\end{cases} \qquad (27)$$

$$H_r = -E_\varphi/Z_0 \qquad (28)$$

$$H_\varphi = E_r/Z_0 \qquad (29)$$

$$H_z = 0 \qquad (30)$$

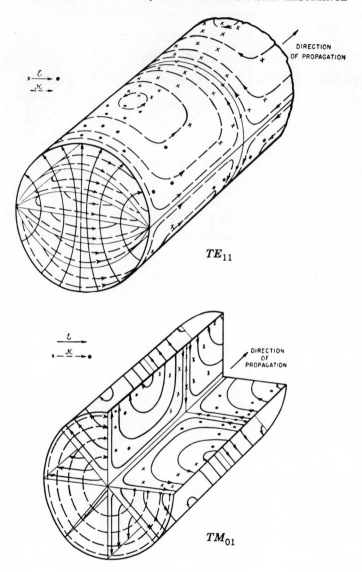

Fig. 4–15.   Several mode configurations in cylindrical waveguides [Reintjes and Coate (1952), pp. 608, 609, 610].

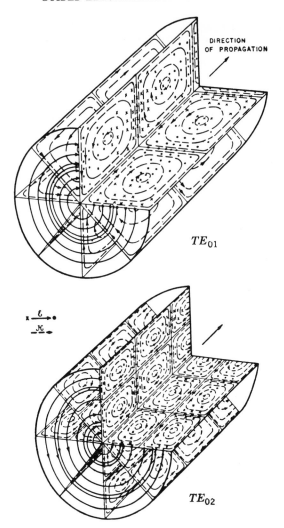

TE_{01}

TE_{02}

where again the term exp $(j\omega t - \gamma z)$ is understood, and several modes are sketched on Figs. 4-14 and 4-15. In addition

$$Z_{TM} = (\mu/\epsilon)^{1/2} [1 - (f_c/f)^2]^{1/2} \tag{31}$$

The boundary condition requires the transverse electric field to be zero at the boundary, so that

$$J_m(k_c a) = 0 \tag{32}$$

with the roots $(k_c a)_{mn} = k_c a$ listed in Table 8-1. Therefore

$$\lambda_c = 2\pi a/(k_c a)_{mn} = 1/[f_c(\mu\epsilon)^{1/2}] \tag{33}$$

and

$$\alpha_R = \frac{R_s}{a(\mu/\epsilon)^{1/2}} \frac{1}{[1 - (f_c/f)^2]^{1/2}} \quad \text{Np/m} \tag{34}$$

$$= \frac{8.686 R_s}{a(\mu/\epsilon)^{1/2}} \frac{1}{[1 - (f_c/f)^2]^{1/2}} \quad \text{dB/m} \tag{34a}$$

As in the case of rectangular waveguides, frequencies which exceed the cutoff frequency f_c are propagated while others are exponentially attentuated (cf. Sec. 4G). The TE_{11} mode is the dominant mode because it has the lowest cutoff frequency. It is the circular analog of the rectangular waveguide TE_{10} mode, as may be seen by comparing Figs. 4-7, 4-9, 4-14, and 4-15. When a centered circular iris is placed in a rectangular TE_{10} mode waveguide one may consider it as propagating the circular TE_{11} mode, and if the iris diameter is less than $0.293 \lambda_c$ cm, as in a resonant cavity iris, then the iris waveguide will be operating below cutoff.

F. Miscellaneous Types of Waveguides

The preceding sections contained a detailed treatment of waveguides with rectangular and cylindrical cross sections. These are the principal waveguides to be encountered in both ESR and radar applications. Nevertheless, it is useful for ESR spectroscopists to be acquainted with other types of guiding systems. [Ramo, Whinnery, and Van Duzer (1965); Pierce (1950)]. Webb (1962) has discussed the use of traveling wave helices in ESR spectrometers.

Elliptic Waveguides: Several wave configurations in waveguides of elliptical cross section are shown graphically in Fig. 4-16. They are expressed mathematically by means of Mathieu functions [Stratton (1941); *RLS*-10, p. 80], which employ elliptic coordinates [see Margenau and Murphy (1956), Sec. 5.9)]. In the limit of small ellipticity the elliptic modes degenerate into the cylindrical modes discussed in the previous section.

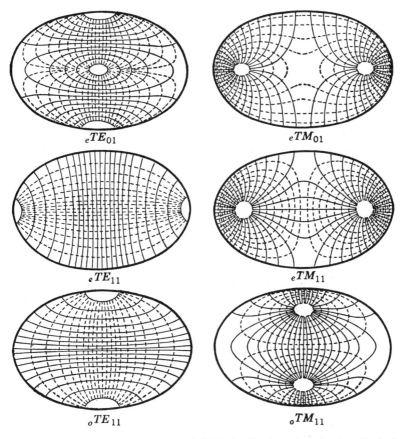

$_eTE_{01}$ $_eTM_{01}$

$_eTE_{11}$ $_eTM_{11}$

$_oTE_{11}$ $_oTM_{11}$

Fig. 4–16. Cross sectional view of field distribution of modes in elliptical waveguide (*RLS*-10, p. 84).

Radial Transmission Lines: These consist of two plane concentric circular parallel conductors separated by a dielectric. The generator is placed in the center, and the microwave energy is propagated radially. The sectorial horn antenna discussed in Sec. 7-Q is a wedge-shaped waveguide which may be considered as an intermediate case between a rectangular and a radial transmission line.

Conical Waveguides: Microwaves may be propagated along a conical waveguide with and without the outer conductor, and such a waveguide is shown in Fig. 4-17. When the conical solid angle is 4π, the waveguide becomes all space and spherical waves propagate radially in all directions (see *RLS*-10, p. 98).

Single and Double Ridge Waveguides: These have the cross sections shown on Fig. 4-18 and are discussed in *RLS*-10, p. 399.

Helical Waveguides: A wire wound in the form of a helix can propagate microwaves with a phase velocity less than the velocity of light. They are used for antennae, and are employed in traveling wave tubes as slow wave structures [Ramo, Whinnery, and Van Duzer (1965); Pierce (1950); Webb (1960)].

Inclined Plane Waveguides: It was mentioned earlier that microwaves can propagate between parallel plane conductors. Propagation can also occur when the planes are not parallel.

Guidance by a Single Cylindrical Conductor: Stratton (1941, p. 524) discusses the propagation of a *TEM* wave along a wire, and mentions that *TE* and *TM* modes are rapidly attenuated.

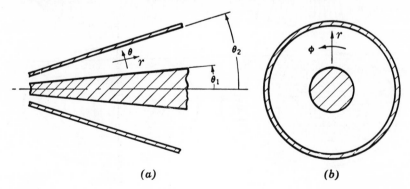

(a)   (b)

Fig. 4–17.   Conical waveguide.   (a) Longitudinal view;   (b) cross sectional view (*RLS*-10, p. 98).

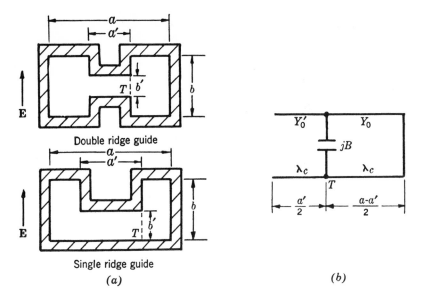

Fig. 4–18. Ridge waveguides. (a) Cross sectional view; (b) equivalent
network (RLS-10, p. 399).

Dielectric Rod Waveguide: The dielectric rod waveguide is known
in optics as the light pipe. The dielectric constant of the rod is
assumed to exceed that of the dielectric outside, and while the microwaves (or light) pass down the rod they undergo multiple reflections
at an angle which exceeds the critical angle θ_c. As a result, total
internal reflection occurs, and none of the energy is lost from the rod.
There is a critical frequency f_c below which energy is lost to the outside medium. For $f > f_c$ there are no losses to the outside, and for a
perfect dielectric ($\epsilon'' = 0$) the wave propagates unattenuated. In
practice the dielectric will have a finite loss tangent which results in
attenuation. For the TM_{0n} mode in a dielectric rod characterized
by the parameters μ_r, ϵ_r, and radius a, one has

$$f_c = \frac{X_{0n}}{2\pi a (\mu_r \epsilon_r - \mu_e \epsilon_e)^{1/2}} \tag{1}$$

where μ_e and ϵ_e characterize the external medium. From eq.
(4-E-33) expression (1) reduces to that of a cylindrical waveguide
bounded by a conductor when $\mu_r \epsilon_r \gg \mu_e \epsilon_e$.

When $f \gg f_c$ the electromagnetic fields attenuate very rapidly in the external medium, and are only appreciable near the interface. This is the case with a light pipe. When f is only slightly above f_c, the microwaves energy storage extends far into the external medium, but for perfect dielectrics inside and outside, none is lost from the rod to this medium.

A dielectric slab with a dielectric constant exceeding that of the external medium can conduct electromagnetic radiation in a manner analogous to the dielectric rod. The rod and slab waveguides are discussed by Ramo, Whinnery, and Van Duzer (1965), p. 448, and by Subrahmaniam (1962). Brackett, Kasai, and Myers (1957) have made use of dielectric waveguide cells in their microwave spectrometer.

G. Waveguides beyond Cutoff

When the microwave frequency f is less than the cutoff frequency f_c then the phase constant β becomes imaginary and is given by

$$\beta = -j(2\pi/\lambda_c) \, [1 - (f/f_c)^2]^{1/2} \tag{1}$$

Under these conditions the propagation constant γ becomes real and is denoted by

$$\gamma = \alpha + j\beta \tag{2}$$

$$= \alpha + \alpha_c \tag{3}$$

where $\alpha_c = j\beta$. Since both α and α_c are positive definite when $f < f_c$ it follows that the electromagnetic energy is exponentially attenuated. When $f \ll f_c$ one obtains the simplified expression

$$\alpha_c = 2\pi f_c(\mu\epsilon)^{1/2} = 2\pi/\lambda_c \tag{4}$$

A typical application of these formulae is the estimation of the insertion loss of a thick centered circular iris of radius a and thickness l across a rectangular waveguide which propagates the TE_{10} rectangular mode. This iris will sustain the circular TE_{11} mode for which

$$\alpha_c = (k_c a)'_{11}/a \tag{5}$$

from eq. (4-E-23) where $(k_c a)'_{11}$ is the Bessel function root and $f \ll f_c$ in the iris. Therefore the iris exponentially attenuates the microwaves in accordance with the relation $\exp(-\alpha_c l)$.

H. Phase, Group, and Signal Velocity

The propagation constant of either a plane wave or a guided wave may be represented by the propagation factor $\exp[j(\omega t - \beta z)]$ where the propagation constant γ is purely imaginary in the absence of attenuation.

$$\gamma = j\beta \tag{1}$$

The surfaces of constant phase are determined by

$$\omega t = \beta z + \text{const} \tag{2}$$

and these surfaces move forward at the phase velocity v_p

$$v_p = \omega/\beta \tag{3}$$

For a plane wave the group velocity v_g equals the phase velocity since

$$v_g = dz/dt = \omega/\beta \tag{4}$$

Consider two harmonic waves E_1 and E_2 of slightly differing frequency ω and $\omega + \Delta\omega$, where

$$E_1 = \cos(\omega t - \beta z) \tag{5}$$

$$E_2 = \cos[(\omega + \Delta\omega)t - (\beta + \Delta\beta)z] \tag{6}$$

They superpose to give

$$E_1 + E_2 = 2 \cos \tfrac{1}{2}(z\Delta\beta - t\Delta\omega)$$
$$\cos[(\beta + \Delta\beta/2)z - (\omega + \Delta\omega/2)t] \tag{7}$$

and produce a combination of a carrier oscillation at the frequency $(\omega + \tfrac{1}{2}\Delta\omega) \sim \omega$ and a modulation oscillation at the frequency $\Delta\omega$,

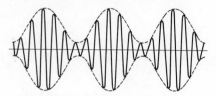

Fig. 4–19.   A modulated waveform.

as shown on Fig. 4-19.   The modulation envelope forms surfaces of constant phase defined by

$$t\Delta\omega = z\Delta\beta + \text{const} \tag{8}$$

and the envelope moves forward at the group velocity v_g

$$v_g = dz/dt = \Delta\omega/\Delta\beta \tag{9}$$

This may be considered the definition of group velocity $(d\omega/d\beta)$. In a nondispersive medium the group and phase velocities are equal. A wave packet ψ may be considered the superposition of a large number of frequencies in the neighborhood of a particular frequency ω.

$$\psi = \int_{\beta_0 - \Delta\beta}^{\beta_0 + \Delta\beta} A_{(\beta)} \exp\left[j(\omega t - \beta z)\right] d\beta \tag{10}$$

where $A_{(\beta)}$ is the amplitude of the wave at the propagation constant β.   It may be shown [cf. Stratton (1941), p. 332] that the wave-packet propagates at the group velocity v_g

$$v_g = (d\omega/d\beta)_{\beta_0} \tag{11}$$

The concepts of phase and group velocity may be clarified by a consideration of the relationship between the wavelength λ and the angular frequency ω

$$\beta = 2\pi/\lambda \tag{12}$$

$$\omega = \beta v_p \tag{13}$$

It follows that

$$v_g = d\omega/d\beta = v_p + \beta(dv_p/d\beta) = v_p - \lambda \, (dv_p/d\lambda) \tag{14}$$

In regions of normal dispersion the phase velocity increases with increasing wavelength and

$$v_g < v_p \qquad (15)$$

Anomalous dispersion results in the group velocity exceeding the phase velocity, and there are instances where v_g may exceed c, the velocity of light *in vacuo*. A more subtle analysis [Stratton (1941), p. 333] indicates that for both normal and abnormal dispersion the maximum velocity at which a signal can travel before actuating a measuring instrument is the velocity of light c *in vacuo*.

In waveguides

$$v_p = c/[1 - (f_c/f)^2]^{1/2} \qquad (16)$$

and

$$v_g = c[1 - (f_c/f)^2]^{1/2} \qquad (17)$$

which corresponds to normal dispersion.

References

Included in this list are several books that are not referred to in the text, and the entire *MIT Radiation Laboratory Series* (*RLS*) which was published by the McGraw-Hill Book Co., Inc., New York and recently reprinted by Boston Technical Publishers, Inc., Boston, Mass., 1964.

American Institute of Physics Handbook, 2nd Ed., McGraw-Hill, N. Y., 1963.

Bell Labs Staff, *Radar Systems and Components*, Van Nostrand, N. Y., 1949.

E. B. Brackett, P. H. Kasai, and R. J. Myers, *RSI*, **28**, 699 (1957).

J. G. Brainerd, Ed., G. Koehler, and H. J. Reich, *Ultra-High-Frequency Techniques*, Van Nostrand, Princeton, N. J., 1942.

A. R. Bronwell and R. E. Beam, *Theory and Application of Microwaves*, McGraw-Hill, N. Y., 1947.

E. L. Ginzton, *Microwave Measurements*, McGraw-Hill, N. Y., 1957.

E. I. Green, F. A. Leibe, and H. E. Curtis, *Bell System Tech. J.*, **15**, 248 (1936).

A. F. Harvey, *Microwave Engineering*, Academic Press, N. Y., 1963.

J. D. Jackson, *Classical Electrodynamics*, Wiley, N. Y., 1962.

H. Margenau and G. M. Murphy, *The Mathematics of Physics and Chemistry*, Vol. 1, 2nd Ed., Van Nostrand, Princeton, N. J., 1943.

T. Moreno, *Microwave Transmission Design Data*, McGraw-Hill, N. Y., 1948.

L. S. Nergaard and M. Glicksman, Ed., *Microwave Solid State Engineering*, Van Nostrand, Princeton, N. J., 1964.

J. R. Pierce, *Travelling Wave Tubes*, Van Nostrand, Princeton, N. J., 1950.

S. Ramo, J. R. Whinnery, and T. Van Duzer, *Fields and Waves in Communication Electronics*, Wiley, N. Y., 1965.

J. F. Reintjes and G. T. Coate, *Principles of Radar*, 3rd Ed., The Technology Press, MIT, and McGraw-Hill, N. Y., 1952.

RLS-1, L. N. Ridenour, Ed., *Radar System Engineering*, 1947.

RLS-2, J. S. Hall, Ed., *Radar Aids to Navigation*, 1947.

RLS-3, A. Roberts, Ed., *Radar Beacons*, 1947.

RLS-4, J. A. Pierce, A. A. McKenzie, and R. H. Woodward, Eds., *Long Range Navigation*, (*Loran*), 1948.

RLS-5, G. N. Glasoe and J. V. Lebacqz, Eds., *Pulse Generators*, 1948.

RLS-6, G. B. Collins, Ed., *Microwave Magnetrons*, 1948.

RLS-7, D. R. Hamilton, J. K. Knipp, and J. B. H. Kuper, Eds., *Klystrons and Microwave Triodes*, 1948.

RLS-8, C. G. Montgomery, R. H. Dicke, and E. M. Purcell, Eds., *Principles of Microwave Circuits*, 1948.

RLS-9, G. L. Ragan, Ed., *Microwave Transmission Circuits*, 1948.

RLS-10, N. Marcuvitz, Ed., *Waveguide Handbook*, 1951.

RLS-11, C. G. Montgomery, Ed., *Technique of Microwave Measurements*, 1947.

RLS-12, S. Silver, Ed., *Microwave Antenna Theory and Design*, 1949.

RLS-13, D. E. Kerr, Ed., *Propagation of Short Radio Waves*, 1951.

RLS-14, L. D. Smullin and C. G. Montgomery, Eds., *Microwave Duplexers*, 1948.

RLS-15, H. C. Torrey and C. A. Whitmer, Eds., *Crystal Rectifiers*, 1948.

RLS-16, R. V. Pound, Ed., *Microwave Mixers*, 1948.

RLS-17, J. F. Blackburn, Ed., *Components Handbook*, 1949.

RLS-18, G. E. Valley and H. Wallman, Eds., *Vacuum Tube Amplifiers*, 1948.

RLS-19, B. Chance, V. W. Hughes, E. F. MacNichol, D. Sayre, and F. C. Williams, *Waveforms*, 1949.

RLS-20, B. Chance, R I. Hulsizer, E. F. MacNichol, and F. C. Williams, *Electronic Time Measurements*, 1949.

RLS-21, I. A. Greenwood, J. V. Holdan, and D. MacRae, *Electronic Instruments*, 1948.

RLS-22, T. Soller, M. A. Starr, and G. E.Valley, *Cathode Ray Tube Displays*, 1948.

RLS-23, S. N. Van Voorhis, Ed., *Microwave Receivers*, 1948.

RLS-24, J. L. Lawson and G. E. Uhlenbeck, Eds, *Threshold Signals*, 1950.

RLS-25, H. M. James, N. B. Nichols, and R. S. Phillips, Eds., *Theory of Servomechanisms*, 1947.

RLS-26, W. M. Cady, M. B. Karelitz, and L. A. Turner, Eds., *Radar Scanners and Radomes*, 1948.

RLS-27, A. Svoboda and H. M. James, Eds., *Computing Mechanisms and Linkages*, 1948.

RLS-28, K. Henney, *Index*, 1953.

A. Sommerfeld, *Vorlesungen über Theoretische Physik*, 2 Auflage, Band III, Dieterich'sche Verlagsbuchhandlung, Inh. W. Klemm, Wiesbaden, 1948.

G. C. Southworth, *Principles and Applications of Waveguide Transmission*, Van Nostrand, Princeton, N. J., 1950, p. 689.

J. A. Stratton, *Electromagnetic Theory*, McGraw-Hill, N. Y., 1941.

V. Subrahmaniam, *J. Indian Inst. Sci.*, **44**, 148 (1962).

M. Sucher and J. Fox, Eds., *Handbook of Microwave Measurements*, 3rd Ed., Interscience, N. Y., 1963.

R. H. Webb, *RSI*, **33**, 732 (1962).

J. Weber, *Am. J. Phys.*, **22**, 618 (1954).

CHAPTER 5

Microwave Network Theory

A. Networks

This chapter considers the microwave analog of classic networks. A network may be considered as an assembly of microwave components provided with several inputs and outputs, and placed in a black box so that only the input and output terminals are accessible. These terminals may be waveguides or coaxial lines in a typical case, and when the network is in use, each will be attached to a generator, detector, load, or other microwave component. In the remainder of this chapter and throughout the book, each input and output will be referred to as a terminal pair in accordance with conventional engineering terminology.

The easiest way to explain the nature of a network is to discuss an example, and the example selected is shown on Fig. 5-1. The admittance formulation presupposes that at each terminal pair the voltage is shown and the current is unknown. For simplicity assume that the voltage V_1 is impressed on terminal pair number one, and the other two terminal pairs are short-circuited, so that

$$V_2 = V_3 = 0 \tag{1}$$

as shown in Fig. 5–2a. Let the generator internal impedance $R_G = 0$. In this case

$$I_2 = I_3 \tag{2}$$

and

$$I_1 = (1/R_0 + 1/R_1)V_1 \tag{3}$$

$$I_2 = I_3 = (1/R_0)V_1 \tag{4}$$

125

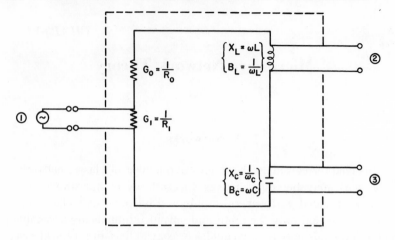

Fig. 5–1. A series RLC circuit as an example of a passive three-terminal pair network.

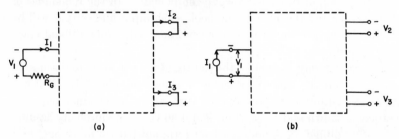

Fig. 5–2. Three-terminal pair network: (a) a voltage source V is impressed on one terminal pair and the other two are short-circuited; (b) a current source I is impressed on one terminal and the other two terminals are open-circuited.

If terminal pair number two is activated with the voltage V_2 and the other two are short-circuited, then

$$I_1 = I_3 = (1/R_0)V_2 \tag{5}$$

$$I_2 = (1/R_0 + 1/j\omega L)V_2 \tag{6}$$

where ω is the angular frequency.

By repeating this process of successively activating one terminal pair and short-circuiting the remainder, one obtains the information required to evaluate each term in the admittance matrix

$$
\begin{bmatrix} I_1 \\ I_2 \\ I_3 \end{bmatrix} = \begin{bmatrix} Y_{11} & Y_{12} & Y_{13} \\ Y_{21} & Y_{22} & Y_{23} \\ Y_{31} & Y_{32} & Y_{33} \end{bmatrix} \begin{bmatrix} V_1 \\ V_2 \\ V_3 \end{bmatrix}
\tag{7}
$$

which in tensor notation is written as follows

$$
\mathbf{I} = \mathbf{YV}
\tag{8}
$$

The admittance matrix Y is given explicitly by

$$
Y = G_0 \begin{bmatrix} 1 + \dfrac{G_1}{G_0} & -1 & -1 \\ -1 & 1 - j\dfrac{B_L}{G_0} & -1 \\ -1 & -1 & 1 + j\dfrac{B_C}{G_0} \end{bmatrix}
\tag{9}
$$

where the conductances G and susceptances B are defined in Fig. 5–1. In general, the admittance Y has the form

$$
Y = G \mp jB
\tag{10}
$$

and the impedance Z is defined in terms of the resistance R and reactance X:

$$
Z = 1/Y = R \pm jX
\tag{11}
$$

By definition G, B, R, and X are real. For an inductance

$$
X_L = \omega L \qquad B_L = 1/\omega L
\tag{12}
$$

and for a capacitance

$$
X_C = 1/\omega C \qquad B_C = \omega C
\tag{13}
$$

For completeness it should be mentioned that some authors define the inverse inductance $1/L$ and the elastance S

$$
S = 1/C
\tag{14}
$$

but these two quantities will not be used in this book.

Equation (7) means that if the voltages at the three-terminal pairs are known, then the ith current may be calculated from the equation

$$I_i = Y_{i1} V_1 + Y_{i2} V_2 + Y_{i3} V_3 \tag{15}$$

where $i = 1$, 2, or 3. As mentioned above, this is known as the admittance formulation. When the currents through the three terminals are known, the three voltages may be computed from the three equations of the form

$$V_i = Z_{i1}I_1 + Z_{i2}I_2 + Z_{i3}I_3 \tag{16}$$

or, in matrix notation

$$\mathbf{V} = \mathbf{ZI} \tag{17}$$

The elements Z_{ij} of the impedance matrix

$$Z = \begin{bmatrix} Z_{11} & Z_{12} & Z_{13} \\ Z_{21} & Z_{22} & Z_{23} \\ Z_{31} & Z_{32} & Z_{33} \end{bmatrix} \tag{18}$$

are computed by successively open-circuiting two terminal pairs and impressing a known current I_i into the remaining element. For example, in the setup of Figs. 5–1 and 5–2b

$$I_2 = I_3 = 0 \tag{19}$$

$$V_1 = \frac{R_1(Z_S - R_1)}{Z_S} I_1 \tag{20}$$

and

$$V_2 = \frac{j\omega L R_1}{Z_S} I_1 \tag{21}$$

$$V_3 = \frac{R_1}{j\omega C Z_S} I_1 \tag{22}$$

where the denominator common to all the terms is

$$Z_S = R_0 + R_1 + j\omega L + 1/j\omega C \tag{23}$$

The entire impedance matrix is

$$Z = \frac{1}{Z_S} \begin{bmatrix} R_1(Z_S - R_1) & j\omega LR_1 & \dfrac{R_1}{j\omega C} \\[2ex] j\omega LR_1 & j\omega L(Z_S - j\omega L) & \dfrac{L}{C} \\[2ex] \dfrac{R_1}{j\omega C} & \dfrac{L}{C} & \dfrac{1}{j\omega C}\left(Z_S - \dfrac{1}{j\omega C}\right) \end{bmatrix} \tag{24}$$

and its derivation is left as an exercise for the reader.

B. Network Characteristics

There are several important network theorems which apply to lumped constant circuits, and they may be extended to microwave networks by defining the voltage V and current I in terms of the waveguide electric and magnetic fields E and H, respectively. This entails (*RLS–8*, p. 83): (*1*) choosing the voltage V proportional to the transverse electric field E_t in the waveguide; (*2*) selecting the current I proportional to the transverse magnetic field H_t; (*3*) normalizing the constants of proportionality so that $\frac{1}{2} V - I$ equals the complex power flow. In other words,

$$\mathbf{E}_t(x,y,z) = V(z) \, \mathbf{f}(x,y) \tag{1}$$

$$\mathbf{H}_t(x,y,z) = I(z) \, \mathbf{g}(x,y) \tag{2}$$

with the normalization condition over the waveguide cross section

$$\int \mathbf{f} \times \mathbf{g} \cdot d\mathbf{S} = 1 \tag{3}$$

The equivalence between the electromagnetic quantities (E_t, H_t) and the lumped circuit quantities (V, I) enables one to write lumped constant equivalent circuits for microwave networks. For example, a resonant cavity may be represented by an RLC circuit, and an iris coupling hole is the analog of a transformer. These equivalent circuits will be encountered frequently throughout the remainder of the book.

Now that the relevance of classical network theory to microwave components has been established, it is expedient to mention several theorems and characteristics of networks. It will be assumed that all the networks under discussion are passive, which means that they contain no internal sources of voltage or current. In addition, only linear networks will be discussed; e.g., when the applied emf's are doubled, all the currents will double. Also each element is assumed to be nondirectional so that interchanging its two terminals has no effect on the currents and voltages in the network. Ferrite isolators and circulators do not behave the same in each direction, and so they cannot be treated by elementary network theory.

Kirchhoff's First Law: The algebraic sum of the voltage drops around a closed path vanishes. This is equivalent to saying that the energy of a charge is unchanged after being carried around a circuit, and that the line integral of the electric field is independent of the path.

Kirchhoff's Second Law: The algebraic sum of the currents flowing into each branch point equals zero. This law results from the conservation of charge.

Superposition Theorem: Each applied emf produces its corresponding currents through all the terminals of the network, irrespective of the simultaneous presence of other applied voltages at the same or other terminals. The corresponding statement is true for applied current generators and the resulting voltages.

Reciprocity Theorem: Both the impedance matrix Z and the admittance matrix Y are symmetrical, so the off-diagonal elements satisfy the relations

$$Z_{ij} = Z_{ji} \qquad (4)$$

and

$$Y_{ij} = Y_{ji} \qquad (5)$$

Physically, reciprocity means that the positions of an impedanceless generator and an impedanceless ammeter may be interchanged without effecting the ammeter reading. This theorem results from the symmetry of Maxwell's equations. Isolators, circulators, and other unidirectional devices do not obey the reciprocity theorem.

Thévenin's Theorem: A network having one accessible terminal pair and containing one or more internal sources of emf may be replaced by an electromotive force V in series with an impedance Z. The magnitude of the emf is that which would appear across the two terminals when they are open-circuited, and the impedance Z is that appearing across the terminals where all the emf's in the network are replaced by their internal impedances. Figure 5-3 shows an equivalent network which illustrates Thévenin's theorem.

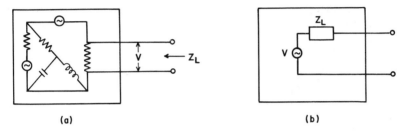

(a)   (b)

Fig. 5-3. (a) Network containing voltage sources, and (b) its Thévenin's equivalent network.

Foster's Theorem: Foster (1924) showed that the reactance $(Z = jX)$ of a lossless one-terminal pair network must continuously increase with frequency, although it can go through infinities, as shown in Fig. 5-4. A similar behavior is exhibited by the susceptance $(Y = jB)$. These slopes may be expressed in terms of the electric and magnetic stored energy U_E and U_H, respectively [Ramo, Whinnery, and Van Duzer (1965)]

$$dX/d\omega = 4(U_E + U_H)/|\,I\,|^2 \qquad (6)$$

$$dB/d\omega = 4(U_E + U_H)/|\,V\,|^2 \qquad (7)$$

Kramers-Kroniglike Impedance Relations: It is well known to students of magnetic resonance that the real and imaginary parts of the magnetic susceptibility obey the Kramers-Kronig relations (1926, 1927). Similar relations are sometimes satisfied by the

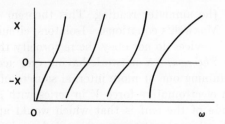

Fig. 5–4.   Example of susceptance X vs. frequency ω for a lossless one-terminal pair network.

frequency dependence of the resistance R and the reactance X of a lumped constant circuit.

$$R(\omega) = -\frac{2}{\pi} \int_0^\infty \frac{\omega' X(\omega')d\omega'}{\omega'^2 - \omega^2} + R_0 \qquad (8)$$

$$X(\omega) = \frac{2\omega}{\pi} \int_0^\infty \frac{R(\omega')d\omega'}{\omega'^2 - \omega^2} + X_0(\omega) \qquad (9)$$

where $X_0(\omega)$ is the reactance function of a lossless two-terminal pair network, and the resistance R_0 is independent of frequency [Ramo, Whinnery, and Van Duzer (1965), p. 624].

C. Properties of n-Terminal Pair Networks

This section will consider one-, two-, three-, four-, and multi-terminal pair networks.

One-Terminal Pair Networks: The reactance in a lossless one-terminal pair network is a constantly increasing function of the frequency, in accordance with Foster's reactance theorem. Any lossy one-terminal pair network can be represented by a lossless two-terminal pair network terminated by a frequency-independent resistance R, as shown in Fig. 5–5. Two important microwave one-

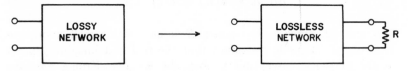

Fig. 5–5.   Two equivalent representations of a lossy one-terminal pair network.

terminal pair circuits are a resonant cavity, which may be represented by an RLC-tuned circuit, and a matched load which is equivalent to a resistor.

Two-Terminal Pair Networks: The most common microwave network is the transducer or two-terminal pair network. Since the impedance matrix Z is symmetrical,

$$\mathbf{Z} = \begin{bmatrix} Z_{11} & Z_{12} \\ Z_{12} & Z_{22} \end{bmatrix} \tag{1}$$

a transducer may be represented by three parameters. Several transducers may be connected together in cascade, and the resulting cascaded network may itself be represented by only three parameters. General two-terminal pair π and T networks are shown on Figs. 5-6a and 5-6b, respectively, while a T network of loosely coupled coils is presented in Fig. 5-6c.

The impedance matrix of the T network is given by eq. (1) and the analogous admittance matrix for the π network is

$$\mathbf{Y} = \begin{bmatrix} Y_{11} & Y_{12} \\ Y_{12} & Y_{22} \end{bmatrix} \tag{2}$$

These matrices are reciprocals

$$\mathbf{YZ} = \mathbf{ZY} = 1 \tag{3}$$

with the relations

$$Y_{11} = Z_{22}/(Z_{11}Z_{22} - Z_{12}{}^2) \tag{4}$$

$$Y_{12} = - Z_{12}/(Z_{11}Z_{22} - Z_{12}{}^2) \tag{5}$$

$$Y_{22} = Z_{11}/(Z_{11}Z_{22} - Z_{12}{}^2) \tag{6}$$

and the determinates of the two matrices are also reciprocals

$$(Z_{11}Z_{12} - Z_{12}{}^2)\ (Y_{11}Y_{22} - Y_{12}{}^2) = 1 \tag{7}$$

(a)

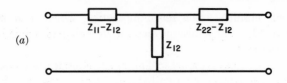

(b)

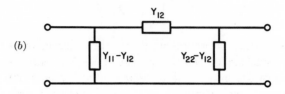

(c)

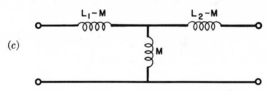

Fig. 5–6.   (a) T network; (b) its dual π network; (c) T network equivalent of loosely coupled coils.

When a two-terminal pair network is terminated by a load Z_L, the impedance Z_{in} looking into the network is

$$Z_{\text{in}} = Z_{11} - Z_{12}{}^2/(Z_{22} + Z_L) \tag{8}$$

$$= Z_{11}\left(1 - \frac{k^2}{1 + (Z_L/Z_{22})}\right) \tag{9}$$

where the coupling constant k

$$k = Z_{12}/(Z_{11}Z_{22})^{1/2} \tag{10}$$

expresses the degree of coupling between the two-terminal pairs of the network.

No impedance or admittance network exists for an ideal (lossless) transformer. It is possible, however, to relate the input and output voltages V_1 and V_2 and currents I_1 and I_2, respectively, to each other as follows

$$\begin{bmatrix} V_1 \\ I_1 \end{bmatrix} = \begin{bmatrix} \dfrac{1}{n} & 0 \\ 0 & n \end{bmatrix} \begin{bmatrix} V_2 \\ -I_2 \end{bmatrix} \tag{11}$$

where n is the turns ratio of the transformer. A transformer may be used as the equivalent circuit of an iris.

The impedance and admittance matrices for several transmission line two-terminal pair networks are shown in Fig. 5-7. These figures are discussed in RLS-8, Sec. 4-5. The matrix defined by the equation

$$\begin{bmatrix} V_1 \\ I_1 \end{bmatrix} = \begin{bmatrix} \mathcal{A} & \mathcal{B} \\ \mathcal{C} & \mathcal{D} \end{bmatrix} \begin{bmatrix} V_2 \\ -I_2 \end{bmatrix} \tag{12}$$

is listed in Table 5-1 for four simple two-terminal pair networks.

TABLE 5-1

Simple Circuit Components and Their Corresponding Matrices (RLS-9, p. 547)

Component	Circuit	$\mathcal{ABCD}$ matrix
Series impedance		$\begin{bmatrix} 1 & Z \\ 0 & 1 \end{bmatrix}$
Shunt admittance		$\begin{bmatrix} 1 & 0 \\ Y & 1 \end{bmatrix}$
Section of line		$\begin{bmatrix} \cosh \gamma l & Z_0 \sinh \gamma \\ \dfrac{\sinh \gamma l}{Z_0} & \cosh \gamma l \end{bmatrix}$
		$Z_0 = $ Characteristic impedance
		$\gamma = $ Propagation function
Ideal transformer		$\begin{bmatrix} 1/n & 0 \\ 0 & n \end{bmatrix}$

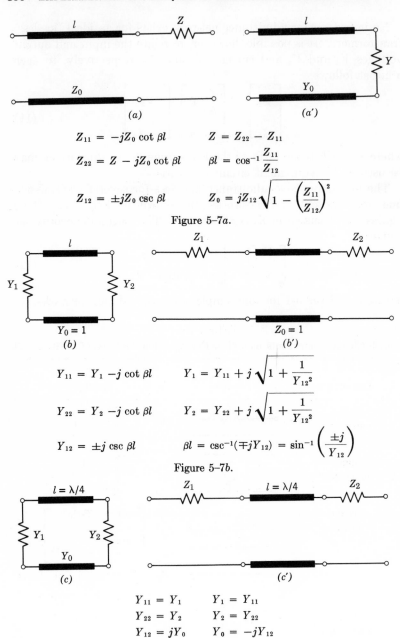

$$Z_{11} = -jZ_0 \cot \beta l \qquad Z = Z_{22} - Z_{11}$$

$$Z_{22} = Z - jZ_0 \cot \beta l \qquad \beta l = \cos^{-1} \frac{Z_{11}}{Z_{12}}$$

$$Z_{12} = \pm jZ_0 \csc \beta l \qquad Z_0 = jZ_{12}\sqrt{1 - \left(\frac{Z_{11}}{Z_{12}}\right)^2}$$

Figure 5–7a.

$$Y_{11} = Y_1 - j \cot \beta l \qquad Y_1 = Y_{11} + j\sqrt{1 + \frac{1}{Y_{12}{}^2}}$$

$$Y_{22} = Y_2 - j \cot \beta l \qquad Y_2 = Y_{22} + j\sqrt{1 + \frac{1}{Y_{12}{}^2}}$$

$$Y_{12} = \pm j \csc \beta l \qquad \beta l = \csc^{-1}(\mp jY_{12}) = \sin^{-1}\left(\frac{\pm j}{Y_{12}}\right)$$

Figure 5–7b.

$$Y_{11} = Y_1 \qquad Y_1 = Y_{11}$$

$$Y_{22} = Y_2 \qquad Y_2 = Y_{22}$$

$$Y_{12} = jY_0 \qquad Y_0 = -jY_{12}$$

Figure 5–7c.

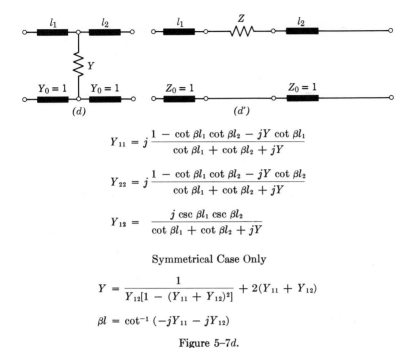

$$Y_{11} = j \frac{1 - \cot \beta l_1 \cot \beta l_2 - jY \cot \beta l_1}{\cot \beta l_1 + \cot \beta l_2 + jY}$$

$$Y_{22} = j \frac{1 - \cot \beta l_1 \cot \beta l_2 - jY \cot \beta l_2}{\cot \beta l_1 + \cot \beta l_2 + jY}$$

$$Y_{12} = \frac{j \csc \beta l_1 \csc \beta l_2}{\cot \beta l_1 + \cot \beta l_2 + jY}$$

Symmetrical Case Only

$$Y = \frac{1}{Y_{12}[1 - (Y_{11} + Y_{12})^2]} + 2(Y_{11} + Y_{12})$$

$$\beta l = \cot^{-1} (-jY_{11} - jY_{12})$$

Figure 5–7d.

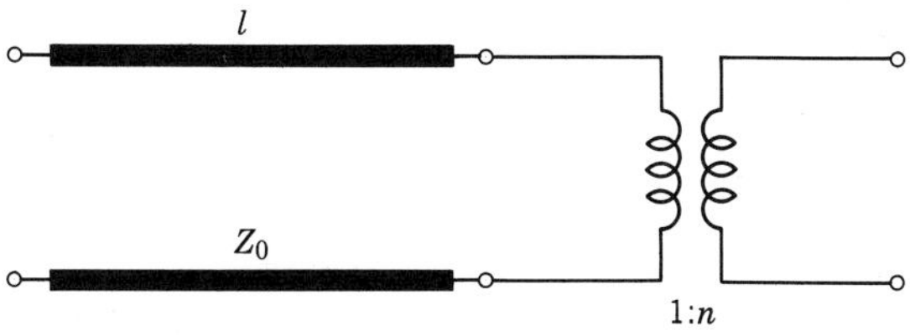

$$Z_{11} = -jZ_0 \cot \beta l \qquad \beta l = \cos^{-1} \frac{\sqrt{Z_{11}Z_{22}}}{Z_{12}}$$

$$Z_{22} = -jn^2 Z_0 \cot \beta l \qquad Z_0 = -jZ_{11} \sqrt{\frac{Z_{12}^2}{Z_{11}Z_{22}} - 1}$$

$$Z_{12} = jnZ_0 \csc \beta l \qquad n = \sqrt{\frac{Z_{22}}{Z_{11}}}$$

Figure 5–7e.

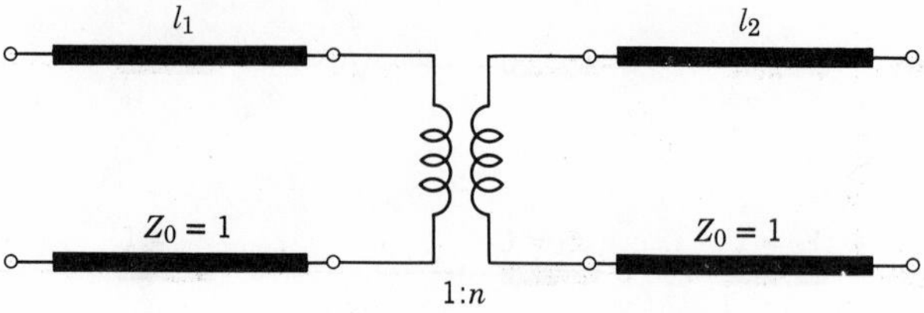

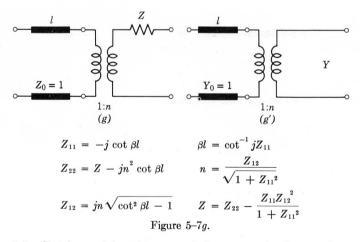

$$Z_{11} = j \tan [\beta l_1 + \tan^{-1} (n^2 \tan \beta l_2)]$$

$$Z_{22} = j \tan \left[\beta l_2 + \tan^{-1} \left(\frac{\tan \beta l_1}{n^2} \right) \right]$$

$$Z_{11}Z_{22} - Z_{12}^2 = \frac{n^2 \tan \beta l_1 \tan \beta l_2 - 1}{\tan \beta l_1 \tan \beta l_2 - n^2}$$

$$\tan \beta l_1 = \frac{1 + c^2 - a^2 - b^2}{2(bc - a)} \pm \sqrt{\left[\frac{1 + c^2 - a^2 - b^2}{2(bc - a)} \right]^2 + 1}$$

$$\tan \beta l_2 = \frac{b + c\alpha}{-\alpha + a} = \frac{1 + \alpha a}{c - \alpha b}$$

$$n^2 = \frac{-c\alpha - b}{1 + \alpha a} = -\frac{a - \alpha}{c - \alpha b}$$

$$a = -jZ_{11}$$
$$b = Z_{11}Z_{22} - Z_{12}^2$$
$$c = -jZ_{22}$$
$$\alpha = \tan \beta l_1$$

Figure 5–7f.

$$Z_{11} = -j \cot \beta l \qquad \beta l = \cot^{-1} jZ_{11}$$

$$Z_{22} = Z - jn^2 \cot \beta l \qquad n = \frac{Z_{12}}{\sqrt{1 + Z_{11}^2}}$$

$$Z_{12} = jn \sqrt{\cot^2 \beta l - 1} \qquad Z = Z_{22} - \frac{Z_{11}Z_{12}^2}{1 + Z_{11}^2}$$

Figure 5–7g.

Fig. 5–7. Sketches and impedance or admittance matrix elements for seven transmission line networks (RLS–8, pp. 105–107).

When several two-terminal pair networks are connected together or "cascaded" the entire group may be considered as a single two-terminal pair network or filter characterized by the matrix (1) or (2). When an infinite number of these identical networks is cascaded, the input impedance Z_{in} must equal the load impedance Z_L, and so

$$Z_{in} = Z_{11} - Z_{12}^2/(Z_{22} + Z_{in}) \qquad (13)$$

where Z_{11}, Z_{12}, and Z_{22} correspond to a single network. The current in the nth individual network is

$$I_{n+1}/I_n = e^{-\Gamma} \qquad (14)$$

where Γ is the propagation constant given by

$$\cosh \Gamma = (Z_{11} + Z_{22})/2Z_{12} \qquad (15)$$

Of course, two-terminal pair networks may also be connected in other ways besides cascading, as indicated on Fig. 5-8.

Three-Terminal Pair Networks: A three terminal pair network has six independent parameters

$$\mathbf{Z} = \begin{bmatrix} Z_{11} & Z_{12} & Z_{13} \\ Z_{12} & Z_{22} & Z_{23} \\ Z_{13} & Z_{23} & Z_{33} \end{bmatrix} \qquad (16)$$

Most of the microwave three-terminal pair networks encountered in radar and ESR applications have two identical pairs, so that the

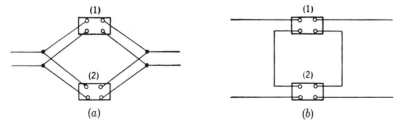

Fig. 5–8. Two-terminal pair networks connected (a) in parallel and (b) in series $(RLS$–8, p. 120).

impedance (or admittance) matrix has only four independent elements

$$\mathbf{Z} = \begin{bmatrix} Z_{11} & Z_{12} & Z_{13} \\ Z_{12} & Z_{11} & Z_{13} \\ Z_{13} & Z_{13} & Z_{33} \end{bmatrix} \tag{17}$$

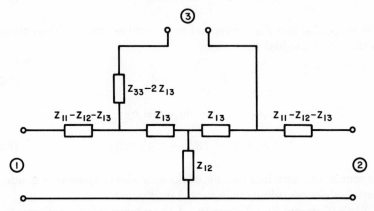

Fig. 5–9. Equivalent circuit for a symmetrical three-terminal pair network.

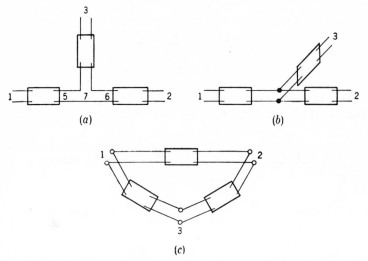

Fig. 5–10. Combination of three two-terminal pair networks to give a three-terminal pair network: (a) series T; (b) shunt T; (c) delta (RLS-8, p. 123).

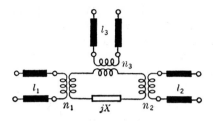

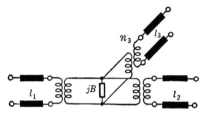

Fig. 5–11. Transformer representation of series (top) and shunt (bottom) T junctions (RLS-8, p. 122).

as shown on Fig. 5-9. Examples of such symmetric circuits are a waveguide tee, a symmetrical directional coupler, a resonant reaction cavity coupled symmetrically to a waveguide, and a slotted section. Figure 5-10 indicates how several two-terminal pair networks may be combined to form a three-terminal pair network and Fig. 5-11 presents the transformer representation for series and shunt T junctions.

D. Dual Networks

The current–voltage equations corresponding to the T network shown on Fig. 5-6a are

$$V_1 = Z_{11}I_1 + Z_{12}I_2 \tag{1a}$$

$$V_2 = Z_{12}I_1 + Z_{22}I_2 \tag{1b}$$

and the analogous equations for the π network of Fig. 5-6b are

$$I_1 = Y_{11}V_1 - Y_{12}V_2 \tag{2a}$$

$$I_2 = -Y_{12}V_1 + Y_{22}V_2 \tag{2b}$$

Equations (1) become very complicated when expressed in terms of admittances and eqs. (2) become complex in terms of impedances, as is evident from the transformation relations presented in Sec. 5-C. Thus the T network is the simple, logical representation of eqs. (1) and the π network plays the same role for eqs. (2). Excluding their internal structure there is no way to tell the difference between these two networks by external current, voltage, or impedance measurements, so they are indeed equivalent.

Mathematically the T and π networks are referred to as duals of each other. Current I is the dual of voltage V, impedance Z is the dual of admittance Y, resistance R is the dual of conductance G, and reactance X is the dual of susceptance B, as shown in Table 5-2.

TABLE 5–2

List of Dual Circuit Elements

Current	I	V	Voltage
Current generator	—	—	Voltage generator
Impedance	Z	Y	Admittance
Resistance	R	G	Conductance
Reactance	X	B	Susceptance
Inductance	L	C	Capacitance
Series circuit	—	—	Parallel circuit
T network	T	π	Pi network
Y network	Y	Δ	Delta network

In general one may write

$$Z = R + jX \tag{3}$$

and

$$Y = G + jB \tag{4}$$

For a series circuit

$$X = \omega L - 1/\omega C \tag{5}$$

and for a parallel circuit

$$B = \omega C - 1/\omega L \tag{6}$$

which indicates that "series" is the dual of "parallel." The impedance Z of a parallel circuit with admittance Y is

$$Z = 1/Y = (G - jB)/(G^2 + B^2) \tag{7}$$

and the admittance of a series circuit is

$$Y = 1/Z = (R - jX)/(R^2 + X^2) \tag{8}$$

When using the Smith chart it is customary to work with per unit or normalized impedances z and admittances y by setting

$$z = Z/Z_0 \tag{9}$$

and

$$y = Y/Y_0 \tag{10}$$

where the denominators $Z_0 = 1/Y_0$ are the characteristic impedance and admittance, respectively. For a more general viewpoint on dual circuits consider the network on Fig. 5-12a and its dual on Fig. 5-12b. The two loop equations for network (a) are

$$V = (R_1 + j\omega L_1)I_1 + (1/j\omega C_{12}) (I_1 - I_2) \tag{11}$$

$$0 = (1/j\omega C_{12}) (I_2 - I_1) + (R_2 + 1/j\omega C_2)I_2 \tag{12}$$

and the two corresponding node equations for network (b) are

$$I = (G_1 + j\omega C_1)V_1 + (1/j\omega L_{12}) (V_1 - V_2) \tag{13}$$

$$0 = (1/j\omega L_{12}) (V_2 - V_1) + (G_2 + 1/j\omega L_2)V_2 \tag{14}$$

If each quantity in eqs. (11) and (12) is replaced by its dual, then one obtains eqs. (13) and (14), respectively. This indicates that the two networks are duals of each other. The two loops with circulating currents I, and I_2 are analogs of the two nodal points V_1 and V_2.

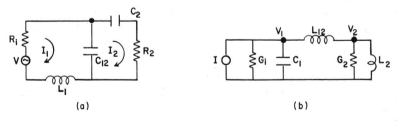

(a)   (b)

Fig. 5–12. The network (a) has an applied voltage source V and two unknown currents I_1 and I_2 and its dual (b) has an applied current source I and two unknown voltages V_1 and V_2.

The capacitance C_{12} is common to both loops and its dual the inductance L_{12} is common to both nodes. Aside from these common circuit elements, loop I_1 has V, R_1, and L_1, while node V_1 has the duals I, G_1, and C_1 associated with it. Similarly loop I_2 has elements R_2 and C_2 while node V_2 has the duals G_2 and L_2. A voltage generator is the dual of a current generator, and each is shown on Fig. 5-13 with its internal impedance (admittance). A more detailed discussion of dual networks may be found in Chap. 2 of *Transients in Linear Systems*, Vol. 1, by Gardner and Barns (1942).

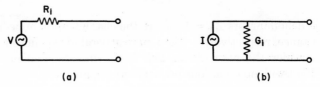

(a)   (b)

Fig. 5–13. (a) A voltage generator and (b) its dual, a current generator. The former has a series internal impedance R_i and the latter has a shunt internal admittance G_i.

The networks discussed in this chapter are assumed to be planar, i.e., they can be drawn on a piece of paper without any lines crossing other lines. A planar network always has a topological dual and conversely. Those networks which are their own dual are called self-dual. The twin T network discussed in Sec. 12-E is an example of a nonplanar network.

E. Microwave Networks or Junctions

A waveguide junction is defined as a region of space completely enclosed by a perfectly conducting metal surface except for one or more transmission lines that perforate the surface. The medium within has time-independent ϵ, μ, and σ, and generally only one mode will be present in each transmission line. The present section will discuss general characteristics of waveguide junctions.

Termination of a Single Transmission Line: This is a waveguide junction with only one transmission line perforating the surface as shown on Fig. 5-14, and both the transmission line and junction support an electromagnetic field configuration. It was mentioned in Sec. 5-B that the transverse electric and magnetic fields ($\mathbf{E}_t$ and

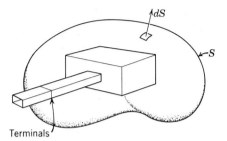

Fig. 5–14. A waveguide terminal in its enveloping surface (*RLS*-8, p. 132).

$\mathbf{H}_t$) may be defined in terms of a properly normalized current and voltage (V and I) as follows:

$$\mathbf{E}_t(x,y,z) \ = \ V(z)\ \mathbf{f}(x,y) \tag{1}$$

$$\mathbf{H}_t(x,y,z) \ = \ I(z)\mathbf{g}(x,y) \tag{2}$$

As a result, each solution of Maxwell's equations leads to a definite voltage and current at a particular waveguide termination. The inverse of this statement is also true, and it is usually formulated as the Uniqueness theorem: "For a particular value of voltage (or current) there corresponds a unique electromagnetic field distribution inside a termination." A short proof is given in *RLS*-8, p. 134. The theorem breaks down for completely lossless enclosures, but such enclosures are not physically realizable.

The ratio of the terminal voltage to the terminal current is given by the load impedance

$$V/I \ = \ Z_L(\omega) \ = \ 1/Y_L(\omega) \tag{3}$$

which is a function of the frequency ω. The impedance and admittance may be defined by

$$Z_L \ = \ \frac{2j\omega(U_H - U_E) + P}{\frac{1}{2}\,|\,I\,|^2} \tag{4}$$

$$Y_L \ = \ \frac{2j\omega(U_E - U_H) + P}{\frac{1}{2}\,|\,V\,|^2} \tag{5}$$

where U_E and U_H are the mean stored electric and magnetic energies respectively, and P is the power dissipated in the termination. The impedance (and admittance) is purely imaginary when $P = 0$, as expected. When the stored electric and magnetic energies are equal then resonance occurs, and both Z_L and Y_L are real. For a lossless termination both the reactance and susceptance are odd functions of the frequency, and the electric field is 90° out of phase with the magnetic field.

In the above discussion the termination was represented by the ratio of the voltage V to the current I,

$$Z_L = V/I \tag{6}$$

An alternative representation employs the ratio of the incident wave A to the reflected wave B which is defined as the reflection coefficient Γ

$$\Gamma = B/A \tag{7}$$

These two representations are related as follows

$$V = K(A + B) = KA(1 + \Gamma) \tag{8}$$

$$I = (1/K)\,(A - B) = (A/K)\,(1 - \Gamma) \tag{9}$$

and

$$Z = K^2(1 + \Gamma)/(1 - \Gamma) \tag{10}$$

where K is the proportionality constant.

The reflection coefficient Γ and its complex conjugate Γ^* are related to the stored energy by the relation

$$(1 + \Gamma)(1 - \Gamma^*) = \frac{2j\omega(U_H - U_E) + P}{\frac{1}{2}\,|\,A\,|^2} \tag{11}$$

which is analogous to eqs. (4) and (5). In general,

$$\Gamma\Gamma^* \leqslant 1 \tag{12}$$

and for a lossless termination,

$$\Gamma\Gamma^* = 1 \qquad (13)$$

so that in this case,

$$| \, U_H - U_E \, | \leqslant | \, A \, |^2/2\omega \qquad (14)$$

In other words the difference between the electric and magnetic stored energy in the termination is less than or equal to $1/\omega$ J when 1 W is incident on the termination. At resonance the stored electric energy equals the stored magnetic energy.

Multiterminal Junctions: The results of the previous section may be easily extended to the n-terminal pair junction such as the one shown on Fig. 5-15. The Uniqueness theorem has the form "to a particular value of the current or voltage at the n-terminal pairs there corresponds a unique electromagnetic field distribution within the junction." As before, the theorem breaks down for an idealized lossless junction, but it may be extended to cover this case also. It follows from this theorem and the linearity of Maxwell's equations that the electric and magnetic fields at any point inside the network are linear functions of the currents or voltages applied to the n junctions. Furthermore, the n-terminal currents are linearly related to the n-terminal voltages, and for the ith voltage V_i,

$$V_i = \sum_{j=1}^{n} Z_{ij} I_j \qquad (15)$$

and ith current

$$I_i = \sum_{j=1}^{n} Y_{ij} V_j \qquad (16)$$

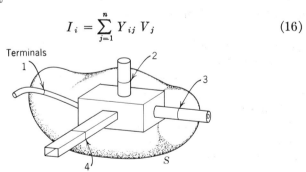

Fig. 5–15.   Example of a four-terminal junction (*RLS*–8, p. 139).

In matrix notation $\mathbf{V} = \mathbf{Z}\,\mathbf{I}$ or

$$
\begin{bmatrix} V_1 \\ V_2 \\ \cdot \\ \cdot \\ \cdot \\ V_n \end{bmatrix}
=
\begin{bmatrix}
Z_{11} & Z_{12} & \cdots & \cdots \\
Z_{21} & Z_{22} & \cdots & \cdots \\
\cdots & \cdots & \cdots & \cdots \\
\cdots & \cdots & \cdots & \cdots \\
\cdots & \cdots & \cdots & \cdots \\
\cdots & \cdots & \cdots & Z_{nn}
\end{bmatrix}
\begin{bmatrix} I_1 \\ I_2 \\ \cdot \\ \cdot \\ \cdot \\ I_n \end{bmatrix}
\tag{17}
$$

and similarly for the admittance form $\mathbf{I} = \mathbf{Y}\,\mathbf{V}$. The matrices $\mathbf{Z}$ and $\mathbf{Y}$ are symmetrical (see RLS-8, p. 142) since

$$
Z_{ij} = Z_{ji} \tag{18}
$$

and

$$
Y_{ij} = Y_{ji} \tag{19}
$$

For a multiterminal pair network

$$
\sum_i V_i \cdot I_i{}^* = 4j\omega(U_H - U_E) + 2P \tag{20}
$$

and using eq. (15) one obtains

$$
\sum_{i,j} I_i{}^* Z_{ij} I_j = 4j\omega(U_H - U_E) + 2P \tag{21}
$$

which requires that the determinate of the real part of the impedance or admittance matrix (and also the determinate of each of the minors obtained by sucessively removing diagonal elements in any order) be greater than or equal to zero (RLS-8, p. 143).

Most practical microwave junctions with more than one terminal pair are essentially lossless. Examples of such low-loss devices are waveguides, T junctions, tuners, irides, directional couplers, hybrid tees, etc. For these essentially lossless junctions, all the terms in both the impedance and admittance matrices may be considered as purely imaginary.

The Scattering Matrix: The voltage V_i and current I_i of the ith terminal pair are related to the incident and reflected electric field amplitudes A_i and B_i, respectively, by the relations

$$
V_i = (Z_{0i})^{1/2}\,(A_i + B_i) \tag{22}
$$

and

$$I_i = [1/(Z_{0i})^{1/2}] (A_i - B_i) \qquad (23)$$

where Z_{0i} is the characteristic impedance of the ith transmission line. It is assumed that $\frac{1}{2}|A|^2$ and $\frac{1}{2}|B|^2$ are normalized to be equal to the average incident and reflected power, respectively. For simplicity, normalize I_i and V_i so that $Z_{0i} = 1$. Then

$$V_i = A_i + B_i \qquad (24)$$

$$I_i = A_i - B_i \qquad (25)$$

$$A_i = \tfrac{1}{2}(V_i + I_i) \qquad (26)$$

$$B_i = \tfrac{1}{2}(V_i - I_i) \qquad (27)$$

The impedance matrix Z_{ij} is defined by

$$V_i = \sum_{j=1}^{n} Z_{ij}I_j \qquad (28)$$

and as a result

$$A_i = \tfrac{1}{2}\sum_{j=1}^{n} (Z_{ij} + \delta_{ij})I_j \qquad (29)$$

$$B_j = \tfrac{1}{2}\sum_{j=1}^{n} (Z_{ij} - \delta_{ij})I_j \qquad (30)$$

where the Kronecker delta is defined by

$$\delta_{ij} = \begin{cases} 0 & i \neq j \\ 1 & i = j \end{cases} \qquad (31)$$

In matrix notation

$$\mathbf{A} = \tfrac{1}{2}(\mathbf{Z} + \mathbf{I})\mathbf{I} \qquad (32)$$

$$\mathbf{B} = \tfrac{1}{2}(\mathbf{Z} - \mathbf{I})\mathbf{I} \qquad (33)$$

where I is the unit tensor which has all its diagonal matrix elements equal to one, and all its off-diagonal matrix elements equal to zero. For example, in four dimensions

$$I = \begin{bmatrix} 1 & 0 & 0 & 0 \\ 0 & 1 & 0 & 0 \\ 0 & 0 & 1 & 0 \\ 0 & 0 & 0 & 1 \end{bmatrix} \tag{34}$$

One may also write down the inverse of the above formulae

$$I = 2(Z + I)^{-1}A \tag{35}$$

$$V = 2Z(Z + I)^{-1}A \tag{36}$$

and

$$B = (Z - I)(Z + I)^{-1}A \tag{37}$$

$$= SA \tag{38}$$

where S is the scattering matrix (RLS-8, p. 148)

$$S = (Z - I)(Z + I)^{-1} = (I - Y)(I + Y)^{-1} \tag{39}$$

The scattering matrix relates the electric-field amplitudes incident on a waveguide junction to the reflected amplitudes, and its defining relation (38) has the explicit form

$$\begin{bmatrix} B_1 \\ B_2 \\ \cdot \\ \cdot \\ \cdot \\ B_n \end{bmatrix} = \begin{bmatrix} S_{11} & S_{12} & \cdots & S_{1n} \\ S_{21} & S_{22} & \cdots & S_{2n} \\ \cdots & \cdots & \cdots & \cdots \\ \cdots & \cdots & \cdots & \cdots \\ \cdots & \cdots & \cdots & \cdots \\ S_{n1} & S_{n2} & \cdots & S_{nn} \end{bmatrix} \begin{bmatrix} A_1 \\ A_2 \\ \cdot \\ \cdot \\ \cdot \\ A_n \end{bmatrix} \tag{40}$$

For a general waveguide junction the determinant of the scattering matrix obeys the condition

$$\det (I - S^*S) \geqslant 0 \tag{41}$$

and the same relation holds for each of the scattering matrix's principal minors, where $\mathbf{S}^*$ is the complex conjugate of $\mathbf{S}$. The matrix $\mathbf{S}^*$ is formed by replacing each element of $\mathbf{S}$ by its complex conjugate. In the particular case of a lossless junction

$$\mathbf{S}^*\mathbf{S} = \mathbf{I} \tag{42}$$

Since $\mathbf{S}$ is symmetrical it equals its transpose $\widetilde{\mathbf{S}}$, and its reciprocal $\mathbf{S}^{-1}$ is given by

$$\mathbf{S}^{-1} = \widetilde{\mathbf{S}}^* = \mathbf{S}^* \tag{43}$$

which means that the scattering matrix $\mathbf{S}$ is unitary. More explicitly, for a unitary matrix

$$\sum_{j=1}^{n} S_{ij}S_{jk}^* = \delta_{ik} \tag{44}$$

where δ_{ij} is the Kronecker delta defined by eq. (31). Thus the scattering matrix for a lossless junction is both symmetrical and unitary.

Sometimes it is desired to relate A_1 and B_1 at the input of a two-terminal pair junction to the output values A_2 and B_2. This may be done by transforming eq. (38).

$$\begin{bmatrix} B_1 \\ B_2 \end{bmatrix} = \begin{bmatrix} S_{11} & S_{12} \\ S_{12} & S_{22} \end{bmatrix} \begin{bmatrix} A_1 \\ A_2 \end{bmatrix} \tag{45}$$

to the T matrix form

$$\begin{bmatrix} B_2 \\ A_2 \end{bmatrix} = \begin{bmatrix} T_{11} & T_{12} \\ T_{21} & T_{22} \end{bmatrix} \begin{bmatrix} A_1 \\ B_1 \end{bmatrix} \tag{46}$$

The transmission coefficients T_{ij} may be expressed in terms of the matrix elements S_{ij}

$$\mathbf{T} = \begin{bmatrix} S_{12} - \dfrac{S_{22}S_{11}}{S_{21}} & \dfrac{S_{22}}{S_{21}} \\ -\dfrac{S_{11}}{S_{21}} & \dfrac{1}{S_{12}} \end{bmatrix} \tag{48}$$

For a lossless junction ($S_{12} = S_{21}$), this simplifies to

$$S = \frac{1}{T_{22}} \begin{bmatrix} T_{21} & 1 \\ 1 & T_{12} \end{bmatrix} \tag{49}$$

where, in general, $T_{12} \neq T_{21}$. If n two-terminal pair junctions are connected in cascade the output values of (B_{out}, A_{out}) are related to the input values (B_{in}, A_{in}) by the overall $\mathbf{T}$ matrix

$$\mathbf{T} = \mathbf{T}_n \mathbf{T}_{n-1} \ldots \mathbf{T}_1 \tag{50}$$

Both the $\mathbf{T}$ matrix and the scattering matrix will be found useful in analyzing the properties of microwave junctions, and use will be made of them later in the book.

F. The Symmetry of Waveguide Junctions

Scientists working in the field of electron spin resonance are doubtless familiar with ligand or crystal field theory which makes use of group theory in order to determine the energy level splittings of atoms in crystalline electric fields of various symmetries. A similar approach may be employed to characterize the electromagnetic fields, currents, and voltages of waveguide junctions in terms of their symmetries. Several waveguide junctions with planes and axes of symmetry are shown in Fig. 5-16. The junctions in these figures are classified by the symmetry operators which leave them unchanged. The symmetry characteristics of Fig. 5-16 are given in Table 5-3, and some important symmetry operators are defined in Table 5-4. Herzberg (1945) has an excellent table of point groups at the beginning of his introduction to *Infrared and Raman Spectra of Polyatomic Molecules*.

The successive application of two identical reflections leaves the space coordinates, x, y, z and the electromagnetic vectors unchanged, so in operator notation one may write

$$\mathbf{\delta}_{x,y}\, \mathbf{\delta}_{x,y} = \mathbf{\delta}_{y,z}\, \mathbf{\delta}_{y,z} = \mathbf{\delta}_{z,x}\, \mathbf{\delta}_{z,x} = 1 \tag{1}$$

where I is the identity operator. The successive application of the three reflections $\mathbf{\delta}_{x,y}$, $\mathbf{\delta}_{y,z}$, and $\mathbf{\delta}_{z,x}$ corresponds to an inversion i

$$\mathbf{\delta}_{x,y}\, \mathbf{\delta}_{y,z}\, \mathbf{\delta}_{z,x} = i \tag{2}$$

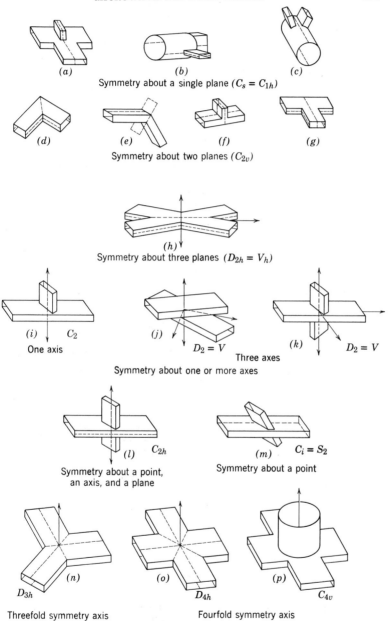

Fig. 5–16. Symmetries of waveguide junctions (*RLS*–8, pp. 401–403).

TABLE 5–3

Symmetry Elements of the Common Point Groups

Point group		Symmetry elements[a]	Examples
Schoenflies symbol	International symbol		
C_1	1	No symmetry	Human ear, Cathedral of Notre Dame
$C_i = S_2$	$\bar{1}$	Inversion i	
C_2	2	One C_2	7/2 turn helix
$C_s = C_{1v} = C_{1h}$	m	One $\sigma = \sigma_h$	*Homo sapiens* (external)
C_{2v}	mm	One C_2, two σ_v	Arrow
C_{2h}		One C_2, one σ_h, i	
C_{3v}	$3m$	One C_3, three σ_v	Three-sided pyramid
C_3	3	One C_3	Propeller with pointed front center
C_{4v}	$4mm$	One C_4, one C_2 (coincident with C_4) two σ_v, two σ_d	Great Pyramid of Egypt, Eifel Tower
S_4	4	Coincident C_2 and S_4	
$D_2 = V$	222	Three mutually perpendicular C_2	Directional coupler of Fig. 5–20
$C_{\infty v}$	∞m	One C_∞, any C_p, infinite number of σ_v	Baseball bat (excluding label)
$D_{2h} = V_h$	$\dfrac{2\,2\,2}{mmm}$	Three mutually $\perp$ C_2, three mutually $\perp$ σ, i	Chanel No. 5 symbol

TABLE 5–3 (*continued*)

Point group		Symmetry elements[a]	Examples
Schoenflies symbol	International symbol		
D_3	32	Three $C_2 \perp$ to C_3	Propeller (center is same in front and back)
D_{3h}	$\bar{6}m2$	One C_3, three $C_2 \perp$ to C_2, three $\eth_v$, one $\eth_h$	Ballentine beer symbol
D_{4h}	$\dfrac{4\,2\,2}{mmm}$	Coincident C_4, S_4 and C_2, four $C_2 \perp$ to C_4, two $\eth_v$, two σ_d, one $\eth_h$, i	Perfect square
C_{6v}	$6mm$	Coincident C_6, C_3, and C_2, three $\eth_v$, three σ_d	Wooden lead pencil
$D_{2d} = V_d$	$\bar{4}2m$	Three mutually $\perp$ C_2, one S_4 (coincident with one C_2), two $\eth_d$ through S_4	Baseball, including stitching; tennis ball
$D_{\infty h}$	∞/mm	C_∞, infinite number of $C_2 \perp$ to C_∞, infinite number of $\eth_v$, one $\eth_h$, any C_p and any S_p coincident with C_∞, i	Symmetric dumb-bell
O_h	$\dfrac{4}{m}\,\bar{3}\,\dfrac{2}{m}$	Three mutually $\perp$ C_4, four coincident S_4 and C_2, four coincident S_6 and C_3, six C_2, nine $\eth$, i	Dice sans dots, cube, octahedron

[a] All groups also contain the identity element I. Cyclically generated rotations such as $(C_3)^2$ and $(C_6)^5$ are not listed.

TABLE 5-4

Definition of Several Important Symmetry Elements

Symmetry element	Symmetry operation
I	Identity $\begin{Bmatrix} x \to x \\ y \to y \\ z \to z \end{Bmatrix}$ leaves figure unchanged
i	Inversion $\begin{Bmatrix} x \to -x \\ y \to -y \\ z \to -z \end{Bmatrix}$ inverts coordinates
$\sigma_h = \sigma_{x,y}$	Reflection in x,y plane $\begin{matrix} x \to x \\ y \to y \\ z \to -z \end{matrix}$
σ_v	Reflection in plane parallel to z-axis [e.g., $\sigma_{y,z}$ and $\sigma_{z,x}$]
σ_d	Diagonal reflection plane, e.g., $\begin{Bmatrix} x \to y \\ y \to x \\ z \to z \end{Bmatrix}$
C_p	p-fold symmetry axis. Rotation by $360/p$ degrees leaves figure unchanged, where p is a positive integer.
C_2	Twofold symmetry axis. If the z direction is the twofold symmetry axis then $\begin{Bmatrix} x \to -x \\ y \to -y \\ z \to \ \ z \end{Bmatrix}$ and the symmetry element may be called $C_2\ (z)$.
S_p	A rotation by $360/p$ degrees followed by a reflection at a plane perpendicular to the axis of rotation.

Other important relations are

$$\sigma_{x,y}\, \mathbf{C_2}(z) = \mathbf{i} \tag{3}$$

$$\sigma_{x,y}\, \mathbf{C_p}(z) = \mathbf{S_p}(z) \tag{4}$$

An inspection of Maxwell's equations indicates that their form is invariant under rotations and reflections, but particular solutions of these equations need not be invariant. For example, the reflection $\mathbf{d}_{y,z}$ in the y,z plane corresponds to the transformation

$$x \to - x$$
$$y \to y \qquad\qquad (5)$$
$$z \to z$$

and such a symmetry operation leads to the even and odd solutions of Maxwell's equations shown in Table 5-5. Corresponding solutions may be easily written down for the $\mathbf{d}_{x,y}$ and $\mathbf{d}_{z,x}$ planes.

If the symmetry plane does not contain a metallic sheet then the solutions shown in Table 5-5 must be symmetrical at the $\mathbf{d}_{y,z}$ symmetry plane and at this plane.

Even solution	Odd solution
$E_x = 0$	$E_y = 0$
$H_y = 0$	$E_z = 0$
$H_z = 0$	$H_x = 0$

The field distribution in the odd solution is the same as it would be if the symmetry plane were replaced by a perfectly conducting metallic film, and so it corresponds to an electric wall, while the even solution corresponds to a magnetic wall at the symmetry plane.

TABLE 5-5

Even and Odd Solutions of Maxwell's Equations with a Reflection Plane of Symmetry $\mathbf{d}_{y,z}$ (adapted from RLS-8, p. 413)

Even	Odd
$E_x(x,y,z) = -E_x(-x,y,z)$	$E_x(x,y,z) = E_x(-x,y,z)$
$E_y(x,y,z) = E_y(-x,y,z)$	$E_y(x,y,z) = -E_y(-x,y,z)$
$E_z(x,y,z) = E_z(-x,y,z)$	$E_z(x,y,z) = -E_z(-x,y,z)$
$H_x(x,y,z) = H_x(-x,y,z)$	$H_x(x,y,z) = -H_x(-x,y,z)$
$H_y(x,y,z) = -H_y(-x,y,z)$	$H_y(x,y,z) = H_y(-x,y,z)$
$H_z(x,y,z) = -H_z(-x,y,z)$	$H_z(x,y,z) = H_z(-x,y,z)$
$J_x(x,y,z) = -J_x(-x,y,z)$	$J_x(x,y,z) = J_x(-x,y,z)$
$J_y(x,y,z) = J_y(-x,y,z)$	$J_y(x,y,z) = -J_y(-x,y,z)$
$J_z(x,y,z) = J_z(-x,y,z)$	$J_z(x,y,z) = -J_z(-x,y,z)$
$\rho(x,y,z) = \rho(-x,y,z)$	$\rho(x,y,z) = -\rho(-x,y,z)$

A reflection in the z axis corresponds to a 180° or a twofold rotation $C_2(z)$ about the z axis, which produces the transformation

$$x \to - x$$
$$y \to - y \tag{6}$$
$$z \to z$$

The two solutions of Maxwell's equation for this symmetry are shown in Table 5-6. The labels even and odd are somewhat arbitrary.

Table 5-7 lists the two solutions which leave Maxwell's equations invariant under an inversion i,

$$x \to - x$$
$$y \to - y \tag{7}$$
$$z \to - z$$

It should be noted from these tables that the components of the current density J behave like the corresponding components of E under spatial symmetry.

The symmetry of several important waveguide junctions has been discussed in detail by Dicke, (RLS-8, Chap. 12) and the results will

TABLE 5–6

Solutions of Maxwell's Equations Symmetrical under Reflection in the z Rotation Axis $C_2(z)$ (adapted from RLS–8, p. 416)

Even		Odd	
$E_x(x,y,z) =$	$-E_x(-x,-y,z)$	$E_x(x,y,z) =$	$E_x(-x,-y,z)$
$E_y(x,y,z) =$	$-E_y(-x,-y,z)$	$E_y(x,y,z) =$	$E_y(-x,-y,z)$
$E_z(x,y,z) =$	$E_z(-x,-y,z)$	$E_z(x,y,z) =$	$-E_z(-x,-y,z)$
$H_x(x,y,z) =$	$-H_x(-x-y,z)$	$H_x(x,y,z) =$	$H_x(-x,-y,z)$
$H_y(x,y,z) =$	$-H_y(-x,-y,z)$	$H_y(x,y,z) =$	$H_y(-x,-y,z)$
$H_z(x,y,z) =$	$H_z(-x,-y,z)$	$H_z(x,y,z) =$	$-H_z(-x,-y,z)$
$J_x(x,y,z) =$	$-J_x(-x,-y,z)$	$J_x(x,y,z) =$	$J_x(-x,-y,z)$
$J_y(x,y,z) =$	$-J_y(-x,-y,z)$	$J_y(x,y,z) =$	$J_y(-x,-y,z)$
$J_z(x,y,z) =$	$J_z(-x,-y,z)$	$J_z(x,y,z) =$	$-J_z(-x,-y,z)$
$\rho(x,y,z) =$	$\rho(-x,-y,z)$	$\rho(x,y,z) =$	$-\rho(-x,-y,z)$

TABLE 5-7

Solutions of Maxwell's Equations Symmetrical under an Inversion i (adapted from RLS-8, p. 416)

Even			Odd		
$E_x(x,y,z)$	$=$	$E_x(-x,-y,-z)$	$E_x(x,y,z)$	$=$	$-E_x(-x,-y,-z)$
$E_y(x,y,z)$	$=$	$E_y(-x.-y,-z)$	$E_y(x,y,z)$	$=$	$-E_y(-x,-y,-z)$
$E_z(x,y,z)$	$=$	$E_z(-x,-y,-z)$	$E_z(x,y,z)$	$=$	$-E_z(-x,-y,-z)$
$H_x(x,y,z)$	$=$	$-H_x(-x,-y,-z)$	$H_x(x,y,z)$	$=$	$H_x(-x,-y,-z)$
$H_y(x,y,z)$	$=$	$-H_y(-x,-y,-z)$	$H_y(x,y,z)$	$=$	$H_y(-x,-y,-z)$
$H_z(x,y,z)$	$=$	$-H_z(-x,-y,-z)$	$H_z(x,y,z)$	$=$	$H_z(-x,-y,-z)$
$J_x(x,y,z)$	$=$	$J_x(-x,-y,-z)$	$J_x(x,y,z)$	$=$	$-J_x(-x,-y,-z)$
$J_y(x,y,z)$	$=$	$J_y(-x,-y,-z)$	$J_y(x,y,z)$	$=$	$-J_y(-x,-y,-z)$
$J_z(x,y,z)$	$=$	$J_z(-x,-y,-z)$	$J_z(x,y,z)$	$=$	$-J_z(-x,-y,-z)$
$\rho(x,y,z)$	$=$	$-\rho(-x,-y,-z)$	$\rho(x,y,z)$	$=$	$\rho(-x,-y,-z)$

be summarized below.   They illustrate the value of utilizing symmetry properties when analyzing the characteristics of a waveguide junction.

Thick Iris: Let V_1 and V_2 be measures of the transverse electric field, and I_1 and I_2 be measures of the transverse magnetic field

$$\mathbf{V} = \begin{bmatrix} V_1 \\ V_2 \end{bmatrix}, \text{ and } \mathbf{I} = \begin{bmatrix} I_1 \\ I_2 \end{bmatrix} \tag{8}$$

appearing at the junctions 1 and 2 of the iris shown in Fig. 5-17. The reflection operator $\mathbf{\delta}_h$ at the plane of symmetry

$$\mathbf{\delta}_h = \begin{bmatrix} 0 & 1 \\ 1 & 0 \end{bmatrix} \tag{9}$$

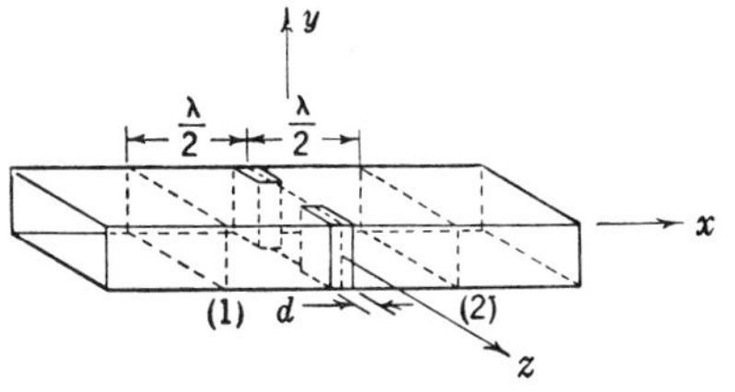

Fig. 5-17.   The thick iris (RLS-8, p. 417).

gives

$$\mathbf{d}_h \mathbf{V} = \mathbf{V}' \text{ and } \mathbf{d}_h \mathbf{I} = \mathbf{I}' \tag{10}$$

The impedance matrix Z of the junction satisfies the equation

$$\mathbf{V} = \mathbf{ZI} \tag{11}$$

and it is related to the reflection operator by

$$\mathbf{d}_h \mathbf{Z} = \mathbf{Z} \mathbf{d}_h \tag{12}$$

The even and odd solutions are

Even	Odd
$V_1 = V_2$	$V_1 = - V_2$
$I_1 = I_2$	$I_1 = - I_2$

and the impedance matrix has the form [see eq. (5-D-9); RLS-8, p. 420]

$$\mathbf{Z} = \tfrac{1}{2} \begin{bmatrix} z_1+z_2 & z_1-z_2 \\ z_1-z_2 & z_1+z_2 \end{bmatrix} \tag{14}$$

which corresponds to the T section equivalent circuit shown in Fig. 5-18. When the iris thickness d is small compared to the guide wavelength λ_g, then the capacitive reactance z_z satisfies the inequality

$$0 < jz_2 < \pi(d/\lambda_g) \tag{15}$$

The impedance matrix may be written as a similarity transformation

$$\mathbf{Z} = \mathbf{M} \begin{bmatrix} z_1 & 0 \\ 0 & z_2 \end{bmatrix} \mathbf{M}^{-1} \tag{16}$$

where $\mathbf{M}$ is a unitary matrix

$$\mathbf{M} = \frac{1}{(2)^{1/2}} \begin{bmatrix} 1 & 1 \\ 1 & -1 \end{bmatrix} \tag{17}$$

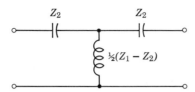

Fig. 5–18.   The equivalent circuit of a thick iris.

Symmetrical T Junction: The symmetrical T junctions shown in Fig. 5-19 have the operators (RLS-8, p. 431)

$$\mathbf{\delta} = \begin{bmatrix} 0 & 1 & 0 \\ 1 & 0 & 0 \\ 0 & 0 & 1 \end{bmatrix} \qquad \text{shunt } T \qquad (18)$$

$$\mathbf{\delta'} = \begin{bmatrix} 0 & 1 & 0 \\ 1 & 0 & 0 \\ 0 & 0 & 1 \end{bmatrix} \begin{bmatrix} 1 & 0 & 0 \\ 0 & 1 & 0 \\ 0 & 0 & -1 \end{bmatrix} \qquad (19)$$

$$= \begin{bmatrix} 0 & 1 & 0 \\ 1 & 0 & 0 \\ 0 & 0 & -1 \end{bmatrix} \quad \begin{cases} \text{series } T \\ \\ \text{axial } T \end{cases} \qquad (20)$$

The scattering matrix **S** is related to these operators by

$$\mathbf{S} = \mathbf{\delta S}[\mathbf{\delta}]^{-1} = \mathbf{\delta S \delta} \qquad (21)$$

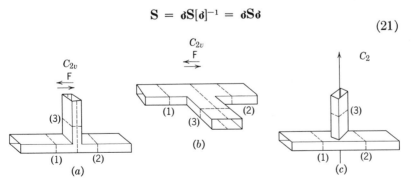

Fig. 5–19.   Symmetrical T junction: (a) series; (b) shunt; (c) axial (RLS-8, p. 431).

and

$$\mathbf{S} = \mathbf{d}'\mathbf{S}[\mathbf{d}']^{-1} = \mathbf{d}'\mathbf{S}\mathbf{d}' \tag{22}$$

for the shunt T and series T (axial T) cases, respectively.

The elements of S must satisfy the relations

$$\left.\begin{array}{c} S_{11} = S_{22} \\ S_{13} = S_{23} \end{array}\right\} \quad \text{shunt } T \tag{23}$$

$$\left.\begin{array}{c} S_{11} = S_{22} \\ S_{13} = S_{23} \end{array}\right\} \quad \text{series } T \text{ and axial } T \tag{24}$$

For a shunt T junction the scattering matrix may be expressed in terms of three parameters

$$\mathbf{S} = \tfrac{1}{4} \begin{bmatrix} (1 + s_2 + 2s_3) & (1 + s_2 - 2s_3) & 2^{1/2}(1 - s_2) \\ (1 + s_2 - 2s_3) & (1 + s_2 + 2s_3) & 2^{1/2}(1 - s_2) \\ 2^{1/2}(1 - s_2) & 2^{1/2}(1 - s_2) & 2(1 + s_2) \end{bmatrix} \tag{25}$$

From the unitary properties of this matrix [eq. (5-E-44)] it may be shown that

$$s_2{}^2 = s_3{}^2 = 1 \tag{26}$$

The scattering matrix is derivable from a similarity transformation

$$\mathbf{S} = 4\mathbf{M} \begin{bmatrix} s_1 & 0 & 0 \\ 0 & s_2 & 0 \\ 0 & 0 & s_3 \end{bmatrix} \mathbf{M}^{-1} \tag{27}$$

where $s_1 = 1$, and the unitary matrix $\mathbf{M}$ has the form

$$\mathbf{M} = \tfrac{1}{2} \begin{bmatrix} 1 & 1 & 2^{1/2} \\ 1 & 1 & -2^{1/2} \\ 2^{1/2} & -2^{1/2} & 0 \end{bmatrix} \tag{28}$$

A perfectly matched T junction has the property that an electromagnetic wave incident on any terminal produces no reflected wave at the same terminal. Since the scattering matrix relates the incident amplitudes A_i to the scattered amplitudes B_i in accordance with eq. (5-E-40), the mathematical definition of a completely matched microwave junction is one whose scattering matrix has all of its diagonal elements equal to zero. Thus a matched T junction would satisfy the relation $s_2 = -1$ and $s_3 = 0$, and the latter condition is incompatible with eq. (26). As a result it is not possible to completely match a T junction. One may match the first two arms alone $(s_2 = 1, s_3 = -1)$

$$S = \begin{bmatrix} 0 & 1 & 0 \\ 1 & 0 & 0 \\ 0 & 0 & 1 \end{bmatrix} \tag{29}$$

or the third arm alone $(s_2 = -1)$

$$S = \tfrac{1}{2} \begin{bmatrix} s_3 & -s_3 & 2^{1/2} \\ -s_3 & s_3 & 2^{1/2} \\ 2^{1/2} & 2^{1/2} & 0 \end{bmatrix} \tag{30}$$

and the former condition decouples the third arm from the other two since

$$\begin{bmatrix} B_1 \\ B_2 \\ B_3 \end{bmatrix} = \begin{bmatrix} 0 & 1 & 0 \\ 1 & 0 & 0 \\ 0 & 0 & 1 \end{bmatrix} \begin{bmatrix} A_1 \\ A_2 \\ A_3 \end{bmatrix} = \begin{bmatrix} A_2 \\ A_1 \\ A_3 \end{bmatrix} \tag{31}$$

Directional Coupler: A directional coupler is designed to couple a small amount of microwave energy out of a waveguide without appreciably disturbing the main power flow. If the wave A_1 is incident in arm 1, then an ideal three-terminal pair directional coupler will transmit most of this signal as the outgoing wave B_2 in arm two and a small signal B_3 in arm three, without producing any reflected wave B_1 in arm one. Thus ideally the scattering matrix

$$S = \begin{bmatrix} S_{11} & S_{12} & S_{13} \\ S_{12} & S_{22} & S_{23} \\ S_{13} & S_{23} & S_{33} \end{bmatrix} \tag{32}$$

will have $S_{11} = S_{22} = 0$, $|S_{12}|$ close to unity, S_{13} very small, and $S_{23} = 0$. The last condition means that microwaves traversing the directional coupler in the reverse direction from terminal 2 to terminal 1 will not couple to the side arm (terminal 3). The coupling C is defined by

$$C = -20 \log_{10} | S_{12} | \tag{33}$$

and the directivity D is

$$D = 20 \log_{10} | S_{13}/S_{23} | \tag{34}$$

It is customary to characterize directional couplers by their coefficients C and D, as discussed in Sec. 7-D.

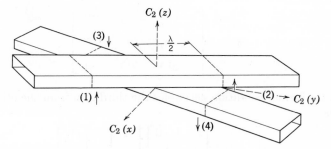

Fig. 5–20. Directional coupler with $D_2 = V$ symmetry. The three mutually perpendicular C_2 axes and the four terminals are labeled (RLS–8, p. 438).

The four-terminal pair directional coupler shown on Fig. 5-20 has three mutually perpendicular C_2 symmetry axes, lacks planes of symmetry, and belongs to point group $D_2 \equiv V$. Its scattering matrix is a function of four parameters.

$$\mathbf{S} = \begin{bmatrix} \alpha & \beta & | & \gamma & \delta \\ \beta & \alpha & | & \delta & \gamma \\ --- & | & --- \\ \gamma & \delta & | & \alpha & \beta \\ \delta & \gamma & | & \beta & \alpha \end{bmatrix} \tag{35}$$

and these parameters may be expressed as linear combinations of four others

$$\left.\begin{array}{l} \alpha = 1/4 \ (s_1 + s_2 + s_3 + s_4) \\ \beta = 1/4 \ (s_1 - s_2 + s_3 - s_4) \\ \gamma = 1/4 \ (s_1 + s_2 - s_3 - s_4) \\ \delta = 1/4 \ (s_1 - s_2 - s_3 + s_4) \end{array}\right\} \tag{36}$$

Magic T: The magic T is defined as a directional coupler which appears matched looking into all arms, and which produces equal power division. Arms 1 and 2 couple only to arms 3 and 4. As a result the scattering matrix has the form

$$\mathbf{S} = \begin{bmatrix} 0 & 0 & | & \alpha & \beta \\ 0 & 0 & | & \gamma & \delta \\ --- & | & --- \\ \alpha & \beta & | & 0 & 0 \\ \gamma & \delta & | & 0 & 0 \end{bmatrix} \tag{37}$$

with the unitary conditions

$$\left.\begin{array}{l} \alpha\beta^* + \gamma\delta^* = 0 \\ \alpha\gamma^* + \beta\delta^* = 0 \\ |\alpha|^2 + |\beta|^2 = |\gamma|^2 + |\delta|^2 = 1 \\ |\alpha|^2 + |\gamma|^2 = |\beta|^2 + |\delta|^2 = 1 \end{array}\right\} \tag{38}$$

and the equal coupling conditions

$$|\alpha| = |\beta| = |\gamma| = |\delta| \tag{39}$$

By the proper choice of reference terminals any magic T may be made to have one of the two following scattering matrices (*RLS-8,* p. 448).

$$\mathbf{S} = 1/2^{1/2} \begin{bmatrix} 0 & 0 & | & j & j \\ 0 & 0 & | & j & -j \\ ---- & | & ---- \\ j & j & | & 0 & 0 \\ j & -j & | & 0 & 0 \end{bmatrix} \tag{40}$$

$$\mathbf{S} = 1/2^{1/2} \begin{bmatrix} 0 & 0 & | & 1 & j \\ 0 & 0 & | & j & 1 \\ -- & -- & | & -- & -- \\ 1 & j & | & 0 & 0 \\ j & 1 & | & 0 & 0 \end{bmatrix} \tag{41}$$

The operation of a magic T is illustrated by the relationship between the incident wave amplitudes A_i and the reflected wave amplitudes B_i which is given by

$$\begin{bmatrix} B_1 \\ B_2 \\ B_3 \\ B_4 \end{bmatrix} = 1/2^{1/2} \begin{bmatrix} 0 & 0 & | & j & j \\ 0 & 0 & | & j & -j \\ -- & -- & | & -- & -- \\ j & j & | & 0 & 0 \\ j & -j & | & 0 & 0 \end{bmatrix} \begin{bmatrix} A_1 \\ A_2 \\ A_3 \\ A_4 \end{bmatrix} \tag{42}$$

$$= j/2^{1/2} \begin{bmatrix} A_3 + A_4 \\ A_3 - A_4 \\ A_1 + A_2 \\ A_1 - A_2 \end{bmatrix} \tag{43}$$

from eq. (40), and analogously by

$$\begin{bmatrix} B_1 \\ B_2 \\ B_3 \\ B_4 \end{bmatrix} = 1/2^{1/2} \begin{bmatrix} A_3 + jA_4 \\ A_4 + jA_3 \\ A_1 + jA_2 \\ A_2 + jA_1 \end{bmatrix} \tag{44}$$

from eq. (41). Thus the microwaves incident on terminals 1 and 2 appear with equal intensity at terminals 3 and 4, and the microwaves incident on terminals 3 and 4 appear with equal intensity at terminals 1 and 2. The two types of magic T differ in the phase relations between the two waves that super-impose at each terminal. An example of a magic T is shown in Fig. 5-21 and several varieties of magic T's are discussed in Sec. 7-F.

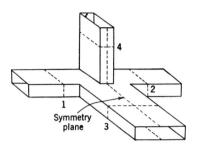

Fig. 5–21.   Magic T (RLS–8, p. 452).

References

R. M. Foster, *Bell System Tech. J.*, **3**, 259 (1924)

M. G. Gardner and J. L. Barnes, *Transients in Linear Systems*, Wiley, N. Y., 1942.

G. Herzberg, *Molecular Spectra and Molecular Structure, II. Infrared and Raman Spectra of Polyatomic Molecules*, 2nd Ed., Van Nostrand, N. Y., 1945.

H. A. Kramers, *Atti Congr. Fis. Como*, **1927**, 525.

R. Kronig, *J. Opt. Soc. Am.*, **12**, 547 (1926).

RLS-8.   We have discussed in detail Chapters 5 and 12 by R. H. Dicke.

RLS-9.

S. Ramo, J. R. Whinnery, and T. Van Duzer, *Fields and Waves in Communication Electronics*, Wiley, N. Y., 1965.

CHAPTER 6

Microwave Generators

A. Frequency Limitations of Conventional Vacuum Tubes

The "very high frequency" or vhf region of the electromagnetic spectrum extends from 300 to 3000 Mc, and it may be considered as a boundary region between radio frequency and microwave techniques. This boundary region corresponds to free space wavelengths between 100 and 10 cm. At radio frequencies, ordinary lumped constant circuit components are employed, while in the microwave region use is made of distributed constant circuits.

Conventional vacuum tubes have an upper limit to their useful frequency range, and this upper limit in the vhf region is set by one of the following factors: (a) the interelectrode capacitance cannot be conveniently decreased; (b) the inductance of the leads to the tube elements cannot be conveniently reduced; (c) the transit time of the electrons in the space between the electrodes approaches a significant fraction of the radio frequency period; (d) appreciable radiation of radio frequency power occurs because the tube structure and connecting leads act as antennae; (e) the foregoing reasons require the use of small tube structures, and these do not dissipate heat efficiently.

These limiting factors have been circumvented by employing new approaches for the design of microwave tubes. It is customary to incorporate cavity resonators to obviate the difficulties arising from radiation, and from lumped inductive and capacitive effects. In a microwave tube the interaction between electromagnetic fields and the electron beam in the "interaction gaps" is of crucial importance, while the collection of the electrons is of only minor importance. The finite transit time of the electrons, which ordinarily has a deleterious effect at high operating frequencies, is actually utilized as an essential factor in klystrons and magnetrons.

Microwave triodes, klystrons, and magnetrons were the microwave tubes which enjoyed widespread use during the wartime and

169

postwar period.   More recently, other types of tubes such as backward wave oscillators (traveling wave tubes) and masers have been developed. Most of these will be discussed in turn.   Since workers in the field of electron spin resonance are interested in using commercially available tubes rather than in designing their own tubes, the emphasis in this chapter will be on the operating principles and applications of these tubes.   Pierce (1962) and Coleman (1963) have reviewed the present status of the microwave tube art.

B. Microwave Triodes

Microwave triodes or space charge limited tubes are widely employed as generators at S band (3000 Mc).   Although most ESR measurements are made between 10,000 and 35,000 Mc, it is sometimes helpful to employ S band to check the frequency dependence of a spectrum, to reduce the effects of dielectric loss in water-containing samples, to accommodate larger sample volumes, to facilitate the use of coaxial transmission lines, etc.   A microwave triode is a convenient source of S band energy, although klystrons are also available for this frequency band.

The electrodes of microwave triodes are frequently planar rather than cylindrical, and disk-seal triodes are popularly referred to as "lighthouse tubes" because of their shape.   The mechanical details of the 2C40 S band tube are shown in Fig. 6–1.   This tube contains an oxide-coated cathode mounted on the end of a cylindrical post situated about 0.1 mm from a mesh grid, and the anode is the end of a similar cylindrical post about 0.3 mm on the other side of the grid. This tube supplies a power output of 1 W at 1000 Mc and 0.1 W at 3000 Mc.   When in use, the lighthouse tube may be inserted in a coaxial resonator.   In this arrangement the vacuum tube electrodes become integral parts of the resonant cavity, and as a result the lead inductance is practically removed, and radiation losses are eliminated.   Thus microwave triodes represent a logical adaption of conventional triode designs to very high frequencies.   These triodes become impractical above 4000 Mc because of the mechanical difficulties associated with the accurate maintenance of closer electrode spacings.

In the upper half of the very high frequency band (1000–4000 Mc) both triodes and klystrons are available for use.   At these

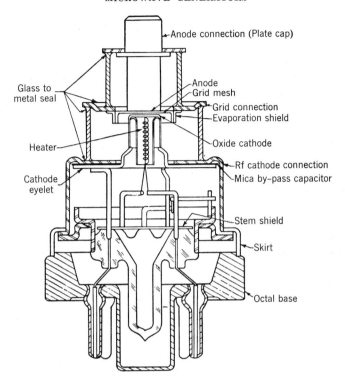

Fig. 6–1.   Mechanical details of the 2C40 tube (*RLS*–7, p. 10).

frequencies, microwave triodes require fewer and lower supply voltages and tend to be more stable in frequency, while it is difficult to achieve wide band tuning with triode tubes.   Microwave triodes may be employed both as oscillators (frequency generators) and as amplifiers.   An extended discussion of triode amplifiers may be found in *RLS*–7, Reintjes and Coate (1952), and Ginzton (1957).

C. Magnetrons

The principal application of magnetrons is to systems which require the generation of very high microwave power outputs, particularly if the power is pulsed rather than continuous.   Some magnetrons furnish in excess of 1 MW of peak output power during the pulse.   In a typical case the pulse will be 0.1 or 1 μsec long, and the duty cycle will be 10^{-3}.   The latter means that the magnetron is only producing microwave power 0.1% of the time.

In a magnetron, the electrons that are emitted by the central cathode execute cycloids in a magnetic field until they either return to the cathode or reach the outer anode.   An example of a cycloid-like electron path is shown in Fig. 6–2.   In this figure the anode is in the center and eight resonators are arranged radially around it. The electrons moving in the magnetic field may be made to travel in suitable orbits and interact with a resonant cavity so as to supply energy to the cavity, thereby sustaining oscillations.   Table 6–1 lists the characteristics of several typical magnetrons.

D. Traveling Wave Tubes and Backward Wave Oscillators

The traveling wave tube is a special type of microwave tube which has a much broader band-width than a klystron or magnetron.   An example of a traveling wave tube is shown in Fig. 6–3.   The cathode

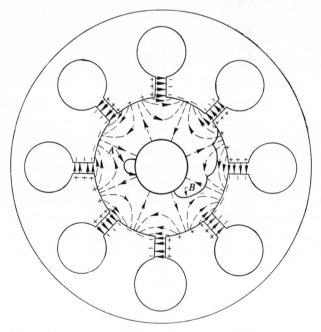

Fig. 6–2.   Paths followed by electrons in oscillating magnetron (*RLS*–6, p. 26).

TABLE 6-1
Characteristics of Several Magnetrons

Tube	Frequency, Gs	Average power, kW	Pulse power, kW	Pulse duration, μsec
4J21[a]	1.0	0.8	800	6
4J39[a]	3.0	0.6	1000	2.5
MA209A	9.6		7	1.0
5780	9.0		250	0.3
MA210B	35		32	0.25
BL-221	70		10	0.03

[a] World War II vintage.

emits electrons which are accelerated and focused by the electron gun. These electrons pass down the helix to the collector at 1/13 of the velocity of light when a 15,000-V accelerating potential is employed. The actual length of the wire in the helix is thirteen times as long as the distance along the axis of the helix. As a result the electromagnetic wave which travels along the wire at the velocity of light actually progresses along the helical axis at 1/13 of the

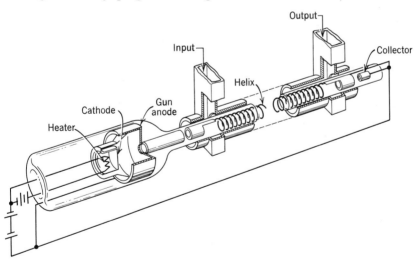

Fig. 6-3. Schematic of traveling wave amplifier [Pierce (1950), p. 7].

velocity of light while it interacts with the electron beam.   The helix may thus be referred to as a slow wave structure, and it operates over a very wide frequency band because it is nonresonant.   The electromagnetic wave interacts with the electrons in such a way that it bunches them, and extracts energy from them.

When the traveling wave tube is employed as an amplifier, the electromagnetic wave enters by the input waveguide in Fig. 6–3. Subsequently, it travels along the helix while interacting with the electronic beam, extracting energy from it, and gradually growing in amplitude.   When it reaches the output waveguide, the wave will be perhaps 20 or 30 dB stronger, which means that the output power from the traveling wave tube may be 100 or 1000 times the input power.

Aside from their high power gain and wide band-width, traveling wave tubes also have desirable noise figures [Hok (1956)], a wide range of design frequencies [200 to 50,000 Mc according to Pierce (1950)], and simplicity of construction.   Their most important feature, however, is their wide band-width.   When a traveling wave tube is converted to an oscillator, it is referred to as a backward wave oscillator or carcinotron.   It may be tuned in frequency by adjusting the beam voltage.   Uchida and Buyle-Bodin (1962) discuss the band-widths and noise characteristics of several types of microwave oscillators.   Wilmshurst, Gambling, and Ingram (1962) compare the sensitivity of resonant cavity and traveling wave tube spectrometers and Webb (1962) discusses the use of traveling wave helixes in ESR and Overhauser (double resonance) studies.   Mock (1960) used a backward wave oscillator and harmonic conversion to operate between 50 and 150 kMc.   See also, Dreizler, Maier, and Rudolph (1960), Kondrat'ev (1963), Sloan, Ganssen, and LaVier (1964), Mouthaan (1965), Ober (1965), and Gittins (1965).

E. Klystrons

Introduction: Klystrons [(*RLS*–7; Harrison (1947)] are employed as generators of microwave power in the frequency range from 500 to 35,000 Mc.   Some have been made to produce continuous wave or CW power up to 25 kW, and others to supply pulsed power up to 10^4 kW, but in electron spin resonance spectrometers the klystron usually provides less than 1 W of CW output.   Since the klystron finds more widespread use in ESR than any other generator of micro-waves, it will be discussed in somewhat more detail than the other microwave sources.

In comparison with lighthouse tubes and conventional low-frequency tubes there are two innovations which characterize a klystron. The first combines the process of velocity modulating and bunching the electron stream to generate the rf (i.e., microwave) oscillations. This means that the finite transit time of the electrons is harnessed to produce the microwave power. Hitherto, this finite transit time had been one of the major hinderances that stood in the way of increasing the usable frequency of vacuum tubes.

The second novel aspect of a klystron is the application of the velocity-modulated rf control voltage to the electrons after they have been accelerated by the full applied plate voltage. This feature of klystrons is so closely connected with the first that it will not be discussed further in itself.

Reflex Klystron: A schematic diagram of a reflex klystron is shown in Fig. 6–4. The cathode supplies electrons by thermionic emission just as in a conventional vacuum tube, and these electrons are accelerated toward the rf gap (anode) by the beam or resonator voltage V_B. In the rf gap the electron beam is subjected to an rf

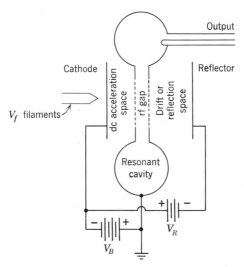

Fig. 6–4. Schematic diagram of a reflex klystron (*RLS*–11, p. 25).

electric field which alternately slows down and speeds up the electrons in the beam, thereby velocity-modulating them. After traversing the rf gap the velocity-modulated electron beam enters the drift space in which the fast electrons move away from the slower ones behind them and catch up with the slower ones in front of them. The net effect is the formation of groups or bunches of electrons. Since the reflector is negative relative to the anode or rf gap, the bunched electron beam is turned around and returned to the gap. When the radio frequency, beam voltage, and reflector voltage are properly adjusted, the bunched electrons will return to the gap with the proper phase, and as a result they will be "debunched" in the process of giving up energy to the resonant cavity. This cavity is coupled to a transmission line in such a way that the energy extracted from the electron beam is made to propagate down the transmission line. If the reflector voltage is not properly chosen, then the electrons will reenter the rf gap with incorrect phases, and no energy will be extracted from them. A necessary condition for a reflex klystron to oscillate is that the transit time in the reflection drift space be in the vicinity of $(n + \frac{3}{4})$ rf periods, where n is an integer. This insures that the electrons are properly bunched when they arrive back at the rf gap. In addition, the dc beam current I_B must exceed a minimum value called the "starting current" to insure that the power extracted from the electron beam is greater than the circuit and load losses involved in maintaining the gap voltage. When these two conditions are satisfied, oscillations will occur.

For a given beam voltage V_B there are definite values of the reflector voltage V_R which correspond to stable oscillations. This is illustrated in Fig. 6–5 for the 2K25 klystron. The various modes which are labeled with their n values are characterized by different transit times (not by different frequencies as in resonant cavity modes), and usually they extend through zero to positive values of the reflector voltage. However, the figure only gives the regions of stable oscillation that correspond to zero reflector current. This is because the current collected by the reflector at positive and at slightly negative values of V_R may cause excessive heating and permanently damage the klystron. To obviate this possibility, it is advisable to install a diode which will short-circuit the reflector to the anode in the event that the negative voltage supply to the reflector fails to operate.

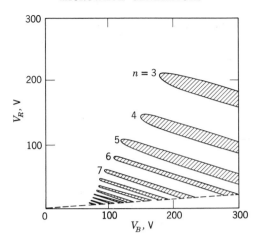

Fig. 6–5. Reflector-mode pattern of the type 2K25 reflex klystron operating at 3.2 cm. The shaded areas correspond to those combinations of beam voltage V_B and reflector voltage V_R at which oscillation occurs (*RLS*–11, p. 27).

In routine use, a klystron is operated at a predetermined beam voltage, and often this voltage is a value recommended by the manufacturer. For a particular value of beam voltage V_B and klystron cavity frequency f_0, the klystron frequency f and power output P will vary in the manner shown in Fig. 6–6. When the cavity frequency f_0 is altered, the mode patterns of Fig. 6–5 will shift to the right or left corresponding to variations of the transit time with frequency. A typical reflex klystron has a mechanical tuning range

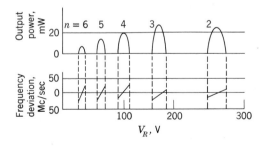

Fig. 6–6. Output power and frequency of oscillation as functions of reflector voltage in the type 2K25 (732A/B) reflex klystron. Beam voltage = 300 V; λ = 3.2 cm (*RLS*–11, p. 27).

between 5 and 50%, which means that the klystron cavity frequency f_0 may be varied within this range. The electronic tuning range is the deviation from f_0 that may be obtained through variations in the reflector voltage only, as shown in Fig. 6–6. Typical electronic tuning ranges are from 0.2 to 0.8% of the frequency f_0. For example, the Varian X-13 klystron may be tuned mechanically from 8100 to 12,400 Mc and has an average electronic tuning range of 60 Mc at 8100 kMc and 45 Mc at 12,400 Mc. It is normal for both the electronic tuning range and the power output to be frequency dependent.

Reflector Modulation: The effect of square-wave and sawtooth reflector voltage modulation on the klystron power output is shown in Fig. 6–7. The particular square wave illustrated has the effect of producing pulses of microwave power. If the amplitude of the sawtooth in Fig. 6–7b were increased to a value that extended from 20 to 300 V for the 2K25 klystron, then the entire mode pattern shown on the upper part of Fig. 6–6 would be displayed on the oscilloscope. This is a convenient technique to employ when tuning a klystron to an external resonant cavity. Often a low amplitude sine-wave reflector voltage modulation is employed as an integral part of an automatic frequency control (AFC) system. Anomalous modulation effects occur at very high frequencies when the period of the modulation frequency $(1/f_m)$ becomes comparable to the decay time of the loaded klystron resonant cavity, or when f_m itself becomes comparable to the cavity band-width. Sushkov and Meos (1965) generated nanosecond pulses with a klystron.

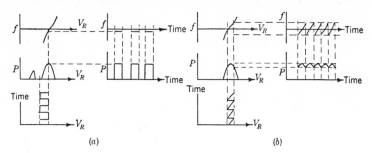

(a)   (b)

Fig. 6–7. Amplitude and frequency modulation characteristics of the reflex klystron: (a) for square-wave amplitude modulation; (b) for sawtooth frequency and amplitude modulation (*RLS*-11, p. 28).

Rieke Diagram: For fixed filament and beam voltages the power output of a klystron depends upon the load. Figure 6–8 shows the variation in the power output for three loads when the frequency is changed by varying the reflector voltage. The maximum power output is obtained with the optimum load which corresponds to terminating the transmission line with the complex conjugate of the generator impedance. A greater range of frequencies may be obtained with a lighter load. There are some loads which prevent the klystron from oscillating. A complete picture of the dependence of the power output on load may be obtained by plotting lines of constant power on a Smith chart, as illustrated in *RLS*-7, p. 434. Such a plot is called a Rieke diagram, and it includes the regions of nonoscillation. Of particular note is the fact that a reflex klystron has a greater power output at its optimum load than at the matched load which occurs in the center of the Smith chart or Rieke diagram.

Hysteresis: When the output power and frequency at a given reflector voltage depend on the direction of approach to this reflector voltage, then the phenomenon of electronic tuning hysteresis occurs. An example of this is shown in Fig. 6–9, which presents the oscilloscope trace of a klystron mode produced by a sinusoidal sweep. The first half of the cycle *A* traces out the mode from right to left, and the retrace *B* fails to produce the extreme left side of the mode. Equally spaced frequency markers are shown. Electronic hysteresis may be caused by electrons making multiple transits through the rf gap, by transit angles varying with the rf voltage, and by an appreciable variation of the small-signal electronic transconductance across the width of a low mode. The double-valued sinks which result from the long line effect also constitute a type of hysteresis (*RLS*-7).

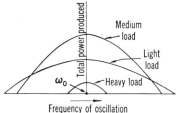

Fig. 6–8. Total rf power produced during electronic tuning for three types of loads (*RLS*-7, p. 316).

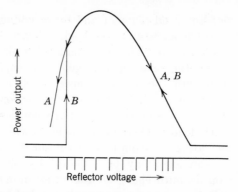

Fig. 6–9. The oscilloscope traces A, B show the hysteresis in the dependence of the klystron power on the reflector voltage $-V_R$. Equally spaced frequency markers are shown below (RLS-7, p. 391).

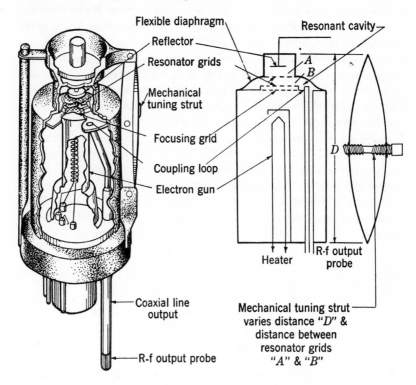

Fig. 6–10. Schematic diagram of 723 klystron construction (RLS-11, p. 38).

Specific Reflex Klystrons: The 2K25 (723A/B) klystron is illustrated in Fig. 6–10 because so many of the pioneer electron spin
resonance studies were made with this wartime vintage tube. The
characteristic curves of the more modern VA–6312 klystron are
shown in Fig. 6–11. Table 6–2 gives the electrical characteristics
of some frequently used klystrons. The tubes in the first half of the
table are obsolete and should not be used for new equipment. They
are included because much of the experimental work in ESR has
been carried out with them. Some are now available at low cost.

A worn-out klystron may frequently be diagnosed by the following
simple test. First, the filament voltage is raised to 6.6 V and the
reflector voltage is set at a value where the klystron is not oscillating
(low resonator current and no signal at detector). The filament
voltage is now decreased to 5.7 V, and if this lowers the resonator
current by more than 15%, the klystron may be replaced. Another
characteristic of a worn out klystron is an unusually low power
output combined with a subnormal beam current.

F. Frequency Multiplication and Other
Millimeter Wave Sources

At present, klystrons and magnetrons are limited to the production
of microwave frequencies below 200,000 Mc ($\lambda = 4$ mm), and most
microwave generators are designed for much lower frequencies. For
studies in the neighborhood of g factor two a frequency of 75,000
Mc corresponds to a magnetic field strength of 27,000 G (2.7 Wb/m),
and many electromagnets equipped with tapered pole caps are
capable of obtaining this field in magnet gaps of the order of 1 cm
or less. The use of such high frequencies and fields can help to
resolve field-dependent effects such as slightly anisotropic g factors
and complex spectra resulting from overlapping paramagnetic species.
Equipment for 2-mm microwaves is described by van Es, Gevers, and
de Ronde (1960-61). See also, Rubin (1955), Zimmerer (1962),
Burrus (1963), Rodrigue (1963), Davis, Clarke, and Morris (1964),
and the reviews by Willshaw (1961), and Coleman (1963).

It is possible to produce high microwave frequencies by starting
with a low-frequency klystron and multiplying the fundamental to a
high harmonic by means of a nonlinear device such as a crystal diode.
For example, Gordy and his co-workers [(Gordy 1948); Smith,

TABLE 6-2

Summary of Reflex Klystron Characteristics (Reproduced in part from *RLS*-11, pp. 35 and 36)

Type No.	Frequency range, Gc	Beam voltage, V	Beam current, mA	Reflector voltage,[a] V	Power output, mW	Electronic tuning range, Mc	Electronic tuning rate, Mc per reflector V	Mfr.	Notes[b]
2K25 (723A/B)	8.5-9.66	300	22	110-170	23	45	2.2	BTL WL	"160-volt mode"
				60-110	23	65	4.2	Raytheon —	"100-volt mode"
726C	2.7-2.96	300	22	90-130	120-200	30	0.9	WE	
726B	2.88-3.175	300	22	90-130	70-155	35	—	WE	
726A	3.175-3.41	300	22	130-165	110	30	—	WE	
2K29	3.4-3.9	300	22	90-172	75-150	48-34	1.7-0.7	BTL WE	
2K22	4.3-3.9	300	22	—	(75)	—	—	BTL WE	
2K27	5.2-5.57	300	22	—	(40)	—	—	BTL WE	
2K26	6.25-7.06	300	22	—	(25)	—	—	BTL WE	
2K28	1.2-3.75	250	25	110	70	21	0.85	Raytheon	3500-
2K41	2.65-3.32	1000	50	380	450	6	0.04	Sperry	$V_G = +40$
2K39	7.5-10.3	1250	45	600	350	20	0.26	Sperry	
		700	19	40	70	6	0.6	—	
2K42	3.3-4.2	1250	45	<750	600	12	0.07	Sperry	

2K45	8.5–9.66	300	25	95–145	30	45	0.7	BTL, WE	Thermally tuned
2K33	23.6–24.4	1800	8	100	20	40	1.5	Raytheon	—
2K50	23.5–24.5	300	22	60–80	10	55	—	BTL, WE	Thermally tuned
2K48	3.0–5.0	1000	10	75–300	20	—	—	BTL	—
2K49	5.0–10.0	1250	12	50–350	10	—	—	Sperry	—
X–13	8.1–12.4	500	55	285–500	200	43		BTL	
V–58	8.5–10.0	500	60	20–1000	600	50		Sperry	
V153–6315	8.5–10.0	250	30	20–300	200	90		Varian	
V270/6312	8.5–10.0	300	25	85–500	60	30		Varian	
VA 92C	12.4–14.5	600	58	230	400	50		Varian	
VA 94	16.0–17.0	300	38	100–150	40	55		Varian	
VA 96B	22.0–25.0	750	32	125–225	40	120		Varian	
VA 98	23.6–24.4	375	32	20–500	45	80		Varian	
VA 97	34.0–35.6	400	35	75–170	16	60		Varian	
VA 97B	32.6–34.0							Varian	
35V11	32–37	2000	12	330	200	90	2.0	OK1	$E_c = -90$
50V10	46–54	2500	25	180	50	140	4.5	OK1	$E_c = -100$
70V11A	65–75	2700	25	205	125	165	5.5	OK1	$E_c = -125$
90V11	85–95	2500	20	155	60	300	20	OK1	$E_c = -125$
100V10A	95–105	2500	20	205	25	250	8	OK1	$E_c = -100$
120V10	107–122	2500	17	220	10	350	20	OK1	$E_c = -150$

[a] The reflector voltage is negative.
[b] E_c is the electrode control voltage.

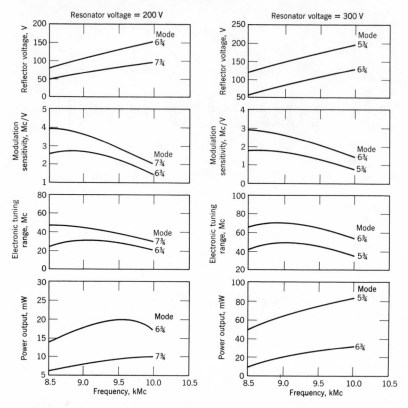

Gordy, Simmons, and Smith (1949); Gilliam, Johnson, and Gordy (1950)] employ a 1N26 silicon crystal multiplier driven by a QK–142 or QK–226 klystron for the 2–5 mm region, and they obtained usable power in the second, third, and fourth harmonics. These two klystrons supply 10 and 5 mW, respectively, and the power output from the frequency tripler was about 1 μW. Subsequently, King and Gordy (1953, 1954) [see also, Burrus and Gordy (1954, 1956)] employed pieces of silicon broken from commercial 1N26 crystals to produce frequencies in the range 1–2 mm. They emphasize the importance of obtaining a good contact point, and the fine tungsten wire or cat's whisker (0.005 cm diameter) may have its point sharpened by electrolytic etching [King and Gordy (1951); RLS–15]. In addition, a bias voltage of 3.5 V was found helpful. One should exercise care to avoid exposing the crystal contacts to high humidity.

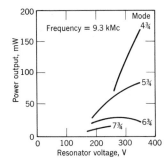
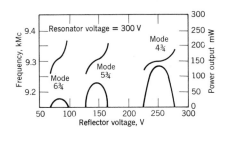

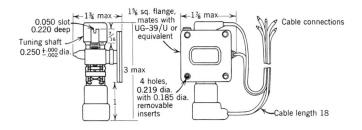

Fig. 6–11. Typical characteristic curves for Varian VA–6312 klystron. The dimensions are in inches (courtesy of Varian Associates, Palo Alto, California).

Johnson, Slager, and King (1954) give an excellent discussion of millimeter wave harmonic generators. Table 6–3 summarizes some of these data, Fig. 6–12 shows the details of their harmonic generator, and Fig. 6–13 gives the variation in harmonic output as a function of fundamental power. Trambarulo and Burrus (1960, 1961) achieved 103 Gc (λ = 2.9 mm) with a tunnel diode.

It should be possible to obtain 1 mW of power at the second harmonic when a K band fundamental frequency is used. From the third to the sixth harmonic the power output decreases by about a factor of 10 per harmonic, and for the next two harmonics a smaller decrease occurs. [(Townes and Schawlow (1955); see also, Nethercot, Klein, and Townes (1952)].

Millimeter microwaves may be generated by other means [(Townes and Schawlow (1953), Chap. 16; Deb and Daw (1959); Coleman

TABLE 6–3

Typical Values of Harmonic Signals Using a Silicon Crystal Multiplier[a] Driven by
a Reflex Klystron [Reproduced from Johnson, Slager, and King (1954)]

Driver klystron (Raytheon)	Measured power output, mW	Fundamental wavelength, mm	Harmonic number	Wavelength of harmonic, mm	Conversion loss, dB	Signal-to-noise ratio for weakest harmonic[b]
2K33A	35	12.5	2	6.25	18	
			3	4.17	35	
			4	3.12	45	
			5	2.50	60	350
QK290	35	9.5	2	4.75	20	
			3	3.17	40	
			4	2.38	55	
			5	1.90	70	30
QK291	12	8.5	2	4.25	21	
			3	2.83	40	
			4	2.12	60	100
QK294	3	7.5	2	3.75	33	
			3	2.5	45	900

[a] The multiplier crystal was operated open-circuited.

[b] This ratio was obtained using 1000-cps square-wave modulation on the klystron reflector, a silicon detector crystal, and a 15-cps band-width amplifier.

(1963); Sen (1964)] such as: (a) a spark or arc oscillator [Froome
(1960); Kneubühl, Moser, and Steffan (1964)]; (b) direct harmonic
output from klystrons, magnetrons, and traveling wave tubes
[Barchukov and Prokhindeev (1959)]; (c) hot bodies [Dicke (1946)];
(d) electron beams [Brannen, Froelich, and Stewart (1960); Froelich
and Brannen (1963); Coleman and Enderby (1960); Poynter and
Steffensen (1963)]; (e) masers [Foner, Momo, and Mayer (1959);
Gordy and Cowan (1960)]; (f) optical frequency mixing [Fontana and
Pantell (1962)]; (g) ferrites [Ayres, Vartanian, and Melchor (1956,
1957); Ayres (1959); Skomal and Medina (1959); Elliott, Schaug-
Pettersen, and Shaw (1960); Kumagi, Nakanishi, and Okamoto
(1960); Auld, Shaw, and Winslow (1961); Jepsen (1961); Auld
(1962); Risley, Deuthett, and Kaufman (1962); Zinchenko and

Zhigailo (1964)]; (h) parametric amplifiers [Deloach (1963)]; (i) tunnel diodes [Oguey (1963)]; (j) laddertrons [Fujisawa (1964)]; (k) cyclotron radiation [Bott (1965)]; (l) Cherenkov radiation [Coleman (1963); Sen (1964)]. Pierce (1950 and 1962) reviewed millimeter microwaves and summarized limits on the available output power from thermal sources, as shown on Fig. 6–14. This graph shows

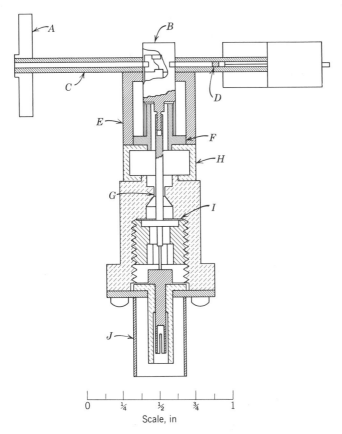

Scale, in

Fig. 6–12. Details of harmonic generator which utilizes cutout 1N26 or 1N31 crystals. (A) Coupling flange; (B) crystal cartridge; (C) waveguide with inner dimensions, 0.191 x 0.087 mm; (D) shorting plunger; (E) cylindrical housing; (F) crystal mount; (G) chokes; (H) K band waveguide with inner dimensions 1.07 x 0.43 mm; (I) mica washers; (J) BNC cable connector [Johnson, Slager, and King (1954)].

that at sufficiently low wavelengths, thermal sources become more efficient than tube sources. In 1954, the microwave spectroscopists, Burrus and Gordy (1954, 1956) detected several OCS rotational transitions between 0.77 and 1.0 mm, while Genzel and Eckhardt (1954) used a heat source and grating to detect a rotational transition of H_2S at wavelengths up to 0.99 mm. Thus the experimental techniques of the microwave and infrared spectral regions overlapped just below a wavelength of 1 mm. The microwave infrared gap has been discussed by Coleman (1962). Jones and Gordy (1964) recently extended high-resolution microwave spectroscopy to $\lambda = 0.43$ mm.

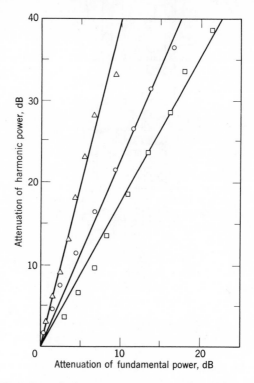

Fig. 6–13. Variation of the output power in the (□) second harmonic, (○) third harmonic, and (△) fourth harmonic of a silicon crystal with the incident fundamental power. The wavelength of the fundamental is 9.5 mm, and zero attentuation corresponds to an output power of 50 mW from the klystron [Johnson, Slager, and King (1954)].

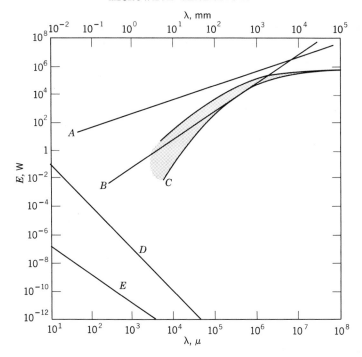

Fig. 6–14. Limits on the power available from several sources: (A) Conduction through a cube λ on a side, 1000°K temperature difference; (B) radiation from a square λ on a side, 1000°K; (C) (shaded) power from electron tubes; (D) radiation per cm,² 5000°K, 1% band; (E) radiation per cm², 5000°K, 1 Mc bandwidth [Pierce (1950)].

A millimeter ESR spectrometer is described by Elliston, Troup, and Hutton (1963), and a millimeter microwave spectrometer which uses a Fabry-Perot interferometer is discussed by Lichtenstein, Gallagher, and Cupp (1963). Mock (1960) used a backward wave oscillator and harmonic conversion as a microwave source for an ESR spectrometer which operates in the range from 50 to 150 Gc. A number of conferences have been devoted to millimetric microwaves [e.g., see Selected Bibliography and Brown (1963)].

G. Klystron Power Supplies

Power Supply Requirements: There are three basic power supplies required for a klystron: (1) the filament voltage V_f, (2) the beam (resonator) voltage V_B, and (3) the reflector voltage V_R. The functions of these power supplies are shown diagrammatically on Fig. 6–4. The filament voltage heats the cathode and causes it to emit electrons thermionically, the beam voltage accelerates the electrons, and the reflector voltage reverses their direction. The reflector voltage is by far the most critical of the three voltages, and requires the most stable source, while the filament supply is the least critical. Some klystrons also require an additional supply voltage for the focus grid.

The Filament Power Supply: The simplest way to obtain a constant filament voltage is to use a lead storage ("automobile") battery. This source of V_f is electrically more stable and ripple-free than most electronic sources of V_f now in use. The only liability is the necessity of periodically checking the level of the acid in the battery cells, and charging them perhaps once or twice a week. One hazardous aspect of using a storage battery arises when the resonant cavity grid (anode) is grounded and the cathode is operated at the potential $-V_B$. In this case it is necessary to connect one terminal of the battery to the cathode in order to avoid damaging the klystron. This means that the storage battery may be riding at a lethal voltage, and it should be kept in an insulated box made of wood or other insulating material. It would be a wise precaution to provide the cover of the box with an interlock which automatically turns off the klystron power supply when it is opened. A typical electronic filament power supply consists of a full-wave rectifier followed by a π filter. It is certainly not as ripple-free as a storage battery, but it does render satisfactory service. In general, increasing the filament voltage increases the klystron power output, but it also shortens the klystron's lifetime. It is best to employ the value of V_f that is recommended by the manufacturer. The fact that the output power increases with the filament voltage is merely mentioned in case one needs extra power and cannot obtain a more powerful klystron, since this is a convenient source of increased power. If the filament voltage is increased too much, one runs the risk of permanently damaging the klystron. Case and Larsen (1963) describe the circuit shown on Fig. 6–15 which protects a klystron against overvoltage and undervoltage on its filament. This circuit also provides thermal protection against failure of the klystron water cooling system.

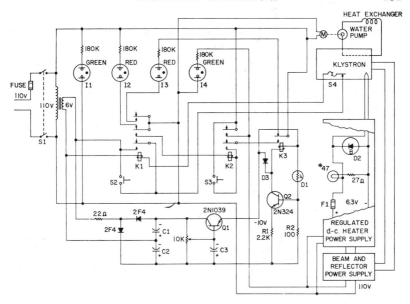

Fig. 6–15.   Circuit for protection of klystron from overheating and abnormal heater voltage.   (*11, 12, 13, 14*) NE51; (*K1*) 6 V, ac, 3PDT; (*K2*) 110 V, ac, DPDT; (*K3*) sensitive relay, 1000 Ω, 2.3 mA, SPDT; (*F1*); (*S2, S3*) momentary, normally off; (*S4*) thermostat, adjustable, opens on temperature rise; (*C1, C2, C3*) tantalum electrolytic 68 µf, 15 V; (*D1*) CdSe photoconductive cell, ¼-in. diameter, 160–K light resistance at 2-ft-C; (*D2*) Zener diode, 6.8 V, 10 W; (*D3*) IN270; (*M*) small ac motor [Case and Larsen (1963)].

The Beam Voltage Power Supply: It is desirable to have a beam or resonator voltage V_B with at most one or two millivolts of ripple. When the grid (anode) is grounded, V_B must be obtained from a negative power supply with the transistors or vacuum tubes operating "upside down," while when the cathode is grounded a standard or positive power supply may be employed.   One simple type of beam supply consists of several large B batteries connected in series.   This becomes inconvenient for use with klystrons that require 1 or 2 kV, but it is quite satisfactory for low-voltage klystrons like the older 2K25 and the newer V–153/6315 tubes.   A disadvantage of B batteries is the necessity of replacing them occasionally. Toward the end of their lifetime they tend to become noisy.   Nevertheless, they constitute a very simple way to set up a klystron beam voltage power supply if one is in a hurry to build a spectrometer.

Several examples of electronically regulated beam power supplies are shown in Figs. 6–16 and 6–17. The circuit on Fig. 6–16 was designed by Bennett (1947) and later was modified by Crable and Anderson. The 110-V input 60-cps voltage is increased to the kilovolt range by means of the transformer and rectified (full wave) by the bridge arrangement of four 1616 tubes. The π filter UTC-S-27 removes much of the ripple, and the regulator or pass tube 812 plus the dc amplifier 2C53 regulate the voltage output. The beam voltage output appears across the 120-kΩ resistor and two OD3 (VR 150) voltage regulator tubes in the upper righthand part of Fig. 6–16, with the anode grounded through the 0–25 mA meter. The magnitude of the beam voltage is set by the autotransformer, while the reflector and focus voltages are adjusted by 100-kΩ potentiometers. Further details on the principles behind the operation of stabilized power supplies are given in Sec. 9-F.

The power supply of Strandberg, Johnson, and Eshbach (SJE) (1954) shown in Fig. 6–17 is more sophisticated than the one previously described. It is capable of producing output voltages from 1.5 to 3.0 kV with less than 1 mV ripple, which is significantly below the ripple output of Bennett's circuit. In the same article, SJE give a similar circuit for producing a regulated output from 0.5 to 1.5 kV.

In the high-voltage SJE circuit the alternating current enters a full wave rectifier followed by a filter, and these are housed in a separate chassis. The output of the filter goes to the 807 regulator or pass tube. The dc amplifier consists of two stages of amplification. The voltage is varied by means of a Variac, and this is ganged to two steatite switches which adjust the tap point for the inverse feedback, and maintain a constant regulator tube current. Heavy rubber 5 kV test probe leads are required for all high-voltage wiring to prevent random spikes in the output voltage. The components of the regulator chassis are mounted on $\frac{1}{4}$-in. Micarta panel. The lower voltage range SJE power supply is similar to the one shown in Fig. 6–17 and so will not be discussed separately.

The klystron power output increases and the klystron lifetime decreases with an increase in beam voltage. In this respect the beam voltage behaves like the filament voltage, and again too high a value can damage the tube.

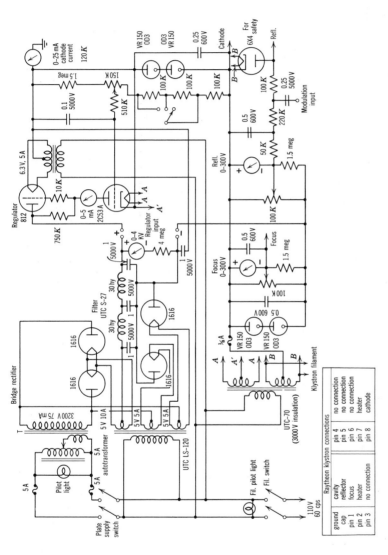

Fig. 6-16. Circuit of a klystron power supply [Gordy, Smith, and Trambarulo (1953), p. 54]. This circuit was designed by Bennett (1947) and later modified by G. F. Crable and R. S. Anderson.

The Reflector Voltage Power Supply: The reflector voltage may be obtained from B batteries, and these will have a long lifetime since the reflector does not draw current. Such a battery supply will be discussed in the next section. The reflector voltage in Bennett's circuit shown in Fig. 6–16 is provided by two OD3 (VR-150) tubes in series, and a 100 kΩ potentiometer is employed for altering this voltage. The 6X4 diode is a protective device because it will conduct and short-circuit the reflector to the cathode if the reflector begins drawing current. Provision is made for modulating the reflector.

Each of the SJE circuits provides an electronically regulated reflector voltage, and the principle of operation of these regulator circuits is the same as that of the corresponding beam voltage supplies. Again, provision is made for a sweep or modulation input. The high voltage SJE circuit is designed for two klystrons, and so has two separate reflector voltage outputs. This is convenient for use with a superheterodyne spectrometer which employs two klystrons.

Additional Voltage Supplies: Some of the older klystrons have focusing grids and require an additional voltage supply. The Bennett circuit on Fig. 6–16 provides for such a focus output voltage.

H. Frequency Stabilization of Klystrons

The principal function which an electron spin resonance spectrometer must perform is to measure accurately the ratio of the frequency to the magnetic field strength corresponding to a resonance absorption. To attain high precision in such a measurement, it is necessary to stabilize both the frequency and the magnetic field to a sufficient extent so that uncertainties in these two quantities are less than the desired uncertainty in the g factor determination. Regulated power supplies alone do not produce sufficient stability. This section will discuss how to stabilize the frequency, and Sec. 9–F will cover magnetic field stabilization. Most of the general stabilization techniques to be described may be used with several types of rf oscillators, but for simplicity only the klystron will be discussed.

The object of a frequency stabilizer is to respond to all frequency changes by a mechanism which returns the frequency to its initial value. For example, the klystron frequency may be compared to

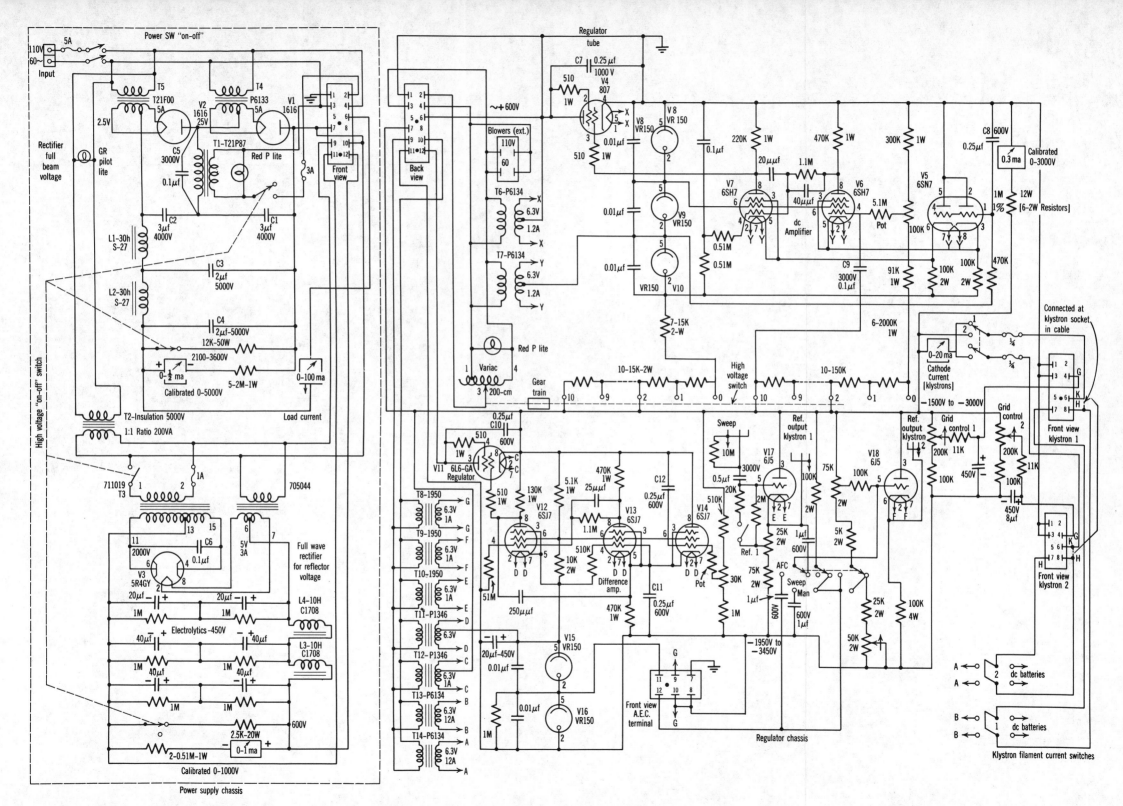

Fig. 6–17. 1.5 to 3.0–kV klystron power supply [Strandberg, Johnson, and Eshback (1954)].

the resonant frequency of a cavity, and when a change occurs in the klystron frequency a small error voltage may be produced which has a positive polarity for a frequency decrease, and a negative polarity for an increase (or vice versa). This error signal may be amplified and applied to the klystron reflector voltage supply in such a way as to bring the frequency back to its initial value. In the remainder of this section several practical ways of performing this stabilizing action will be described. It is difficult to stabilize a klystron to better than one part in 10^6.

The original articles on klystron stabilizers [Pound (1946, 1947); RLS–11, p. 58; Tuller, Galloway, and Zaffarano (1948)] presented the fundamental principals of stabilization, and Miessner (1949) and Dayhoff (1951) designed simplified stabilizers. More recent modifications are described by Zimmerer (1959), Bruin and van Ladesteyn (1959), Jung (1960), Smith (1960), Radford (1963), and Kester (1965). Khaikin (1961) stabilized a traveling wave tube in a lead superconducting cavity to one part in 10^9. Narath and Gwinn (1962) and Olivier (1962) describe klystron phase stabilization systems.

Pound Stabilizers: The Pound stabilizer [Pound (1946, 1947); RLS–11, p. 58] is designed to maintain the klystron at a minimum difference in frequency from a standard reference cavity. In addition, it removes the frequency deviations occurring at audiofrequencies and higher which are normally found in the output power of a microwave oscillator. The long-term stability of the stabilized oscillator is almost completely determined by the stability of the reference cavity. It is possible to increase long-term stability by employing cavities with temperature-compensated tuning mechanisms, or by making the cavity walls of Invar, or even of fused quartz lined with a metallic film.

A block diagram of an electronic frequency-stabilization system is shown in Fig. 6–18. The discriminator produces a signal which is a measure of the difference between the klystron and the cavity frequencies. This error voltage is amplified and applied to the klystron reflector to return its frequency to the proper value. To avoid "singing" around the amplifier loop, rigid requirements are imposed on the phase and amplitude characteristics of the amplifier. These requirements are discussed in the references cited above.

The operating principle of the stabilizer may be explained as follows. When the amplifier is disconnected from the klystron

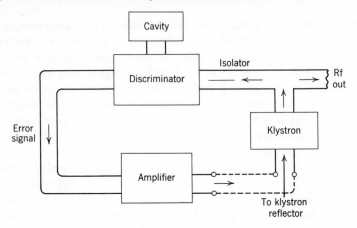

Fig. 6–18. Block diagram of electronic frequency stabilization system (RLS–11, p. 60).

(dotted lines on Fig. 6–17) let the klystron frequency deviate slightly by $\Delta\omega_0$, and when the error signal amplifier is reconnected this frequency shift will be reduced to $\Delta\omega_S$. The stabilization factor S is then defined by the ratio of the frequency shifts that occur during unstabilized and stabilized operation

$$S = \Delta\omega_0/\Delta\omega_S \qquad (1)$$

$$= 1 + AB \qquad (2)$$

where A is the change in the error signal amplifier output voltage per unit frequency change, and B is the klystron's electronic tuning rate (frequency change per unit reflector voltage change). A depends on the amplifier gain, the characteristics of the cavity and associated microwave circuit, and the microwave power, while B depends on the klystron, its effective load, and in particular, on the line length between the klystron and reference cavity. The best absolute stability results when this line length minimizes B at the resonant frequency since the cavity coupling and amplifier gain can be increased to give the maximum electronic stabilization factor compatible with the negative feedback stability condition.

There are two versions of the Pound stabilizer: the dc system and the i.f. system. Each will be discussed in turn.

The dc Pound Stabilizer: The dc Pound circuit is the microwave equivalent of the frequency discriminator employed at low frequencies. An example of a microwave discriminator is shown in Fig. 6–19, where the resonant cavity terminates a magic T arm (*2*) which is $1/8\lambda_g$ shorter than the short-circuited arm (*1*) opposite it. Far off resonance, the cavity acts as a short circuit and the reflected waves from arms 1 and 2 return to the T $\pi/2$ out of phase. As a result, they excite equal amplitude waves in the other two arms of the T. These waves induce the voltages V_A and V_B in the two crystals A and B, and these two voltages are subtracted to give a zero error voltage V_e, where

$$V_e = V_B - \tfrac{1}{2}V_A \tag{3}$$

At resonance, the reference cavity acts like a pure conductance and the error voltage is again zero, although V_A and V_B individually differ from their off-resonance values. At frequencies slightly removed from resonance, the cavity admittance contains an inductive or capacitive term so that the phase of the reflected wave from the cavity is advanced or retarded, and each detector receives a different signal. On one side of resonance, $\tfrac{1}{2}V_A > V_B$ and on the other side,

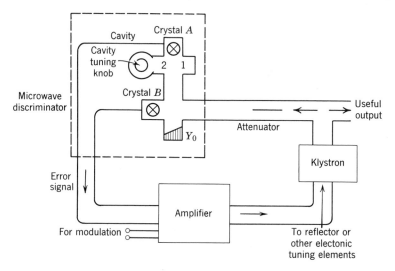

Fig. 6–19. Block diagram of a dc stabilizer (*RLS*–11, p. 68).

$\frac{1}{2}V_A < V_B$ so the error voltage has the frequency dependence shown schematically in Fig. 6–20, and more quantitatively in Fig. 6–21. In an alternative experimental setup the discriminator may be made with only one magic T, (see RLS–11, p. 63). The dc amplifier shown in RLS–11, p. 67 may be employed to amplify V_e. It consists of two direct coupled push-pull stages of amplification, with an overall gain of 600.

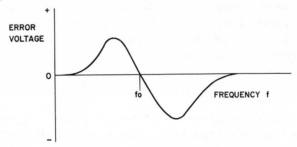

Fig. 6–20.   Discriminator output voltage or error voltage V_e as a function of the microwave frequency f incident on the discriminator.

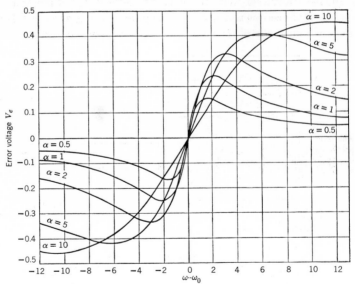

Fig. 6–21.   Discriminator output voltage V_e vs. deviation of frequency from reference value ω_o for various cavity-coupling factors α of a balanced magic T discriminator (RLS–11, p. 66).

The i.f. Pound Stabilizer: The i.f. Pound stabilizer was designed to circumvent the need for a dc amplifier, which is at best troublesome, and to eliminate the use of crystals as detectors since they have poor noise figures in this application. A block diagram of the i.f. system is shown in Fig. 6–22. The i.f. oscillator produces the modulation frequency ω_2 which supplies the reference signal for the lock-in mixer, and which also enters the waveguide at the modulator crystal B. The high Q cavity and magic T are matched in such a way that at resonance the microwaves ω_1 from the klystron impinge on the magic T and split equally between the cavity and mixer crystal arms of the T without entering the modulator crystal arm. As a result of the electrical match at resonance, the mixer crystal A receives no sidebands of the rf carrier frequency ω_1. When ω_1 deviates from the reference frequency ω_0, the cavity arm of the magic T reflects a signal which depends in sign on, and is proportional in amplitude to, the imaginary part of the cavity reflection coefficient Γ_C. Half of the signal reflected from the cavity enters the modulator crystal arm where it is mixed with the i.f. frequency to produce the two sideband frequencies $(\omega_1 \pm \omega_2)$ in addition to the fundamental ω_1. These three frequencies are then reflected to the mixer crystal A, which receives the voltage V_A

$$V_A = \frac{V_0}{2^{1/2}} \sin \omega_1 + \frac{V_e |\Gamma_C| m}{4 (2)^{1/2}} \left\{ \sin [(\omega_1 + \omega_2)t + \delta] \right.$$

$$\left. + \sin [(\omega_1 - \omega_2)t + \delta] \right\} \qquad (4)$$

where V_0 is the voltage incident on the T; m is the modulation coefficient; and δ is a phase factor which depends on the line lengths in the T, the phase characteristics of the T, and the phase of Γ_C.

The crystal output voltage V_e contains terms found in the envelope of the superposition of the incident waves, and this i.f. error voltage V_e is proportional to $|\Gamma_C| \cos \delta$ (see *RLS*–11, p. 70):

$$V_e \approx \frac{V_0 |\Gamma_C| m}{2 (2)^{1/2}} \cos \delta \cos \omega_2 t \qquad (5)$$

The product $|\Gamma_C| \cos \delta$ is the imaginary part of the cavity reflection coefficient, and as a result the form of eq. (4) is identical with the

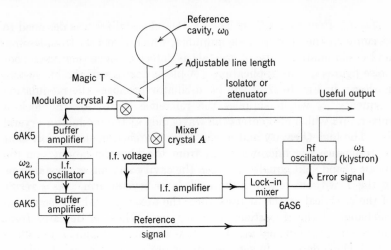

Fig. 6–22.　Block diagram of i.f. Pound stabilizer (*RLS*-11, p. 70).

output voltage of the dc discriminator shown in Figs. 6–20 and 6–21. The i.f. voltage is amplified and then compared to the i.f. reference signal in the lock-in mixer. Finally it arrives at the klystron to return its output to the desired frequency ω_0.

When $\omega_1 = \omega_0$ the i.f. voltage becomes zero since $\Gamma_C = 0$, while just off resonance this voltage differs from zero and has opposite phases on either side of resonance. The sense can be reversed by changing the cavity-to-T line-length by a quarter of a guide wavelength, since mathematically this changes δ by π radians. By this method the sign of the error voltage produced by the lock-in mixer can be adjusted to provide stabilization. If the phase is incorrect by π radians, antistabilization results. The electronic circuits which may be employed in the i.f. Pound stabilizer are shown in *RLS*–11, p. 74.

Frequency Modulation: Both types of Pound stabilizers may be adapted to allow for frequency modulation of the output power.

The Reflector Modulation Stabilizer: A simpler automatic frequency control system than the Pound stabilizer puts a modulation (~ 10 kc) on the klystron reflector which substitutes for the i.f. frequency in the i.f. Pound stabilizer. The block diagram of such a stabilizer which employs batteries for the reflector voltage is shown in Fig. 6–23. The oscillator modulates the klystron output by impressing a 13-kc voltage on the reflector, and it also provides the reference signal on the grid of the 6AS6 mixer tube. The error signal is detected at the crystal detector, amplified, and impressed on the control grid of the mixer tube. This error signal interacts with the reference signal in such a way as to change the amount of plate current i_p through the tube. The voltage drop across the resistor R is $i_p R$, and it is in series with the reflector batteries so it provides part of the total reflector voltage. The error signal changes this voltage drop in such a way as to counteract a frequency deviation and return the klystron to its proper frequency. Thus the electronics of the reflector modulation stabilizer are similar to those of the i.f. Pound stabilizer, with the principal differences being (1) the manner in which the i.f. frequency acquires the error signal information, and (2) the actual frequency employed for the error signal. Details of the electronic circuits incorporated in the reflector modulation stabilizer are shown in Figs. 6–24 through 6–26. In many ways they resemble the i.f. stabilizer circuitry, and so will not be discussed further.

The mechanism whereby the error signal is produced is shown in Fig. 6–27 where the U-shaped part of the diagram is a spread-out picture of the bottom of the cavity pip shown in Fig. 6–28c. On

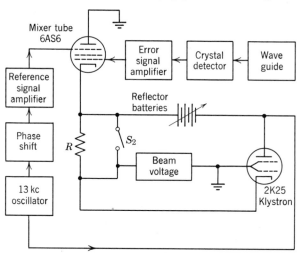

Fig. 6–23. Block diagram of klystron stabilizer [Poole (1958)].

resonance, the 13-kc reflector modulation signal produces a 26-kc output, and close to resonance, one obtains a 13-kc output plus a 26-kc signal with the 13-kc component having the opposite phase on the two sides of resonance, as indicated by Fig. 6–27b and Fig. 6–27d. The greater the deviation from resonance, the larger the amplitude of the 13-kc error signal. The phase of the reference signal can be adjusted by the phase reversal switch and phase shifting 100kΩ potentiometer between the two stages of reference signal amplification on Fig. 6–25. The RLC tuned circuit which constitutes the load of the preamplifier of Fig. 6–26 is designed to reject the 26-kc component of the error signal. As a result, the 13-kc error signal mixes with the 13-kc reference signal in the 6AS6 mixer, and a properly adjusted phase shift results in frequency stabilization.

Jung (1960) has described the fully transistorized klystron stabilizer shown in Figs. 6–29, 6–30, and 6–31. It is the reflector type and uses a 50–kc reflector modulation. The system employs a dc gain of

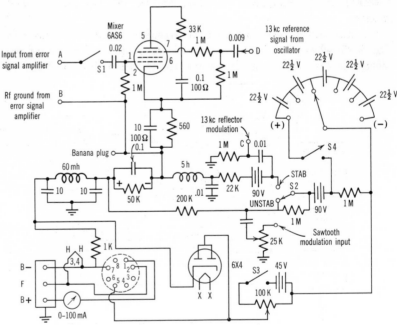

Fig. 6–24. Klystron stabilizer. The capacitors are in microfarads, and the approximate capacitive reactance at 13 kc is given for several of them [Poole (1958)].

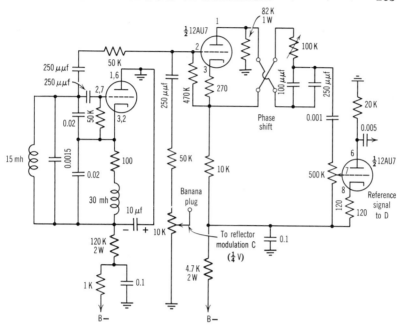

Fig. 6–25. Oscillator for klystron stabilizer. Capacitors are in μf [Poole (1958)].

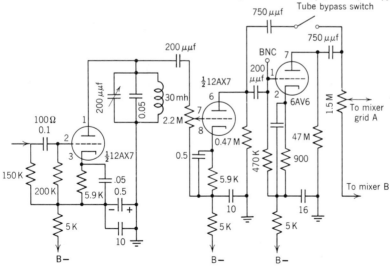

Fig. 6–26. Error signal amplifier for klystron stabilizer. The capacitors are in microfarads [Poole (1958)].

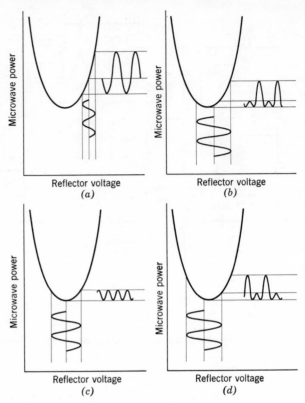

Fig. 6-27.   Error signal klystron stabilizer in the neighborhood of resonance: (a) far off resonance $(f \gg f_0)$; (b) close to resonance $(f > f_0)$; (c) on resonance $(f = f_0)$; (d) close to resonance $(f < f_0)$ [Poole (1958)].

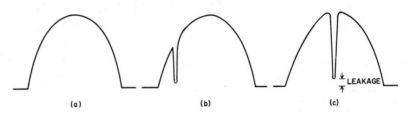

Fig. 6-28.   Klystron mode (a) far removed from cavity frequency, (b) with cavity frequency on side of mode, and (c) with cavity frequency centered on mode. The ordinate is klystron power and the abscissa is reflector voltage.

1000, and a 50 cps band-width. The circuits of Fig. 6–30 may be operated with either a B battery supply, or the electronic supply shown in Fig. 6–31. The latter delivers 20 mA with a ripple of 2.5 mV.

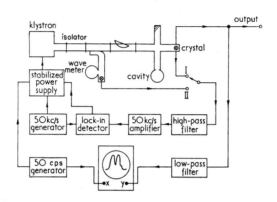

Fig. 6–29. Block diagram of 50-kc reflector modulation stabilizer [Jung (1960)].

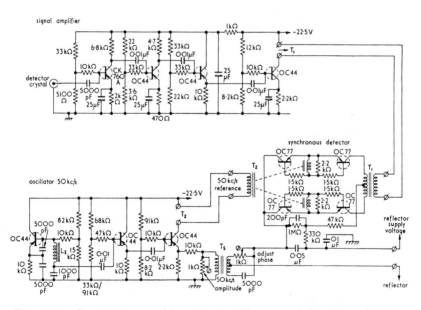

Fig. 6–30. Circuit diagram of transistorized klystron stabilizer [Jung (1960)].

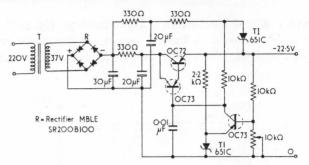

Fig. 6-31. Circuit diagram of stabilized power supply [Jung (1960)].

The Pound stabilizer is intrinsically superior to the reflector type because it puts out one frequency rather than a frequency band. However, the Pound systems are much more difficult to build and put in operation than the reflector modulation system.

Miscellaneous Types of Stabilizers: Sirkis and Coleman (1954) describe a frequency stabilizer which employs a reference cavity, a slotted line, and a Tektronix Model 512 oscilloscope. It contains a discriminator with two detecting probes [Pircher (1951)] located on a transmission line which is terminated by a high Q reference cavity. The direct coupled difference amplifier of the oscilloscope is employed to amplify the discriminator output. The original article should be consulted for further details. Dušek (1961) describes an AFC system for use with ferromagnetic samples which absorb strongly at resonance. Hervé, Pescia, and Sauzade (1959) and Sauzade (1961) present a stabilizer for a high power carcinotron.

Redhardt (1961) reduced the effect of klystron noise with the ESR cavity and a second nearly equivalent cavity both coupled to a microwave bridge. He showed both mathematically and experimentally that the system will tolerate fluctuations in the source frequency up to 10^3–10^4 times as high as in the single cavity case before producing a noticeable change in the wave reflected from the ESR cavity. By means of this method, it is possible to compensate for frequency fluctuations greater than the width of the resonator response. Mehlkopf and Smidt (1961) describe a similar system.

Peter and Strandberg (1958) describe a phase stabilizer which can lock the klystron to a high harmonic of a quartz-controlled oscillator. Phase stabilization is capable of producing a more monochromatic output than other stabilizing schemes discussed above.

Waring (1963) designed the simple automatic frequency control shown on Fig. 6–32. The frequency of the TE_{011} mode cylindrical reference cavity is modulated by an alternating electric current which passes along a wire located in the cavity. The cavity is placed in a 1000-G magnetron magnet which produces vibrations in the wire, thereby modulating its resonant frequency. This produces an error signal which provides the automatic frequency control. The correction circuit shown in Fig. 6–33 employs a balanced version

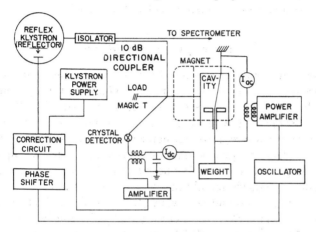

Fig. 6–32. Frequency stabilizer using a frequency modulated reference cavity [Waring (1963)].

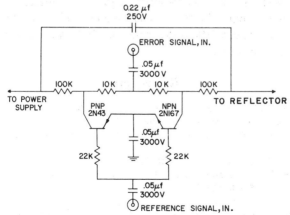

Fig. 6–33. Correction circuit for AFC system [Waring (1963)].

of the phase-sensitive detector described by Bennett, Hoell, and Schwenker (1958). This AFC system is useful for dispersion mode studies because it does not use a frequency modulated source of microwaves. Several recent articles [Gambling and Wilmshurst (1961); Bouthinon and Coumes (1964); Owston (1964); Berry and Benton (1965)] describe klystron stabilizers. Payne (1964) designed an "electron oscillator" ESR spectrometer which achieves high sensitivity without a frequency stabilizer [see also, Price and Anderson (1957) and Sloan, Ganssen, and LaVier (1964)].

I. Frequency Standards

A cavity wavemeter is ordinarily employed for measuring a microwave frequency to about one part in 20,000, but Bussey and Estin (1960) have reported a precision of one or two parts in 10^6 [see also, van den Bosch and Bruin (1953)]. If the microwave frequency is mixed with the appropriate harmonic of a crystal oscillator, the beat or intermediate frequency may be measured. This is capable of determining the microwave frequency to within one part per million. Frequency standards for obtaining considerably more accuracy are reviewed by Townes and Schawlow (1955) in Chap. 17 of their book. Rogers, Cox, and Braunschweiger (1950), Takahashi, Okaya, and Ogawa (1952), Hedrick (1953), and Beers (1959) have presented detailed treatments of frequency standards. Essen and Parry (1959) describe an X band cesium frequency standard with a precision of a few parts in 10^{11}. Wertheimer, Bellet, Caille, Carlier, Messelyn, and Specq (1963) describe a 5-Mc frequency standard for microwave spectroscopy.

References

M. Anderegg, P. Cornaz, and J. P. Borel, *J. Angew. Math. Phys.*, **14**, 201 (1963).

B. A. Auld, *J. Appl. Phys.*, **33**, 112 (1962).

B. A. Auld, H. J. Shaw, and D. K. Winslow, *J. Appl. Phys. Suppl.*, **32**, 317S (1961).

W. P. Ayres, *Trans. IRE, MTT-7*, **1959**, 62.

W. P. Ayres, P. H. Vartanian, and J. L. Melchor, *J. Appl. Phys.*, **27**, 188 (1956); *Proc. IRE*, **45**, 643 (1957).

V. Baláš, *Cesk. Casopis Fys. A*, **15**, 203 (1965).

A. I. Barchukov and A. V. Prokhindeev, *Radiotekhn. i Elektron.*, **4**, 1173 (1959).

Y. Beers, *RSI*, **30**, 9 (1959).

R. G. Bennett, P. C. Hoell, and R. P. Schwenker, *RSI*, **29**, 659 (1958).

W. S. Bennett, Master's Thesis, Duke University, 1947.

J. E. Berry, Jr. and A. Benton, *RSI*, **36**, 958 (1965).

I. B. Bott, *Phys. Letters*, **14**, 293 (1965).

M. Bouthinon and A. Coumes, *J. Phys. Suppl.*, **25**, 41A (1964).

E. Brannen, H. Froelich, and T. W. W. Stewart, *J. Appl. Phys.*, **31**, 1829 (1960).

M. R. Brown, *Nature*, **200**, 1270 (1963).

F. Bruin and D. van Ladesteyn, *Physica*, **25**, 1 (1959).

C. A. Burrus, Jr., *IEEE Trans. MTT-11*, **1963**, 357.

C. A. Burrus and W. Gordy, *Phys. Rev.*, **93**, 896 (1954); **101**, 599 (1956).

H. E. Bussey and A. J. Estin, *RSI*, **31**, 410 (1960).

W. E. Case and N. T. Larsen, *RSI*, **34**, 809 (1963).

P. D. Coleman, *Proc. IRE*, **50**, 1219 (1962); *IEEE Trans.*, *MTT-11*, 271 (1963).

P. D. Coleman and C. Enderby, *J. Appl. Phys.*, **31**, 1695 (1960).

Q. V. Davis, J. L. Clarke, and R. G. T. Morris, *RSI*, **35**, 561 (1964).

E. S. Dayhoff, *RSI*, **22**, 1025 (1951).

S. Deb and A. N. Daw, *J. Sci. Instr. Res.*, **18A**, 510 (1959).

B. C. Deloach, *Proc. IEEE*, **51**, 1153 (1963).

R. H. Dicke, *RSI*, **17**, 268 (1946).

H. Dreizler, W. Maier, and H. D. Rudolph, *Arch. Sci.*, **13**, 137 (1960).

H. O. Dressel, S. M. Stone, and G. E. Weibel, *Fourth International Congress, Microwave Tubes*, Schereningen, Holland, Sept. 1962.

J. Dušek, *Czech. J. Phys.*, **B11**, 528 (1961).

B. J. Elliott, T. Schaug-Pettersen, and H. J. Shaw, *J. Appl. Phys.*, *Suppl.*, **31**, 400S (1960).

P. R. Elliston, G. J. Troup, and D. R. Hutton, *JSI*, **40**, 586 (1963).

L. Essen and J. V. L. Parry, *Nature*, **184**, 1791 (1959).

S. Foner, L. R. Momo, and A. Mayer, *Phys. Rev. Letters*, **3**, 36 (1959).

J. R. Fontana and R. H. Pantell, *Proc. IRE*, **50**, 1796 (1962).

H. Froelich and E. Brannen, *IRE Trans.*, *MTT-11*, 288 (1963).

K. D. Froome, *Nature*, **184**, 808 (1959); **188**, 43 (1960).

K. Fujisawa, *IEEE Trans. Electron Devices*, *ED-11*, **1964**, 381.

W. A. Gambling and T. H. Wilmshurst, *JSI*, **38**, 334 (1961).

L. Genzel and W. Eckhardt, *Z. Phys.*, **139**, 592 (1954).

O. R. Gilliam, C. M. Johnson, and W. Gordy, *Phys. Rev.*, **78**, 140 (1950).

E. L. Ginzton, *Microwave Measurements*, McGraw-Hill, N. Y., 1957.

J. F. Gittins, *Power Travelling Wave Tubes*, American Elsevier, N. Y., 1965.

W. Gordy, *Rev. Mod. Phys.*, **20**, 668 (1948).

W. Gordy and M. Cowan, *J. Appl. Phys.*, **31**, 941 (1960).

W. Gordy, W. V. Smith, and R. F. Trambarulo, *Microwave Spectroscopy*, Wiley, N. Y., 1953.

A. G. Gurevich, *Proc. Intern. Conf. on Magnetism*, London, 1965, p. 615.

A. E. Harrison, *Klystron Tubes*, McGraw-Hill, N. Y. 1947.

L. C. Hedrick, *RSI*, **24**, 565 (1953).

J. Hervé, J. Pescia, and M. Sauzade, *C. R. Acad. Sci.*, **249**, 1486 (1959).

G. Hok, *Proc. IRE*, **44**, 1061 (1956).

R. L. Jepsen, *J. Appl. Phys.*, **32**, 2627 (1961).

C. M. Johnson, D. M. Slager, and D. D. King, *RSI*, **25**, 213 (1954).

G. Jones and W. Gordy, *Phys. Rev.*, **135**, A295 (1964).

P. Jung, *JSI*, **37**, 372 (1960).

T. Kester, *JSI*, **42**, 442 (1965).

W. C. King and W. Gordy, *Phys. Rev.*, **90**, 319 (1953); **93**, 407 (1954).

M. S. Khaikin, *PTE*, **3**, 103 (1961).

F. K. Kneubühl, J. F. Moser, and H. Steffen, *Helv. Phys. Acta*, **37**, 596 (1964).

B. V. Kondrat'ev, *Ukr. Fiz. Zh.*, **8**, 1203 (1963).

S. Kumagi, Y. Nakanishi, and N. Okamoto, *Tech. Rept. Osaka Univ.*, **10**, 69 (1960).

M. Lichtenstein, J. J. Gallagher, and R. E. Cupp, *RSI*, **34**, 843 (1963).

A. F. Mehlkopf and J. Smidt, *RSI*, **32**, 1421 (1961).

B. F. Miessner, *Proc. IRE*, **37**, 1445 (1949).

J. B. Mock, *RSI*, **31**, 551 (1960).

K. Mouthaan, *Intern. J. Electron.*, **18**, 301 (1965).

A. Narath and W. D. Gwinn, *RSI*, **33**, 79 (1962).

A. H. Nethercot, J. A. Klein, and C. H. Townes, *Phys. Rev.*, **86**, 789 (1952).

J. Ober, *Philips Res. Rept.*, **20**, 357 (1965).

H. J. Oguey, *IEEE Trans. Microwave Theory Tech.*, *MTT-11*, **1963**, 412.

M. Olivier, *J. Phys. Radium*, **23**, 144A (1962).

C. N. Owston, *JSI*, **41**, 698 (1964).

J. B. Payne, *IEEE Trans. Microwave Theory Tech.*, *MTT-12*, **1964**, 48.

M. Peter and M. W. P. Strandberg, *Proc. IRE*, **43**, 869 (1958).

J. R. Pierce, *Traveling Wave Tubes*, Van Nostrand, N. Y., 1950; *Physics Today*, **3**, 24 (1950); *Proc. IRE*, **50**, 978 (1962).

G. Pircher, *Onde Élect.*, **31**, 144 (1951).

C. P. Poole, Jr., Ph.D. Thesis, Department of Physics, University of Maryland, 1958.

R. V. Pound, *RSI*, **17**, 490 (1946); *Proc. IRE*, **35**, 1405 (1947); *RLS*-11, pp. 58–78.

R. L. Poynter and G. R. Steffensen, *RSI*, **34**, 77 (1963).

V. G. Price and C. T. Anderson, *IRE Nat. Conv. Record, Part 3*, **5**, 57 (1957).

H. E. Radford, *RSI*, **34**, 304 (1963).

A. Redhardt, *Z. Angew. Phys.*, **13**, 108 (1961).

J. F. Reintjes and G. T. Coate, Eds., *Principles of Radar*, McGraw-Hill, N. Y., 1952.

A. S. Risley and I. Kaufman, *J. Appl. Phys. Suppl.*, **33**, 1269 (1962); D. D. Douthett, I. Kaufman, and A. S. Risley, *J. Appl. Phys.*, **33**, 1395 (1962).

RLS-6.

RLS-7.

RLS-11.

RLS-15.

G. P. Rodrigue, *IEEE Trans. Microwave Theory Tech.*, *MTT-11*, **1963**, 351.

J. R. Rogers, H. L. Cox, and P. G. Braunschweiger, *RSI*, **21**, 1014 (1950).

S. W. Rubin, *PRD Rept.*, **4**, No. 3, October 1955.

M. Sauzade, *Ann. Phys. (France)*, **6**, 595 (1961).

S. N. Sen, *J. Sci. Ind. Res.*, **23**, 416 (1964).

M. D. Sirkis and P. D. Coleman, *RSI*, **25**, 401 (1954).

E. N. Skomal and M. A. Medina, *J. Appl. Phys. Suppl.*, **30**, 161S (1959).

E. L. Sloan, III, A. Ganssen, and E. C. LaVier, *Appl. Phys. Letters*, **4**, 109 (1964).

A. G. Smith, W. Gordy, J. A. Simmons, and W. V. Smith, *Phys. Rev.*, **75**, 260 (1949).

M. I. A. Smith, *JSI*, **37**, 398 (1960).

M. W. P. Strandberg, H. R. Johnson, and J. R. Eshbach, *RSI*, **25**, 776 (1954).

A. D. Sushkov and V. A. Meos, *Zh. Tekh. Fiz.*, **35**, 723 (1965).

I. Takahashi, A. Okaya and T. Ogawa, *J. Inst. Commun. Engrs. Japan*, **35**, 462 (1952).

C. H. Townes and A. L. Schawlow, *Microwave Spectroscopy*, McGraw-Hill, N. Y., 1955.

R. Trambarulo and C. A. Burrus, *Proc. IRE* (*Corresp.*), **48**, 1776 (1960; **49**, 1075 (1961).

W. G. Tuller, W. C. Galloway, and F. P. Zaffarano, *Proc. IRE*, **36**, 794 (1948).

T. Uchida and M. Buyle-Bodin, *Ampére Colloquium*, Eindhoven, 1962, p. 726.

J. C. van den Bosch and F. Bruin, *Physica*, **19**, 705 (1953).

C. W. van Es, M. Gevers, and F. C. de Ronde, *Philips Tech. Rev.*, **22**, 113, 181 (1960–61).

B. B. van Iperen and W. Kuypers, *Philips Res. Rept.*, **20**, 462 (1965).

R. K. Waring, Jr., *RSI*, **34**, 1228 (1963).

R. H. Webb, *RSI*, **33**, 732 (1962).

R. Wertheimer, J. Bellet, F. Caille, J. Carlier, J. Messelyn and A. Specq, *J. Phys.* (*France*) *Suppl.*, **24**, 3, 9A (1963).

W. E. Willshaw, *Nachrichtentech.* (*NTF*), **22**, 6 (1961).

J. H. Wilmshurst, W. A. Gambling, and D. J. E. Ingram, *J. Electron. Control*, **13**, 339 (1962).

R. W. Zimmerer, *RSI*, **30**, 1052 (1959); **33**, 858 (1962).

N. S. Zinchenko and B. A. Zhigailo, *Zh. Tekh. Fiz.*, **34**, 164, (130) (1964).

CHAPTER 7

Waveguide Components

A. Spectrometer Waveguide Components

The block diagram of a typical unsophisticated electron spin resonance spectrometer is shown in Fig. 7-1. The waveguide components may be considered as bounded by the klystron, resonant cavity, and two crystals. They are connected to the electronic circuits by means of the cable from the klystron stabilizer-power supply, and through the two coaxial (or parallel wire) cables from the crystals. The magnet system is not connected to the waveguide, but modulation coils often are mounted on the cavity.

The purpose of the present chapter is to describe the operating principles and practical application of the various waveguide components that one customarily incorporates into ESR spectrometers. An attempt will be made to provide enough information to assist in the design of new equipment, and in the assembly of novel spectrometer arrangements. No mention will be made of those waveguide components such as *TR* (transmit-receive) or *ATR* (anti-transmit-receive) tubes which are widely used in radar (cf. *RLS*-14), but are almost never used in ESR spectrometers.

Much of the information contained in this chapter may be found in Volumes 8, 9, 10, 11, and 14 of the *MIT Radiation Laboratory Series* (*RLS*). A number of more recent developments, such as isolators and circulators, will also be described. General background material may be found in Southworth (1962); van Es, Gevers, and de Ronde (1960–61); and Wheeler (1962).

B. Attenuators

An attenuator is a circuit element which, when inserted between a generator and a load, reduces the amplitude and changes the phase of the radio frequency signal incident on the load. [Fulford and Blackwell (1956)]. Usually the phase change is disregarded.

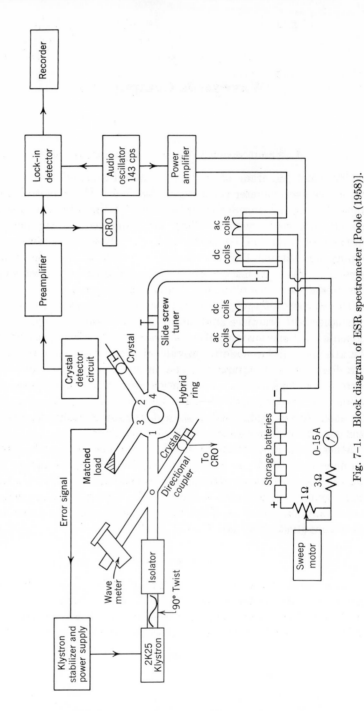

Fig. 7–1. Block diagram of ESR spectrometer [Poole (1958)].

Definitions: The insertion loss L is defined in terms of the power P_1 delivered by a generator of arbitrary internal impedance to an arbitrary load divided by the power P_2 delivered by the same generator to the same load when an attenuator or other microwave network is inserted between them in the transmission line:

$$L = 10 \log_{10} (P_1/P_2) \text{ dB} \tag{1}$$

The insertion loss is not an intrinsic property of the attenuator, but depends on the generator and load impedances. The attenuation α

$$\alpha = 10 \log_{10} (P_1/P_2) \text{ dB} \tag{2}$$

is the insertion loss measured when both the generator and load ends of the transmission line are terminated in matched impedances. Under these conditions P_1 is the maximum available power from the generator and P_2 is the power delivered through the attenuator to a matched load.

A reflective attenuator is one which produces attenuation without internal dissipation of power. For example, a dissipationless metallic obstruction in a transmission line will change the power delivered from a generator to a load. If the generator or load is not matched, the change could be either an increase or a decrease in the power delivered to the load. Thus the insertion loss can either be positive or negative. However, reflective attenuation α_r can only be positive because under matched conditions such a metallic obstruction can only set up a reflected wave and thereby reduce the power transmitted to a load. A section of waveguide beyond cutoff is a commonly used reflective attenuator. Many attenuators are unsymmetrical, i.e., have different input and output impedances, and as a result they are partly dissipative and partly reflective.

The dissipative attenuation α_d is defined in terms of Fig. 7-2 by

$$\alpha_d = 10 \log_{10} \left[\frac{Re(V_1 I_1^*)}{Re(V_2 I_2^*)} \right] \text{ dB} \tag{3}$$

The difference between the total attenuation α, the dissipative attenuation α_d, and the reflective attenuation α_r is illustrated by the

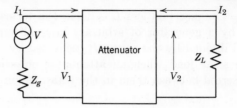

Fig. 7–2. Two-terminal pair attenuator activated by the voltage generator V with internal impedance Z_g and terminated by the load Z_L (RLS-11, p. 681).

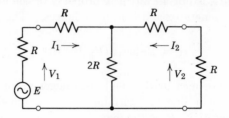

Fig. 7–3. The T network equivalent circuit for a particular attenuator (RLS-11, p. 681).

T network attenuator in Fig. 7–3. The input power to the attenuator is $2E^2/9R$ and the output power is $E^2/36R$. Therefore

$$\alpha_d = 10 \log_{10} 8 = 9.03 \text{ dB} \tag{4}$$

and since the output power in the absence of the attenuator is $E^2/4R$ one obtains

$$\alpha = 10 \log_{10} 9 = 9.54 \text{ dB} \tag{5}$$

Finally the resistive attenuation α_r is

$$\alpha_r = 0.51 \text{ dB} \tag{6}$$

The attenuation α should not be confused with the attenuation constant α. The latter is the dissipative part of the propagation constant γ

$$\gamma = \alpha + j\beta \tag{7}$$

which measures the amplitude $e^{-\gamma z}$ along the z direction in a transmission line.

Design Considerations: A calibrated attenuator is one which has a dial and can be set for a predetermined attenuation constant α. Most attenuators are designed to be broadband devices, and they are rated in terms of the maximum voltage standing wave ratio (VSWR) which they produce when inserted in a matched line at any frequency within the predetermined frequency band. An attenuator frequently possesses a maximum power capacity, and it may be burned out if this input power is exceeded. The attenuator calibration curve (dB versus displacement) is ordinarily furnished by the manufacturer.

Resistive Attenuators: Almost all commercial broadband attenuators or pads are of the resistive type. A simple type of fixed coaxial line attenuator has its inner conductor fabricated from high resistance wire or coated with Aquadag. This is a colloidal suspension of fine carbon powders which may be painted on the inner conductor and dried in a baking oven at 100°C. Theoretically, the attenuation constant α of a coaxial cable should have the form

$$\alpha = p/\lambda^{1/2} + q/\lambda \tag{8}$$

where p takes into account the conductor losses and q arises from the dielectric losses. The values of p and q for two typical coaxial cables are given in Table 7–1.

A simple waveguide antenna may be constructed from an IRC resistance card, which is a phenol fiber 0.08 cm thick on which is sprayed a mixture of graphite and a binder. The latter volatilizes at about 100°C, and leaves a carbon coating which absorbs microwave power. These resistance cards are discussed in Sec. 7-I. Uskon cloth and Polyiron may also be employed as attenuating materials.

TABLE 7–1

Coaxial Cable Attenuation as Function of Wavelength (RLS-11, p. 744)

Kind of cable	Type	$\lambda =$ 10 cm	$\lambda =$ 3.30 cm	p	q
Low-loss cable	RG-9/U	0.16	0.326	0.392	0.360
High-loss cable	RG-21/U	0.83	1.60	2.40	0.81

Measured attenuation in dB/ft — Coefficients of eq. (8)

A waveguide flap attenuator is shown in Fig. 7–4. It consists of a single strip of 200 Ω/square IRC resistance card cut in a circle to minimize the VSWR. The design in Fig. 7–4 provides 10–15 dB at X band. For greater rigidity, two 200 Ω/square resistance cards may be glued back to back, and this results in a combined film resistivity of 100 Ω/square, and greater attenuation. The resistance card is inserted into the broad side of the waveguide so that the **E** vector will be parallel to the card. One liability of the flap attenuator is that the calibration curve of dB/insertion is very nonlinear. The rotating spiral attenuator described on RLS-11, p. 749, has a linear calibration curve.

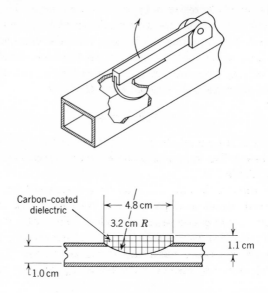

Fig. 7–4.   Variable waveguide attenuator of the flap type.

Another attenuator which is easy to build is the vane type shown in Fig. 7–5. The attenuation is small when the vane is at the waveguide edge because the E field is very small there, and it is a maximum in the center of the waveguide where the E field reaches a maximum. Metalized plate attenuators are made from dielectrics coated with metal films that are thin relative to the skin depth δ (cf. p. 73).

$$\delta = (2/\omega\sigma\mu)^{1/2} \tag{9}$$

as discussed in *RLS*-11, p. 751.   Design specifications and calibration curves for several types of attenuators are found in *RLS*-11, Chap. 12.

Decoupling Attenuators: It used to be customary to employ 10 dB of attenuation between the klystron and the remainder of the transmission line in order to prevent the waveguide system from "pulling" or interacting with the klystron, and affecting its power and frequency output.   The isolator to be described next has almost uni-

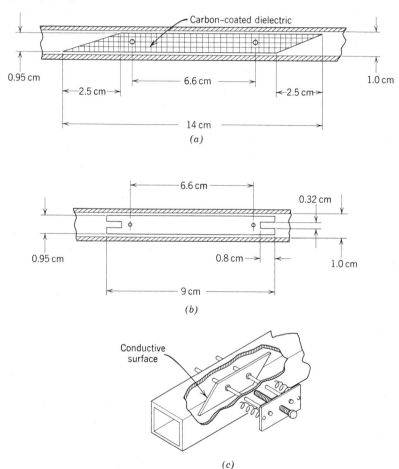

Fig. 7-5.   Variable waveguide attenuator of the vane type: (*a*) tapered vane; (*b*) notched vane; (*c*) perspective of assembly (*RLS*-11, p. 750).

versally replaced the attenuator in this function. This means that it is no longer necessary to waste 90% or more of the microwave power in order to match the microwave generator to the transmission line.

C. Isolators

An isolator or gyrator is a two-terminal pair microwave ferrite device which makes use of the Faraday effect to permit the transmission of microwaves in one direction, and prevents their transmission in the opposite direction [Hogan (1952); Rowen (1953)]. Ferrites are magnetic materials with resistivities from 10^6 to 10^{13} times that of iron [Owens (1956)]. As a result, no skin depth difficulties hinder the propagation of microwaves through them. The ferrite is placed in a circular waveguide, and the electron spins in the ferrite are aligned by a magnetic field directed along the microwave axis of propagation. As the microwaves propagate through the ferrite they interact with the spins, and the result of this interaction is that the plane of polarization of the microwaves is rotated. Another way of viewing this rotation is to consider the incident linearly polarized wave as resolved into a positive and a negative circularly polarized component. These two circular components travel at different velocities in the ferrite, and on emerging they unite to form a plane wave that is polarized in a different direction from the incident wave.

The most significant feature of this Faraday rotation is its antireciprocal character. Assume that a microwave plane wave traverses an isolator, and has its plane of polarization rotated by the angle θ. If it is reflected and traverses the isolator in the opposite direction, its plane of polarization will be rotated by another angle θ for a total rotation of 2θ. If the isolator obeyed the reciprocity theorem the rotation of the returning wave would cancel that of the incident one, instead of adding to it.

Two examples of isolators are shown in Fig. 7–6. The input and output waveguides on the right are oriented at angles of 45° with respect to each other, and they are separated by a circular waveguide containing the ferrite. The longitudinal magnetic field is adjusted to the value that rotates the microwave plane of polarization by 45° so that in one direction the output wave is polarized properly relative to the waveguide, while in the other direction, it is 90° out of phase with the waveguide, and cannot propagate. The resistor cards help to match the ferrite by reducing reflections. A waveguide twist may be employed to rotate one of the waveguides back so it is parallel to the other, since it is convenient to be able to insert the isolator in a transmission line without having to rotate the source waveguide components relative to the remainder of the waveguide system. Another method is to orient the two rectangular waveguide terminals of the isolator at $\pm 22.5°$, respectively, relative to the waveguide transmission line into which it is inserted. In this case the H field from the source waveguide will be reduced to $H \cos (\pi/8)$ or $0.924H$ when it enters the isolator waveguide input, and after undergoing the Faraday rotation the H field will be farther reduced to $H (\cos \pi/8)^2$ or $0.854H$ when it leaves the isolator.

The amount of attenuation provided by the isolator in the backward direction is varied by changing the strength of the longitudinal magnetic field. The magnetic field may be produced by a coil and supplied by a storage battery in series with a potentiometer that varies the magnetic field strength. There is a very nonlinear relation between the strength of the magnetic field and the current in the

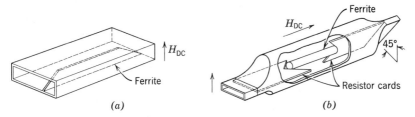

(a)   (b)

	f, Mc	Loss, dB Forward	Loss, dB Return
Isolator (a)	10,000	0.7	22
	6,000	0.8	22
	4,000	—	—
Isolator (b)	10,000	0.1	25–30
	6,000	—	—
	4,000	0.2	25–30

Fig. 7–6. Two types of X band isolators. (a) The rectangular type has a forward loss of 0.75 dB and a return loss of 22 dB, while (b) the cylindrical type has a forward loss of 0.15 dB and a return loss of about 28 dB [Rowen (1953)].

coils. In addition, isolators exhibit a pronounced hysteresis because the amount of attenuation depends on the previous history of the applied current. A typical isolator hysteresis curve is shown in Fig. 7-7.

A nonvariable isolator is usually placed between the klystron and the rest of the waveguide components to prevent the waveguide network from acting back on and influencing the frequency stability of the klystron. The isolator is said to decouple or match the klystron to the transmission line. Such a nonvariable isolator usually employs a permanent magnet, and care must be exercised not to store it near ferromagnetic objects (e.g., on a steel shelf) where it may become demagnetized.

A variable isolator may be employed to adjust the amount of microwave power that is incident on the sample resonant cavity when very low power studies are being made. Such low power levels are often required for studies at liquid helium temperature. Crystal detectors do not function well when the overall microwave power drops below 1 or 2 mW because under these conditions sufficient leakage (crystal current) cannot be provided. Thus it is often desirable to use an isolator to lower the power incident on the cavity, but not the power incident on the crystal detector. This can be accomplished by placing the isolator between the microwave bridge (magic T) and the resonant cavity. In this position it will attenuate the incident microwave power, but will not attenuate the reflected signal. When using this experimental setup, the isolator current may be

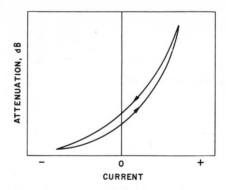

Fig. 7-7. Typical isolator hysteresis loop showing attenuation as a function of the direct current through the coil.

turned off while the klystron frequency (and reference cavity) are adjusted to the sample cavity frequency, since during this procedure it is desirable to display the cavity "pip" on the oscilloscope. Too much isolator attenuation will decouple the cavity from the rest of the waveguide system, and prevent such oscilloscopic observation of the sample cavity.

Since the isolator is a nonreciprocal device it cannot be represented by an equivalent circuit consisting of resistors, inductors, and capacitors. The scattering matrix for an ideal isolator is

$$\begin{bmatrix} B_1 \\ B_2 \end{bmatrix} = \begin{bmatrix} 0 & S_{12} \\ 0 & 0 \end{bmatrix}\begin{bmatrix} A_1 \\ A_2 \end{bmatrix} = \begin{bmatrix} 0 & 1 \\ 0 & 0 \end{bmatrix}\begin{bmatrix} A_1 \\ A_2 \end{bmatrix} \tag{1}$$

In other words, when the microwave amplitudes A_1 and A_2 are incident on the two terminals, the respective transmitted amplitudes B_1 and B_2 are given by

$$B_1 = A_2 \tag{2}$$

$$B_2 = 0 \tag{3}$$

The impedance and admittance matrices are antisymmetric and have the form

$$Z = \begin{bmatrix} 0 & R \\ -R & 0 \end{bmatrix} \tag{4}$$

and

$$Y\begin{bmatrix} 0 & -1/R \\ 1/R & 0 \end{bmatrix} \tag{5}$$

which leads to the relations

$$V_1 = RI_2 \tag{6}$$

$$V_2 = RI_1 \tag{7}$$

There is a very extensive literature on isolators, and only several selected references will be mentioned. Gyorgy and Hagedorn (1960) discuss microwave absorption in ferrites, DeGrasse (1959) considers single crystal garnets, Imamutdinov (1961) describes the rotation of the plane of polarization in ruby, Vartanian, Melchor, and Ayres (1956) describe a broadband ferrite isolator, and Swartz (1961) describes a uhf isolator.

Microwave applications of ferrites are discussed by Sakiotis and Chait (1953), Lax and Button (1962), Schweizerhof (1963), and in a number of articles in the October 1956 issue of *Proc. IRE*, Vol. 44.

D. Directional Couplers

A directional coupler is usually employed to monitor the power P_i in the incident or forward traveling wave of a transmission line by extracting a small amount of it. The total power P is the difference between the powers P_i and P_r in the forward and backward (reflected) traveling waves, respectively,

$$P = P_i - P_r \qquad (1)$$

$$= P_i(1 - |\Gamma|^2) \qquad (2)$$

where Γ is the complex voltage reflection coefficient of the terminating load.

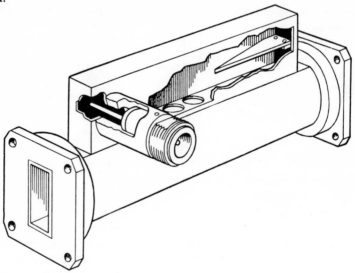

Fig. 7–8. Two-hole directional coupler (*RLS*-8, p. 312).

A small probe or hole in the waveguide is sensitive to the total electric (or magnetic) field strength. If two holes are placed a quarter of a wavelength apart as shown on Fig. 7–8, then only the forward traveling wave in the main guide will be coupled to the coaxial output. The power coupled from the backward traveling wave is dissipated in the matched load shown in the upper right of Fig. 7–8. The amount of power coupled from the main waveguide increases with increasing hole diameter (RLS-11, p. 875). Directional couplers may also be made with one hole (the Bethe-hole coupler) and many holes. Sometimes other types of coupling techniques are used. The design specifications for a large number of directional couplers are given in Chap. 14 of RLS-11.

Directional couplers are usually characterized by their directivity, D, which is a measure of the rejection of the backward traveling wave

$$D = 10 \log_{10} (P_f/P_b) \qquad (3)$$

and the coupling C which characterizes the amount of power extracted by the side or auxiliary arm

$$C = 10 \log_{10} (P_i/P_f) \qquad (4)$$

The quantities in the arguments of the logarithms are defined in Fig. 7–9. The directivity of the two-hole coupler shown in Fig. 7–8 is

$$D = -20 \log_{10} (2\pi\Delta l/\lambda_g) \qquad (5)$$

where Δl is the departure of the hole spacing from a quarter of a guide wavelength and

$$\Delta l \ll \lambda_g \qquad (6)$$

The expression for the coupling C is considerably more complicated (RLS-11, p. 877).

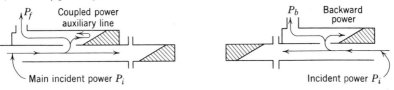

Fig. 7–9. Powers used to define coupling and directivity (RLS-11, p. 859).

The branched guide coupler shown in Fig. 7–10 is susceptible to an exact mathematical analysis (RLS-11, p. 866 ff). The phase relations are such that a traveling wave in either guide will only generate in the other guide a pure traveling wave moving in the same direction. The branched guide coupler may be represented by the transformer equivalent circuit of Fig. 7–11, where n is the transformer ratio of the T junction and Z_0 and Z' are characteristic impedances. The impedance matrix is

$$
\begin{bmatrix} V_1 \\ V_2 \\ V_3 \\ V_4 \end{bmatrix} = \begin{bmatrix} 0 & j & jZ'/n^2 & 0 \\ j & 0 & 0 & jZ'/n^2 \\ jZ'/n^2 & 0 & 0 & j \\ 0 & jZ'/n^2 & j & 0 \end{bmatrix} \begin{bmatrix} I_1 \\ I_2 \\ I_3 \\ I_4 \end{bmatrix} \tag{7}
$$

One can show that the coupling C and directivity D are given by

$$
C = 20 \log_{10} (n^2/Z' + Z'^3/4n^6) \tag{8}
$$

$$
D = 20 \log_{10} (2n^4/Z'^2) \tag{9}
$$

and both improve as n increases. Both quantities depend upon the frequency.

The scattering matrix for a directional coupler is (RLS-8, p. 302)

$$
S = \begin{bmatrix} 0 & (1 - S_0^2)_{1/2} & 0 & jS_0 \\ (1 - S_0^2)_{1/2} & 0 & jS_0 & 0 \\ 0 & jS_0 & 0 & (1 - S_0^2)_{1/2} \\ jS_0 & 0 & (1 - S_0^2)_{1/2} & 0 \end{bmatrix} \tag{10}
$$

where S_0 is real and positive. This scattering matrix may be regarded as the standard form for a directional coupler. An important microwave network theorem states that any completely matched junction of four terminal pairs is a directional coupler.

In electron spin resonance spectrometers, a directional coupler is often employed to couple a little power (C $\sim$ 20 dB) from the main waveguide to an auxiliary arm equipped with a wavemeter and detector. To measure the frequency one may use a crystal detector in series with a microammeter. When the wavemeter is tuned to the proper frequency, it will absorb energy and decrease the detected current. The setting for the minimum current gives the microwave frequency. If power is to be measured, the auxiliary arm may be terminated by a bolometer or thermistor associated with a power bridge. When the directional coupler has a coupling of less than 20 dB the auxiliary arm may couple back into the main waveguide arm and produce interference and noise. In any event, it is best to minimize these effects and establish uniform experimental conditions by setting the detector-tuning plunger for zero detector currents in the sidearm. Sometimes more than one directional coupler is employed in a spectrometer [e.g., see Hirshon and Fraenkel (1955); Frait (1957); Figs. 13–7, 13–10, 13–18].

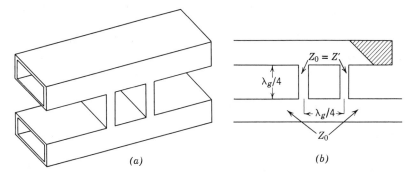

Fig. 7–10. (a) Branched guide coupler and (b) its schematic representation (*RLS*-11, p. 867).

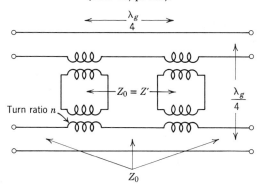

Fig. 7–11. Equivalent circuit of branched guide coupler (*RLS*-11, p. 868). Two alternate equivalent circuits are given in *RLS*-11, p. 868.

A directional coupler may be used as a substitute for a magic T. This has the principal benefit of rendering the bridge more compact in size.   A circulator is to be preferred, however.

E. T Junctions

A T junction is a three-terminal pair network which consists of a main transmission line plus a sidearm which comes out from it at right angles. T junctions are discussed in detail in RLS-8, Chap. 9, RLS-10, Chap. 6, and RLS-14, Chap. 7.   There are three important theorems that apply to T junctions (RLS-8, Sec. 9-1).

Theorem I.   It is always possible to place a short circuit in one arm of a T junction in such a position that there is no transmission of power between the other two arms.

Theorem II.   If a T junction is symmetrical, then a short circuit can be so placed in the arm of symmetry that reflectionless transmission is possible between the other two equivalent arms.

Theorem III.   A general T junction cannot be matched completely.   A completely matched T junction is one whose input impedance at any arm is a matched load when the other two arms are terminated in matched loads.   Because of this inability to match a three-terminal pair T junction, ESR spectrometers ordinarily employ a circulator or a four-terminal pair magic T to couple power to and from the resonant cavity.

A waveguide E-plane T junction shown on Fig. 7–12 is equivalent to a series connection, and the waveguide H-plane T junction shown on Fig. 7–13 is equivalent to a shunt or parallel connection to the

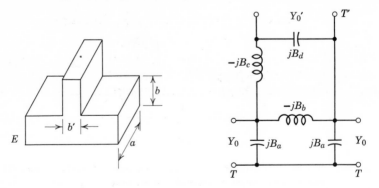

Fig. 7–12. An E plane T junction and its equivalent circuit (RLS-10, p. 337).

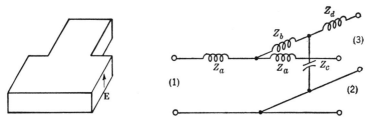

Fig. 7–13.   An H plane T junction and its equivalent circuit (RLS-8, p. 295 and RLS-10, p. 355).

main waveguide.   One should remember that the E-plane T junction branches off in the direction of the electric vector $\mathbf{E}$, and the H-plane T junction branches off in the direction of the transverse magnetic vector $\mathbf{H}$ of the dominant TE_{01} mode.   The transformer representations of T junction equivalent circuits are found in RLS-8, pp. 122 and 285, and in RLS-11, p. 867.   Figure 7–11 illustrates E-plane or series transformer equivalent circuits.

A coaxial-line T junction employs magnetic coupling, and resembles a shunt junction with the equivalent circuit shown in Fig. 7–13.   At very high frequencies, a junction effect is appreciable and a more complex equivalent circuit is required.   Ordinarily, in ESR one employs coaxial T junctions at wavelengths much greater than the coaxial cable radius, and so one does not have to be concerned about the matching problems associated with the T.   This is the case with a coaxial cable carrying a 100 kc modulation signal.   In special applications the match may be important.

F. Magic T or Microwave Bridge Networks

General Characteristics: A magic T is a directional coupler with equal power division, as discussed in RLS-8, Cháps. 9 and 12, RLS-10, Chap. 7, RLS-11, Chap. 9, and RLS-14, Chap. 8.   Its low-frequency analog is the hybrid coil of Fig. 7–14, and a sketch of

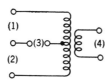

Fig. 7–14.   Circuit of a hybrid coil (RLS-8, p. 307).

the side outlet magic T is shown in Fig. 7–15. Arm 1 (sidearm) is opposite to arm 2 (side arm), and arm 3 (H or shunt arm) is opposite to arm 4 (E or series arm), while arms 1 and 2 are adjacent to arms 3 and 4. The magic T is matched by terminating each arm with its characteristic impedance. It has the property that at match, a wave incident on any arm will split equally between the two adjacent arms, while no power will be reflected back or enter the opposite arm. Thus, at match the opposite arms of a magic T are decoupled from each other. If A_1, A_2, A_3, and A_4 are the wave amplitudes incident on the four junctions, then at match the respective reflected wave amplitudes B_1, B_2, B_3, and B_4 are given by the scattering matrix

$$
\begin{bmatrix} B_1 \\ B_2 \\ B_3 \\ B_4 \end{bmatrix} = \frac{j}{2^{1/2}} \begin{bmatrix} 0 & 0 & 1 & 1 \\ 0 & 0 & 1 & -1 \\ 1 & 1 & 0 & 0 \\ 1 & -1 & 0 & 0 \end{bmatrix} \begin{bmatrix} A_1 \\ A_2 \\ A_3 \\ A_4 \end{bmatrix} \tag{1}
$$

which is equivalent to the four equations:

$$
\begin{aligned}
B_1 &= (j/2^{1/2})(A_3 + A_4) \\
B_2 &= (j/2^{1/2})(A_3 - A_4) \\
B_3 &= (j/2^{1/2})(A_1 + A_2) \\
B_4 &= (j/2^{1/2})(A_1 - A_2)
\end{aligned} \tag{2}
$$

These four equations are a mathematical statement of the magic T property mentioned above.

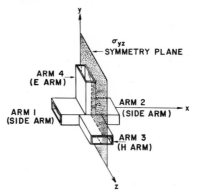

Fig. 7–15. A magic T.

The lack of coupling between arms 3 and 4 results from symmetry because the TE_{10} mode in arm 3 has even symmetry (i.e., is symmetric) and that in arm 4 has odd symmetry (i.e., is antisymmetric) with reference to the y,z symmetry plane σ_{yz}. To show this, consider the TE_{01} electromagnetic vectors in the two arms in question with x set equal to zero at the σ_{yz} symmetry plane. The electromagnetic fields transform in the manner shown on Table 7–2 where the arrow points to the sign that results from reflection at σ_{yz}. From a comparison with Table 5–4, one sees that the solution in arm 3 is even while that in arm 4 is odd. An incoming even wave cannot produce an outgoing odd wave and vice versa. The waveforms in arms 1 and 2 may be either symmetric or antisymmetric depending, respectively, on whether the symmetry plane occurs at the center of the **H** vector loops where H_x is maximum and H_z and E_y are zero, or between two such loops where H_z and E_y are maxima, and H_x is zero. More explicitly for arms 1 and 2 one has the two solutions shown in Table 7–2. It should be noted that the even and odd solution in arms 1 and 2 are $\lambda_g/4$ or 90° out of phase with respect to each other. This phase difference is responsible for the two negative signs in eq. (1). (The forbidden solutions correspond to higher order modes.)

The lack of coupling between arms 1 and 2 results from the use of matching devices to match the magic T into arms 3 and 4. This matching may be accomplished by means of an iris and post as shown in Fig. 7–16, or by other methods (e.g., *RLS*-14, p. 365).

TABLE 7–2

Symmetry Properties of the TE_{10} Mode Solutions of Maxwell's Equations in the Magic T Shown in Fig. 7–15 with Respect to the $\sigma_{y,z}$ Reflection Plane

Arm	Symmetric (even) solution	Antisymmetric (odd) solution
1 and 2	$H_x(x,z) \rightarrow H_x(-x,z)$ $E_y(x,z) \rightarrow E_y(-x,z)$ $H_z(x,z) \rightarrow -H_z(-x,z)$	$H_x(x,z) \rightarrow -H_x(-x,z)$ $E_y(x,z) \rightarrow -E_y(-x,z)$ $H_z(x,z) \rightarrow H_z(-x,z)$
3	$H_x(x,z) \rightarrow H_x(-x,z)$ $E_y(x,z) \rightarrow E_y(-x,z)$ $H_z(x,z) \rightarrow -H_z(-x,z)$	Forbidden
4	Forbidden	$E_x(y,z) \rightarrow E_x(y,z)$ $H_y(y,z) \rightarrow H_y(y,z)$ $H_z(y,z) \rightarrow H_z(y,z)$

An alternative type of magic T consists of the ring circuit, hybrid T or "rat race," and an example of one is shown in Fig. 7–17. This circuit may be analyzed by considering that the input from arm 1 splits, with half of the incident power going around the ring counterclockwise and the other half going around clockwise. At arm 2 the two paths correspond to $\lambda_g/4$ and $5\lambda_g/4$ and at arm 4 they both correspond to $3\lambda_g/4$, so in each case the signals add. However, at arm 3, the two paths correspond to $\lambda_g/2$ and λ_g, so the signals arrive out of phase, and cancel. A similar analysis may be made for inputs to the other arms. One concludes that the rat race resembles the side outlet magic T in that a signal incident on any arm splits equally between the two adjacent arms and does not couple at all to the

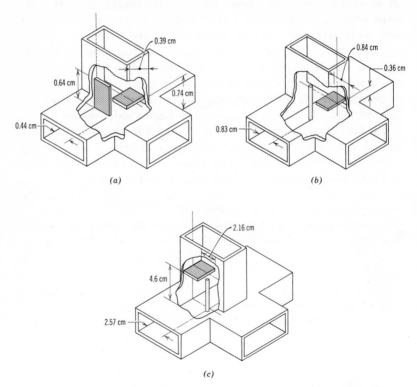

(a) (b)

(c)

Fig. 7–16. Positions of irides and posts for matching waveguide T"s. Waveguides (a) 0.64 × 1.27 cm (¼ × ½ in.); (b) 1.27 × 2.54 cm (½ × 1 in.); (c) 3.81 × 7.62 cm (1½ × 3 in.) (RLS-11, pp. 526–528; RLS-14, pp. 361, 362).

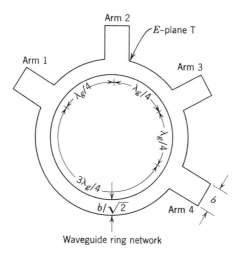

Waveguide ring network

Fig. 7–17. Waveguide ring network (rat race) (*RLS*-11, p. 529; *RLS*-14, p. 359).

opposite arm. In the waveguide case the ring is matched to the four-terminal waveguides by making the ring dimensions equal to $1/\sqrt{2}$ times the small dimensions of the waveguide, as indicated on Fig. 7–17 (cf. Sec. 7-O). The rat race is frequency sensitive since the arms are a quarter of a wavelength apart at only one frequency.

A right-angle ring circuit magic *T* can also be analyzed in terms of the two possible paths from each input to output junction. (See *RLS*-8, p. 309 and *RLS*-14, p. 367.) Both the ring and right-angle ring circuits may be employed for coaxial magic *T*'s as shown in Fig. 7–18. Section 4-C discusses the relationship between the radii and characteristic impedance of a coaxial line. A magic *T* with one waveguide and three coaxial terminations is shown in *RLS*-8, p. 308 and *RLS*-11, p. 529. Kesselring (1962) describes a coaxial bridge.

The magic *T* forms an integral part of many ESR spectrometers, and in this application one ordinarily places the resonant cavity and klystron in opposite arms, with the detector and a matched load terminating the remaining two arms, as suggested in Fig. 7–19. The function of the load is to match the magic *T* and dissipate half of the power from the klystron. The bridge is usually operated near match so that the incident klystron power splits equally between the cavity and load, and the reflected signal splits between the signal source and detector. Usually an isolator is placed in front of the source, and it acts as a matched load for the signal reflected into the klystron arm. Thus one of the inefficiencies of a magic T is the factor of two loss every time the microwaves pass through the T. More recently, the circulator has been employed instead of a magic T since it does not entail such a loss. It will be described in the next section. Magic T junctions are also employed in balanced mixers, the Pound frequency stabilizer (microwave discriminator), balanced duplexers, and other applications.

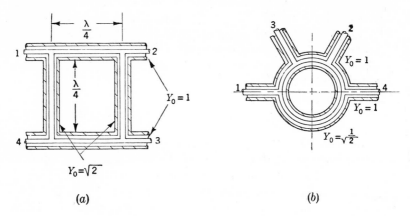

(a)   (b)

Fig. 7–18. Coaxial ring circuit magic T's: (a) rectangular form and (b) circular form (*RLS*-14, p. 368).

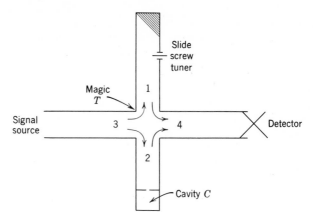

Fig. 7–19. The use of a magic T in an ESR spectrometer [Feher (1957)].

G. Circulators

A circulator is a nonreciprocal multiterminal pair network which transmits power from one terminal to the next in sequence [Truehaft (1956)]. In other words, a signal entering the ith arm of the circulator leaves by the $(i + 1)$th arm. In addition, a circulator appears matched looking into each arm. [Rowen (1953); Truehaft (1956); Fox, Miller, and Weiss (1955)].

Fig. 7–20 shows two types of circulators: The rectangular circulator on the left has a device (π) that changes the phase of the microwaves by π or 180° when they traverse it in one direction. If the path length from terminals 1 and 2 to 3 and 4 is the same around both paths, and equal to an even number of guide wavelengths, then in the absence of the unidirectional element, a signal entering 1 will leave by 4 and one entering 3 will leave by 2. This device will be reciprocal and have the scattering matrix

$$\begin{bmatrix} B_1 \\ B_2 \\ B_3 \\ B_4 \end{bmatrix} = \begin{bmatrix} 0 & 0 & 0 & 1 \\ 0 & 0 & 1 & 0 \\ 0 & 1 & 0 & 0 \\ 1 & 0 & 0 & 0 \end{bmatrix} \begin{bmatrix} A_1 \\ A_2 \\ A_3 \\ A_4 \end{bmatrix} \tag{1}$$

where A_i and B_i are the input and output waves, respectively, at the ith junction. When the unidirectional π phase shift is inserted, the signals entering terminals 2 and 4 will be unaffected, but these entering 1 and 3 will now leave by 2 and 4, respectively, which corresponds to

$$\begin{bmatrix} B_1 \\ B_2 \\ B_3 \\ B_4 \end{bmatrix} = \begin{bmatrix} 0 & 0 & 0 & 1 \\ 1 & 0 & 0 & 0 \\ 0 & 1 & 0 & 0 \\ 0 & 0 & 1 & 0 \end{bmatrix} \begin{bmatrix} A_1 \\ A_2 \\ A_3 \\ A_4 \end{bmatrix} \tag{2}$$

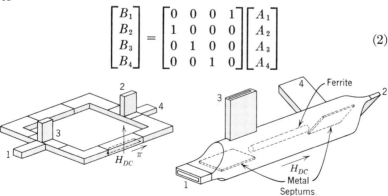

Fig. 7–20. Two types of circulators [Rowen (1953)].

As a result $B_{i+1} = A_i$, and the wave that enters the ith arm leaves by the $(i + 1)$th arm.

The circulator on the righthand side of Fig. 7–20 may be analyzed by considering that the ferrite rotates the microwaves counterclockwise through $\pi/4$ or 45° relative to the direction looking along the magnetic field H_{DC}. The signal that enters terminal 1 cannot leave 3 as a result of symmetry. It traverses the ferrite and is rotated to the proper angle to leave by terminal 2. Similarly, the signal that enters by 3 is rotated into line with 4, where it leaves the isolator. One can similarly reason that the signals entering terminals 2 and 4 will leave by 3 and 1, respectively. In matrix notation one has

$$
\begin{bmatrix} B_1 \\ B_2 \\ B_3 \\ B_4 \end{bmatrix} = \begin{bmatrix} 0 & 0 & 0 & 1 \\ 1 & 0 & 0 & 0 \\ 0 & 1 & 0 & 0 \\ 0 & 0 & 1 & 0 \end{bmatrix} \begin{bmatrix} A_1 \\ A_2 \\ A_3 \\ A_4 \end{bmatrix} \tag{3}
$$

so the two circulators shown on Fig. 7–18 have the same scattering matrix.

One may recall from eqs. (5-F-40) and (5-F-41) that the magic T has two types of scattering matrices which differ in the phases of the output waves B_i. The same situation is true with circulators, and if phases were taken into account, some of the scattering matrix elements of unity would have general values $e^{j\phi}$ which reduce to ± 1 and $\pm j$ when ϕ assumes integral multiples of $\pi/2$. For simplicity the phase relations were not considered.

In an ESR spectrometer one may make use of a three-terminal pair circulator by placing the klystron in arm 1, the resonant cavity in arm 2, and the detector in arm 3, as shown on Fig. 7–21. This arrangement allows the klystron power to go directly to the cavity, and the signal reflected at resonance to go directly to the detector in accordance with the relation

$$
\begin{bmatrix} B_1 \\ B_2 \\ B_3 \end{bmatrix} = \begin{bmatrix} 0 & 0 & 1 \\ 1 & 0 & 0 \\ 0 & 1 & 0 \end{bmatrix} \begin{bmatrix} A_1 \\ A_2 \\ A_3 \end{bmatrix}
$$

In practice, A_1 will be large, A_2 will be small, and A_3 will be zero if the detector presents a matched load to the transmission line. The last condition is not ordinarily satisfied (cf. following section and 14-C).

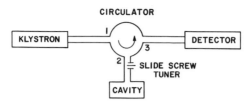

Fig. 7-21. The use of a circulator in an ESR spectrometer.

Circulators have small insertion losses, just as their isolator counterparts do. This will usually be specified by the manufacturer.

A number of circulators have been described in the literature, such as Y junction circulators [Chait and Curry (1959); Clark (1961)], X circulators [Yoshida (1959)], a tetrahedral circulator [Weiss (1960)], a Hall effect circulator [Grubbs (1959)], a coaxial circulator [Clark (1961)], an L band circulator [Arams and Krayer (1958, 1959)], and circulators for the frequency range 70 to 140 Gc [Thaxter and Heller (1960)].

H. Tuners

A tuner is a device which introduces reactance or susceptance into a transmission line. This has the effect of altering the impedance match and changing the standing wave ratio. The most important tuning adjustment in an ESR spectrometer is provided by the slide screw tuner shown in Figs. 7–19 and 7–21. Ideally, before insertion of the tuner in Fig. 7–19, the entire microwave network consisting of the various magic T arms will be matched, and as a result, all of the klystron power from arm 3 will split between arms 1 and 2 with none reaching the detector in arm 4. Since a crystal works best with a finite microwave power incident upon it the slide screw tuner is introduced to mismatch the magic T slightly, and thereby allow a little klystron power to reach the detector. The present section will describe the principle of tuning and discuss the details of several types of tuners (RLS-8, Chap. 5; see also RLS-9, Chap. 8; RLS-14, Chap. 2). If one employs the circulator shown on Fig. 7–21, the slide screw tuner may be put in the cavity arm (terminal 2) and adjusted for the proper crystal current.

Single Screw Tuner: Several types of tuners insert obstacles into the transmission line. These obstacles reflect the microwaves, and thereby alter the impedance match and VSWR. When a screw is inserted into the center of the broad side of a rectangular waveguide as shown in Fig. 7–22, it first acts like a shunt capacitance across the waveguide, with the susceptance $B = \omega C$ increasing with insertion in accordance with the curve of Fig. 7–23. When the length of the screw approximates a quarter of a guide wavelength, it becomes resonant and the susceptance becomes infinite. Greater insertions produce an inductive effect $B = -1/\omega L$. Since rf electrical currents flow along the screw it is necessary for it to make good electrical contact with the waveguide. At X band a number two copper (or brass) screw is satisfactory.

Double and Triple Screw Tuner: The single screw tuner may be employed to match over a wide range of loads, but it suffers from the drawback that it does not cover much of the inductive range of

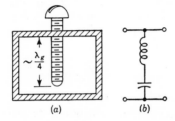

$$(a) \qquad (b)$$

Fig. 7–22. (a) A single screw tuner and (b) its equivalent circuit (*RLS*-9, p. 705).

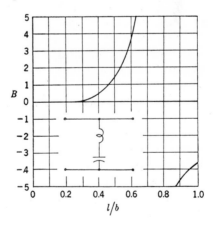

Fig. 7–23. The susceptance B of a tuning screw 0.13 cm in diameter as a function of the depth of insertion l in X band waveguide of width $b = 1$ cm when $\lambda = 3.2$ cm (*RLS*-8, p. 169).

susceptance. A pair of tuning screws separated by $\lambda_g 8$ (or $5\lambda_g 8$ will allow tuning over a much wider range of susceptances (*RLS*-9, p. 507). Such a double screw tuner is often employed to match a crystal mount.

Another frequently used tuner is the triple screw tuner in which the three screws are separated from each other by intervals of $\lambda_g/4$ (*RLS*-8, p. 182). Each pair of this triplet matches on opposite sides of a Smith chart representation of the transmission line. Both the double and triple screw tuners are capable of achieving a VSWR < 2.

Slide Screw Tuner: A single screw that may be moved along the waveguide for at least a half of a guide wavelength will also match a transmission line over a wide range of susceptance. Such a device is illustrated on Fig. 7–24. To a first approximation the magnitude of the reflection from the screw depends on its insertion, and the phase of the reflection depends on its position. In the two- and three-screw tuners the magnitude–phase relationship was adjusted by the multiple reflections off different screws. From Figs. 7–19 and 7–21 it may be seen that a slide screw tuner is customarily employed as an integral part of the ESR bridge. To use the tuner in this application, its longitudinal position is varied until one obtains a maximum signal (leakage) on the crystal, and its insertion is adjusted for the desired leakage. For small insertions this produces an undercoupled cavity match. It is possible to overcouple the cavity by adjusting the longitudinal position for a minimum in the leakage.

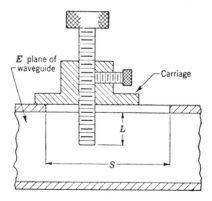

Fig. 7–24. Slide screw tuner capable of moving a distance S along the waveguide (*RLS*-9, p. 486).

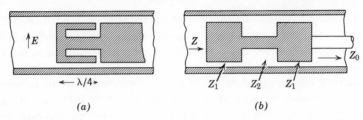

Fig. 7–25.   Plungers for use in rectangular waveguide; (a) folded back type; (b) dumbbell type (*RLS*-8, p. 198).

Tuning Plunger: Impedance matching is frequently accomplished by placing a tuning plunger at the end of a waveguide (*RLS*-8, p. 198). Two examples of such plungers are shown on Fig. 7–25.   The plunger on the left of the figure has a folded-back coaxial linelike arrangement or choke joint that consists of two $\lambda_g/4$ line lengths, and it has the effect of reflecting a short circuit at the end of the plunger.   The other plunger uses three quarter-wave-length sections (*RLS*-8, p. 198). A tuning plunger is frequently employed in conjunction with a detector mount in order to shift the maximum in the electric vector to the position of the detector.

E-H Tuner: This type of tuner consists of an unmatched magic *T* with plungers in arms 3 and 4.   These plungers are used to match the impedance of the main transmission line formed by the other two arms (1 and 2, respectively, of the *T*).   *E-H* tuners are not used very often in ESR spectrometers because they are large in size and cannot be conveniently adjusted to a null or matched position.

I. Matched Loads

A load is a resistive impedance (admittance) which terminates a transmission line.   Short-circuit terminations or plungers were discussed in the last section.   A transmission line which is terminated in its characteristic impedance Z_0 is equivalent to a transmission line of infinite length, and is said to be matched.   The physical significance of a matched transmission line is that it dissipates all of the incident microwave power without producing any reflected wave. In other words it produces a voltage standing wave ratio (VSWR) of 1.   In an ESR spectrometer a matched load is placed in one arm of the magic *T*, as shown on Fig. 7–19, and this helps to match the entire waveguide network.   A resonant cavity with a properly matched iris is said to be critically coupled, and at its resonant frequency it becomes a matched load when placed at the end of a transmission line. Such a cavity is also shown in Fig. 7–19. Matched loads are discussed in the first few sections of *RLS*-11, Chap. 12.

Matched loads employed in resonance spectroscopy are ordinarily of the low power variety. The polyiron matched load shown in Fig. 7–26 produces a VSWR of 1.01 over the 3.13 to 3.53-cm band. Polyiron is capable of withstanding higher microwave powers than the other-low power loads to be discussed.

A fairly simple matched load may be constructed from an IRC resistance card, and several designs are shown in Fig. 7–27. The resistance card may be easily damaged by soldering operations and excessive power levels, but the latter limitation is not important at the

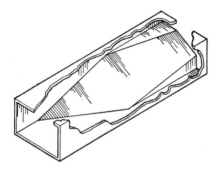

Fig. 7–26.   A well-matched polyiron termination for 1.27 × 2.54 cm (½ × 1 in.) waveguide (*RLS*-11, p. 726).

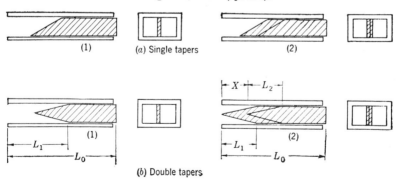

Fig. 7–27.   Various designs of IRC resistance loads for rectangular waveguides: (a) single tapers; (b) double tapers (*RLS*-11, p. 729).

ESR power levels currently in use ($P < 1$W). It is fairly easy to construct a homemade matched load. Metalized glass may also be employed for the construction of matched loads. Another simple matched load is constructed from a wooden wedge two or three guide wavelengths long which is coated with graphite (i.e., Glyptal). Loads are ordinarily tapered to insure a low VSWR.

In radar applications it is frequently necessary to employ high power loads, and these may often be recognized by their cooling fins. Coaxial matched loads are constructed on the same principles, and from the same materials as waveguide loads, as discussed in *RLS*-11, Sec. 12-1.

J. Resonant Cavities

In electron spin resonance spectroscopy, a resonant cavity ordinarily forms an integral part of an ESR spectrometer because it houses the sample. Other ESR applications include a reference cavity for a low-power bridge, and a frequency meter. The reader is referred to Chap. 8 for a detailed discussion of resonant cavities.

K. Irides (Irises)

An iris may be defined as a metallic partition extending partially across the waveguide in a plane perpendicular to the direction of propagation. Four commonly used irides are shown in Fig. 7–28.

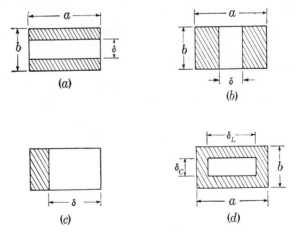

Fig. 7–28. Windows for rectangular guides: (a) symmetrical capacitive; (b) symmetrical inductive; (c) asymmetrical inductive; (d) resonant (*RLS*-12, p. 230).

The two inductive irides have an inductance connected across the transmission line as their equivalent circuit, and the capacitive iris has a capacitance connected across the transmission line as its equivalent circuit. The resonant iris receives its name from the fact that its equivalent circuit is a combination of inductive and capacitive elements in parallel. The electrical characteristics of the symmetrical and asymmetrical shunt irides are shown graphically in *RLS*-9, p. 212 and *RLS*-10, p. 222.

The circular iris is frequently employed as a coupling hole from a waveguide to a resonant cavity, and it is discussed in detail in Sec. 8-F. A circular iris across a waveguide may be employed as a narrow-band filter as shown in Fig. 7–29. This iris resonates when the periphery of the opening is equal to approximately half a wavelength, and the frequency dependence of the voltage standing wave ratio from such a filter is shown in *RLS*-9, p. 690. The capacitive screw is only a trimmer for small frequency adjustments. When a thin resonant iris is employed to couple energy into a resonant cavity, a tuning screw such as the one shown in Fig. 7–29 may be used to match the

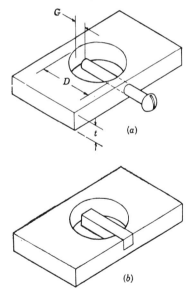

Fig. 7–29. Centered circular irides suitable for narrow band filters matched by (a) screw and (b) rectangular post (*RLS*-9, p. 690).

cavity over a wide range of Q values. The equivalent circuit for a resonant iris used in this manner is a transformer, as shown in Figs. 8–21a, 8–22a, and 14–20.

L. Mode Transducers

A mode transducer is a device to transform a guided electromagnetic wave from one mode to another. This may take the form of a waveguide iris to transform from one rectangular waveguide mode to another, as Fig. 7–30 illustrates, or it may be a device to transform from a rectangular to a cylindrical waveguide mode, such as the ones illustrated on Figs. 7–31 and 7–32.

M. Slotted Sections

In Sec. 7-H it was mentioned that slide screw tuners accomplish their task by moving a probe along the broad section of the wave-

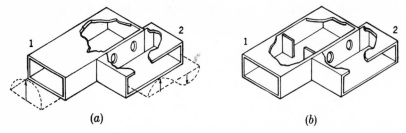

(a)   (b)

Fig. 7–30. Coupling from the TE_{10} mode in one waveguide to the TE_{20} mode in another by means of small holes: (a) shows **E** vector and (b) shows inductive iris (RLS-8, p. 337).

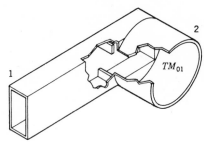

Fig. 7–31. Transducer from the TE_{10} rectangular mode to the TM_{01} cylindrical mode (RLS-8, p. 339).

guide to vary its coupling with the electric field vector.   A slotted line or slotted section is a slide-screw tuner which is provided with a mechanism for measuring the strength of the microwave electric field at the probe.   Figure 7–33 shows a sketch of a coaxial section and another of a waveguide slotted section.   The probe insertion may be

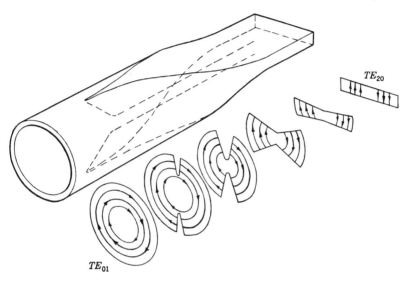

Fig. 7–32.   Transducer for converting from the TE_{20} mode in rectangular guide to the TE_{01} mode in round guide (*RLS*-8, p. 340).

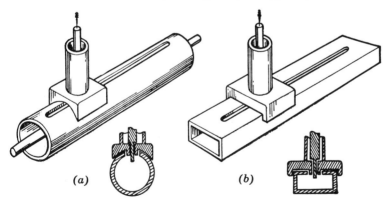

Fig. 7–33.   Slotted section with probe: (*a*) coaxial line; (*b*) waveguide (*RLS*-11, p. 479).

varied, and it is best to insert it as little as is feasible in order to avoid disturbing the electromagnetic field configuration. Ordinarily one employs an electric probe such as the one illustrated on the figure, but a magnetic probe consisting of a small loop antenna could also be used. The slot itself acts as a waveguide beyond cutoff, and so does not appreciably radiate energy to the exterior. When making use of the slotted section, one assumes that the slotted line itself may be treated as a lossless transmission line, and that the presence of the probe does not seriously modify the electromagnetic field configurations in the transmission line. The latter is often minimized through the use of a probe shield.

The probe of the slotted section extracts a small fraction of the power flowing in the transmission line, and it is connected to an external circuit containing a rectifier or detector. When the microwave source is unmodulated, the crystal detector may be followed by a dc meter or by a dc amplifier and a meter. A more sensitive system employs a superheterodyne receiver equipped with a crystal mixer, local oscillator, and second detector. When the microwave source is modulated, then a crystal or bolometer followed by a narrow band amplifier may be employed. When working into a low impedance load, a crystal detector produces about 1 μA of rectified current for 1 μW of incident rf power. At this and lower power levels the crystal is a square law detector with the rectified current proportional to the microwave power.

By moving the probe along the slot, one may measure the power P_{max} and P_{min} at the maximum and minimum positions along the line, and deduce the VSWR from the formula

$$\text{VSWR} = \left(\frac{P_{max}}{P_{min}}\right)^{1/2} = \frac{|A| + |B|}{|A| - |B|} \tag{1}$$

where A and B are the amplitudes of the incident and reflected waves, respectively. The ratio P_{max}/P_{min} is sometimes referred to as the power standing wave ratio. The magnitude of the reflection coefficient of the load $|\Gamma_L|$ may be deduced from the expression

$$|\Gamma_L| = \frac{|B|}{|A|} = \frac{\text{VSWR} - 1}{\text{VSWR} + 1} \tag{2}$$

The complex reflection coefficient Γ_L of the load is defined by

$$\Gamma_L = |\Gamma_L| e^{j\theta} \tag{3}$$

and the phase angle θ may be determined by observing the distance $x_{\min}$ of the nearest minimum from the load. One obtains

$$\theta = 2\beta x_{\min} \pm \pi \tag{4}$$

where β is the phase constant (imaginary part of the propagation constant γ). Equation (2) may be reformulated in terms of the load impedance or admittance

$$\Gamma_L = \frac{Z_L - 1}{Z_L + 1} = \frac{1 - Y_L}{1 + Y_L} \tag{5}$$

Figure 7–34 gives a plot of the probe power P_S versus probe position x for several load reflection coefficients Γ_L. It is important to determine the phase of the reflection coefficient from the position of a minimum because the maxima are slightly shifted when the probe susceptance is not equal to zero, as is normally the case.

A detailed discussion of slotted sections and voltage standing wave ratio measurements is given in RLS-11, Chap. 8, and several particular references are Oliner (1954), El'kind (1961), and Nunn (1961).

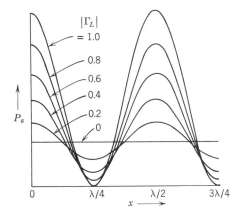

Fig. 7–34. Variation of probe power P_S with position of probe. The parameter Γ_L is the load reflection coefficient, and the origin is taken at the point where Γ_L is a maximum (RLS-11, p. 475).

N. Waveguide Bends and Twists

Waveguide bends are designed to minimize reflections. A circular bend such as the one shown on Fig. 7-35 should either have a radius R much greater than the guide wavelength, or it should have the mean length L equal to $\lambda_g/2$. Such a bend may be constructed by filling the waveguide with Cerrobend or Wood's metal, bending it, and then melting out the filler. This method of bending usually produces excessive distortions in a small-dimension waveguide, and in this case electroforming is preferable. Bends with cut-off corners may be fabricated by sawing and then soldering. Design data are given in RLS-8, Chap. 6 and RLS-9, Chap. 4.

Waveguide twists are employed to change the angular orientation of a rectangular waveguide about the direction of propagation without altering this direction of propagation. If the cross-sectional dimensions of the twisted section equal those in the straight waveguide, then the guide wavelength λ_g in the twist will nearly equal that in the straight waveguide. Twists are best matched when their

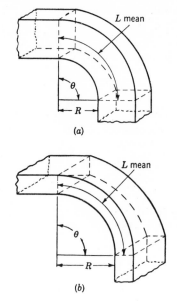

Fig. 7-35. Waveguide bends: (a) H plane bend; (b) E plane bend (RLS-9, p. 208).

length is an integral number of $\lambda_g/2$. They may be constructed by filling a section of waveguide with Cerrobend on Wood's metal and twisting it on a lathe or other machine. Several design data for twists are presented in RLS-9, p. 209.

O. Quarter-Wavelength Transformers

A transmission line of characteristic impedance Z_1 may be matched to a transmission line of characteristic impedance Z_2 by interposing between them a quarter of a wavelength of a transmission line with the characteristic impedance Z_{12} given by (RLS-9, pp. 90 and 217)

$$Z_{12} = (Z_1 Z_2)^{1/2} \tag{1}$$

Quarter-wavelength transformers of this type were employed to match the magic T illustrated in RLS-11, p. 528 and RLS-14, p. 365. The characteristic impedance Z_0 of a coaxial line given by eq. (4-C-2) may be employed in designing coaxial quarter-wavelength transformers.

If two waveguides operating in the TE_{10} mode have the same wide dimension a but different small dimensions b_1 and b_2, respectively, they will each have the same characteristic impedance Z_0 (cf. eq. 4-D-32) if they are filled with the same medium (e.g., air) since Z_0 is independent of b. Nevertheless, when they are joined together, reflections will be set up at their interface, and a large VSWR will result. Their junction may be matched by an intervening quarter wavelength section of length λ_g 14 and width b given by

$$b = (b_1 b_2)^{1/2} \tag{2}$$

Thus for the TE_{10} mode, the narrow dimension of the waveguide acts like an effective characteristic impedance. This principle is applied in Sec. 7-F to match the rat race.

P. Detector Mounts

Waveguide mounts for crystals, bolometers, and thermisters are discussed in Sec. 11-H. They frequently incorporate tuning devices such as a plunger and tuning screws, as shown in Fig. 11–14.

Q. Antennae

Microwave antenna theory is discussed at great length in RLS-12. There are a large number of different types of microwave antennae, such as electric and magnetic dipoles, linear arrays, horns, parabolas, and especially shaped antennae. The electric and magnetic dipoles have electromagnetic field amplitudes that vary as r^{-3} (static field), r^{-2} (induction field), and the r^{-1} (radiation field) (RLS-12, p. 93). The radiation field dominates for distances $r \gg \lambda$ away from the dipole, and produces an inverse-square dependence of the radiated power on the distance. At distances less than a wavelength, the other nonradiative field configurations dominate. The existence of these near-field r^{-3} and r^{-2} terms is important in microwave setups in the laboratory, because radiation effects that result from faulty apparatus design or assembly will frequently manifest themselves in the near-field region. For example, if one failed to place the matched load on the rat race of Fig. 7–1, and then walked past the waveguide opening, the effect on the recorder or oscilloscope display would result from disturbing the near-field electromagnetic configurations emanating from the waveguide. One might have to go to the other side of the room to reach the far-field (radiation-field) region.

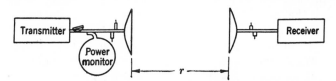

Fig. 7–36. Arrangement of antennae for transmitting microwaves over a short distance r (RLS-11, p. 907).

Sometimes it is desirable to do an ESR or microwave spectroscopy experiment by arranging two antennae as in Fig. 7–36 and placing the sample in the space between them. In such an experimental arrangement it is convenient to place the magnet and sample between two sectoral horns [RLS-12, Chap. 10; De Grasse, Hogg, Ohm, and Scovil (1959); Bottreau and Marzat (1964)] such as those shown in Fig. 7–37. Paraffin or polystyrene lenses may be used to focus the microwaves [Costain (1957)].

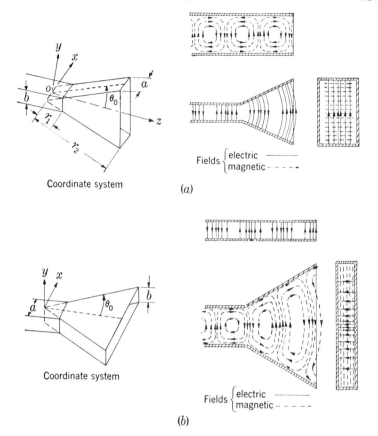

Fig. 7–37. Lowest mode field configurations in sectoral horns: (a) E plane and (b) H plane (RLS-12, p. 351).

R. Phase Shifters

The guide wavelength λ_g in a waveguide depends upon the guide dimensions, and for a rectangular waveguide operating in the TE_{10} mode it is given explicitly by

$$\lambda_g = \lambda/[1 - (\lambda/2a)^2]^{1/2} \tag{1}$$

where λ is the free-space wavelength (for an air-filled waveguide) and a is the wide dimension of the waveguide. If some mechanism is employed to change this dimension, then the result is equivalent to changing the effective length of the waveguide, and the phase of the wave configuration in the waveguide system will be altered. Physically this means that the positions of the maxima and minima in the standing wave pattern will be shifted, and these positions may be measured by means of a slotted line, as discussed in Sec. 7-M.

A phase shifter or squeeze section may be constructed by cutting a slot in the two broad sides of the waveguide and employing a mechanical device to vary the broad waveguide dimension a. Unfortunately, the change in phase is not a linear function of the change in a (see RLS-11, Sec. 8–9).

A phase shifter is useful in an ESR low power bridge. In this application it may be placed between the circulator (or magic T) and sample cavity for adjusting the phase of the microwaves incident on the resonant cavity. This will have the effect of producing absorption, dispersion, or a combination of both. In other words, it permits one to observe either the real part χ' or the imaginary part χ'' of the magnetic susceptibility.

Ferrite phase shifters are discussed by Geiszler and Henschke (1960), Kovtun and Tereshchenko (1961), and Scharfman (1956); Tremblay (1961) discusses a dielectric prism phase shifter.

S. Flexible Couplings and Rotary Joints

It is axiomatic that coaxial cables are flexible and waveguides are rigid. Sometimes one requires a nonrigid waveguide connection, and for this purpose one may employ flexible waveguide (RLS-9, p. 287; RLS-11, p. 244). Flexible waveguides may be constructed from a spirally wrapped metal or from a series of choke and flange joints, called vertebrae, held in a rubber envelope. One ESR application for flexible waveguides is to connect a waveguide network to a resonant cavity suspended in a Dewar flask under close tolerances. This prevents one from tightening waveguide screws in a way that will strain or fracture the glassware.

Rotary joints which permit two transmission lines to rotate relative to each other about their common direction of propagation are important in radar applications for rotating antennae. In ESR single-crystal studies it is useful to be able to rotate a resonant cavity about its axis. This is feasible when the sample is placed in

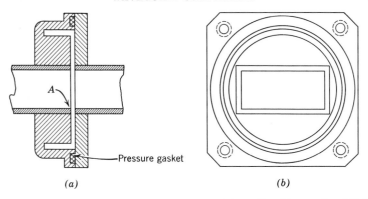

Fig. 7–38. Choke flange waveguide coupling: (a) profile; (b) anterior (RLS-9, p. 194; RLS-11, p. 14).

the center of a cylindrical cavity operating in the TE_{011} mode and coupled with its symmetry axis along the waveguide propagation direction. To provide a proper impedance match, it is best to make the waveguide junction with the choke flange combination shown in Fig. 7–38. The cavity coupling may be a circular slot located at the junction, and concentric with the cavity symmetry axis.

T. Flanges

In electron spin resonance studies, waveguides are usually coupled together by soldering the ends to flat flanges, and screwing the flanges together in order to obtain a good electrical contact. Satisfactory contact may be ensured by moving one flange back a few mils from the end of the waveguide and applying a greater pressure as shown in RLS-9, p. 193, but this is normally not resorted to in ESR since contact couplings are ordinarily satisfactory. An ESR bridge cannot be matched sans good waveguide couplings. It is best to silver solder flanges, although soft soldering can also be satisfactory.

A choke flange such as the one shown in Fig. 7–38 is electrically equivalent to a series-branching transmission line one-quarter wavelength long which ends in a short circuit. Therefore a short circuit is reflected to the point A, and it is not necessary to have good electrical contact at the waveguide joint in order to achieve a low standing wave ratio. The outer groove in the choke flange may be considered as a low-impedance coaxial line. A choke flange is usually threaded,

TABLE 7-3

Standard Rectangular Waveguides and Couplings (*RLS*-11, p. 15)

RMA designation	Waveguide Army-Navy type no.	OD, in. (1 in. = 2.54 cm)	Wall, in.	Wavelength band, cm	Wavelength for P_{max} and loss, cm	P_{max} MW	Loss for copper, dB/m	Choke coupling	Flange coupling	Design wavelength, cm	Bandwidth for VSWR > 1.05, %
WR 284	RG-48/U	3 × 1.5	0.080	7.3 –13.0	10.0	10.5	0.020	UG-54/U	UG-53/U	10.7	±15
		ID2.75 × 0.375	0.049	7.0 –12.6	10.0	2.77	0.058	-200/U	-214/U	9.0	±15
WR 187	RG-49/U	2 × 1	0.064	4.8 – 8.5	6.5	4.86	0.031	-148/U	-149/U		
WR 137	RG-50/U	1.5 × 0.75	0.064	3.6 – 6.3	5.0	2.29	0.063				
WR 112	RG-51/U	1.25 × 0.625	0.064	2.9 – 5.1	3.2	1.77	0.072	-52/U	-51/U	3.20	
WR 90	RG-52/U	1.0 × 0.5	0.050	2.3 – 4.1	3.2	0.99	0.117	-40/U	-39/U	3.20	±6
WR 42	RG-53/U	0.5 × 0.25	0.040	1.07– 1.9	1.25	0.223	0.346	-117/U	-116/U	1.25	> ± 2
WR 34		0.42 × 0.25	0.040	0.9 – 1.4							
WR 28	RG-96/U	0.36 × 0.22	0.040	0.75– 1.1			0.56	-600/U	-599/U		
WR 22		0.304 × 0.192	0.040	0.6 – 0.9							
WR 19		0.268 × 0.174	0.040	0.5 – 0.75							
WR 15		0.228 × 0.154	0.040	0.4 – 0.6							
WR 12		0.202 × 0.141	0.040	0.33– 0.5							
WR 10		0.180 × 0.130	0.040	0.27– 0.4							

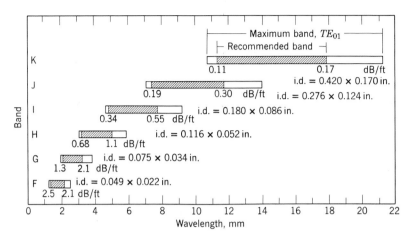

Fig. 7–39. The inner dimensions and losses for the TE_{01} mode in rectangular coin silver waveguide at wavelengths between 1.3 and 18 mm. One inch equals 2.54 cm [Gilliam, Johnson, and Gordy (1950)].

and it is always mated with a flat or cover flange with the screw holes drilled through. Two choke flanges should never be joined together. Other choke flange designs are discussed in *RLS*-9, Chap. 4. Both choke and waveguide flanges are listed in Table 7–3.

U. Waveguides

Waveguides have been extensively discussed in this and preceding chapters, and a large number of formulae, graphs, tables, etc., have been presented to elucidate their properties. The present section will refrain from repeating this material, but instead will merely fill in several practical details which have been overlooked earlier in the book. Table 7–3 lists the physical and electrical characteristics of some common waveguides. Gilliam, Johnson, and Gordy (1950) give the dimensions and wavelength ranges of the special wave-guides developed at Duke University for use in the millimeter wave region.

References

F. R. Arams and G. Krayer, *Proc. IRE*, **46**, 912 (1958); **47**, 442 (1959).
A. Bottreau and C. Marzat, *C. R. Acad. Sci.*, **259**, 758 (1964).
H. N. Chait and T. R. Curry, *J. Appl. Phys. Suppl.*, **30**, 152S (1959).

J. Clark, *J. Appl. Phys. Suppl.*, **32**, 323S (1961).

C. C. Costain, *Can. J. Phys.*, **35**, 241 (1957).

R. W. DeGrasse, *J. Appl. Phys. Suppl.*, **30**, 155S (1959).

R. W. DeGrasse, D. C. Hogg, E. A. Ohm, and H. E. D. Scovil, *J. Appl. Phys.*, **30**, 2013 (1959).

A. I. El'kind, *PTE*, **2**, 116 (323) (1961).

A. G. Fox, S. E. Miller, and M. T. Weiss, *Bell System Tech. J.*, **34**, 5 (1955).

Z. Frait, *Czech. J. Phys.*, **7**, 222, 577 (1957).

J. A. Fulford and J. H. Blackwell, *RSI*, **27**, 956 (1956).

T. D. Geiszler and R. A. Henschke, *J. Appl. Phys.*, **31**, 174S (1960).

O. R. Gilliam, C. M. Johnson, and W. Gordy, *Phys. Rev.*, **78**, 140 (1950).

W. J. Grubbs, *Proc. IRE*, **47**, 528 (1959).

E. M. Gyorgy and F. B. Hagedorn, *J. Appl. Phys.*, **31**, 1775 (1960).

J. M. Hirshon and G. K. Fraenkel, *RSI*, **26**, 34 (1955).

C. L. Hogan, *Bell System Tech. J.*, **31**, 1 (1952).

F. S. Imamutdinov, *Zh. Tekh. Fiz.*, **31**, 1472 (1961).

P. Kesselring, *Helv. Phys. Acta*, **35**, 532 (1962).

N. M. Kovtun and A. I. Tereschenko, *Zh. Tekh. Fiz.*, **31**, 834 (602) (1961).

B. Lax and K. J. Button, *Microwave Ferrites and Ferrimagnetics*, McGraw-Hill, N. Y., 1962.

W. M. Nunn, Jr., *RSI*, **32**, 1106 (1961).

A. A. Oliner, *RSI*, **25**, 13 (1954).

C. D. Owens, *Proc. IRE*, **44**, 1234 (1956).

RLS-8.

RLS-9.

RLS-10.

RLS-11.

RLS-14.

J. H. Rowen, *Bell System Tech. J.*, **32**, 1333 (1953).

N. G. Sakiotis and H. N. Chait, *Proc. IRE*, **41**, 87 (1953).

H. Scharfman, *Proc. IRE*, **44**, 1456 (1956).

S. Schweizerhof, *Z. Angew. Phys.*, **16**, 61 (1963).

G. C. Southworth, *Proc. IRE*, **50**, 1199 (1962).

D. B. Swartz, *J. Appl. Phys. Suppl.*, **32**, 319S (1961).

J. B. Thaxter and G. S. Heller, *Proc. IRE*, **48**, 110 (1960).

R. Tremblay, *Can. J. Phys.*, **39**, 409 (1961).

M. A. Treuhaft, *Trans. IRE*, *CT-3*, No. 2, 127 (1956).

C. W. van Es, M. Gevers, and F. C. de Ronde, *Philips Tech. Rev.*, **22**, 113, 181 (1960–61).

P. H. Vartanian, J. L. Melchor, and W. P. Ayers, *Trans. IRE*, *MTTT-4*, **1956**, 8.

J. A. Weiss, *J. Appl. Phys. Suppl.*, **31**, 168S (1960).

H. A. Wheeler, *Proc. IRE*, **50**, 1207 (1962).

S. Yoshida, *Proc. IRE*, **47**, 1150, 2017, 2018 (1959).

CHAPTER 8

Resonant Cavities

A resonant cavity is an integral part of almost all electron spin resonance spectrometers, and therefore, the present chapter will be devoted to an extensive study of the theory, design, and use of cavities. Resonant cavities have also been used in microwave spectrometers [Townes and Schawlow (1955); Verdier (1958); Beers (1959); Dymanus (1959); Dymanus, Dijkerman, and Zijderveld (1960)] in place of the usual waveguide cell. Stevens (1959) and Stevens and Josephson (1959) have discussed the coupling of a spin system to a cavity mode.

Some investigators such as Hausser and Reinhold (1961), Webb (1962), and Werner (1964) have used helices instead of cavities. Wilmshurst, Gambling, and Ingram (1962) have compared the sensitivities obtained with spectrometers which employ cavities to those using helices, and their conclusions are discussed in Sec. 14-G. Recent theoretical discussions of cavity resonators have been given by Heer (1964), Sloan, Ganssen, and La Vier (1964), and Lawson (1965).

A. The Series RLC-Tuned Circuit

A resonant cavity is the microwave analog of an rf-tuned circuit, and so the latter will be considered first. In Fig. 8–1 we see the series RLC-tuned circuit fed by the voltage V. The differential equation for the voltage V and current I in this circuit is given by

$$V = L(dI/dt) + RI + q/C \tag{1}$$

where I is the current and q is the charge on the condenser. For a sinusoidally varying voltage $V = V_m e^{j\omega t}$ we have the steady-state solution

$$I = (V_m/Z)e^{j(\omega t - \theta)} \tag{2}$$

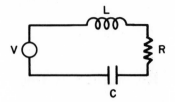

Fig. 8–1.   Series RLC circuit.

where $V_m = I_m |Z|$. The impedance Z has the magnitude

$$Z = [R^2 + (\omega L - 1/\omega C)^2]^{1/2} \tag{3}$$

and the phrase angle θ is

$$\theta = \tan^{-1}\left[\frac{(\omega L - 1/\omega C)}{R}\right] \tag{4}$$

At very low frequencies we may approximate

$$V \cong - jI/\omega C \tag{5}$$

and at very high frequencies

$$V \cong j\omega L I \tag{6}$$

In either case the current is very small and leads or lags the voltage by 90°.   At the resonant frequency f_0

$$\omega_0 = 2\pi f_0 = 1/(LC)^{1/2} \tag{7}$$

we have

$$V = RI \tag{8}$$

so that the current flow reaches a maximum, and is in phase with the voltage.

The quality factor Q is defined as

$$Q = \omega_0 L/R = 1/R\omega_0 C \tag{9}$$

and this Q is very important in the theory of resonant cavities. Using the relation $V = ZI$ and the approximation $(\omega + \omega_0)/\omega \sim 2$ which is valid for a high Q, we can write

$$Z/R = 1 + 2jQ\ (\omega - \omega_0)/\omega_0 \qquad (10)$$

For ω close to ω_0 we let

$$Q = \omega_0/\Delta\omega \qquad (11)$$

and

$$Z/R = 1 + j\ [(\omega - \omega_0)/\tfrac{1}{2}\Delta\omega] \qquad (12)$$

Physically, $\tfrac{1}{2}\Delta\omega$ is the value of $\omega - \omega_0$ which makes the real part of the impedance equal to the imaginary part. At this value the current flow through the circuit of Fig. 8-1 falls to $1/2^{1/2}$ of its value at resonance, and the power dissipated (I^2R) is one half the value at resonance. Another important way of defining Q is

$$Q = \frac{2\pi\,(\text{energy stored})}{\text{energy dissipated per cycle}} = 2\pi\left[\frac{\tfrac{1}{2}LI_m^2}{RI_m^2/2f}\right] \qquad (13)$$

When the energy source of a resonator is turned off the stored energy U decays exponentially from the initial value U_0 according to the relation

$$U = U_0 e^{-\omega_0 t/Q} = U_0 e^{-t\Delta\omega} \qquad (14)$$

B. The Microwave Resonant Cavity

At microwave frequencies it is not feasible to employ lumped-circuit elements such as the RLC circuit just discussed because the skin effect results in a very high effective resistance in ordinary copper wires, and the dimensions of the circuit elements become comparable to the wavelength, which causes them to lose energy by radiation. A microwave resonant cavity is a box fabricated from high conductivity metal with dimensions comparable to the wavelength. At resonance, the cavity is capable of sustaining microwave oscillations which form an interference pattern (standing wave configuration) from superposed microwaves multiply reflected from the cavity walls.   Each particular cavity size and shape can sustain oscillations in a number of different standing wave configurations called modes, and these will be discussed in the next few sections. The modes of rectangular and cylindrical resonant cavities may be derived from the waveguide modes discussed in Chap. 4.

When a waveguide is terminated in its characteristic impedance Z_0, the transverse electric field and transverse magnetic field vectors reach their maxima at the same longitudinal or z position.   In other words they are in phase with respect to both space and time, as shown on Figs. 4–7, 4–9, 4–10, 4–14, and 4–15.   This maximizes the time averaged Poynting's vector $\mathbf{P}$ or vector rate of energy flow given by

$$\mathbf{P} = \tfrac{1}{2}\,\mathbf{E} \times \mathbf{H} \tag{1}$$

In a resonant cavity, on the other hand, the electromagnetic field configurations are the result of standing waves with the transverse electric field maximum occurring $\lambda_g/4$ from the transverse magnetic field maximum, so they are in space quadrature.   This makes Poynting's vector vanish, and consequently there is no net energy flow, but merely energy storage and dissipation.   The wave configurations on Figs. 4–7, 4–9, 4–10, 4–14, and 4–15 may be applied to resonant cavities by displacing the electric field configuration $\lambda_g/4$ along the waveguide so that the righthand rule is obeyed, as shown in Fig. 8–2 (e.g., by curling the fingers in the direction of circular H field lines of force and having the thumb point in the direction of the enclosed $\mathbf{E}$ vector).   In resonant cavities the H field lines of force always form loops which enclose E field lines of force, and the E field lines of force either form loops which enclose H fields, or they terminate on induced surface charges.

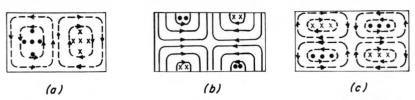

(a)   (b)   (c)

Fig. 8–2.   Electromagnetic field patterns in several rectangular and cylindrical cavity resonators.   (a) Cyl. TE_{112}; rect. TE_{102}; (b) cyl. TM_{012}; (c) cyl. TE_{012}; rect. TE_{202}.   (●) Direction up from the paper; (×) direction down into the paper; (– –) H lines of force; (—) E lines of force.

Before discussing particular cases it will be helpful to say a few words about the general properties of electromagnetic waves confined in a metallic box. In a high Q resonator the electric and magnetic fields are 90° out of time phase with each other. When the electric fields are maximum, the magnetic fields are zero, and vice versa. Hence the stored energy in the electric fields U_E

$$U_E = \frac{\epsilon}{2} \int |E_m|^2 d\tau \qquad (2)$$

equals the stored energy in the magnetic fields U_H

$$U_H = \frac{\mu}{2} \int |H_m|^2 d\tau \qquad (3)$$

when each is evaluated at the part of the cycle corresponding to the maximum value denoted by the subscript m. The losses in a cavity arise from the dissipation of heat by the surface current density J in the skin effect resistance R_s, and this ohmic power loss P_L is given by

$$P_L = \frac{R_s}{2} \int |H_{tm}|^2 dS \qquad (4)$$

where the maximum tangential field H_{tm} along the surface is integrated over all the cavity walls. H_t is numerically equal to and vectorially perpendicular to J, and both H_t and J are parallel to the surface. There may be additional energy dissipation arising from a lossy dielectric such as water, or a paramagnetic sample with a large loss tangent (see Sec. 3-H). In addition, there will be losses from radiation out of a cavity coupling hole. These topics will be elaborated upon later.

When the Q of a resonant cavity arises only from the ohmic losses in the walls it is called the unloaded Q, denoted by the symbol Q_u, and is given by

$$Q_u = \frac{\omega\mu}{R_s} \frac{\int |H_m|^2 d\tau}{\int |H_{tm}|^2 d\tau} \qquad (5)$$

The overall or loaded Q (denoted by Q_L) may be computed by summing the reciprocals of the Q_ϵ due to dielectric losses, the Q_r due to the cavity coupling hole, and Q_u, and hence it has the form

$$1/Q_L = 1/Q_u + 1/Q_\epsilon + 1/Q_r \tag{6}$$

where the individual quality factors are defined by eq. (5) and

$$Q_r = \frac{2\pi \text{ (stored energy)}}{\text{energy lost through coupling holes per cycle}} \tag{7}$$

$$Q_\epsilon = \frac{2\pi \text{ (stored energy)}}{\text{energy lost in dielectric per cycle}} = \frac{\mu \int |H_m|^2 d\tau}{\int \epsilon'' |E_m|^2 d\tau} \tag{8}$$

For the dielectric Q, the numerator is integrated over the regions of the cavity where the imaginary part of the dielectric constant is non-vanishing. At room temperature, Q values usually vary between a few thousand and 50,000, while superconducting cavities give Q's of many million [Maxwell (1964), a review; Verkin, Dmitrenko, Dmitriev, Churilov, and Mende (1963); Viet (1964)]. For example, Wilson (1963) observed a Q of 2×10^8 in a lead-plated TE_{011} mode cylindrical cavity at 2856 Mc and 1.75°K.

Methods of measuring the Q of a microwave cavity resonator are given by RLS-11, Reed (1951), Alaeva and Karasev (1961), and Teodoresku (1962). A microwave pulse experiences a time delay in traversing a transmission cavity [Mungall and Morris (1960); see also Ruthberg (1958)].

The next three sections will be devoted to a detailed discussion of rectangular, cylindrical, and coaxial resonant cavities, respectively. Culshaw (1961), Boyd, Gordon, and Kogelnik (1961, 1962), Wagner and Birnbaum (1961), and Lichtenstein, Gallagher, and Cupp (1962), Ulrich, Renk, and Genzel (1963), Krupnov and Skvortsov (1964), Strauch, Cupp, Lichtenstein, and Gallagher (1964), and Lotsch (1965) discuss the use of the millimeter wave Fabry-Perot interferometer as a resonator. Many other shapes exist including a type without side walls [Szulkin (1960); Vainstein (1963)], a Π-shaped resonator [Patrushev (1956); Dunn, Sabel, and Thompson (1956)], one with nonorthogonal boundaries [Ledinegg and Urgan (1955)], a millimeter wave disk resonator [Barchukov and Prokhorov (1961)], and the "echo box" type with dimensions much greater than the wavelength [see, e.g., Meyer, Helberg, and Vogel (1960); Kahn, Bergstein, Gamo, Goubau, La Tourrette, and Di Francia (1964)]. A number of recent articles treat the interaction between a plasma and a resonant cavity [see, e.g., Agdur and Enander (1962); Thomassen (1963)]. Zimmerer (1962) describes a 50 to 75-Gc wavemeter which uses a confocal resonator and Reichert and Townsend (1965) discuss the line resonator [cf. Sec. 8-N]. Resonant cavities designed for use at high and low temperatures are discussed in Chap. 16, and those that are suitable for irradiation studies are described in Chap. 17. A dual cavity designed to hold both the sample under study and a standard sample [Kohnlein and Müller (1961); Thompson, Persyn, and Nolle (1963)] is described in Secs. 8-K and 14-K. Vetter and Thompson (1962) designed a servo-controlled cavity to follow frequency changes in another cavity, and Erickson (1966) sweeps the ESR frequency by moving the cavity wall with a clock motor. Bimodal cavities are discussed in Sec. 8-J.

Resonant cavities may be employed to generate ultrasonic vibrations in piezoelectric crystals, as discussed in Sec. 19-F [see Baranskii (1957); Jacobsen, Shiren, and Tucker (1959); Bömmel and Dransfeld (1960); Bolef, de Klerk, and Gosser (1962); Dorland (1963)].

Lewis and Carver (1964) studied electron spin transmission through a 30-μ thick lithium sample using two rectangular TE_{101} transmission cavities in series. The reflected and transmitted ESR signals differed considerably, and this was attributed to spin diffusion.

In the magnetic resonance literature it is customary to denote the microwave or rf magnetic field at the sample by H_1, and we shall often adhere to this convention. Thus, we shall talk about the average value of $H_1^2 = \langle H_1^2 \rangle_c$ within the cavity, and the average value of $H^2 = \langle H^2 \rangle_w$ in the waveguide outside the cavity. This is a somewhat inconsistent notation, and the symbol H_1 would not be employed in this manner if usage did not sanction it.

C. Rectangular Resonant Cavities

Rectangular resonant cavities can support both TE_{mnp} modes and TM_{mnp} modes, where the subscripts m, n, and p are the number of half wavelength variations in the standing wave pattern in the x, y, and z directions, respectively, as defined on Fig. 8-3. These modes

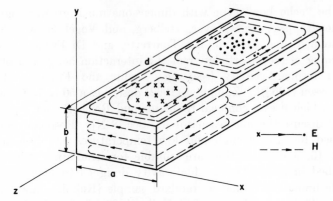

Fig. 8-3. Electromagnetic field configurations in a TE_{102} mode rectangular resonant cavity of dimensions a, b, and d.

are derived from the TE_{mn} and TM_{mn} waveguide modes, respectively, by making the resonant cavity $p/2$ guide wavelengths long. The cavity dimensions are a, b, and d in the x, y, and z directions, with the propagation constant k

$$k = j\beta = (k_x^2 + k_y^2 + k_z^2)^{1/2} \qquad (1)$$

which has the components

$$k_x = m\pi/a, \quad k_y = n\pi/b, \quad k_z = p\pi/d \qquad (2)$$

The resonant frequency $2\pi f_0 = \omega_0$ is given by

$$\omega_0 (\mu\epsilon)^{1/2} = k = 2\pi/\lambda = \pi (m^2/a^2 + n^2/b^2 + p^2/d^2)^{1/2} \qquad (3)$$

where λ is the free space wavelength. The guide wavelength λ_g and cut-off wavelength λ_c were discussed in Chap. 4. The dependence of the frequency on the dielectric constant allows the cavity to be used as a refractometer [Vetter and Thompson (1962)].

Keeping in mind the quantities defined in eqs. (1)–(3) we may write down the wave configuration for the general TE_{mnp} mode with $p > 0$ and either m or $n > 0$.

$$H_x = - H_0 \left(\frac{k_x k_z}{k_x^2 + k_y^2} \right) \sin k_x x \cos k_y y \cos k_z z \qquad (4)$$

$$H_y = - H_0 \left(\frac{k_y k_z}{k_x{}^2 + k_y{}^2} \right) \cos k_x x \sin k_y y \cos k_z z \qquad (5)$$

$$H_z = H_0 \cos k_x x \cos k_y y \sin k_z z \qquad (6)$$

$$E_x = j H_0 (\mu/\epsilon)^{1/2} \left(\frac{k k_y}{k_x{}^2 + k_y{}^2} \right) \cos k_x x \sin k_y y \sin k_z z \qquad (7)$$

$$E_y = - j H_0 (\mu/\epsilon)^{1/2} \left(\frac{k k_x}{k_x{}^2 + k_y{}^2} \right) \sin k_x x \cos k_y y \sin k_z z \qquad (8)$$

$$E_z = 0 \qquad (9)$$

The general TM_{mnp} mode with $m > 0$, $n > 0$ is

$$E_x = - H_0 (\mu/\epsilon)^{1/2} \left(\frac{k_x k_z}{k_x{}^2 + k_y{}^2} \right) \cos k_x x \sin k_y y \sin k_z z \qquad (10)$$

$$E_y = - H_0 (\mu/\epsilon)^{1/2} \left(\frac{k_y k_z}{k_x{}^2 + k_y{}^2} \right) \sin k_x x \cos k_y y \sin k_z z \qquad (11)$$

$$E_z = H_0 (\mu/\epsilon)^{1/2} \sin k_x x \sin k_y y \cos k_z z \qquad (12)$$

$$H_x = j H_0 \left(\frac{k k_y}{k_x{}^2 + k_y{}^2} \right) \sin k_x x \cos k_y y \cos k_z z \qquad (13)$$

$$H_y = - j H_0 \left(\frac{k k_x}{k_x{}^2 + k_y{}^2} \right) \cos k_x x \sin k_y y \cos k_z z \qquad (14)$$

$$H_z = 0 \qquad (15)$$

TE_{mnp} and TM_{mnp} modes of the same order are degenerate because they have identical frequencies, and other cases of so called accidental degeneracy may occur for certain ratios of the cavity dimensions. To increase the frequency in a resonant cavity of a given size, it is necessary to fit additional half waves in one or more dimensions, which means that the order of the mode must increase. If the cavity dimensions are decreased and the mode type is unchanged, then the frequency increases.

The dimensionless quantity $Q_u \delta / \lambda$ for TE modes with m and $n > 0$ is (RSL-11, p. 296)

$$Q_u \frac{\delta}{\lambda} = \frac{\dfrac{abd}{4\pi}(k_x^2 + k_y^2)(k_x^2 + k_y^2 + k_z^2)^{3/2}}{ad[k_x^2 k_z^2 + (k_x^2 + k_y^2)^2] + bd[k_y^2 k_z^2 + (k_x^2 + k_y^2)^2]}$$

$$+ abk_z^2(k_x^2 + k_y^2) \qquad (16)$$

while for $m = 0$, it is

$$Q_u \frac{\delta}{\lambda} = \frac{\dfrac{abd}{2\pi}(k_y^2 + k_z^2)^{3/2}}{k_y^2 d(b + 2a) + k_z^2 b(d + 2a)} \qquad (17)$$

and for $n = 0$

$$Q_u \frac{\delta}{\lambda} = \frac{\dfrac{abd}{2\pi}(k_x^2 + k_z^2)^{3/2}}{k_x^2 d(a + 2b) + k_z^2 a(d + 2b)} \qquad (18)$$

For TM modes and $p > 0$ we have

$$Q_u \frac{\delta}{\lambda} = \frac{\dfrac{abd}{4\pi}(k_x^2 + k_y^2)(k_x^2 + k_y^2 + k_z^2)^{3/2}}{k_x^2 b(a + d) + k_y^2 a(b + d)} \qquad (19)$$

while when $p = 0$ the quality factor for TM modes is given by

$$Q_u \frac{\delta}{\lambda} = \frac{\dfrac{abd}{2\pi}(k_x^2 + k_y^2)^{3/2}}{k_x^2 b(a + 2d) + k_y^2 a(b + 2d)} \qquad (20)$$

When using these formulae it should be recalled that the skin depth δ is defined in Sec. 3-I by

$$\delta = (2/\omega\mu\sigma)^{1/2} \qquad (21)$$

Figure 3–4 shows the dependence of δ on ω for several materials.

The TE_{102} mode (sometimes called TE_{012}) is the dominant mode, and is also the most important one used in ESR spectrometers [see Heuer (1965)]. If we set $m = 1$, $n = 0$, and $p = 2$ in eqs. (4)–(8) we obtain for the only nonvanishing field components

$$H_x = \frac{H_0}{[1 + (d/2a)^2]^{1/2}} \sin \frac{\pi x}{a} \cos \frac{2\pi z}{d} \tag{22}$$

$$H_z = \frac{-H_0}{[1 + (2a/d)^2]^{1/2}} \cos \frac{\pi x}{a} \sin \frac{2\pi z}{d} \tag{23}$$

$$E_y = j(\mu/\epsilon)^{1/2} H_0 \sin \frac{\pi x}{a} \sin \frac{2\pi z}{d} \tag{24}$$

where $k_y = 0$, and the quantity H_0 is slightly redefined to make the equations appear more symmetical. Essentially the same mode configurations may be obtained by letting $p = 0$, and then interchanging the roles of y and z in eqs. (10)–(14). The coefficients of these wave configurations [eqs. (22)–(24)] are related through the characteristic impedance Z_{TE} of the corresponding waveguide with width a

$$Z_{TE} = \frac{(\mu/\epsilon)^{1/2}}{[1 - (f_c/f)^2]^{1/2}} = (\mu/\epsilon)^{1/2} [1 + (d/2a)^2]^{1/2}$$

$$= (\mu/\epsilon)^{1/2} \lambda_g / \lambda \tag{25}$$

The resonant frequency f is independent of the (narrow) b dimension of the cavity, although, of course, the unloaded Q is a function of all of the three cavity dimensions. The lack of dependence of b on f means that the resonant cavity may be made as narrow as one wishes to accommodate a small magnet gap. This is not possible with cylindrical cavities, so that in general a cylindrical cavity requires a considerably wider gap. The b dimension may be increased to accommodate variable temperature apparatus within the cavity.

For a TE_{102} mode, the unloaded Q has the form

$$Q_u \frac{\delta}{\lambda} = \frac{4b[a^2 + (\frac{1}{2}d)^2]^{3/2}}{d^3(a + 2b) + 4a^3(d + 2b)} \tag{26}$$

For the TE_{011} mode, the unloaded Q is

$$Q_u\frac{\delta}{\lambda} = \tfrac{1}{2}\frac{b(a^2 + d^2)^{3/2}}{d^3(a + 2b) + a^3(d + 2b)} \tag{27}$$

and for a square cavity $(a = d)$, this simplifies to

$$Q_u\frac{\delta}{\lambda} = \frac{1}{2^{1/2}}\frac{b}{a + 2b} \tag{28}$$

Figure 8–3 gives the configurations of the electric and magnetic fields in the TE_{102} mode, and Fig. 8–4 shows the current flow in the cavity walls.   The electric field begins and ends on induced charges on the broad face of the cavity, and the magnetic field H_t tangential to the cavity walls induces currents in the walls perpendicular to the H_t direction, as shown in Fig. 8–4.   The circuit for the electric current flow is completed by the displacement current which flows through the centers of the magnetic field loops, and induces charges on the wide surface (xz plane) near the centers of these loops.   These charges reverse polarity every half cycle, and the ohmic losses result from electrons rushing back and forth through the cavity walls every half cycle to build them up.

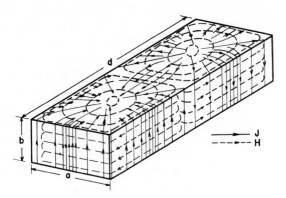

Fig. 8–4.   Current distribution J in a TE_{102} mode rectangular resonant cavity with dimensions a, b, and d.

It is desirable to design the sample cavity in such a way that (1) the rf magnetic field H_1 in the sample is perpendicular to the applied steady magnetic field H_0, (2) the sample is located at a point of maximum H_1, and (3) it is placed at a position of minimum E. The first requirement arises from the nature of the resonance condition for allowed transitions; the second requirement is because below saturation the amount of rf energy absorbed by the sample is proportional to H_1^2, and the greater the H_1, the greater the signal to noise ratio, while the third requirement minimizes the dielectric power loss which has a deleterious effect on the signal to noise ratio. These three requirements are met by the arrangement shown in Fig. 8–5, when the constant magnetic field is in the y direction of Fig. 8–3. Such a cavity may be provided with a mount for orienting single crystal samples and for variable temperature studies (see Chap. 16). Longer cavities are sometimes used with aqueous and other lossy samples [Estin (1962); Wilmshurst (1963); Stoodley (1963)].

A knowledge of mode configurations and current flow in resonant cavities is particularly useful for designing special purpose resonators without appreciably decreasing their Q. For example, it is possible to cut slots in the bottom of the rectangular TE_{10p} cavity parallel to the directions of current flow shown in Fig. 8–4 and these slots may be used for uv irradiation. In another arrangement a split cavity may be used as shown in Fig. 8–6 [Poole and Anderson 1959)], where it is not necessary to achieve good electrical contact along the split when the cavity is assembled.

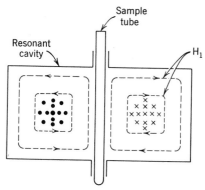

Fig. 8–5. ESR sample tube in rectangular TE_{102} resonant cavity.

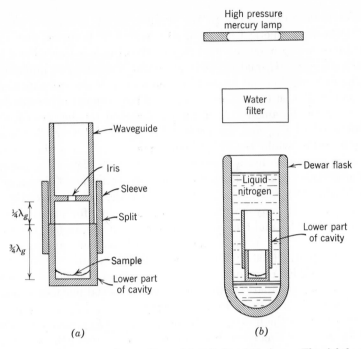

(a)   *(b)*

Fig. 8–6. Split rectangular cavity and irradiation technique. The righthand illustration shows the cavity disassembled from the waveguide. (a) Resonant cavity assembled; (b) resonant cavity irradiated [Poole and Anderson (1959)].

D. Cylindrical Resonant Cavities

In analogy to rectangular resonant cavities, cylindrical cavities can support both TE_{mnp} and TM_{mnp} modes, where the subscripts m, n, and p refer to the number of half cycle variations in the angular (ϕ), radial (r), and longitudinal (z) directions, respectively. These modes may be derived from the TE_{mn} and TM_{mn} cylindrical waveguide modes discussed in Chap. 4 [see Wilson, Schramm, and Kinzer (1946)].

Let the resonant cavity radius be a, and let the length be d. In analogy to the rectangular cavity case, we have

$$k = j\beta = \omega_0(\mu\epsilon)^{1/2} = (k_c^2 + k_z^2)^{1/2} = \left[\frac{(k_c a)_{mn}^2}{a^2} + \left(\frac{p\pi}{d}\right)^2\right]^{1/2} \quad (1)$$

where $(k_c a)_{mn}$ is a Bessel function root since cylindrical waveguide modes have Besseloid radial variations and $k_z = p\pi/d$. For transverse magnetic waves TM_{mnp}, the quantity $(k_c a)_{mn}$ is the nth root of the mth order Bessel function $J_m(k_c r)$

$$J_m(k_c a) = 0 \qquad (2)$$

For transverse electric modes the first derivative of the Bessel function $J_m(k_c r)$ must vanish at the surface

$$\frac{d}{dr} J_m(k_c r)\big|_{r=a} = J_m{}'(k_c a) = 0 \qquad (3)$$

and the nth root of this equation for the mth order Bessel function is denoted by $(k_c a)_{mn}'$. The most useful Bessel roots $(k_c a)_{mn}'$ and $(k_c a)_{mn}$ are listed in columns 2 and 4, respectively, of Table 8–1. For TE modes, $(k_c a)_{mn}'$ replaces $(k_c a)_{mn}$ in eq. (1).

TABLE 8–1

The nth Roots of the mth Order Bessel Functions $J_m{}'(k_c a)$ and $J_m(k_c a)$, and the Corresponding TE_{mnp} and TM_{mnp} Cylindrical Cavity Modes (RLS-11, p. 299)

TE_{mnp} mode	nth root of $J_m{}'(k_c a)$	TM_{mnp} mode	nth root of $J_m(k_c a)$
11p	1.841	01p	2.405
21p	3.054	11p	3.832
01p	3.832	21p	5.136
31p	4.201	02p	5.520
41p	5.318	31p	6.380
12p	5.332	12p	7.016
51p	6.415	41p	7.588
22p	6.706	22p	8.417
02p	7.016	03p	8.654
61p	7.501	51p	8.772
32p	8.016	32p	9.761
13p	8.536	61p	9.936
71p	8.578	13p	10.174
42p	9.283		
81p	9.648		
23p	9.970		
03p	10.174		

The mode configurations for the general cylindrical TE_{mnp} mode with $n > 0$ and $p > 0$ are

$$H_r = \frac{k_z H_0}{(k_c{}^2 + k_z{}^2)^{1/2}} J_m{}'(k_c r) \cos m\phi \cos k_z z \tag{4}$$

$$H_\phi = - \frac{m k_z H_0}{(k_c{}^2 + k_z{}^2)^{1/2}} \frac{J_m(k_c r)}{k_c r} \sin m\phi \cos k_z z \tag{5}$$

$$H_z = \frac{k_c H_0}{(k_c{}^2 + k_z{}^2)^{1/2}} J_m(k_c r) \cos m\phi \sin k_z z \tag{6}$$

$$E_r = - m(\mu/\epsilon)^{1/2} H_0 \left[J_m(k_c r)/k_c r \right] \sin m\phi \sin k_z z \tag{7}$$

$$E_\phi = - (\mu/\epsilon)^{1/2} H_0 J_m{}'(k_c r) \cos m\phi \sin k_z z \tag{8}$$

$$E_z = 0 \tag{9}$$

The mode configurations for the TE_{011} mode are given in Sec. 8–H. For the TM_{mnp} modes with $m > 0$ we have

$$E_r = - \frac{(\mu/\epsilon)^{1/2} H_0 k_z}{(k_c{}^2 + k_z{}^2)^{1/2}} J_m{}'(k_c r) \cos m\phi \sin k_z z \tag{10}$$

$$E_\phi = \frac{(\mu/\epsilon)^{1/2} H_0 m k_z}{(k_c{}^2 + k_z{}^2)^{1/2}} \frac{J_m(k_c r)}{k_c r} \sin m\phi \sin k_z z \tag{11}$$

$$E_z = \frac{(\mu/\epsilon)^{1/2} H_0 k_c}{(k_c{}^2 + k_z{}^2)^{1/2}} J_m(k_c r) \cos m\phi \cos k_z z \tag{12}$$

$$H_r = - m H_0 [J_m(k_c r)/k_c r] \sin m\phi \cos k_z z \tag{13}$$

$$H_\phi = - H_0 J_m{}'(k_c r) \cos m\phi \cos k_z z \tag{14}$$

$$H_z = 0 \tag{15}$$

The dependence of the frequency f on the radius a and the length d of a cylindrical cavity in a vacuum (or air) is easily presented graphically by rearranging eq. (1) to the form

$$(2af)^2 = \left(\frac{c(k_c a)_{mn}}{\pi} \right)^2 + \left(\frac{cp}{2} \right)^2 \left(\frac{2a}{d} \right)^2 \tag{16}$$

where $c = 1/(\mu_0\epsilon_0)^{1/2}$ is the velocity of light *in vacuo*. For convenience one plots $(2af)^2$ against $(2a/d)^2$ as shown on Fig. 8–7. In designing a resonant cavity it is best to select values of a and d so that there are no extraneous modes which have resonant frequencies near the design point. In TE modes, $(k_c a)_{mn}'$ replaces $(k_c a)_{mn}$ in eq. (16).

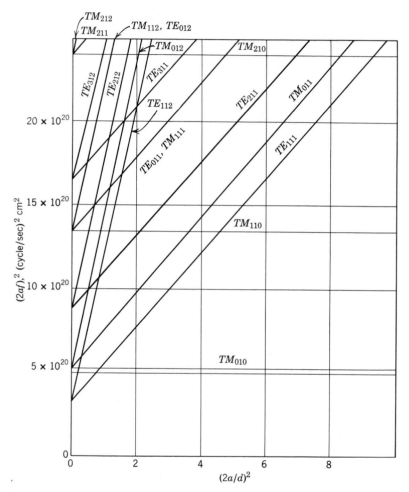

Fig. 8–7. Mode chart for right circular cylinder of radius a, length d, and resonant frequency f (*RLS*–11, p. 298).

The Q factor for the TE_{mnp} cylindrical mode is (RLS-11, Sec. 5-5)

$$Q_u\frac{\delta}{\lambda} = \frac{(1/2\pi)[1 - m/(k_ca)'^2_{mn}]\,[(k_ca)'^2_{mn} + (p\pi a/d)^2]^{2/3}}{(k_ca)'^2_{mn} + (2a/d)\,(p\pi a/d)^2 + (1 - 2a/d)\,[mp\pi a/d(k_ca)_{mn}']^2}$$

$$(17)$$

and the corresponding formula for the TM_{mnp} mode is

$$Q_u\frac{\delta}{\lambda} = \frac{[(k_ca)^2_{mn} + (p\pi a/d)^2]^{1/2}}{2\pi(1 + 2a/d)} \tag{18}$$

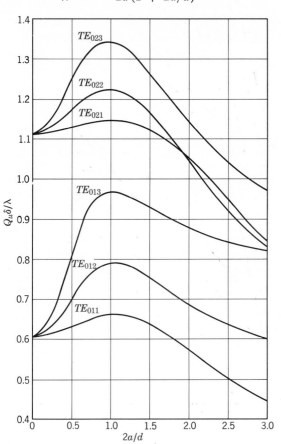

Fig. 8–8. $Q_u\delta/\lambda$ vs. $2a/d$ for several TE_{0np} modes in a right circular cylinder (RLS–11, p. 300).

These formulae are plotted in Figs. 8–8 to 8–10.   One should note from Fig. 8–8 that a TE_{0np} mode has a maximum value of $Q\delta/\lambda$ when the cavity length d equals the diameter $2a$.

As Fig. 8–7 indicates, the dominant mode in a cylindrical cavity is the TE_{111} mode.   Its configuration corresponds to half of the TE_{112} mode which is sketched in Fig. 8–11.   It is analogous to the TE_{101} rectangular cavity mode, and the two may be derived from one another by deforming the cylinder into a rectangular parallelopiped, and vice versa.   Since this mode is dominant, it may be used in situations where the magnet pole gap is too small to support higher order modes.   Unfortunately, the TE_{111} mode has the lowest Q factor of any transverse electric mode, as Fig. 8–9 indicates.   If it is desired

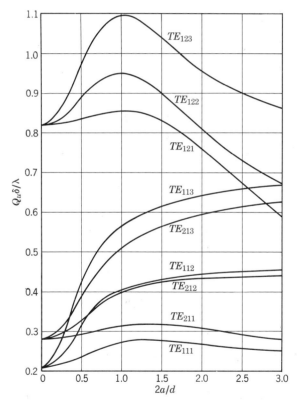

Fig. 8–9. $Q_u\delta/\lambda$ vs. $2a/d$ for several TE_{mnp} modes in a right circular cylinder [RLS–11, p. 301].

to employ a TE_{11p} cylindrical resonator for a sample cavity, the sketch of the TE_{112} mode in Fig. 8–11 may be used as a guide in positioning the sample. Rieckhoff and Weissbach (1962) use the TE_{112} mode for optical studies at liquid helium temperatures.

If one provides a tuning plunger on one end of a TE_{111} cavity, then it is necessary to build into the plunger a quarter wave choke which reflects a short circuit to the gap between the end of the plunger and the cavity walls. Such a plunger allows the rf current to flow at the gap, and this current flow is necessary for a high Q.

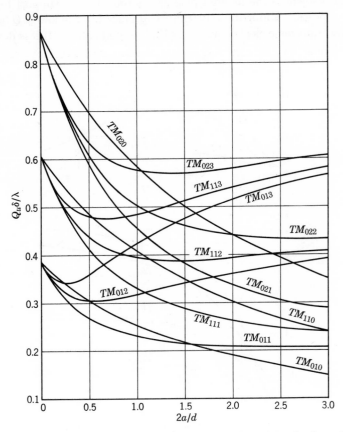

Fig. 8–10. $Q_u\delta/\lambda$ vs. $2a/d$ for several TM_{mnp} modes in a right circular cylinder (RLS–11, p. 302).

Most frequency meters [e.g., RLS-11; Rogers, Cox, and Braun-schweiger (1950); Bussey and Estin (1960)] employ the cylindrical TE_{011} mode because it has a fairly high Q factor, and because there is no rf current flow between the cylinder walls and the end plate. In fact, there is no electric current flow in either the radial (r) or longitudinal (z) direction, but only in the angular (ϕ) direction. This property enables one to use a pistonlike tuning plunger on the end plate, as shown in Fig. 8–12, so that the frequency may be varied by screwing the end plate in and out. The current flow property renders it unnecessary to achieve good electrical contact between the end plate and the cylinder. If one deliberately leaves the finite gap between the piston edges and the walls as shown in Fig. 8–12, then other modes will be suppressed because they require rf current to

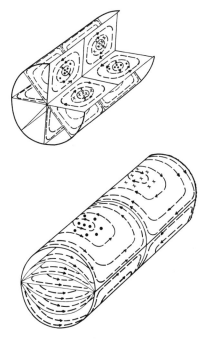

Fig. 8–11. Diagrammatic sketch of the TE_{012} (above) and TE_{112} (below) cylindrical resonant cavity modes [adapted from Reintjes and Coate (1952), p. 608 and p. 610].

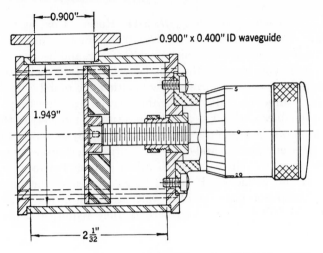

Fig. 8–12. Wavemeter for 10,000-Mc region (*RLS*-11, p. 323).

flow across this gap. In particular, this will suppress the TM_{111} mode which is degenerate with the TE_{011} mode (see Fig. 8–7). The cylindrical TE_{011} mode is particularly useful for a sample cavity since H_z is very strong along the cavity axis. More efficient mode suppression is obtained by means of a helical line of epoxy on the side wall [Estin (1962)]. It is possible to have a very large hole in the end plate [e.g., see Fig. 8–13] without appreciably decreasing the Q. When employed as a sample cavity its plunger may be easily tuned for use at the same frequency with and without a Dewar insert or a quartz linear [Estin (1962)]. This cavity may be used with a larger sample than the rectangular TE_{101} cavity, and in addition it has a considerably higher Q. Two disadvantages of this cavity are its large size (large magnet gap requirement) and the slight inconvenience of adapting it to 100-kc modulation.

E. Coaxial Resonant Cavities

Coaxial resonators are less important than waveguide resonators for ESR applications, and the reader is referred to other sources (e.g., *RLS*-11) for background information and design data. The TE_{mnp} and TM_{mnp} modes are labeled with the same convention that is employed in the cylindrical case. The resonant frequencies depend

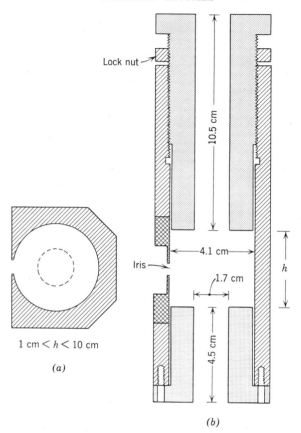

Fig. 8-13. Tunable TE_{011} mode cylindrical resonant cavity. This X band copper cavity was provided with a tunable iris, and a scale plus a vernier for setting the frequency. Spacers may be used with the bottom end plate to properly center the iris. (a) Top view; (b) side view.

upon Bessel functions of both the first and the second kind. *TEM* modes also exist here. Sometimes reentrant cavities are employed as coaxial type cavities, and they are used with microwave triodes (see Sec. 6-B). Raoult and Fanguin (1960) describe a coaxial resonator which is excited by probes from a circular TE_{11} mode waveguide inside its center conductor while Rajangam, Hai, and Mackenzie (1965) frequency-modulated a reentrant coaxial cavity. Decorps and Fric (1964) designed a meter wave spectrometer which uses a coaxial cavity.

F. Coupling to Resonators

The resonant cavity may be coupled to the waveguide by means of a coupling hole or iris, so this section will be prefaced by a few words about coupling holes or irides. Consider a waveguide with a generator at one end, a load at the other, and a thin copper sheet placed perpendicular to the waveguide axis blocking the passage of microwave power to the load. If a slot is cut in the center of the copper sheet parallel to the long waveguide dimension, a capacitive iris is formed, while if the slot is cut parallel to the short dimension, an inductive iris is formed. The voltage reflection coefficient Γ at the iris is defined as the ratio of the amplitude of the incident **E** vector to the amplitude of the reflected **E** vector. Thus Γ is a measure of the amount of power that fails to pass through the iris and enter a resonant cavity. Figure 8–14 shows the reflection coefficient Γ for inductive and capacitive irides as a function of the slot width. Figure 8–15 shows the effect of iris width on the cavity Q. When the hole thickness increases, the size of the coupling hole must be increased to maintain a constant coupling. The resonant cavity illustrated on Fig. 8–6 was used with a symmetrical inductive iris 5.3 mm wide and

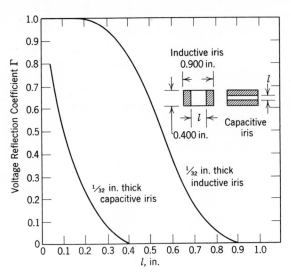

Fig. 8–14.   Reflection coefficient of inductive and capacitive irides in waveguide 1.02 × 2.29 cm. at λ = 3.2 cm. (*RLS*–14, p. 52).

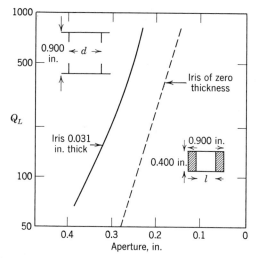

Fig. 8–15.   Loaded Q as a function of iris width l for rectangular cavity in 1.02 × 2.29 cm guide (*RLS*-9, p. 655).

0.5 mm thick.   Further details on inductive and capacitive irides are found in Sec. 7-K.

Of somewhat wider application is the centered circular iris shown in Fig. 8–16.   The relationship between the iris diameter and thickness and its electrical properties (susceptance) are shown in Fig. 8–17 and *RLS*-14, p. 53.   These data are useful for designing coupling holes according to the procedure outlined in *RLS*-8, Sec. 7-10.

An equivalent circuit for the centered circular iris is shown in Fig. 8–18, where the reflection (reaction) resonant cavity near its resonant frequency ω_0 is represented by a series RLC circuit with the usual conditions

$$\omega_0 = 1/(LC)^{1/2} \tag{1}$$

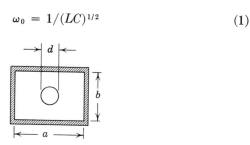

Fig. 8–16.   Centered circular iris.

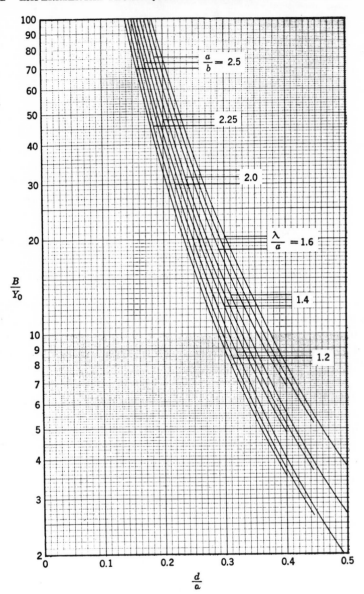

Fig. 8–17. The relative susceptible B/Y_0 of a centered circular iris of zero thickness, where d is the iris diameter, a and b are the waveguide dimensions defined in Fig. 8–16 and λ is the free space wavelength (RLS–10, p. 240).

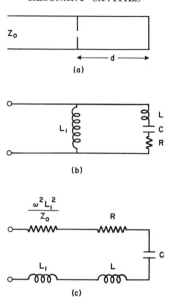

Fig. 8–18. (a) A waveguide reflection cavity and iris; (b) its equivalent circuit; (c) an alternative equivalent circuit (see *RLS*-8, p. 232; see also, Fig. 8–2).

and

$$Q = \omega_0 L/R = 1/R\omega_0 C \tag{2}$$

and Z_0 is the characteristic impedance of the waveguide given by

$$Z_0 = \frac{1}{Y_0} = \left(\frac{\mu}{\epsilon}\right)^{1/2}\left[1 - \left(\frac{f_c}{f}\right)^2\right]^{-1/2} = \frac{120\pi}{[1 - (f_c/f)^2]^{1/2}} \tag{3}$$

for TE modes.

The cavity loss resistance R may be evaluated by assuming that all the cavity ohmic losses are in the cavity side walls, so the input impedance of the cavity Z_S in the absence of the iris would be (RLS-8, Sec. 7-10)

$$Z_S = Z_0 \tanh (\alpha + j\beta)d \tag{4}$$

$$= \frac{\alpha d + j \tan \beta d}{1 + j\alpha d \tan \beta d} \tag{5}$$

$$\approx Z_0(\alpha d + j \tan \beta d) \tag{6}$$

since $\beta d \approx n\pi$, where n is an integer and both $\alpha d \ll 1$ and $|\tan \beta d| \ll 1$. Near resonance we may write

$$\tan \beta d \approx \tan \pi(1 - \Delta\lambda_g/\lambda_g) \tag{7}$$

$$\approx -\pi\Delta\lambda_g/\lambda_g \tag{8}$$

$$\approx \pi(\lambda_g^2/\lambda^2)(\omega - \omega_0)/\omega_0 \tag{9}$$

and eq. (6) becomes

$$Z_S = Z_0 \left[\alpha d + j(\pi\lambda_g^2/\lambda^2)(\omega - \omega_0)/\omega_0\right] \tag{10}$$

which is the same form as a series RLC circuit input impedance from eq. (8-A-10)

$$Z_S = R \left[1 + 2jQ(\omega - \omega_0)/\omega_0\right] \tag{11}$$

Therefore

$$R = Z_0\alpha d \tag{12}$$

the unloaded Q is given by

$$Q_u = (\pi/2\alpha d)(\lambda_g/\lambda)^2 \tag{13}$$

and

$$L = (\pi/\omega_0)(Z_0/2)(\lambda_g/\lambda)^2 \tag{14}$$

From the equivalent circuit in Fig. 8–18 the radiation Q is

$$Q_r = (Z_0/\omega_0 L_1)(L + L_1)/L_1 \tag{15}$$

$$= (Z_0^2/\omega_0^2 L_1^2)(\pi/2)(\lambda_g/\lambda)^2 \tag{16}$$

using the approximating $L_1 \ll L$. For the case of critical coupling when the resonant cavity is perfectly matched to the waveguide and the voltage standing wave ratio is unity, one has

$$Q_r = Q_u \tag{17}$$

and

$$\alpha d \approx (\omega_0 L_1 / Z_0)^2 = (Y_0 / B)^2 \tag{18}$$

where $Y_0 = 1/Z_0$ is the characteristic admittance and $B = 1/\omega L_1$ is the susceptance.

A cavity $\lambda_g/2$ long constructed from X band ($ab = 2.25 \times 1$ cm) waveguide at $\lambda = 3.2$ cm has $\alpha d \approx 3 \times 10^{-4}$ Np (using α from Table 7–1), so the iris susceptance $B/Y_0 \approx 55$ is required for critical coupling. From Fig. 8–17 this corresponds to an iris diameter $d \sim 0.2a$ giving a hole diameter of 0.45 cm for a zero thickness iris. The apparent susceptance of this hole in a nonzero thickness iris will be greater as shown in *RLS*-14, p. 53, so that a somewhat greater hole size is needed in practice. Since ohmic losses in the cavity ends were ignored, their inclusion tends to require an even larger hole, and a nominal diameter for a rectangular cavity is about 0.6 cm.

The coupling constant of the iris may be made variable by placing a capacitive tuning screw immediately outside the iris. The behavior of such a screw is discussed in Sec. 7-K. Here it will suffice to mention that for small insertions the screw acts like a capacitance in parallel with the equivalent inductance of an inductive or circular iris, and by varying its insertion, a wide range of coupling constants may be obtained. Another way to vary the coupling constant is to gradually insert a piece of dielectric such as Teflon in front of the iris. The Teflon tuner may be inserted perpendicular to the narrow wall of the waveguide, and this allows the iris of a rectangular TE_{101} cavity to be tuned conveniently while the cavity remains in the magnetic field. It does not provide as wide a range of tuning conditions as the screw arrangement. Variable coupling to resonant cavities is discussed by Gould and Cunliffe (1956), Gordon (1961), and Faulker and Holman (1963) [see also, Ager, Cole, and Lambe (1963)].

Two single crystals of Al_2O_3 may be used to produce simultaneously a high pressure seal and an impedance match to a high Q cavity resonator [Lawson and Smith (1959)]. The resonator supports pressures up to 10^4 bars (see Sec. 16–D).

To connect a coaxial line to a resonant cavity several types of coupling devices may be used, such as loops, probes, and irides. Some specific coupling arrangements are illustrated in Figs. 8–19 and 8–20.

Further information on irides will be found in Sec. 7-K.

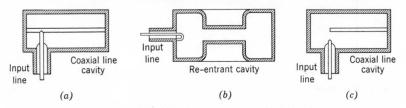

Fig. 8–19.   Methods of connecting a coaxial line to a cavity resonator. (a) Junction coupling; (b) loop coupling; (c) probe coubling [Reintjes and Coate (1952), p. 668].

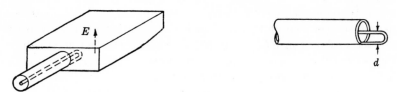

Fig. 8–20.   Loop-coupled rectangular cavity (*RLS*–14, p. 26).

G. Radiation Quality Factor

A resonant cavity without any connecting aperture to the outside world is characterized by its unloaded quality factor Q_u. To be useful it is necessary to connect a cavity to a waveguide by means of an iris or other coupling device, and this entails a lowering of the Q. The extent to which the Q is lowered is characterized by its radiation quality factor Q_r, and so Q_r will be discussed next.

Sometimes it is convenient to represent the circuit of a coupling hole by a transformer with turns ratio n, and the resulting equivalent circuits are shown in Figs. 8–21 and 8–22 for a reaction (reflection) and transmission cavity, respectively. For the reflection cavity circuit, the radiation Q is given by

$$Q_r = L\omega/R_G n^2 \qquad (1)$$

where R_G includes the characteristic impedance of the waveguide plus the generator impedance. The unloaded Q, including ohmic losses in the cavity walls and dielectric losses in the sample, is

$$Q_u = L\omega/R_c \qquad (2)$$

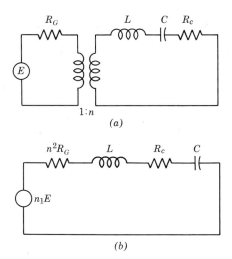

(a)

(b)

Fig. 8–21. (a) Equivalent circuit of a reflection cavity; (b) alternative form for the equivalent circuit of a reflection cavity.

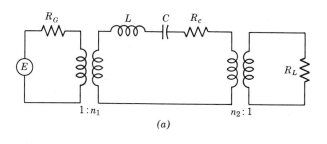

(a)

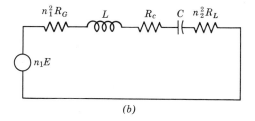

(b)

Fig. 8–22. (a) Equivalent circuit of a transmission cavity; (b) alternative form for the equivalent circuit of a transmission cavity (RLS-11, p. 290).

The ratio of these Q's equals the coupling parameter β

$$\beta = Q_u/Q_r = R_G n^2/R_c \qquad (3)$$

The radiation Q represents losses due to power which may be considered as leaving the cavity through the coupling hole to be dissipated in R_G, while the unloaded Q here represents losses due to the cavity alone. The overall or loaded Q_L is given by

$$1/Q_L = 1/Q_r + 1/Q_u \qquad (4)$$

If the cavity is perfectly coupled or matched to the waveguide, then

$$\beta = \text{VSWR} = 1 \qquad (5)$$

and at resonance the cavity effectively terminates the transmission line in its characteristic impedance Z_0. For the overcoupled cavity

$$Q_u/Q_r > 1 \qquad (6)$$

and the voltage standing wave ratio VSWR is given by

$$\beta = \text{VSWR} \qquad (7)$$

since the transmission line is effectually terminated by a resistance greater than its characteristic impedance Z_0. The inverse is true in the undercoupled case, where

$$Q_u/Q_r < 1 \qquad (8)$$

and

$$1/\beta = \text{VSWR} \qquad (9)$$

The coupling parameter represents the efficacy with which energy stored in the cavity-coupling system is coupled to the external load, and dissipated there (RLS-11, p. 289).

The transmission cavity with the equivalent circuit shown in Fig. 8–22 [see also Roussy and Felden (1965)] may lose power through each coupling hole so the radiation Q has the form

$$Q_r = L\omega/(R_G n_1^2 + R_L n_2^2) \qquad (10)$$

The input and output cavity coupling parameters denoted by β_1 and β_2, respectively, are defined by

$$\beta_1 = R_G n_1^2 / R_c \tag{11}$$

$$\beta_2 = R_L n_2^2 / R_c \tag{12}$$

Therefore the ratio of Q_u to Q_r is given by

$$Q_u / Q_r = \beta_1 + \beta_2 = (R_G n_1^2 + R_L n_2^2)/R_c \tag{13}$$

If both the generator and detector are matched to the waveguide of characteristic impedance Z_0 then

$$R_G = R_L = Z_0 \tag{14}$$

with the result that

$$Q_u / Q_r = (Z_0 / R_c)\,(n_1^2 + n_2^2) \tag{15}$$

and at the optimum operating conditions we have

$$R_G n_1^2 = R_c = R_L n_2^2 \tag{16}$$

When the resonant cavity terminates the waveguide transmission line, the iris is usually located at a point of maximum tangential H field in the waveguide. Maximum coupling to the resonant cavity occurs if the iris is also located at a point in the cavity where the H field is strong and oriented in the same direction as the H field in the waveguide. In a picturesque way we may say that the **H** vector on the cavity side of the iris is a logical continuation of the **H** vector on the waveguide side. Two ways of coupling a TE_{011} cylindrical cavity resonator to the end of a rectangular waveguide operating in the TE_{10} mode are shown on Fig. 8–23. When the iris is inductive or capacitive, it may be considered as transmitting the rectangular TE_{10} mode, and when it is circular, it may be considered as transmitting the cylindrical TE_{11} mode. If the iris location is changed from the optimum locations shown on Fig. 8–23, the coupling constant decreases and a larger opening must be used to preserve the same Q.

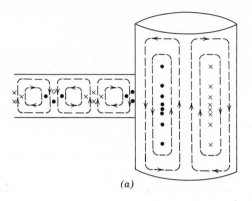

(a)

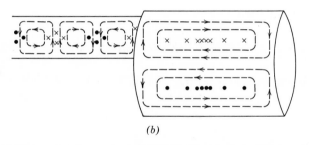

(b)

Fig. 8–23. Two methods of coupling to the TE_{011} mode in a cylindrical resonant cavity: (a) lateral coupling; (b) end plate coupling.

If the resonant cavity in Fig. 8–23a is rotated by 90° about the waveguide axis, it will be properly oriented to excite the cylindrical TM_{111} mode, which is degenerate with the cylindrical TE_{011} mode.

The coupling parameters are of great practical importance because the ESR sensitivity depends upon whether or not the cavity is overcoupled or undercoupled, and also upon the extent of its deviation from perfect coupling or match (cf. Sec. 4-A). Frequently wavemeters (frequency meters) are undercoupled to the sidewall of a waveguide so that when they are off resonance they produce very little disturbance in the waveguide VSWR and mode configurations. This absorption cavity coupling is seldom used for ESR sample cavity applications (see Sec. 14-G).

H. Filling Factors

The ESR signal at resonance is proportional to the amount of power absorbed by the sample, and this in turn is proportional to the average value of the microwave magnetic field $\langle H_1{}^2 \rangle_s$ at the sample, where, in general,

$$\langle H_1{}^2 \rangle = \frac{\int H_1{}^2 dV}{\int dV} = \frac{1}{V} \int H_1{}^2 dV \tag{1}$$

More precisely, H_1 is the component of the rf magnetic field in the direction of the static magnetic field. If the sample has an rf susceptibility χ'' and a volume V_s, then the amount of power absorbed is proportional to $\chi'' V_s \langle H_1{}^2 \rangle_s$. The resonance absorption will decrease the Q of the resonant cavity, and this may be expressed mathematically by adding the sample loss term Q_χ to eq. (8-B-6) as follows:

$$1/Q = 1/Q_u + 1/Q_\epsilon + 1/Q_r \qquad \text{off resonance} \tag{2}$$

$$1/Q = 1/Q_u + 1/Q_\epsilon + 1/Q_r + 1/Q_\chi \qquad \text{at resonance} \tag{3}$$

where Q_χ is the ratio of the power stored in the overall cavity volume V_c to the power dissipated in the sample

$$Q_\chi = \frac{\frac{1}{2}\mu_0 \int_{\text{cavity}} H_1{}^2 dV}{\frac{1}{2}\mu_0 \int_{\text{sample}} \chi'' H_1{}^2 dV} \tag{4}$$

$$= \frac{V_c \langle H_1{}^2 \rangle_c}{\chi'' V_s \langle H_1{}^2 \rangle_s} \tag{5}$$

Equation (5) may be expressed in terms of the filling factor η

$$Q_x = 1/(\chi'' \eta) \tag{6}$$

where η is defined by

$$\eta = \frac{\int_{\text{sample}} H_1{}^2 dV}{\int_{\text{cavity}} H_1{}^2 dV} = \frac{V_s \langle H_1{}^2 \rangle_s}{V_c \langle H_1{}^2 \rangle_c} \tag{7}$$

In the absence of saturation effects the sensitivity of an ESR spectrometer is inversely proportional to Q_x, as explained in Sec. 14-C.

It is usually easy to obtain the volume ratio V_s/V_c, but the ratio $\langle H_1^2 \rangle_s / \langle H_1^2 \rangle_c$ requires the integration of H_1^2 over both the sample and the cavity. This will be done for several cases that commonly arise in ESR experiments.

First consider a very small sample placed in the center of the sample tube shown on Fig. 8-5. The microwave field H_1 has a sinusoidal variation along the axis of the tube with a maximum in the center of the TE_{102} rectangular cavity, and zero at the top and bottom. The microwave magnetic field configurations in this TE_{102} mode resonator [see Heuer (1965)] are given explicitly by eqs. (8-C-22) to (8-C-24)

$$H_x = \frac{H_0}{[1 + (d/2a)^2]^{1/2}} \sin \frac{\pi x}{a} \cos \frac{2\pi z}{d} \tag{8}$$

$$H_z = - \frac{H_0}{[1 + (2a/d)^2]^{1/2}} \cos \frac{\pi x}{a} \sin \frac{2\pi z}{d} \tag{9}$$

$$E_y = (\mu/\epsilon)^{1/2} H_0 \sin \frac{\pi x}{a} \sin \frac{2\pi z}{d} \tag{10}$$

$$H_x = E_x = E_z = 0 \tag{11}$$

where $m = 1$, $n = 0$, and $p = 2$. The x direction is taken along the sample tube, and the z direction along the length of the cavity, in accordance with Fig. 8–3. The sample is located at $x = \frac{1}{2}a$, $y = \frac{1}{2}b$, and $z = \frac{1}{2}d$, and as a result at the sample position, H_z vanishes and $H_1 = H_x$, with the explicit value

$$H_1 = \frac{H_0}{[1 + (d/2a)^2]^{1/2}} \tag{12}$$

Since the sample is small (dimensions $\ll a$, b, and d), H_1 is essentially constant over its volume, and so

$$\langle H_1^2 \rangle_s = H_1^2 = \frac{H_0^2}{1 + (d/2a)^2} \tag{13}$$

To find $\langle H_1^2 \rangle_c$ it is necessary to integrate H_1^2

$$H_1^2 = H_x^2 + H_z^2 \tag{14}$$

over the cavity using the expression (1)

$$\langle H_1^2 \rangle_c = \frac{1}{abd} \left[\int_0^a \int_0^b \int_0^d H_x^2 \, dx \, dy \, dz + \int_0^a \int_0^b \int_0^d H_z^2 \, dx \, dy \, dz \right] \quad (15)$$

$$= \frac{1}{ad} \left[\int_0^a \int_0^d H_x^2 \, dx \, dz + \int_0^a \int_0^d H_z^2 \, dx \, dz \right] \quad (16)$$

since the electromagnetic fields are independent of y, and the cavity volume V_c equals abd. Each integration gives either $a/2$ or $d/2$ so that

$$\langle H_1^2 \rangle_c = \frac{1}{4} H_0^2 \left[\frac{1}{1 + (d/2a)^2} + \frac{1}{1 + (2a/d)^2} \right] \quad (17)$$

$$= \frac{1}{4} H_0^2 \quad (18)$$

independent of the ratio $2a/d$. The filling factor η then becomes

$$\eta = \frac{V_s}{V_c} \frac{4}{1 + (d/2a)^2} = 4 \frac{V_s}{V_c} \left(\frac{\lambda}{\lambda_g} \right)^2 \quad (19)$$

using eq. (7). Usually $d \approx 2a$, and when d actually equals $2a$ then η becomes

$$\eta = 2 V_s / V_c \quad (20)$$

A comparison of eqs. (13) and (18) indicates that, in a TE_{102} rectangular resonant cavity with $d = 2a$, the maximum squared rf field H_x at the sample is about twice the average value in the cavity.

When an ESR spectrometer is used to study samples of fairly high electrical conductivity (e.g., in cyclotron resonance), it is sometimes convenient to construct one wall of the cavity out of the sample itself. If the end of a rectangular TE_{102} cavity (the side opposite the iris) consists of a sample of effective thickness δ, then $z = d$, and eqs. (8) and (9) become

$$H_x = \frac{H_0 \sin \pi x/a}{[1 + (d/2a)^2]^{1/2}} \quad (21)$$

$$H_z = E_x = 0 \quad (22)$$

Consequently, $\langle H_1^2 \rangle_s$ is

$$\langle H_1^2 \rangle_s = \frac{H_0^2}{ab\delta[1 + (d/2a)^2]} \int_0^a \sin^2 \frac{\pi x}{a} \, dx \int_0^b dy \int_{d-\delta}^d dz \qquad (23)$$

$$= \frac{1}{2} \frac{H_0^2}{1 + (d/2a)^2} \qquad (24)$$

As a result

$$\eta = \frac{2V_s}{V_c} \frac{1}{1 + (d/2a)^2} \qquad (25)$$

and if $2a = d$

$$\eta = V_s/V_c \qquad (26)$$

One can easily show that for a "square mode" cavity $(2a = d)$, this result is independent of z [Poole (1958)] since a uniform planar sample located across the waveguide in the xy plane has the filling factor

$$\eta = V_s/V_c \qquad (26)$$

for all z. This case also corresponds closely to a flat quartz aqueous solution cell. Materials of high dielectric loss are efficiently studied with this arrangement. The Hedvig (1959) equation (8-I-17) modifies this result for high dielectric constants.

If the sample tube of radius r in Fig. 8–5 is completely filled, then one has $V_s = \pi r^2 a$, and

$$\langle H_1^2 \rangle_s = \frac{H_0^2}{\pi r^2 a} \left[\frac{1}{1 + (d/2a)^2} \int_0^a \sin^2 \frac{\pi x}{a} \, dx \int_0^r \cos^2 \frac{2\pi z}{d} \, dz \int_{-r \sin \phi}^{r \sin \phi} dy \right.$$

$$\left. + \frac{1}{1 + (2a/d)^2} \int_0^a \cos^2 \frac{\pi x}{a} \, dx \int_0^r \sin^2 \frac{2\pi z}{d} \, dz \int_{-r \sin \phi}^{r \sin \phi} dy \right] \qquad (27)$$

where the relevant coordinate system is shown in Fig. 8–24. The integration over x gives $a/2$ immediately since the sample tube extends uniformly over the entire cavity width from $x = 0$ to $x = a$, and one easily obtains

$$\langle H_1^2 \rangle_s = \frac{H_0^2}{\pi r} \left\{ \frac{1}{1 + (d/2a)^2} \int_{-r}^{r} \left[1 - \left(\frac{z}{r} \right)^2 \right]^{1/2} \cos^2 \frac{2\pi z}{d} \, dz \right.$$
$$\left. + \frac{1}{1 + (2a/d)^2} \int_{-r}^{r} \left[1 - \left(\frac{z}{r} \right)^2 \right]^{1/2} \sin^2 \frac{2\pi z}{d} \, dz \right\} \tag{28}$$

where $\sin \phi = [1 - (z/r)^2]^{1/2}$. If we assume $2a = d$ then this simplifies to

$$\langle H_1^2 \rangle_s = \frac{H_0^2}{\pi r} \int_0^r \left[1 - \left(\frac{z^2}{r} \right) \right]^{1/2} dz \tag{29}$$

$$= \tfrac{1}{4} H_0^2 \tag{30}$$

and the filling factor is

$$\eta = V_s / V_c \tag{31}$$

Note that this result is independent of r (except for the dependence of V_s on r). It is identical to that obtained above in the parallel plane case for the same condition of $2a = d$. Equation (31) will of course be much more complicated when $2a \neq d$. If $2a \neq d$ then an approximate expression may be obtained by assuming $(2a/d)^{\pm 1} = 1 \pm \delta$, where $\delta \ll 1$ and $z/r \ll 1$ over the range of integration, and by

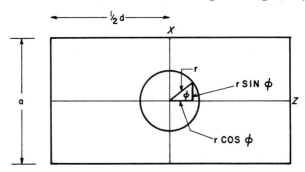

Fig. 8–24. Coordinate system for perturbation theory calculation of the filling factor η of a dielectric rod in a rectangular TE_{102} mode resonant cavity.

expanding the sines and cosines in power series.   This will be left as an *exercitatio lectori.*

All of the above filling factor calculations were for the TE_{102} mode rectangular resonant cavity.   The second most important cavity resonator for use in ESR spectrometers is the cylindrical TE_{011} type, and its electromagnetic wave configurations are (see Sec. 8-D)

$$H_r = \frac{H_0 J_0'(k_c r) \cos(\pi z/d)}{\{1 + [(k_c a)_{01}'d/\pi a]^2\}^{1/2}} \tag{32}$$

$$H_z = \frac{H_0 J_0(k_c r) \sin(\pi z/d)}{\{1 + [\pi a/(k_c a)_{01}'d]^2\}^{1/2}} \tag{33}$$

$$E_\phi = -(\mu/\epsilon)^{1/2} H_0 J_0'(k_c r) \sin(\pi z/d) \tag{34}$$

$$H_\phi = E_r = E_z = 0 \tag{35}$$

where the root of $J_0'(k_c r)$ is given by $(k_c a)_{01}' = 3.832$.   The electric field equations are not needed here, but are merely listed for completeness.   The average value of H_1 over the volume of the cavity of length d and radius a is given by eq. (1).

$$\langle H_1^2 \rangle_c$$

$$= \frac{H_0^2}{\pi a^2 d} \left[\frac{1}{1 + [(k_c a)_{01}'d/\pi a]^2} \int_0^a J_0'^2(k_c r) r\, dr \int_0^d \cos^2 \frac{\pi z}{d}\, dz \int_0^{2\pi} d\phi \right.$$

$$\left. + \frac{1}{1 + [\pi a/(k_c a)_{01}'d]^2} \int_0^a J_0^2(k_c r) r\, dr \int_0^d \sin^2 \frac{\pi z}{d}\, dz \int_0^{2\pi} d\phi \right] \tag{36}$$

The second and third integrals of each pair give $d/2$ and 2π, respectively, so that

$$\langle H_1^2 \rangle_c = \frac{H_0^2}{a^2} \left[\frac{1}{1 + [(k_c a)_{01}'d/\pi a]^2} \int_0^a J_0'^2(k_c r) r\, dr \right.$$

$$\left. + \frac{1}{1 + [\pi a/(k_c a)_{01}'d]^2} \int_0^a J_0^2(k_c r) r\, dr \right] \tag{37}$$

These integrals may be evaluated from the useful general relations [e.g., see Margenau and Murphy (1956); Jahnke and Emde (1933)]

$$\int_0^r J_n^2(k_c r)\, r dr = \frac{r^2}{2}\left[J_n^2(k_c r) - J_{n-1}(k_c r)\, J_{n+1}(k_c r) \right] \quad (38)$$

$$J_n'(k_c r) = (n/k_c r)\, J_n(k_c r) - J_{n+1}(k_c r) \quad (39)$$

$$(2n/k_c r)\, J_n(k_c r) = J_{n-1}(k_c r) + J_{n+1}(k_c r) \quad (40)$$

which give the pertinent particular expressions

$$\int_0^r J_0^2(k_c r)\, r dr = (r^2/2)\, [J_0^2(k_c r) + J_1^2(k_c r)] \quad (41)$$

$$\int_0^r J_0'^2(k_c r)\, r dr = (r^2/2)\, [J_0^2(k_c r) - (2/k_c r)\, J_0(k_c r)\, J_1(k_c r)$$
$$+ J_1^2(k_c r)] \quad (42)$$

$$J_0'(k_c r) = -J_1(k_c r) = J_{-1}(k_c r) \quad (43)$$

$$J_2(k_c r) = (2/k_c r)\, J_1(k_c r) - J_0(k_c r) \quad (44)$$

The application of the boundary conditions for this mode yields

$$J_0'(k_c a) = J_{\pm 1}(k_c a) = 0 \quad (45)$$

with the Bessel function root $(k_c a)_{01}'$ obtained from Table 8–1

$$(k_c a)_{01}' = 3.832 \quad (46)$$

$$J_0(k_c a) = 0.4028 \quad (47)$$

$$J_0(0) = 2 \lim_{r \to 0} \left[\frac{J_1(k_c r)}{k_c r} \right] = 1 \quad (48)$$

The maximum value of $J_0'(k_c r)$

$$\max J_0'(k_c r) = 0.5819 \quad (49)$$

occurs at the radial distance

$$k_c r = 1.84 \tag{50}$$

and the only zero of $J_c(k_c r)$ occurs at the value

$$k_c r = 2.405 \tag{51}$$

which is listed in Table 8-1. Using these expressions and eqs. (17) and (18), eq. (37) is easily evaluated to give

$$\langle H_1{}^2 \rangle_c = \frac{H_0{}^2 J_0{}^2 (k_c a)}{2} = 0.0811 H_0{}^2 \tag{52}$$

a fantastically simple answer for such a complex expression. This derivation was carried out in detail to illustrate the method of handling an equation like (37).

For a small sample located exactly in the center of the resonant cavity one has $r = 0$ and $z = \frac{1}{2}d$ to give $H_1 = H_z$ and

$$\langle H_1{}^2 \rangle_s = \frac{H_0{}^2}{1 + (0.82a/d)^2} \tag{53}$$

since $J_0(0) = 1$, and the filling factor is

$$\eta = \frac{12.33}{1 + (0.82a/d)^2} \frac{V_s}{V_c} \tag{54}$$

This may be expressed in terms of the free space wavelength λ and the cutoff wavelength $\lambda_c = 2\pi a/(k_c a)_{01}{}'$

$$\eta = 12.33 \quad (V_s/V_c) \, (\lambda/\lambda_c)^2 \tag{55}$$

In a typical case $(\lambda/\lambda_c)^2 = 2/3$.

If the sample is contained in a tube of radius r which extends along the axis of the cavity from the top to the bottom it will lie along loops of $H_1 = H_z$, as shown on Fig. 8-11. The filling factor may be obtained from eq. (8-H-36) by integrating from 0 to r instead of from 0 to a. The $H_z{}^2$ integral remains unchanged, while the first $H_r{}^2$

integral is reduced by $\frac{1}{2}$ since only the component $H_r \cos \phi$ is perpendicular to the applied field. In other words, $\langle H_1{}^2 \rangle_s$ is defined as $\langle (\mathbf{H}_1 \cdot \mathbf{H}_{dc})^2 \rangle_s / H_{dc}{}^2$ where H_{dc} is the "constant" applied field. Thus we obtain

$$\langle H_1{}^2 \rangle_s = \frac{H_0{}^2}{2} \left[\frac{J_0{}^2(k_c r) - (2/k_c r) \, J_0(k_c r) \, J_1{}^2(k_c r) + J_1{}^2(k_c r)}{1 + (1.22d/a)^2} \right.$$

$$\left. + \frac{J_0{}^2(k_c r) + J_1{}^2(k_c r)}{2[1 + (0.82a/d)^2]} \right] \qquad (56)$$

When $r \ll a$, then $J_0(k_c r) \gg J_1(k_c r)$ and $(2/k_c r) \, J_1(k_c r) \sim 1$, which renders the first term negligible, so we obtain the approximation

$$\langle H_1{}^2 \rangle_s \approx \frac{J_0 \, (k_c r) H_0{}^2}{2[1 + (0.82a/d)^2]} \qquad (57)$$

The filling factor for $k_c r \ll 1$ is [setting $J_0(k_c r) = 1$]

$$\eta \approx 6.16 \, (V_s/V_c) \, (\lambda/\lambda_c)^2 \qquad (58)$$

which is half the value for a point sample [eq. (52)].

We have been calculating the average value of H_1 in the sample relative to its average value in the cavity itself. Ginzton (1957) describes a metallic disk for determining H_1 in a cavity. However, it is often not convenient to measure directly the average value of H_1 in the cavity, but instead we ordinarily measure the power incident upon the resonant cavity. Thus it will be useful to compute the ratio of H_1 expressed in gauss inside the cavity to Poynting's vector $\frac{1}{2}(\mathbf{E} \times \mathbf{H})$ expressed in watts incident on the cavity. A similar calculation by Meyer (1955) is quoted by Marr and Swarup (1960). Robinson (1963) uses an ESR signal to map out the rf magnetic fields in microwave structures, and other perturbing samples were used by Boudouris (1964) and Scaglia (1965) for this purpose.

For a TE_{10} rectangular waveguide mode the incident power per unit area A is

$$dP_w/dA = \frac{1}{2} |\mathbf{E} \times \mathbf{H}| \qquad \text{W/m} \qquad (59)$$

$$= \frac{1}{2} E_y H_x \qquad \text{W/m} \qquad (60)$$

where the factor of one half results from averaging over time. Since from eq. (4-D-16) [aside from a phase factor]

$$E_y = Z_{TE} H_x \tag{61}$$

with the waveguide impedance Z_{TE} given explicitly by

$$Z_{TE} = (\mu/\epsilon)^{1/2} [1 - (f_c/f)^2]^{-1/2}$$
$$= (\mu/\epsilon)^{1/2} [1 + (d/2a)^2]^{1/2} = (\mu/\epsilon)^{1/2} \lambda_g/\lambda \tag{62}$$

from eq. (4-D-18) we obtain

$$dP_w/dA = \tfrac{1}{2} Z_{TE} H_x{}^2 \tag{63}$$

Using eq. (8) and the notation $H_w = H_0$

$$\frac{dP_w}{dA} = \tfrac{1}{2} Z_{TE} H_w{}^2 \sin^2 \frac{\pi x}{a} \tag{64}$$

where the subscript w denotes the microwaves in the incident waveguide in contrast to the subscript c which refers to analogous quantities within the resonant cavity. The power P_w is a function of y, so we integrate over the waveguide cross section, to give

$$P_w = \frac{Z_{TE} H_w{}^2}{2} \int_0^a \sin^2 \frac{\pi x}{a} \, dx \int_0^b dy \tag{65}$$

$$= \tfrac{1}{4} ab H_w{}^2 Z_{TE} \tag{66}$$

where H_w is in ampere turns and a, b, and d are in meters. For X band, $a = 2.3 \times 10^{-2}$ m, $b = 1.0 \times 10^{-2}$ m, $2a \sim d$, and $(f_c/f)^2 \sim \tfrac{1}{2}$,

$$Z_{TE} = 120\pi/0.5^{1/2} = 533 \quad \Omega \tag{67}$$

and therefore

$$H_w \sim 6 \, P_w{}^{1/2} \quad \text{At} \tag{68}$$

This must be multiplied by $4\pi \times 10^{-7}$ H/m to convert it to the units of magnetic induction B, and then by 10^4 to convert it to gauss (or oersted)

$$H_w \sim 0.08 \, P_w{}^{1/2} \quad \text{G} \tag{69}$$

One should bear in mind that H_w is the maximum value of the **H** vector that is propagating along the waveguide, while the average value of $\langle H^2 \rangle_w$ is

$$\langle H^2 \rangle_w = \tfrac{1}{4} H_w^2 = 2 \times 10^{-3} P_w \tag{70}$$

If the resonant cavity is matched to the transmission line then all of the incident microwave energy will enter the cavity and be dissipated there. Under these conditions the loaded Q is given by [see Zverev (1961)]

$$Q_L = \frac{\omega\mu}{2P_w} \int_{\text{cavity}} H_1^2 dV \tag{71}$$

where the numerator is evaluated at a time when the **E** vector is zero and H_1 is a maximum throughout the cavity. If the microwave cavity is the rectangular TE_{102} type with the same cross section as the waveguide, then one has for the H_1 field in the cavity

$$\langle H_1^2 \rangle_c = Q_L \langle H^2 \rangle_w \tag{72}$$

$$= 2 \times 10^{-3} Q_L P_w \tag{73}$$

Therefore 1 W of power incident upon a TE_{102} mode rectangular resonant cavity with a loaded Q of 4000 produces therein an average rf field of about 3 G. If the resonant cavity is of another type then one has

$$\langle H_1^2 \rangle_c = Q_L (V_w/V_c) \langle H_1^2 \rangle_w \tag{74}$$

where V_w is the volume of a section of waveguide one guide wavelength long. This expression may be employed to redefine the filling factor η so that it relates the average value of H_1 in the resonant cavity to that in the waveguide under matched conditions

$$\eta = (1/Q_L) (V_s/V_w) (\langle H_1^2 \rangle_s/\langle H_1^2 \rangle_w) \tag{75}$$

Equation (70) may be used to obtain the practical formulae

$$\langle H_1^2 \rangle_c = 2 \times 10^{-3} P_w Q_L (V_w/V_c) \tag{76}$$

$$\eta = \frac{5 \times 10^2 \langle H_1^2 \rangle_s}{P_w Q_L} \frac{V_s}{V_w} \tag{77}$$

These formulae are very important because they allow one to deduce the actual magnetic field at the sample when making relaxation time measurements.   For example, one may compute the filling factor η in the manner discussed above, and easily measure the microwave power P_w, cavity Q_L, sample volume V_s, and the volume V_w of the section of waveguide that is one guide wavelength long.   Then it is easy to calculate $\langle H_1{}^2 \rangle_s$ from the relation

$$\langle H_1{}^2 \rangle_s = 2 \times 10^{-3} \, P_w Q_L \eta \, (V_w/V_s) \tag{78}$$

Electron spin resonance spectrometers are usually operated with an intentional slight mismatch in order to produce a finite "leakage" of microwave power at the detector crystal.   To account approximately for this effect, the last few equations must have the term $(1 - |\Gamma|^2)$ added to them where Γ is the reflection coefficient at the cavity. Accordingly,

$$\langle H_1{}^2 \rangle_c = (1 - |\Gamma|^2) \, Q_L \, (V_w/V_c) \, \langle H^2 \rangle_w \tag{79}$$

$$= 2 \times 10^{-3} \, (1 - |\Gamma|^2) \, P_w Q_L \eta \, (V_w/V_c) \tag{80}$$

where $\langle H^2 \rangle_w$ refers to the incident wave only, and therefore satisfies eq. (66).   Similarly,

$$\eta = \frac{1}{(1 - |\Gamma|^2) Q_L} \left(\frac{V_s}{V_w} \right) \frac{\langle H_1{}^2 \rangle_s}{\langle H^2 \rangle_w} \tag{81}$$

$$= \frac{5 \times 10^2 \, \langle H_1{}^2 \rangle_s}{(1 - |\Gamma|^2) \, P_w Q_L} \left(\frac{V_s}{V_w} \right) \tag{82}$$

$$\langle H_1{}^2 \rangle_s = 2 \times 10^{-3} \, (1 - |\Gamma|^2) \, P_w Q_L \eta \, (V_w/V_s) \tag{83}$$

$$= \eta \, (V_c/V_s) \, \langle H_1{}^2 \rangle_c \tag{84}$$

The last equation is repeated for ease of reference.

We will conclude this section by calculating several of these quantities for both a rectangular TE_{102} and two cylindrical TE_{011}

mode X band resonant cavities. This will afford us the opportunity to compare the relative merits of the two cavity types.

For the rectangular cavity let $d = 2a = 4.5$ cm and $b = 1$ cm so that V_c is close to 10 cm^3. Since the cross section of this cavity (1 $\times$ 2.25 cm) is the same as that of the waveguide and $d = \lambda_g$ it follows that $V_w = 10$ cm^3 also [see, however, Fig. 8–25 and Altschuler (1963)]. The cylindrical cavity shown in Fig. 8–13 has $a = 2.05$ cm, and if we let the length $d = 4.1$ cm, then $a/d \sim \frac{1}{2}$ and $V_c \sim 54$ cm^3. For comparison purposes a second cylindrical cavity of the same frequency (9.7 kMc) but with an a/d ratio of 3/2 will also be considered. Its radius may be determined from Fig. 8–7 and the ratio of the Q_L values for the two cylindrical cavities may be deduced from Fig. 8–8. The data on these three cavities are listed in Table 8–2.

We will use three samples. The first will be a small piece of DPPH of volume $V_s = 10^{-3}$ cm^3, the second will fill a cylindrical tube 6 cm

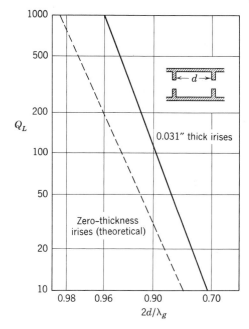

Fig. 8–25. Foreshortening of rectangular waveguide cavity as a function of loaded Q (RLS–9, p. 655).

long with a radius $r = 0.2$ cm; the third will be the entire cavity itself (e.g., filled with gas). The corresponding sample volumes are

$$V_{s_1} = 10^{-3} \text{ cm}^3 \tag{85a}$$

$$V_{s_2} = 4\pi \times 10^{-2} d \tag{85b}$$

$$V_{s_3} = V_c \tag{85c}$$

The effective tube length d differs slightly for the three cavities. The ratios of these sample volumes to each cavity volume are listed in Table 8–2, and the filling factors are included for each case.

TABLE 8–2

Comparison of a Cylindrical TE_{011} Mode Resonator and a Rectangular TE_{102} Mode Resonator at X Band ($V_w = 10$ cm³) with about 100 mW $= P_w$ Incident upon the Cavity

			Cylindrical cavities		Rectangular
	Equation	Sample no. [a]	$a/d = \frac{1}{2}$	$a/d = 3/2$	cavity ($d = 2a$)
Dimensions, cm			$a = 2.05$ $d = 4.1$	$a = 3.0$ $d = 2.0$	$1 \times 2.25 \times 4.5$
V_c, cm³	—	—	54	57	10
Q_L	—	—	12,000	8000	4000
V_w/V_c	—	—	0.19	0.175	1
$(<H_1^2>_c)^{1/2}$, G	8–76	—	0.68	0.53	0.9
V_s/V_c	—	1	1.85×10^{-5}	1.7×10^{-5}	10^{-4}
η	8–54, 8–20	1	1.6×10^{-4}	8.2×10^{-5}	2×10^{-4}
$(<H_1^2>_s)^{1/2}$, G	8–7	1	2.0	1.2	1.3
V_s/V_c	—	2	9.5×10^{-3}	4.3×10^{-3}	2.8×10^{-2}
η	8–58, 8–31	2	4.2×10^{-2}	1×10^{-2}	2.8×10^{-2}
$(<H_1^2>_s)^{1/2}$, G	8–7	2	1.4	0.85	0.9
V_s/V_c	—	3	1.00	1.00	1.00
η	8–56, 8–7	3	0.85	0.69	1.00
$(<H_1^2>_s)^{1/2}$, G	8–7	3	0.63	0.44	0.9

[a] Sample No. 1: small piece DPPH ($V_s = 10^{-3}$ cm³). Sample No. 2: cylindrical tube of radius $r = 0.2$ cm and effective length $= d$. ($V_s = 0.126d$ cm³). Sample No. 3: entire cavity filled ($V_s = V_c$).

Let us assume a klystron power output of 200 mW so that 100 mW are incident on the cavity with the other 100 mW dissipated in the matched load of the magic T. If we work with a leakage of 0.1 mW on the crystal detector, then the power reflected from the resonant cavity will be about 0.2 mW since 50% is lost in each passage through the magic T. This means that at the cavity one may estimate

$$|\Gamma|^2 \sim \frac{H_1{}^2{}_{\text{reflected}}}{H_1{}^2{}_{\text{absorbed}}} \sim \frac{2 \times 10^{-4}\text{W}}{10^{-1}\text{W}} = 2 \times 10^{-3} \qquad (86)$$

and the voltage standing wave ratio VSWR

$$\text{VSWR} = \frac{1 + |\Gamma|}{1 - |\Gamma|} \sim 1 + 2|\Gamma| \qquad (87)$$

is very, very close to one. As a result the term $(1 - |\Gamma|^2)$ in eqs. (79)–(83) may be neglected. Equation (86) is only valid when the cavity is close to match (i.e., $|\Gamma|^2 \ll 1$).

We may estimate that the unloaded Q's of the rectangular and the two cylindrical cavities respectively are 8000, 16,000, and 24,000, so the corresponding loaded Q's will be half of these values, as shown in Table 8–2. If the cavity is not close to match then a more subtle analysis is required.

There are several interesting things to be learned from Table 8–2. In the first place, the cylindrical cavities have much higher Q's than the rectangular cavity, and so they store more microwave energy. However, this energy is spread over a larger volume so that the average microwave magnetic field strength is about the same in all three cases. The cylindrical cavity concentrates H_1 to a greater extent in the center (particularly for a small a/d ratio), but for cylindrical sample tubes extending the length of the cavity some of the total H_1 is ineffective because the radial component is, in general, not perpendicular to the large applied magnetic field. All of the microwave magnetic field components in the rectangular TE_{102} cavity are perpendicular to the applied field. Note that the sensitivity for the cylindrical cavity is improved by decreasing its radius to length ratio a/d. The Q is a maximum when $d = 2a$, so the optimum sensitivity will be obtained with $d > 2a$.

The calculations carried out above neglect the manner in which the real and imaginary parts of the sample's dielectric constant perturb the value of the rf magnetic field (i.e., $\langle H_1{}^2 \rangle_s$) at the sample. this effect may be appreciable in magnitude. Kramer and Müller-Warmuth (1963) took account of the extent to which a sample of high dielectric constant "draws in" the rf field H_1. They defined a dielectric enhancement factor $K_d \geq 1$

$$H_{1\epsilon} = K_d H_1 \qquad (88)$$

where H_1 is the field in the absence of the sample, and $H_{1\epsilon}$ is the field in the sample. Table 8–3 gives some empirically determined dielectric enhancement factors for several commonly used organic solvents. The measurements were carried out at 3000 Mc in flat cells placed in the rectangular TE_{105} resonator shown on Fig. 8–32. It must be emphasized that K_d is strongly dependent on the cell dimensions and shape. The solvents listed in Table 8–3 are frequently employed in electrolytic studies (see Sec. 15-F).

The detailed calculations presented in this section furnish an insight into the manner in which the electromagnetic field distribution in the resonant cavity interacts with the sample. Each paramagnetic spin interacts with its local H_1 field, and so it is the average of the rf magnetic field magnitude which is responsible for the sensitivity. We calculated $(\langle H_1{}^2 \rangle_s)^{1/2}$ as a measure of H_1 at the sample since the

TABLE 8–3

Dielectric Enhancement Factors K_d at 3000 Mc for Several Commonly Used Organic Solvents [see eq. (88)] [Kramer and Müller-Warmuth (1963)]

Inner Dimensions of cell, mm	Solvent	K_d
$1 \times 17 \times 50$	Benzene	1.18
	Dioxane	1.48
	Diethyleneglycoldimethylether (DGDE)	1.61
	Tetrahydrofuran (THF)	1.74
	Dimethylglycol (DMG)	2.35
$2 \times 26 \times 45$	Ethylalcohol	1.05
	Methylalcohol	1.13
	Water	1.46

average $\langle H_1 \rangle_s$ often vanishes from cancellation between oppositely polarized (plus and minus) values of H_1. One may consider $\langle H_1^2 \rangle_s$ as the quantity which is measured in an ESR experiment.

It is shown in Sec. 14-D that for a particular sample and ESR spectrometer the minimum detectable number of spins $N_{\min}$ below saturation obeys the proportionality [eq. (14-D-12)]

$$N_{\min} \propto V_s/[Q_L \eta \omega_0^2 (P_w)^{1/2}] \tag{89}$$

The total number of spins in the sample N_{spin} is related to the minimum detectable number through the signal to noise ratio y_m' [eq. (14-D-9)].

$$N_{\text{spin}} = y_m' N_{\min} \tag{90}$$

The quantities V_s, η, and $P_w^{1/2}$ of eq. (89) may be calculated by methods discussed in this section, and Secs. 8-B through 8-D contain formulae for computing the Q of rectangular and cylindrical cavities. Table 8–2 lists typical values of these quantities.

Muromtsev, Piskunov, and Verein (1962) tabulated parameters for several resonant cavities, and applied the results to ESR studies at high power levels.

The significance of many of the results obtained in this section will become clear after reading Chap. 14, and in particular, Sec. 14-D.

I. Factors Which Effect the Resonance Frequency of Cavities

In performing experiments with an ESR spectrometer it is frequently necessary to introduce a sample, modulation posts, a Dewar, etc. into a resonant cavity. Such objects serve to change both the frequency and the Q of the resonator. To provide an insight into the reasons for these changes, a few words will be said about factors which alter the electromagnetic characteristics of resonators.

The preceding sections of this chapter considered resonant cavities in free space, so that they were characterized by the dielectric constant ϵ_0 and the permeability μ_0. The angular frequency $\omega_0 = 2\pi f_0$ and the wavelength λ_0 in the unbounded dielectric obeyed the relation

$$\lambda_0 \omega_0 = 2\pi(\mu_0 \epsilon_0)^{-1/2} = 2\pi c \tag{1}$$

where c is the velocity of light *in vacuo*. If a second lossless medium is characterized by a different dielectric constant ϵ and the same permeability μ_0 then one has

$$\lambda_1\omega_1 = 2\pi(\mu_0\epsilon_1)^{-1/2} = 2\pi v_1 \qquad (2)$$

where v_1 is the velocity in medium 1. If the electromagnetic waves of the same frequency $\omega_1 = \omega_0$ are propagated in each boundless medium, then the wavelengths will obey the relation

$$\lambda_1/\lambda_0 = (\epsilon_1/\epsilon_0)^{-1/2} \qquad (3)$$

The quantities λ_g, λ_c, and the various k_i are defined geometrically at the beginning of Secs. 8-C and 8-D in terms of the cavity dimensions and type of mode. The wavelength is still the actual distance between successive mode patterns; changing the dielectric constant merely changes the resonant frequency associated with the wavelength.

For a dielectric filled waveguide the lowest frequency that will propagate is called the cutoff frequency $\omega_c = 2\pi f_c$, and it is given by

$$\omega_c = c(\epsilon/\epsilon_0)^{-1/2} (2\pi/\lambda_c) = ck_c/(\epsilon/\epsilon_0)^{-1/2} \qquad (4)$$

where the subscript 1 is omitted for simplicity. This has the explicit values

$$\omega_c = \begin{cases} \dfrac{c}{(\epsilon/\epsilon_0)^{1/2}} \left[\left(\dfrac{\pi m}{a}\right)^2 + \left(\dfrac{\pi n}{b}\right)^2 \right]^{1/2} & \text{rectangular mode} \\[4mm] \dfrac{c}{(\epsilon/\epsilon_0)^{1/2}} \dfrac{(k_c a)_{mn}}{a} & \text{cylindrical } TM \text{ mode*} \end{cases} \qquad (5)$$

The quantity $(k_c a)_{mn}$ is a Bessel function root, and so it takes on only the values listed in Table 8-1. Since k_c increases with increasing values of the relative dielectric constant ϵ/ϵ_0 for a fixed cutoff frequency, it follows that correspondingly smaller values of the guide radius a are required to satisfy the condition $J(k_c a) = 0$ [or $J'(k_c a) = 0$] for a given mode. Therefore, dielectric filled waveguide may be scaled down in the ratio $(\epsilon/\epsilon_0)^{-1/2}$ to propagate the same frequency

* For TE modes, replace $(k_c a)_{mn}$ by $(k_c a)_{mn}'$.

(i.e., to have the same value of ω_c). When space is at a premium, such as in a Dewar, one may use a Teflon-filled waveguide. [A ridge waveguide (cf. Sec. 4-F) is also useful for this application.]

If one scales the dimensions of a waveguide filled with a material of dielectric constant ϵ in the ratio $(\epsilon/\epsilon_0)^{-1/2}$, then the guide wavelength will also change in that ratio. It follows that a resonant cavity filled with a dielectric constant ϵ will have the same frequency as its analog *in vacuo* if all of its dimensions are decreased by the factor $(\epsilon_0/\epsilon)^{1/2}$.

The unloaded Q of a resonator given by eqs. (8-C-26 to 8-C-28) and (8-D-17) and (8-D-18) may be written in terms of the skin depth δ and the wavelength λ in an unbounded region

$$Q_u = [\lambda/\delta] \times \text{geometrical factor} \tag{6}$$

where the dimensionless geometrical factor depends upon the cavity's mode and relative dimensions. The geometric factor is unchanged when the dimensions of the cavity are scaled. Hence, using eq. (3) we obtain for a scaled cavity in a medium of relative dielectric constant ϵ/ϵ_0

$$Q_u = [\lambda_0(\epsilon/\epsilon_0)^{-1/2}] \times \text{geometrical factor} \tag{7}$$

since the skin depth δ of the cavity walls is uneffected by the dielectric medium. In this discussion we assume that the dielectric is lossless. If it is not, they we must take into account the term Q_ϵ due to dielectric losses, as discussed in Sec. 8-B, and illustrated by eqs. (8-B-6) and (8-B-8).

The quantity that one measures in an electron spin resonance experiment is the average rf magnetic field $\langle H_1{}^2 \rangle_s$ at the sample. From eq. (8-H-74) we obtain the average of $H_1{}^2$ in the cavity in terms of its value in the external waveguide under matched conditions

$$\langle H_1{}^2 \rangle_c = Q_L \, (V_w/V_c) \, \langle H_1{}^2 \rangle_w \tag{8}$$

One may determine the ratio of $\langle H_1{}^2 \rangle_c$ for a cavity filled with a lossless dielectric ϵ to its counterpart $\langle H_1{}^2 \rangle_{c0}$ *in vacuo* from eq. (7) and the scale factor for $(V_c/V_{c0}) \sim (\epsilon/\epsilon_0)^{-3/2}$. This gives

$$\langle H_1{}^2 \rangle_c = \langle H_1{}^2 \rangle_{c0} \, (\epsilon/\epsilon_0) \tag{9}$$

for the same frequency and incident power where the ratio Q_L/Q_u is unaffected by the scaling. From eq. (8-H-7) we obtain

$$\langle H_1{}^2 \rangle_s = \langle H_1{}^2 \rangle_{s0} \left(\frac{\epsilon}{\epsilon_0}\right) \left[\frac{\eta_1 V_c/V_s}{\eta_0 (V_{c0}/V_{s0})}\right] \tag{10}$$

We shall compare uniformly scaled samples at the same relative positions in the resonant cavity so that the ratio $\eta V_c/V_s$ remains constant. Consequently for the rf field H_1 at the sample,

$$\langle H_1{}^2 \rangle_s = \langle H_1{}^2 \rangle_{s0} \ (\epsilon/\epsilon_0) \tag{11}$$

As a check on this we may relate the average electric energies within and without the cavity through an expression similar to eq. (8)

$$\epsilon \langle E^2 \rangle_c = Q_L \ (V_w/V_c) \ \epsilon_0 \langle E^2 \rangle_w \tag{12}$$

Therefore,

$$\langle E^2 \rangle_c = \langle E^2 \rangle_{c0} \tag{13}$$

Equations (9) and (13) may be combined to produce the expected result that the energy stored in the electric fields equals the energy stored in the magnetic fields for each cavity.

$$\frac{\epsilon \langle E^2 \rangle_c}{\mu_0 \langle H_1{}^2 \rangle_c} = \frac{\epsilon_0 \langle E^2 \rangle_{c0}}{\mu_0 \langle H_1{}^2 \rangle_{c0}} = 1 \tag{14}$$

The important result of this discussion is eq. (11). It indicates that for a lossless medium the average value of the magnetic field squared at the sample position is proportional to the dielectric constant. A dielectric filled cavity is particularly advantageous when a small single crystal of constant size is under study, since it will fill a larger percentage of the cavity. More explicitly, for this case,

$$\eta = \eta_0 \ (\epsilon/\epsilon_0)^{3/2} \tag{15}$$

If, on the other hand, the sample dimensions are also scaled in the same ratio as the cavity dimensions then V_s/V_c remains constant, and

$$\eta = \eta_0 \tag{16}$$

Hedvig (1959) used a rectangular cavity partially filled with a lossless dielectric ϵ and located the sample at the enhanced field given by eq. (11). The corresponding filling factor η_ϵ is

$$\eta_\epsilon = \frac{\langle H_1{}^2\rangle_{s_\epsilon}V_s}{\langle H_1{}^2\rangle_{c_0}V_{c_0} + \langle H_1{}^2\rangle_{c_\epsilon}V_{c_\epsilon}} \tag{17}$$

where $\langle H_1{}^2\rangle_{c_{\epsilon_0}}V_{c_{\epsilon_0}}$ corresponds to the empty part of the cavity and $\langle H_1{}^2\rangle_{c_\epsilon}\ V_{c_\epsilon}$ corresponds to the dielectric filled part. The sensitivity ratio for this case characterized by Q_ϵ and η_ϵ compared to the "empty cavity" case characterized by Q_0 and η_0 with a constant sample size V_s is given by

$$\text{sensitivity ratio} = \frac{Q_\epsilon}{Q_0}\frac{\eta_\epsilon}{\eta_0} \tag{18}$$

$$= \left(\frac{Q_\epsilon}{Q_0}\right)\left(\frac{\langle H_1{}^2\rangle_{s_\epsilon}}{\langle H_1{}^2\rangle_{s_0}}\right)\left(\frac{\langle H_1{}^2\rangle_{c_0}V_{c_0}}{\langle H_1{}^2\rangle_{c_\epsilon}V_{c_\epsilon} + \langle H_1{}^2\rangle_{c_0}V_{c_0}}\right) \tag{19}$$

Hedvig reported that in his experimental arrangement with a quartz sheet ($\epsilon/\epsilon_0 \sim 6$) the ratio ($Q_\epsilon/Q_0$) was greater than 0.9, and the ratio of the average squared fields in the cavity was 0.93. The enhancement factor $\langle H_1{}^2\rangle_{s_\epsilon}/\langle H_1{}^2\rangle_{s_0}$ is about ϵ/ϵ_0 from eq. (11). The experiments indicated a factor of 4.5 gain in sensitivity.

In Sec. 8-F we saw that the equivalent circuit of an inductively coupled cavity places the iris inductance L_1 in series with the cavity inductance L, and the resonant frequency is given by

$$\omega = 1/[C(L + L_1)]^{1/2} \tag{20}$$

This means that the presence of the iris lowers the resonant frequency somewhat, since in practice $L \gg L_1$. It is shown graphically in Fig. 8–25 that when an iris is introduced into a resonant cavity, the length of the cavity must be reduced to maintain the same resonant frequency. The amount of foreshortening may be plotted against the iris size by using Fig. 8–15 to convert from Q_L to the aperture dimension l.

It is possible to tune a rectangular resonant cavity over a 10% frequency band by means of a capacitive tuning screw placed $\lambda_g/4$ from one end where the rf currents are a minimum, as shown in Fig. 8–26.

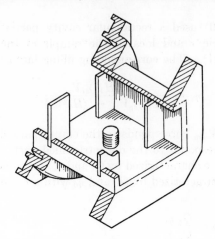

Fig. 8–26. TE_{101} rectangular cavity resonator with frequency tuning screw (*RLS*-9, p. 656).

A rectangular TE_{101} mode cavity may be conveniently varied in frequency over a 4.5% range by the insertion of quartz tubing [Bersohn (1963)]. A metallic post may be used to tune a rectangular cavity over a 3% frequency range [MacDonald (1955)]. If one wall of a resonant cavity is made of ferrite, the application of a magnetic field up to 100 G tangential to the wall will vary the cavity resonant frequency without effectively changing the Q [Tereshchenko, Korobkin, and Kovtun (1961); Tereschenko and Korobkin (1963); see also Gheorghiu and Rodeanu (1963)].

When a dielectric is placed in a resonant cavity, it decreases the resonant frequency. Before discussing small pieces of dielectric material placed in a cavity, it will be instructive to consider the case of a resonant cavity which has a resonant frequency ω_0 when it is completely filled with a lossless material of dielectric constant ϵ_0. Maxwell's equations are

$$\nabla \times \mathbf{E} + j\omega\mu\mathbf{H} = 0 \tag{21}$$

$$\nabla \times \mathbf{H} - j\omega\epsilon\mathbf{E} = 0 \tag{22}$$

and at resonance the stored electric and magnetic energies are

$$U_E = \tfrac{1}{2}\int \epsilon E^2 d\tau = U_H = \tfrac{1}{2}\int \mu H^2 d\tau \tag{23}$$

Allow the dielectric constant to change from ϵ_0 to ϵ_1 and let the new resonant frequency be ω_1 without any change occurring in the permeability μ_0. If the stored energy is maintained constant then $\mathbf{H}_0 = \mathbf{H}_1$ so that

$$\tfrac{1}{2}\int \epsilon_0 E_0{}^2 d\tau = \tfrac{1}{2}\int \epsilon_1 E_1{}^2 d\tau \tag{24}$$

and

$$(\epsilon_0/\epsilon_1)^{1/2} = \mathbf{E}_1/\mathbf{E}_0 \tag{25}$$

From eq. (22)

$$\omega_0 \epsilon_0 \mathbf{E}_0 = \omega_1 \epsilon_1 \mathbf{E}_1 \tag{26}$$

and hence

$$\omega_1/\omega_0 = (\epsilon_0/\epsilon_1)^{1/2} \tag{27}$$

Consider a cylindrical (or rectangular) resonant cavity partially filled with two dielectrics when the interface of the dielectrics is perpendicular to the cavity axis, as shown in Fig. 8–27. The cavity end plates are located at $z = 0$ and $z = d$, and the dielectric surface is at $z = a$. The tangential electric field in Region 1 is $E_1 \sin k_{1z}z$ and that in Region 2 is $E_2 \sin k_2(d - z)$. At the interface the tangential electric field and its first derivitive must be continuous so (RLS-8, Sec. 11-8)

$$E_1 \sin k_{1z}a = E_2 \sin k_{2z} (d - a) \tag{28}$$

$$k_{1z}E_1 \cos k_{1z}a = -k_{2z}E_2 \cos k_{2z} (d - a) \tag{29}$$

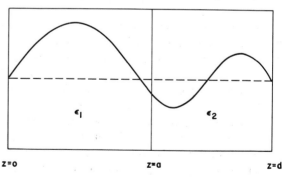

z=0   z=a   z=d

Fig. 8–27. The electric field waveform in a resonant cavity containing two different dielectrics.

and therefore,

$$\cot k_{2z} (d - a) = -(k_{1z}/k_{2z}) \cot k_{1z}a \tag{30}$$

If the two dielectrics have real and imaginary parts

$$\epsilon_1 = \epsilon_1' + j\epsilon_1'' \tag{31}$$

$$\epsilon_2 = \epsilon_2' + j\epsilon_2'' \tag{32}$$

then Q_u is given by

$$\frac{\epsilon_1' \int_0^a E_1^2 \sin^2 k_{1z}zdz + \epsilon_2' \int_a^d E_2^2 \sin^2 k_{2z}(d - z)dz}{\epsilon_1'' \int_0^a E_1^2 \sin^2 k_{1z}zdz + \epsilon_2'' \int_a^d E_2^2 \sin^2 k_{2z}(d - z)dz + (\text{loss in walls})} \tag{33}$$

where

$$\int_0^a \sin^2 k_{1z}zdz = \frac{1}{2} a - (1/4k_{1z}) \sin 2k_{1z}a \tag{34}$$

and

$$\int_a^d \sin^2 k_{2z}(d - z) \, dz = \frac{1}{2} (d - a)$$
$$- (1/4k_{2z}) \sin 2k_{2z} (d - a) \tag{35}$$

The metallic loss term is obtained by intergrating the magnetic field over the surface, as discussed earlier in this chapter.

The resonant frequency of a cavity partly filled with dielectric is given by the solution of a transcendental equation. Graphical solutions of this equation have been obtained, and they are given in the figures in RLS-8, pp. 386–389 for three typical cases of a dielectric slab in a TE_{10} mode rectangular waveguide. Ferrite loaded cavities are discussed by Spencer, LeCraw, and Ault (1957), Steinert (1959), Villeneuve (1959), Okada (1961) and Auld (1963). Perturbations by dielectric and metallic ellipsoids are treated by Mullett (1957).

Sometimes, a resonant cavity will deviate only slightly from an ideal shape, and when this occurs, its frequency shifts by Δf from the unperturbed cavity which has the frequency f_0. This will occur, for example, when a small indentation is put in a cavity wall as illustrated on Fig. 8–28, or when a small piece of dielectric is inserted into the cavity. Such a problem may be solved by the perturbation method which is outlined by Ramo, Whinnery, and Van Duzer [(1965, p. 568] [see also Pozzolo and Zich (1962–63)]. Their method assumes that the perturbed wave configurations differ very little from the ideal solution, and a calculation is made of the energy changes produced by the deviation. If the perturbed cavity only differs appreciably from the ideal one in a small volume change $\Delta\tau$, which is much less than the total volume V, then when $\Delta\tau$ is in a region of strong electric field strength, the electric energy change ΔU_E is assumed to be proportional to the volume change $\Delta\tau$ [Slater (1946); see Callebaut and Vanwornhoudt (1960)]. For the case shown at the bottom of Fig. 8–28 we have

$$\Delta U_E = \tfrac{1}{2}\epsilon E^2 \Delta\tau \qquad (36)$$

where E is the value of the electric field in the volume increment. The energy change ΔU_E may be positive or negative depending on whether or not $\Delta\tau$ represents an increase or a decrease in the cavity volume.

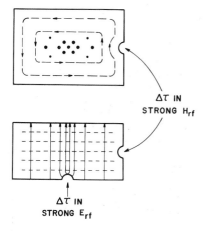

Fig. 8–28.   Diagrammatic representation of the distortion in the microwave magnetic field (– –) and electric field (—) resulting from a small localized change $\Delta\tau$ in the resonant cavity volume.

If the relative dielectric constant in a small region $\Delta\tau$ of strong electric field strength is changed from ϵ_1/ϵ_0 to ϵ_2/ϵ_0 then the change in the electric energy will be

$$\Delta U_E = \tfrac{1}{2}E^2 \, (\epsilon_2/\epsilon_0 - \epsilon_1/\epsilon_0) \, \Delta\tau \qquad (37)$$

In each case the change in magnetic energy ΔU_H results from a frequency change Δf (i.e., dispersion)

$$\Delta U_H = (dU_H/dk) \, \Delta k = (k\Delta f/f) \, (d/dk) \, U_H \qquad (38)$$

If, on the other hand, the small volume change $\Delta\tau$ is in a region of strong magnetic field then we let

$$\Delta U_H = (\mu H^2/2) \, \Delta\tau \qquad (39)$$

for the case shown on Fig. 8–28, and use the expression

$$\Delta U_E = (k\Delta f/f) \, (d/dk) \, U_E \qquad (40)$$

for the change in the stored electrical energy.

Another practical perturbation problem is the effect of scratches on the losses in resonant cavities. Pellegrini (1955) studied this experimentally and found that the measured values of Q agreed with theory [Brown and Ross (1952)] when the size of the scratches was much less than the skin depth. For additional information on resonant cavity perturbation theory, see Price, Reed, and Roberts (1963), Robinson (1963), Boudouris (1964), Brodwin and Parsons (1965), and Scaglia (1965). Saito (1964) used a time-dependent perturbation to modulate the resonant frequency of a cavity.

By using a conductor to perturb the microwave electric field in a resonant cavity one may obtain locally intense microwave magnetic fields [Rodbell (1959)]. This effect may be employed to enhance the intensity of small unsaturated samples.

Variations in the ambient temperature and atmospheric pressure will produce small changes in the frequency of a resonant cavity, and these changes exhibit hysteresis. Crain and Williams (1957) have build pressure and temperature insensitive resonators (see also, Thompson, Freethey, and Waters (1958)].

J. Resonant Cavities Simultaneously Excited in Two Modes

In maser and other applications, it is frequently desirable to excite a resonant cavity simultaneously in two modes. If the two coupling arrangements on Fig. 8–29 are employed, the frequency f_2 in the rectangular resonant cavity will, in a typical case, be approximately 20% greater than the frequency f_1. By proper choice of cavity dimensions, modes, and coupling holes it is possible to excite simultaneously two or more frequencies with any desired power ratio. In the illustrations shown, each frequency is excited from a separate source, and the electromagnetic energy from each source exists in the cavity independently of the other. If the microwave power at one

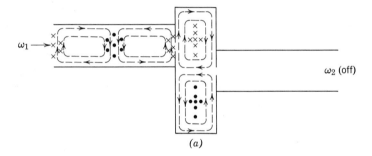

(a)

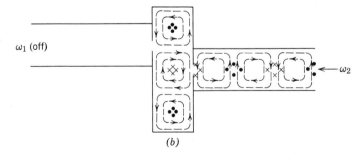

(b)

Fig. 8–29. A rectangular resonant cavity coupled to waveguides. The TE_{102} mode may be excited from the waveguide on the left (a) and the TE_{103} mode from the waveguide on the right (b), where, of course, $\omega_2 > \omega_1$.

exciting frequency is turned off, the other is virtually undisturbed. The coupling holes are shown located at positions of minimum H for the opposite frequency, in order to minimize the radiation of energy out of the cavity and into the waveguide.

Portis and Teaney (1958), Portis (1959), and Teaney, Klein, and Portis (1961) excited two orthogonal TE_{111} modes in a cylindrical resonant cavity, as discussed in Sec. 13-Q. Tinkham and Strandberg (1955) discuss the excitation of circular polarization in microwave cavities. Snowden (1962) also discussed microwave Faraday rotation in a bimodal cavity. Circular polarization can be used to determine the sign of the g factor, as shown in Sec. 8-M.

Maser cavities are described by a number of authors, such as Artman, Bloembergen, and Shapiro (1958), Chang, Cromach, and Siegman (1959), Garstens (1959), Kikuchi, Lambe, Makhov, and Terhune (1959), Bergmann (1960), Maiman (1960), Boyd and Gordon (1961), Wagner and Birnbaum (1961), Boyd and Kogelnik (1962), Troup (1962), Takach and Tot (1963), and Kemeny (1964). Artman, Bloembergen, and Shapiro's cavity oscillates simultaneously at 1373 Mc and 8000 Mc, and a sketch of it is shown in Fig. 8–30. Ganssen and Webster (1965) describe an X band ESR mixer whose two frequencies are separated by 14.55 Mc.

Sometimes it is desired to carry out double resonance experiments with both the saturating frequency and the monitor frequency close together in the microwave region [Moran (1964)]. The bimodal cavity shown in Fig. 8–31 is designed to operate at 3.9 and 4.1 Mc in the liquid helium temperature range. It was designed by Bowers and Mims (1959), and is mentioned in Sec. 19-C.

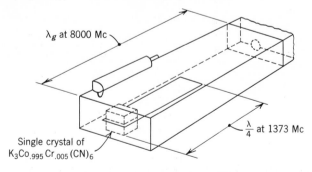

Fig. 8–30.   Maser cavity which simultaneously oscillates at 1373 and 800 Mc [Artman, Bloembergen, and Shapiro (1958)].

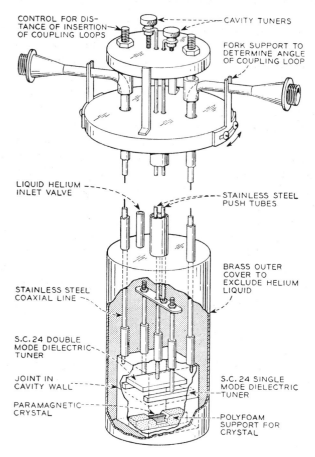

Fig. 8–31. Bimodal cavity showing coupling and tuning arrangements. For experiments above 4.2%, a second cylindrical cover was added, and the intermediate space was evacuated to provide thermal insulation [Bowers and Mims (1959)].

K. Resonant Cavities Containing Two Samples

It is frequently convenient to put a standard sample such as a small piece of DPPH in the same sample tube which contains an unknown specimen in order to place a magnetic field marker on the recording, and thereby facilitate the g factor determination. This is particularly useful if the unknown spectrum is much broader than DPPH, or if it has a different "crossover point" on the recording.

Singer, Smith, and Wagoner (1961) recommend the use of a carefully oriented ruby (Cr^{+3}/Al_2O_3) single crystal as discussed in Sec. 14-K, and shown in Fig. 16–3. The advantage of recording the unknown and the standard sample concurrently is that they each have the same instrumental conditions, and so effects such as Q changes and modulation settings tend to cancel out [Foerster (1960)].

Several authors have suggested the use of a long TE_{10n} rectangular resonator with provision for two sample tubes [Kohnlein and Müller (1960); Kramer and Müller-Warmuth (1963); Thompson, Persyn, and Nolle (1963); and Holz, Köhnlein, Müller and Zimmer (1963)]. A TE_{105} resonator containing a standard and an unknown sample located at positions of maximum H_x is shown in Fig. 8–32. The resonator is moved to place either the reference sample of the unknown sample in the center of the magnet pole caps for the ESR measurement. The sample is located within a double glass wall (glass 1 and glass 2) and double gap (gap 1 and gap 2) arrangement to provide for cooling or heating of the sample in the temperature range from -160 to $+120°C$. Moisture condensation is prevented by a flow of room temperature dry air. One may either place modulation coils on the pole caps or provide each sample with its own set of coils. In a more sophisticated arrangement with a larger magnet, one may modulate each sample at a different frequency, and use a dual recorder to inscribe the two spectra simultaneously.

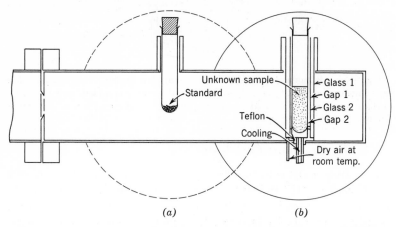

Fig. 8–32. Dual sample cavity for comparing the spectra of an unknown and a standard sample. (a) Magnet for measurement of standard; (b) magnet for measurement of unknown sample [Kramer and Müller-Warmuth (1963)].

L. Resonant Cavities Constructed from Insulating Materials

Sometimes, it is desirable to use resonant cavities with thin walls to facilitate the penetration of the modulation frequency into the interior, or for double resonance experiments. Resonant cavities with very thin conducting walls may be constructed from insulating materials such as epoxy resin [Chester, Wagner, and Castle (1959)] coated with metals of high conductivity. Thompson, Freethey, and Waters (1958) employed low thermal expansion ceramics to minimize the temperature dependence of the frequency. Eisinger and Feher (1958) employed a TE_{011} mode rectangular resonator constructed of Pyrex glass coated with silver on the inside for electron nuclear double resonance (ENDOR) studies. In this arrangement the NMR frequency was supplied by a coil around the cavity, and it entered the cavity through a slit. Bennett, Hoell, and Schwenker (1958) also used a Pyrex cavity. Bakker and Smidt (1962) made use of South African "Wonderstone" as the cavity insulating material while Cook, Matarrese, and Wells (1964) employed epoxide casting resin. Quartz [Vonbun (1960)], ruby [Cross (1959)], and rutile [Okaya and Barash (1962); Chang (1964)] have also been used. Lambe and Ager (1959) and Pipkin and Culvahouse (1957, 1958) used Lucite cavities which may be soft machined from hydrous aluminum silicate, fused at 1000°C, and then coated with a thin film of metal. The Lambe and Ager (1959) design had an unloaded Q of 5000 at 300°K and 20,000 at 4°K. Several of the cavities mentioned in this paragraph have been operated at 4°K. Some of these cavities have been operated in the liquid helium temperature range. Rosenbaum (1964) and Andresen and de Prins (1965) describe a high Q resonator consisting of a dielectric cylinder or rod with metal endplates. Yee (1965) discusses the theory and design of X band dielectric resonators with linear dimensions ~ 1 mm using $SrTiO_3$ which has a relative dielectric constant $\epsilon/\epsilon_0 = 279$.

M. Circular Polarization and the Sign of the g Factor

In most electron spin resonance spectrometers it is only possible to determine the magnitude of the g factor since one measures the product gS_z. In order to determine the sign of g, it is necessary to employ circularly polarized microwaves. The energy level diagram

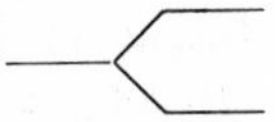

Spin direction

Energy	Positive g	Negative g
$E_+ = \|g\beta HS_z\|$	$S_z = -\frac{1}{2}$	$S_z = \frac{1}{2}$
$E_- = -\|g\beta HS_z\|$	$S_z = \frac{1}{2}$	$S_z = -\frac{1}{2}$

Fig. 8–33.   Energy levels for spin $\frac{1}{2}$ in a magnetic field. The $S_z = \frac{1}{2}$ level lies highest for a positive g factor, while $S_z = -\frac{1}{2}$ has the greatest energy for a negative g factor.

shown on Fig. 8–33 illustrates the physical significance of the sign of the g factor for spin one half.   The state with spin down ($S_z = -\frac{1}{2}$) will be the ground state when the g factor is positive, while the state with spin up ($S_z = \frac{1}{2}$) will be the ground state for a negative g. Both E_+ and E_- equal $-g\beta HS_z$, and the sign comes from the combination of g and S_z.

In an electron spin resonance experiment the spins absorb energy when they interact with a circularly polarized rf field $\mathbf{H}_1 \sin \omega t$ which has the same frequency and the same sense as the spin state's precessional motion.   This behavior may be deduced from the classical equation of motion of a magnetic moment $\boldsymbol{\mu}$ in a magnetic field $\mathbf{H}$ [see, e.g., Abragam (1961)]

$$\frac{d\boldsymbol{\mu}}{dt}\bigg|_L = g\left(\frac{\beta}{\hbar}\right)\,\boldsymbol{\mu} \times \mathbf{H} \tag{1}$$

where the subscript L denotes the fixed or laboratory frame of reference.   If we transform to a frame of reference which is rotating at the frequency ω we obtain

$$\frac{d\boldsymbol{\mu}}{dt}\bigg|_R = g\left(\frac{\beta}{\hbar}\right)\,\boldsymbol{\mu} \times \left(\mathbf{H}_0 + \frac{\omega}{g(\beta/\hbar)}\right) \tag{2}$$

Resonance absorption will occur for the Larmor condition $\omega = \omega_0$ given by

$$\omega_0 = -g\,(\beta/\hbar)\,\mathbf{H}_0 \tag{3}$$

Experimentally, we can induce resonant absorption of rf energy by applying a small amplitude rf magnetic field $H_1 \ll H_0$ confined to a plane perpendicular to the large static field $\mathbf{H}_0$, and oscillating at the

Larmor or resonant frequency ω_0. A further condition for absorption to occur is the necessity that H_1 be circularly polarized so that it satisfies the vector equåtion (3). In other words, for a positive g factor the direction of rotation ω_0 must be opposite to the magnetic field direction H_0 while for a negative g factor, ω_0 must lie along H_0.

In almost all ESR experiments the rf field $H_1 \sin \omega t$ is linearly polarized, and it may be vectorially decomposed into one circularly polarized component which induces rf transitions, and its oppositely rotating component which is ineffective in this respect. If one carries out a more sophisticated experiment with circularly polarized microwaves, then the sign of the g factor may be determined. This section will explain how to produce circular polarization (RLS-8, p. 350; RLS-9, p. 428) in a resonant cavity by both a spacial separation (extrinsic) technique, and a temporal separation (intrinsic) technique.

Eshbach and Strandberg (1952) and Tinkham and Strandberg (1955) discuss several types of extrinsic circular polarization. If either a square or a circular waveguide propagates two perpendicular but otherwise identical modes which are 90° out of time phase with each other, then the microwaves are said to be circularly polarized. Two sets of orthogonal modes are shown on Fig. 8–34. Any waveguide cross section with a fourfold symmetry axis will propagate circularly polarized waves. A linearly polarized wave may be converted to circular polarization by means of a circular polarizer such as the one shown on Fig. 8–35. Its microwave analog is the rhombus waveguide shown in Fig. 8–36, since the two perpendicular modes propagate at different velocities. The length of the deformed waveguide is adjusted until one mode is 90° out of phase with the other.

Another extrinsic method of producing circular polarization employs a conducting vane to short-circuit one of the circularly polarized components a quarter of a wavelength in front of the end plate which

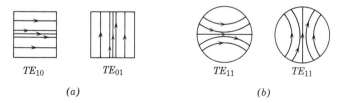

TE_{10} TE_{01} TE_{11} TE_{11}

(a)   (b)

Fig. 8–34.   Degenerate waveguide modes.   (a) Square guide; (b) circular guide
[Eshbach and Strandberg (1952)].

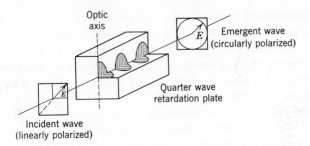

Fig. 8–35.   Birefringent quarter wave plate for producing circular polarization
[Eshbach and Strandberg (1952)].

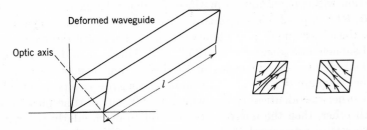

Fig. 8–36.   A rhombic waveguide circular polarizer and its two orthogonal modes
[Eshbach and Strandberg (1952)].

shorts the other component, as shown in Fig. 8–37.   [Tinkham and
Strandberg (1952)].   The incident and reflected waves set up a
circularly polarized standing wave pattern which couples to the
TE_{111} cavity.

The reason why the above polarization schemes are called extrinsic
and spacial is that one part of a linearly polarized wave is physically
separated from the other and retarded in its relative spacial position
by $\lambda_g/4$.   The intrinsic polarization scheme, on the other hand,
makes use of the fact that the magnetic (or electric) fields of a traveling electromagnetic wave appear circularly polarized when viewed
through an aperture properly placed in a waveguide wall [Kastler
(1954)].   The fields in the aperture rotate with time (temporally),
and are circularly polarized, as Fig. 8–38 demonstrates.   An iris
located symmetrically on the other side of the guide centerline will
experience rf magnetic fields rotating in the opposite sense.

Chang (1964) employed the cylindrical TE_{111} absorption cavity
(see Sec. 14-G) shown on Fig. 8–39 to determine the sign of the g

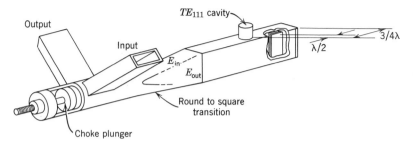

Fig. 8–37. A transition coupler for producing circular polarization [Tinkham and Strandberg (1955)].

factor. It is patterned after a design developed by Galt, Yager, Merritt, Cetlin and Dail (1955), and modified by Hutchison and Weinstock (1960). The circular polarization is produced in the iris by the intrinsic mechanism illustrated on Fig. 8–38. The detector end of the guide is matched to suppress a reflected wave which might interfere with the generation of circular polarization. The best location for the iris in the waveguide may be found empirically by recording DPPH with the regular and reversed magnet polarities. Reversing the magnet polarity is equivalent to reversing the direction of polarization of the microwaves. DPPH has a positive g factor [Chang (1964)], and the condition of optimum coupling occurs where the ESR signal is a maximum for one magnet polarity, and a minimum for the reverse. Chang found that the signal amplitude with the proper polarity is twenty times the amplitude obtained after reversing the magnet, which means that the polarization in the cavity was about 95% circular. The resonant cavity and waveguide combination shown on Fig. 8–39 is suitable for use in the liquid nitrogen and liquid helium temperature ranges. The size, shape, and location of the sample in the cavity are critical. Viewed from the sample it is the radial component of H_1 in the resonant cavity that is circularly polarized, not the longitudinal one. Galt, Yager, Merritt, Cetlin, and Dail (1964), Hutchison and Weinstock (1964), and Chang (1964) all placed their sample in the center of the bottom face of the cavity, as shown on Fig. 8–39.

The use of circular polarization to determine the sign of the g factor is also discussed by Artman and Tannenwald (1955), (1956), Charru (1956), and Battaglia, Iannuzzi, and Polacco (1963). Similar experiments have been carried out by NMR techniques to determine the

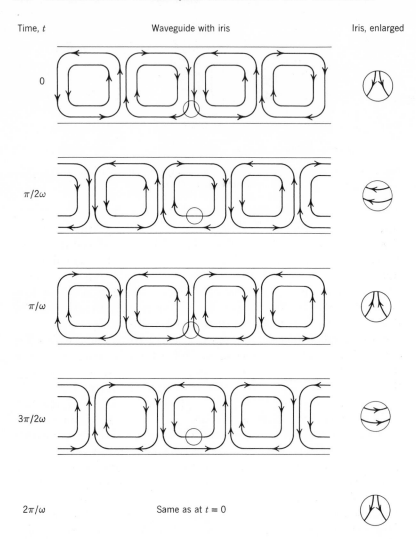

Fig. 8–38. The rf magnetic field loops of a TE_{10} waveguide mode moving past an iris which is placed off center on the broad face of the waveguide. Views are shown for every quarter of a period, and enlargements of the iris fields are presented on the right.

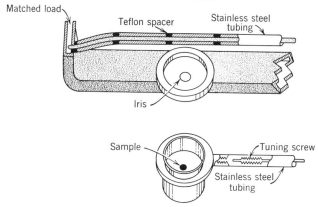

Fig. 8–39. Cylindrical TE_{111} resonant cavity and its waveguide mount. Circular polarization is induced into the cavity by the intrinsic mechanism illustrated on Fig. 8–38 [Chang (1964)].

signs of gyromagnetic ratios [e.g., see Rogers and Staub (1949, 1950); Levinthal (1950); Adler and Yu (1951)]. Dascola, Giori, and Varacca (1965) discuss the Cotton-Mouton effect.

A number of authors have discussed methods of determining the relative signs of hyperfine coupling constants [Heller (1965)]. For this purpose McConnell, Heller, Cole, and Fessenden (1960) and Heller and Cole (1962) used oriented free radicals, McConnell and Holm (1957), Forman, Murrell and Orgel (1959), and Eaton, Josey, Phillips, and Benson (1962) measured NMR shifts in organic complexes of transition elements, while Carrington and Longuet-Higgins (1962) and deBoer and Mackor (1962) deduced the relative signs from the variations in the hyperfine line-widths, and Heller (1965) used zero-field resonance spectra [Cole, Kushida, and Heller (1963)] to evaluate these signs. The fit of high field experimental data with the $A = Q\rho$ relationship of McConnell and Chesnut (1958) and the selfconsistent field treatment of McLachlan (1960) may also be used for this purpose (see Sec. 1-G).

N. Summary and Applications

This chapter is already excessively prolix, so we shall say a few words by way of summary in order to place the various sections in perspective. The first two sections presented some background ma-

terial to give an insight into how resonators work.   The three following sections give detailed discussions of rectangular, cylindrical, and
coaxial cavities.   These sections describe the electromagnetic field
configurations, current distributions, quality factors, etc., of the
individual modes.   This information is important when selecting a
cavity type and modifying its design for a specific experimental
application.   For example, a knowledge of the field distribution is required to properly position the sample, to mount intramural NMR
coils for double resonance experiments, and to incorporate a frequency
changing mechanism into the cavity.   A knowledge of the current
distributions in the walls allows one to cut slots for uv irradiation and
high frequency modulation purposes.   The sensitivity is strongly
dependent on the Q and the impedance match (coupling) between the
resonator and the waveguide.   Sections F and G provide an understanding of this relationship, and prepare the reader for the discussion
of sensitivity that is found in Chap. 14.

   Section 8-H presents a detailed treatment of filling factors.   It
shows one how to calculate the effectiveness of various sample shapes
and orientations, and compares different types of cavities.   This section also provides an understanding of the role that cavities play in the
sensitivity of an ESR spectrometer.   Section I explains how ideal
cavities are perturbed by the insertion of various objects such as
dielectrics and conductors.   Since we frequently insert samples,
dewars, coils, etc., into cavities, it is important to acquire an understanding of the nature of the resultant disturbance.

   Sections J, K, L, and M introduce the reader to specific types of
cavities.   Chapter 14 on sensitivity and Chap. 19 on double resonance
contain several examples of bimodal resonators.   Such cavities find
extensive use in maser and laser applications.

   ESR spectroscopists often find it necessary to design resonators for
special applications such as (1) wavemeters, (2) matched reference
and sample cavities, (3) masers, (4) high and low temperature studies,
(5) irradiation investigations, (6) double resonance, (7) high pressures, (8) refractometers, (9) circular polarization modes, etc.   Diagrams, design data and references for many such cavities will be found
scattered throughout the book.   Birnbaum (1950), Vetter and
Thompson (1962), Roussy (1965), and Verweel (1965) discuss microwave refractometers.   We will conclude this chapter with a discussion of several more cavities designed for specific applications.

A cavity suitable for use in ENDOR experiments [cf. Secs. 19-A and 19-C] was designed by Kramer, Müller-Warmuth, and Schindler (1965), and is shown in Fig. 8–40. The NMR coil is placed within the X band TE_{102} rectangular resonant cavity so that the NMR rf magnetic field, the microwave rf field, and the applied "constant" magnetic field are mutually perpendicular. The coil has two rectangular packets of five turns each around the sample. This arrangement causes an inconsiderable decrease in the NMR filling factor and microwave quality factor. The ESR spectrometer incorporates a Litton L 3503 cw magnetron for saturating the ESR transitions, and a low power (30 mW) klystron to observe the polarization after the saturation. The NMR part of the spectrometer measures the nuclear polarizations and enhancement factors induced by the saturation of the electronic spins. Provision is made for variable temperature studies.

Holton and Blum (1962) used an alternative arrangement to introduce the NMR radio frequency input. They wound their NMR coil around the rectangular TE_{101} cavity, and used a Mylar 0.025-mm

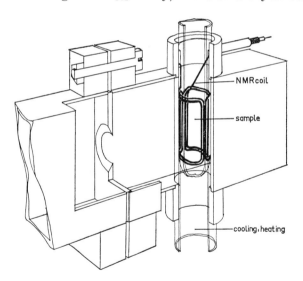

Fig. 8–40. Rectangular TE_{102} mode resonator with internal NMR coil for double resonance studies. Hot or cold nitrogen gas may be introduced from below for variable temperature studies [Kramer, Müller-Warmuth, and Schindler (1965)].

spacer to hold apart the two halves of the cavity which had been cut along the broad face, as shown on Fig. 8–41. The rf input enters the cavity through the slit. The Mylar spacers at the top and bottom of the cavity isolate it electrically at the NMR frequency, and the inductive rf impedence of the cavity permits rf current to flow on the inner surface of the cavity. The 1.25-mm thick cavity walls suppress vibrations. The design was effective at NMR frequencies up to 80 Mc. When the cavity is operated at 1.3°K, it is filled with Styrofoam to exclude liquid helium from the major part of its volume. At this temperature the cavity Q is 110,000. The associated ESR spectrometer is of the superheterodyne type [Feher (1957)].

Mims (1964) studied the effect of exposing a paramagnetic sample

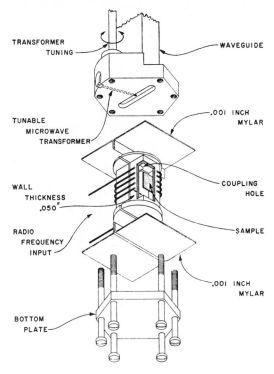

Fig. 8–41. Rectangular TE_{101} mode resonator with external NMR coil (rf input). The radiofrequency enters the cavity through the vertical slit provided by the Mylar spacer. A tunable iris or microwave transformer is incorporated in the design [Holton and Bloom (1962)].

to an electric field while studying its paramagnetic resonance. He used the experimental arrangement shown on Fig. 8–42. The electric field is provided by the aluminum foil electrode which is supplied through a phosphor bronze wire. Provision is made for rotating the sample. A cavity Q of 1000 was maintained, which is the highest value that could be tolerated in view of the 10-Mc band-width of the associated pulsing and detection apparatus. Electric field (Stark) effects in ESR are discussed by Ludwig and Ham (1963) and Kiel (1965).

Electron spin resonance at temperatures up to 1000°K may be carried out using Walsh, Jeener, and Bloembergen's (1965) heated cavity assembly shown on Fig. 8–43. It has a water cooled outer jacket to protect the magnet pole pieces, and is powered by a Variac. The high frequency microwaves were obtained by third harmonic generation from 10 Gc by using a GaAs point-contact diode [Sharpless (1959); see also Sec. 11-E].

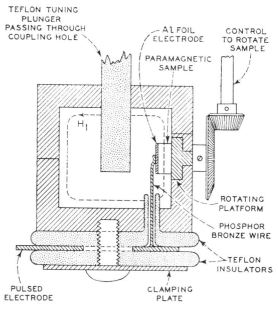

Fig. 8–42. Sample cavity with provision for applying an electric field across the sample. It is introduced into the cavity by phosphor bronze wire mounted on Teflon. Provisions made for rotating the sample [Mims (1964)].

The resonant cavities discussed in this chapter were of the waveguide and coaxial type. Reichert and Townsend (1965) determined that at 1 Gc it becomes prohibitively expensive to generate intense enough uhf or microwave magnetic field amplitudes (e.g., $H_1 \sim 8$ G) in a conventional cavity resonator because the stored energy has to be spread over such a large volume. To circumvent this difficulty for dynamic nuclear enhancement studies, they employed

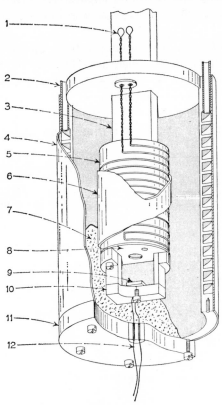

Fig. 8–43. Heated cavity assembly used at 30 kMc/sec: (1) Nichrome heater wire (2) cooling water inlet; (3) stainless steel RG–96/U waveguide; (4) water-cooled outer jacket; (5) copper heat sink with asbestos insulation; (6) Johns-Manville No. 20 refractory cement; (7) Johns-Manville Sil-O-Cel C-3 insulation; (8) copper coupling iris; (9) sample crystal; (10) half-wavelength cavity; (11) OFHC copper cap; (12) platinum-(90% platinum, 10% rhodium) thermocouple [Walsh, Jeener, and Bloembergen (1965)].

the line resonator shown on Fig. 8–44. The mode configuration is discussed qualitatively in the article. It has an effective volume of ~ 60 cm^3 which is two orders of magnitude smaller than the 1 Gc TE_{102} rectangular resonator. The figure shows the 1 Gc ultrahigh frequency input and output coupling arrangement, and the tuning devices. The line resonator (uhf resonator) supported by two Lucite parts is located in the center of the brass box. A 0.025-

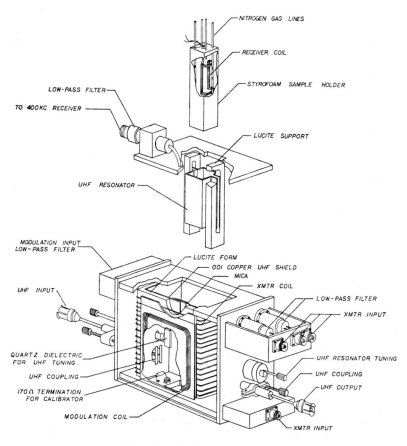

DOUBLE RESONANCE SYSTEM

Fig. 8–44. Exploded view of double resonance system. The line resonator is 8.3 cm long and has a 2.7-cm square cross section and capacitance wings extending 1.6 cm from the main body [Reichert and Townsend (1965)].

mm copper shield prevents the line resonator from radiating. The pulsed NMR transmitter (XTMR) coil surrounds the line resonator, while the corresponding receiver coil is placed within the line resonator [see also Locher and Gorter (1962)].

The remaining chapters of the book contain numerous descriptions of resonant cavities and their uses. We shall mention a few additional ones here. Evenson and Burch (1966) present an X band cavity for studies of paramagnetic gases. Pol'skii (1963, 1964) describes a helically wound cavity with a very homogeneous modulating field. Bil'dyukevich (1964, 1965) designed an 8-mm low temperature resonator with provision for rotating the sample in horizontal and vertical planes, and he also describes a low-temperature X band resonator (1963, 1965). Shaw, Brooks, and Gunton (1965) present an X band cavity with a lithium fluoride window to permit plasma production by ultraviolet irradiation down to 1100 Å. Livingston and Zeldes (1966) used a cavity with a grid on one face for uv irradiating liquids, and their detector was a Philco L4154 backward diode. Noon, Holt, and Reynolds (1965) used a waveguide cell for magnetoplasma studies. Redhardt (1965) discusses accurate measurements on reflection resonators.

References

A. Abragam, *The Principles of Nuclear Magnetism*, Oxford University Press, Oxford, 1961, Chap. 2.

F. Adler and F. C. Yu, *Phys. Rev.*, **82**, 105 (1951).

B. Agdur and B. Enander, *J. Appl. Phys.*, **33**, 575 (1962).

R. Ager, T. Cole, and J. Lambe, *RSI*, **34**, 308 (1963).

T. I. Alaeva and V. Karasev, *PTE*, **5**, 183 (1002) (1961).

H. M. Altschuler, *RSI*, **34**, 1441 (1963).

S. G. Andresen and J. de Prins, *Proc. IEEE*, **53**, 511 (1965).

J. O. Artman, N. Bloembergen, and S. Shapiro, *Phys. Rev.*, **109**, 1392 (1958).

J. O. Artman and P. E Tannenwald, *J. Appl. Phys*, **26**, 1124 (1955).

B. A. Auld, *J. Appl. Phys.*, **34**, 1629 (1963).

M. J. A. Bakker and J. Smidt, *Appl. Sci. Res.*, **B9**, 199 (1962).

K. N. Baranskii, *Dokl. Akad. Nauk, SSSR*, **114**, 517 (1957); transl. *Soviet. Phys. Dokl.*, **2**, 239 (1958).

A. I. Barchukov and A. M. Prokhorov, *Arch. Sci. Spec. No.*, **14**, 494 (1961).

A. Battaglia, M. Iannuzzi, and E. Polacco, *Ricerca Sci. IIA*, **3**, 119 (1963).

Y. Beers, *RSI*, **30**, 9 (1959).

R. G. Bennett, P. C. Hoell, and P. R. Schwenker, *RSI*, **29**, 659 (1958).

S. M. Bergmann, *J. Appl. Phys.*, **31**, 275 (1960).

M. Bersohn, *RSI*, **34**, 107 (1963).

A. L. Bil'dyukevich, *PTE*, **6**, 186 (1194) (1963); **2**, 185 (453) (1964); *Cryogenics*, **5**, 205, 277 (1965).

G. Birnbaum, *RSI*, **21**, 169 (1950).

D. I. Bolef, J. de Klerk, and R. B. Gosser, *RSI*, **33**, 631 (1962); see also D. I. Bolef and J. de Klerk, *IEEE Trans.*, **UE-10**, 19 (1963).

H. E. Bömmel and K. Dransfeld, *Phys. Rev.*, **117**, 1245 (1960).

G. Boudouris, *C. R. Acad. Sci.*, **258**, 2499 (1964).

K. D. Bowers and W. B. Mims, *Phys. Rev.*, **115**, 285 (1959).

G. D. Boyd and J. P. Gordon, *Bell System Tech. J.*, **40**, 489 (1961).

G. D. Boyd and H. Kogelnik, *Bell System Tech. J.*, **41**, 1347 (1962).

M. E. Brodwin and M. K. Parsons, *J. Appl. Phys.*, **36**, 494 (1965).

S. C. Brown and D. J. Ross, *J. Appl. Phys.*, **23**, 711 (1952).

H. E. Bussey and A. J. Estin, *RSI*, **31**, 410 (1960).

D. K. Callebaut and M. C. Vanwormhoudt, *Physica*, **26**, 255 (1960).

A. Carrington and H. C. Longuet-Higgins, *Mol. Phys.*, **5**, 447 (1962).

Te-Tse Chang, *Phys. Rev.*, **136**, A1413 (1964).

W. S. C. Chang, J. Cromach, and A. E. Siegman, *J. Electron. Control*, **6**, 508 (1959).

A. Charru, *C. R. Acad. Sci.*, **243**, 652 (1956).

P. F. Chester, P. E. Wagner, J. G. Castle, and G. Conn, *RSI*, **30**, 1127 (1959).

T. Cole, T. Kushida, and H. C. Heller, *J. Chem. Phys.*, **38**, 2915 (1963).

A. R. Cook, L. M. Matarrese, and J. S. Wells, *RSI*, **35**, 114 (1964).

C. M. Crain and C. E. Williams, *RSI*, **28**, 620 (1957).

L. G. Cross, *J. Appl. Phys.*, **30**, 1459 (1959).

W. Culshaw, *IRE Trans. Microwave Theory Tech.*, **MTT-9**, 2, 135 (1961).

G. Dascola, D. C. Giori, and V. Varacca, *Nuovo Cimento*, **37**, 382 (1965).

E. de Boer and E. L. Mackor, *Mol. Phys.*, **5**, 493 (1962).

M. Decorps and C. Fric, *C. R. Acad. Sci.*, **259**, 1394 (1964).

M. Dorland, *J. Phys. (France), Suppl. No. 10*, **24**, 191A (1963).

P. D. Dunn, C. S. Sabel, and D. J. Thompson, *Atomic Energy Res. Establ. (Harwell, Rept.*, GP/R 1966 (1956).

A. Dymanus, *RSI*, **30**, 191 (1959).

A. Dymanus, H. A. Dijkerman, and G. R. D. Zijderveld, *J. Chem. Phys.*, **32**, 717 (1960).

D. R. Eaton, A. D. Josey, W. D. Phillips, and R. E. Benson, *J. Chem. Phys.*, **37**, 347 (1962).

J. Eisinger and G. Feher, *Phys. Rev.*, **109**, 1172 (1958).

L. E. Erickson, *Phys. Rev.*, **143**, 295 (1966).

J. R. Eshbach, and M. W. P. Strandberg, *RSI*, **23**, 623 (1952).

A. J. Estin, *RSI*, **33**, 369 (1962).

K. M. Evenson and D. S. Burch, *RSI*, **37**, 236 (1966).

E. A. Faulkner and A. Holman, *JSI*, **40**, 205 (1963).

G. Feher, *Bell System Tech. J.*, **36**, 449 (1957).

G. v. Foerster, *Z. Naturforsch.*, **15a**, 1079 (1960).

A. Forman, J. N. Murrell, and L. E. Orgel, *J. Chem. Phys.*, **31**, 1129 (1959).

J. K. Galt, W. A. Yager, F. R. Merritt, B. B. Cetlin, and H. W. Dail, Jr., *Phys. Rev.*, **100**, 748 (1955).

A. Ganssen and J. C. Webster, *Proc. IEEE*, **53**, 540 (1965).

M. A. Garstens, *J. Appl. Phys.*, **30**, 976 (1959).

O. C. Gheorghiu and E. I. Rodeanu, *Stud. Cercetari Fiz.* (*Romania*), **14**, 399 (1963).

E. L. Ginzton, *Microwave Measurements*, McGraw-Hill, N. Y., 1957, p. 445.

J. P. Gordon, *RSI*, **32**, 658 (1961).

R. N. Gould and A. Cunliffe, *Phil. Mag.* (*8th Series*), **1**, 1126 (1956).

K. H. Hausser and F. Reinhold, *Z. Naturforsch*, **16a**, 1114 (1961).

P. Hedvig, *Acta. Phys. Hungaricae*, **10**, 115 (1959).

P. Hedvall and J. Hagglund, *Ericsson Tech.*, **19**, 89 (1963).

C. V. Heer, *Phys. Rev.*, **134**, A799 (1964).

H. C. Heller, *J. Chem. Phys.*, **42**, 2611 (1965).

C. Heller and T. Cole, *J. Chem. Phys.*, **37**, 243 (1962).

K. Heuer, *Jenaer Jahrbuch* (*Germany*), **1965**, 169–179.

W. C. Holton and Y. Blum, *Phys. Rev.*, **125**, 89 (1962).

G. Holz, W. Köhnlein, A. Müller, and K. G. Zimmer, *Strahlentherapie*, **120**, 161 (1963).

C. A. Hutchison and B. Weinstock, *J. Chem. Phys.*, **32**, 56 (1960).

E. H. Jacobsen, N. S. Shiren, and E. B. Tucker, *Phys. Rev. Letters*, **3**, 81 (1959).

E. Jahnke and F. Emde, *Funktionentafln mit Formeln und Kurven*, Teubner, Leipzig, 1933, Vol. 2.

W. K. Kahn, L. Bergstein, H. Gamo, G. J. E. Goubau, J. T. Latourrette, and G. T. Di Francia, *Proc. Symp. Quasi Optics*, Brooklyn Polytechnic Press, 1964, p. 397.

A. Kastler, *C. R. Acad. Sci.*, **238**, 669 (1954).

G. Kemeny, *Phys. Rev.*, **133**, A69 (1964).

M. Kent and J. R. Mallard, *JSI*, **42**, 505 (1965).

A. Kiel, *Proc. Intern. Conf. Magnetism* (*London*), (Inst. Phys. Phys. Soc.), **1965**, 465.

C. Kikuchi, J. Lambe, G. Makhov, and R. W. Terhune, *J. Appl. Phys.*, **30**, 1061 (1959).

W. Köhnlein and A. Müller, *Free Radicals in Biological Systems*, M. S. Blois Jr., H. W. Brown, R. M. Lindblom, M. Weissbluth, and R. M. Lemmon, Eds., Academic Press, N. Y., 1961, p. 113.

K. D. Kramer and W. Müller-Warmuth, *Z. Angew. Phys.* **16**, 281 (1963).

K. D. Kramer, W. Müller-Warmuth, and J. Schindler, *J. Chem. Phys.*, **43**, 31 (1965).

A. F. Krupnov and V. A. Skvortsov, *Zh. Eksperim. i Teor. Fiz.*, **47**, 1605 (1964).

J. Lambe and R. Ager, *RSI*, **30**, 599 (1959).

A. W. Lawson and G. E. Smith, *RSI*, **30**, 989 (1959).

J. D. Lawson, *Am. J. Phys.*, **33**, 1923 (1965).

E. Ledinegg and P. Urgan, *Acta. Phys. Austriaca*, **9**, 335 (1955).

E. C. Levinthal, *Phys. Rev.*, **78**, 204 (1950).

R. B. Lewis and T. R. Carver, *Phys. Rev. Letters*, **12**, 693 (1964).

M. Lichtenstein, J. J. Gallagher, and R. E. Cupp, *RSI*, **34**, 843 (1963).

R. Livingston and H. Zeldes, *J. Chem. Phys.*, **44**, 1245 (1966).

P. R. Locher and C. J. Gorter, *Physica*, **28**, 797 (1962).

H. K. V. Lotsch, *Japan. J. Appl. Phys.*, **4**, 435 (1965).

G. W. Ludwig and F. S. Ham, *Paramagnetic Resonance*, **2**, 620 (1963).

J. R. MacDonald, *RSI*, **26**, 433 (1955).

T. H. Maiman, *J. Appl. Phys.*, **31**, 222 (1960).

H. Margenau and G. M. Murphy, *The Mathematics of Physics and Chemistry*, Vol., 1, 2nd Ed., Van Nostrand, Princeton, N. J., 1956.

G. V. Marr and P. Swarup, *Can. J. Phys.*, **38**, 495 (1960).

E. Maxwell, *Progr. Cryogenics*, **4**, 123 (1964).

H. M. McConnell, C. Heller, T. Cole, and R. W. Fessenden, *J. Am. Chem. Soc.*, **82**, 776 (1960).

H. M. McConnell and C. H. Holm, *J. Chem. Phys.*, **27**, 314 (1957).

H. M. McConnell and D. B. Chesnut, *J. Chem. Phys.*, **28**, 107 (1958).

A. D. McLachlan, *Mol. Phys.*, **3**, 233 (1960).

E. Meyer, H. W. Helberg, and S. Vogel, *Z. Angew. Phys.*, **12**, 337 (1960).

J. W. Meyer, *MIT Lincoln Lab. Rept. M35-46* (1955).

W. B. Mims, *Phys. Rev.*, **133**, A835 (1964).

P. R. Moran, *Phys. Rev.*, **135**, A247 (1964).

L. B. Mullett, *Atomic Energy Res. Establ. (Harwell) Rept. G/R 853* (1957).

A. G. Mungall and D. Morris, *Can. J. Phys.*, **38**, 1510 (1960).

V. Muromtsev, A. K. Piskunov, and N. V. Verein, *Radio Eng. Electron. Phys.*, **7**, 1129 (1962).

J. H. Noon, E. H. Holt, and J. F. Reynolds, *RSI*, **36**, 622 (1965).

F. Okada, *Mem. Defense Acad. (Japan)*, **11**, 52 (1961).

A. Okaya, *Paramagnetic Resonance*, **2**, 687 (1963).

A. Okaya and L. F. Barash, *Proc. IRE*, **50**, 2081 (1962).

V. L. Patrushev, *Dokl. Akad. Nauk.*, **107**, 409 (1956).

U. Pellegrini, *Alta Frequenza*, **24**, 12 (1955).

F. M. Pipkin and J. W. Culvahouse, *Phys. Rev.*, **106**, 1102 (1957); **109**, 319 (1958).

Yu. E. Pol'skii, *PTE*, **3**, 184 (558) (1963); *Cryogenics*, **4**, 141 (1964).

C. P. Poole, Jr., Thesis, University of Maryland, 1958.

C. P. Poole, Jr., and R. S. Anderson, *J. Chem. Phys.*, **31**, 346 (1959).

A. M. Portis, *J. Phys. Chem. Solids*, **8**, 326 (1959).

A. M. Portis and D. T. Teaney, *J. Appl. Phys.*, **29**, 1692 (1958); *Phys. Rev.*, **116**, 838 (1959).

V. Pozzolo and R. Zich, *Atti Accad. Sci. Torino I (Italy)*, **97**, 1056 (1962-3).

R. Price, R. Reed, and C. A. Roberts, *IEEE Trans. Antennas Propagation*, **AP-11**, 587 (1963).

K. B. Rajangam, F. Hai, and K. R. MacKenzie, *RSI*, **36**, 794 (1965).

S. Ramo, J. R. Whinnery, and J. van Duzer, *Fields and Waves in Communication Electronics*, Wiley, N. Y., 1965.

G. Raoult and R. Fanguin, *C. R. Acad. Sci.*, **251**, 1169 (1960).

A. Redhardt, *Z. Angew. Phys.*, **19**, 310 (1965).

E. D. Reed, *Proc. Natl. Electron. Conf.*, **7**, 162 (1951).

J. F. Reichert and J. Townsend, *Phys. Rev.*, **137**, A476 (1965).

J. F. Reintjes and G. T. Coate, *Principles of Radar*, 2nd ed., McGraw-Hill, N. Y., 1952.

K. E. Rieckhoff and R. Weissbach, *RSI*, **33**, 1393 (1962).

RLS-8.

RLS-9.

RLS-10.

RLS-11.

RLS-14.

G. Roberts and W. Derbyshire, *JSI*, **38**, 511 (1961).

L. C. Robinson, *J. Appl., Phys.*, **34**, 1495 (1963).

D. S. Rodbell, *J. Appl. Phys.* **30**, 1845 (1959).

E. H. Rogers and H. H. Staub, *Phys. Rev.*, **76**, 980 (1949); *Helv. Phys. Acta*, **23**, 63 (1950).

J. D. Rogers, H. L. Cox, and P. G. Braunschweiger, *RSI*, **21**, 1014 (1950).

F. J. Rosenbaum, *RSI*, **35**, 1550 (1964).

G. Roussy, *J. Phys. (France)* **26**, 64A (1965).

G. Roussy and M. Felden, *J. Phys. (France)*, **26**, 11A (1965).

S. Ruthberg, *RSI*, **29**, 999 (1958).

T. Saito, *J. Phys. Soc. Japan*, **19**, 1232 (1964).

C. Scaglia, *Electron. Letters*, **1**, No. 7, 200 (1965).

W. M. Sharpless, *Bell System Tech. J.*, **38**, 259 (1959).

T. M. Shaw, G. H. Brooks, and R. C. Gunton, *RSI*, **36**, 478 (1965).

L. S. Singer, W. H. Smith, and G. Wagoner, *RSI*, **32**, 213 (1961).

J. C. Slater, *Rev. Mod. Phys.*, **18**, 441 (1946).

E. L. Sloan III, A. Ganssen, and E. C. LaVier, *Appl. Phys. Letters*, **4**, 109 (1964).

D. P. Snowden, *IRE Trans. Instr.*, **I-11**, 156 (1962).

E. G. Spencer, R. C. LeCraw, and L. A. Ault, *J. Appl. Phys.*, **28**, 130 (1957).

L. A. Steinert, *J. Appl. Phys*, **30**, 1109 (1959).

K. W. H. Stevens, Quantum Electronics Conference, Shawanga Lodge, High View, N. Y., Sept. 1959, p. 545.

K. W. H. Stevens and B. Josephson, *Proc. Phys. Soc.*, **74**, 561 (1959).

L. G. Stoodley, *Nature*, **198**, 1077 (1963).

R. G. Strauch, R. E. Cupp, M. Lichtenstein, and J. J. Gallagher, *Proc. Symposium on Quasi-Optics*, Brooklyn Polytechnic Press, Brooklyn, N. Y., 1964, p. 581.

P. Szulkin, *Bull. Acad. Polon. Sci, Ser. Sci. Tech.*, **8**, 639 (1960).

Sh. Takach and T. Tot, *Acta Tech. Hung.*, **42**, 181 (1963).

D. T. Teaney, W. E. Blumberg, and A. M. Portis, *Phys. Rev.*, **119**, 1851 (1960).

D. T. Teaney, M. P. Klein, and A. M. Portis, *RSI*, **32**, 721 (1961).

I. Teodoresku, *Rev. Phys. (Rumania)*, **7**, 45 (1962).

A. I. Tereshchenko, V. A. Korobkin, and N. M. Kovtun, *Zh. Tech. Fiz.*, **31**, 1388 (1011) (1961).

A. I. Tereshchenko and V. A. Korobkin, *Zh. Tech. Fiz.*, **33**, 214 (154) (1963).

K. I. Thomassen, *J. Appl. Phys.*, **34**, 1622 (1963).

B. C. Thompson, G. A. Persyn, and A. W. Nolle, *RSI*, **34**, 943 (1963).

M. C. Thompson, Jr., F. E. Freethey, and D. M. Waters, *RSI*, **29**, 865 (1958).

M. Tinkham and M. W. P. Strandberg, *Proc. IRE*, **43**, 734 (1955).

C. H. Townes and A. L. Schawlow, *Microwave Spectroscopy*, McGraw-Hill, N.Y., 1955.

G. J. Troup, *Proc. Inst. Radio Engrs. Australia*, **23**, 166 (1962).

J. Uebersfeld, *J. Phys. Radium*, **16**, 78 (1955).

R. Ulrich, K. F. Renk, and L. Genzel, *IEEE Trans.*, **MTT-11, 5**, 363 (1963).

L. A. Vainstein, *Zh. Eksperim. i Teor. Fiz.*, **44**, 1050 (9d63).

P. H. Verdier, *RSI*, **29**, 646 (1958).

J. Verweel, *Philips Res. Rept.*, **20**, 404 (1965).

B. I. Verkin, I. M. Dmitrenko, V. M. Dmitriev, G. E. Churilov, and F. F. Mende, *Zh. Tekh. Fiz*, **34**, 1709 (1320) (1964).

M. J. Vetter and M. C. Thompson, Jr., *RSI*, **33**, 656 (1962).

N. T. Viet, *C. R. Acad. Sci.*, **258**, 4218 (1964).

A. T. Villeneuve, *IRE Trans. Microwave Theory Tech.*, **MTT-7**, 441 (1959).

F. O. Vonbun, *RSI*, **31**, 900 (1960).

W. G. Wagner and G. Birnbaum, *J. Appl. Phys.* **32**, 1185 (1961).

W. M. Walsh, Jr., J. Jeener, and N. Bloembergen, *Phys. Rev.*, **139**, A1338 (1965).

R. H. Webb, *RSI*, **33**, 732 (1962).

K. Werner, *Hochfrequenztech. Elektakust.*, **73**, 115 (1964).

T. H. Wilmshurst, *Nature*, **199**, 477 (1963).

T. H. Wilmshurst, W. A. Gambling, and D. J. E. Ingram, *J. Electron. Control*, **13**, 339 (1962).

I. G. Wilson, C. W. Schramm, and J. P. Kinzer, *Bell System Tech. J.*, **25**, 408 (1946).

P. B. Wilson, *Nucl. Instr. Methods*, **20**, 336 (1963).

H. Y. Yee, *IEEE Trans.* **MTT-13**, 256 (1965).

R. W. Zimmerer, *RSI*, **33**, 858 (1962).

G. M. Zverev, *PTE*, **5**, 109 (930) (1961).

CHAPTER 9

Magnetic Fields

A. Magnetic Field Requirements

In electron spin resonance a large constant magnetic field H is employed for producing resonance absorption in accordance with the resonance condition $H = H_0$ which is usually written

$$h\nu = g\beta H_0 \tag{1}$$

in electron spin resonance studies and

$$\omega = \gamma H_0 \tag{2}$$

in nuclear magnetic resonance studies. In these equations g is the g factor, γ is the gyromagnetic ratio, β is the Bohr magneton, and

$$\hbar\gamma = g\beta \tag{3}$$

When one replaces Planck's constant $h = 2\pi\hbar$ and the Bohr magneton β by their numerical values, then one obtains the functional relationship between the resonant frequency ν and its associated magnetic field H_0

$$\nu = 1.400 \times 10^6 g H_0 \tag{4}$$

where ν is in cycles per second, H is in gauss, and g is a dimensionless factor which is usually close to two. Most ESR work is done in the X band microwave region where the magnetic field $H_0 \sim 3400$ G is required for a typical frequency of 9.5 Gc and $g = 2$. Many ESR experiments are performed in the K band region at 25 Gc (~ 9000 G) and at 35 Gc ($\sim 12{,}500$ G) and it is only in special applications that higher frequencies or fields are employed. Thus for almost all ESR applications a magnet that produces up to 12.5 kG is satisfactory.

The resonant magnetic fields H_0 corresponding to $g = 2$ are listed in Table 9–1 for several ESR frequencies.

Sometimes one encounters a resonance whose width exceeds 1 kG, and when this is the case, it is preferable to use K band, since X band will give a more distorted line-shape, especially at the low field side. The necessity of observing broad resonance lines increases the required upper limit on the magnet since it is desirable to record the resonance line considerably beyond its inflection point ($\frac{1}{2}\Delta H_{pp} + H_0$) on the high field side. A reasonable requirement is the ability to record a K band resonance out to a field of 1.5 H_0 which corresponds to 13,000 G. This upper limit will allow one to record a K band resonance with full width $\Delta H_{pp} = 5000$ G out to a field of $\frac{1}{2}\Delta H_{pp}$ beyond its inflection point (derivative half-width). Broader resonance lines are seldom encountered in ESR.

Several transition elements have g factors which deviate considerably from two (e.g., 0 to 9 for Fe^{+2} and 1.4 to 7 for Co^{+2}), and these deviations are frequently orientation-dependent. A 13,000-G magnet at $f = 24$ Gc will be unable to reach $g < 1.3$, while the same magnet at $f = 9.6$ Gc will have $g < 0.53$ beyond range. These g factor limitations are of practical importance in only a few cases since the overwhelming percentage of the tabulated transition element spectra [Bowers and Owen (1955); Orton (1959)], and all free radicals have $g > 1.3$. Thus both line-width and g factor considerations indicate that a magnet which reaches 13,000 G is adequate for almost all ESR experiments. In NMR studies such a magnet is capable of reaching most nonzero spin nuclei at 2 Mc (K^{39} is an exception), and in addition it will resonate protons up to 55 Mc. These NMR figures can be computed directly from a table of nuclear gyromagnetic ratios since NMR line-widths seldom exceed 50 G, [e.g., see Poole, Swift, and Itzel (1965)] and chemical shifts are rarely greater than one part per thousand [see Pople, Schneider, and Bernstein (1959)].

To detect ESR signals it is not sufficient to have a magnet which will supply the required magnetic field strength; it is also necessary for this magnetic field to be very homogeneous over the sample volume. A rule of thumb is that the variations in the magnetic field strength over the sample ΔH_0 should be less than one tenth of the line-width ΔH_{pp}, and in Table 9–1 values of $\Delta H_0 = \Delta H_{pp}/10$ are tabulated for a typical very narrow ESR line of width 0.1 G. Alkali

TABLE 9-1

Magnetic Field Requirements for Electron Spin Resonance and Nuclear Magnetic Resonance

(ESR sample lengths are for TE_{10}, rectangular resonant cavities)

Resonance experiment	Frequency ν, Mc	Sample length,[a] cm	Coil or waveguide width,[b] cm	Typical width of narrow line, mG	Magnetic field H_0, kG	Magnet homogeneity requirement	
						ΔH_0, mG	$\Delta H_0/H_0$, ppm
ESR–S band	3,000	7.2	3.8	100	1.1	10	10
ESR–X band	10,000	2.3	1.3	100	3.6	10	3
ESR–K band	24,000	1.1	0.63	100	8.6	10	1
ESR–Q band	70,000	0.3	0.35	100	25	10	0.4
ESR– 1mm band	300,000	0.08	0.3	100	110	10	0.1
NMR–H[1]	10	1	1.5	1.0	2.4	0.1	0.04
NMR–C[13]	10	1	1.5	1.0	9.3	0.1	0.01
NMR–K[39]	10	1	1.5	1.0	50	0.1	0.002
NMR–H[1]	100	1	1.5	1.0	24	0.1	0.004

[a] Large inner dimension in waveguide case (limits sample length).
[b] Small outer dimension in waveguide case (limits magnet gap).

metals in ammonia [Hutchison and Pastor (1959)] and some free radical ions [Hausser (1962)] have produced line-widths almost a factor of ten below this value, but at present these are exceptional cases, and so the value of $\Delta H_{pp} = 0.1$ G is used in Table 9–1. From this table it may be seen that a magnet for use at X band should have a magnetic field H which is constant to within 10 mG over the sample volume, and in column three we see that the sample is 0.9 in. or 2.3 cm long when it extends over the entire length of the broad dimension of the waveguide. The X band entry in the last column of the table shows that the relative homogeneity should be

$$\Delta H_0/H_0 = 0.01/3600 = 3 \times 10^{-6} = 3 \text{ ppm} \qquad (5)$$

Since the widths of narrow resonance lines are frequently independent of the microwave frequency, in going from S band to the 1-mm band the absolute homogeneity requirement ΔH_0 remains constant at 10 mG, while the relative homogeneity requirement $\Delta H_0/H_0$ decreases from 10 to 0.1 ppm. This behavior is important in magnet stabilization systems since a magnet current stabilizer usually supplies a current I which is stabilized to deviate by less than a certain $\Delta I/I$ value from the desired current. As a result, for a given stabilizer the absolute current fluctuation will increase with magnetic field strength. Sometimes the homogeneity of a magnet is improved by initially raising the field strength to a high value, and then decreasing it to the desired operating point.

It should be noted that the narrow NMR line-widths listed in Table 9–1 are typically two orders of magnitude below the ESR value, and this puts much more stringent requirements on the NMR magnet stabilization system. In addition, as mentioned above, ESR line-widths almost as narrow as 0.01 G have already been observed, and if still narrower ones are detected, it will become necessary to make use of NMR magnet systems with their increased stability.

This preliminary discussion has outlined the general specifications which must be met by magnet systems for use with ESR spectrometers. The remainder of the chapter will elaborate upon magnet theory, practical magnet systems, methods for measuring magnetic fields, and the repair of magnet systems. Coles (1964) has recently reviewed this field.

B. The Magnetic Circuit

In an electrical circuit, Ohm's law relates the applied electromotive force (emf) or voltage V to the current I in terms of the resistance R

$$\text{emf} = V = IR \tag{1}$$

The resistance of a rod of length l and uniform cross-sectional area A is

$$R = l/\sigma A = \rho(l/A) \tag{2}$$

where the conductivity σ is an intrinsic characteristic of a substance, and of course the reciprocal of the conductivity σ is the resistivity ρ. The electromotive force between two points a and b is the line integral of the electric field E between the points

$$\text{emf} = \int_a^b \mathbf{E \cdot dl} \tag{3}$$

In a magnetic circuit [see, e.g., Page (1949), p. 420] the analog of Ohm's law is

$$\text{mmf} = \mathfrak{R}\phi \tag{4}$$

where the magnetic flux ϕ through the circuit is proportional to the applied magnetomotive force (mmf). The reluctance $\mathfrak{R}$ of a rod of length l and cross sectional area A is related to the permeability μ by the expression

$$\mathfrak{R} = l/\mu A \tag{5}$$

$$= \frac{l \times 10^7}{4\pi A \ (\mu/\mu_0)} \tag{6}$$

where μ_0 is the permeability of free space and μ/μ_0 is relative permeability. Often the magnetic flux ϕ equals the magnetic induction B times the cross-sectional area A

$$\phi = BA \tag{7}$$

If a magnetic circuit such as an iron ring is magnetized by n turns of wire carrying the current I then the magnetomotive force in the circuit is nI

$$\text{mmf} = nI \qquad (8)$$

another definition of mmf is the analog of eq. (3)

$$\text{mmf} = \int_a^b \mathbf{H} \cdot \mathbf{dl} \qquad (9)$$

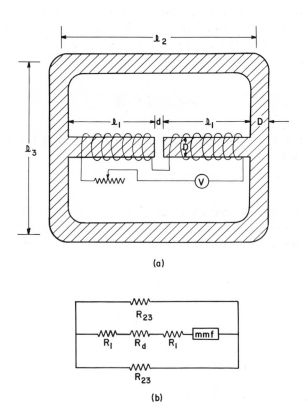

(a)

(b)

Fig. 9–1. Schematic diagram of (a) an electromagnet and (b) its equivalent circuit. The magnet consists of a yoke (l_2, l_3), center iron pieces (l_1), and gap (d).

The magnetic flux ϕ is constant in a series magnetic circuit, so for several successive cross sections A_1, A_2, etc. one has

$$\phi = A_1 B_1 = A_2 B_2, \text{ etc.} \tag{10}$$

and B is constant in a magnet with a constant cross-sectional area which employs cylindrical pole caps as shown on Figs. 9–1 and 9–2a. When tapered pole caps such as the ones shown in Fig. 9–2b are employed, the flux in the air gap is approximated by

$$\phi = (\pi D_2{}^2/4)\, B \tag{11}$$

instead of the cylindrical value

$$\phi = (\pi D_1{}^2/4)\, B \tag{12}$$

If ϕ remains constant in both cases, B, for the tapered case, will increase by the factor $(D_1/D_2)^2$ relative to the cylindrical case. Unfortunately ϕ does not remain constant because the tapered air gap presents a greater reluctance than the cylindrical gap, and this limits ϕ in accordance with the relation

$$\text{mmf} = \phi\, [\Re_{\text{gap}} + \Re_{\text{yoke}}] \tag{13}$$

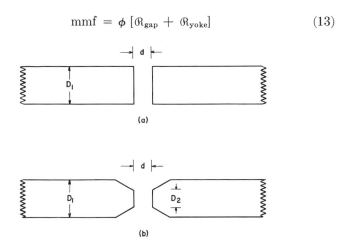

Fig. 9–2. Magnet with (a) cylindrical pole caps and (b) tapered pole caps.

for a constant applied magnetomotive force. When $\mathfrak{R}_{gap} << \mathfrak{R}_{yoke}$ the taper does not change ϕ, but in most practical magnet systems $\mathfrak{R}_{gap}$ is comparable to $\mathfrak{R}_{yoke}$ and the magnitude of the magnetic flux is strongly dependent on the amount of taper.

The preceding paragraph defined the terms employed in a magnetic circuit analysis. These results are summarized on Table 9–2. This presupposes that all of the flux remains in the circuit just as Ohm's law is based on the fact that all of the electrical current remains in the conductor. Unfortunately a considerable amount of flux actually does leak out, so the concept of a magnetic circuit is only an approximation. This is particularly the case when a magnetic circuit has an air gap, since a great deal of flux leakage occurs at the gap, and the greater the gap the more the leakage. Nevertheless some insight can be gained into the way an electromagnet works by analyzing a typical electromagnet from the viewpoint of its magnetic circuit.

TABLE 9–2

Magnetic Circuit Quantities and Their Electrical Analogs.

Magnetic circuit			Electric circuit		
Quantity	Unit, mks	Symbol	Quantity	Unit, mks	Symbol
Magnetomotive force	At	mmf	Electromotive force or voltage	V	emf, V
Magnetic flux	Wb	Φ	Current	A	I
Inverse permeability	M/H	$1/\mu$	Conductivity	$1/M\Omega$	σ
Reluctance	At/Wb	$\mathfrak{R}$	Resistance	Ω	R

Fig. 9–1a shows an electromagnet with a double yoke of permeability μ, and a uniform cross section A in all of its parts. A voltage generator V actuates the coils, and a resistor permits an adjustment of the coil current. The reluctance $\mathfrak{R}_1$ of each center iron piece of length l_1 is

$$\mathfrak{R}_1 = \frac{1}{\mu_0} \frac{l_1}{A(\mu/\mu_0)} \tag{14}$$

and the reluctance $\mathcal{R}_{23}$ of each outer half of the yoke of length $l_2 + l_3$ is

$$\mathcal{R}_{23} = \frac{1}{\mu_0} \frac{l_2 + l_3}{A\,(\mu/\mu_0)} \tag{15}$$

In the air gap $\mu = \mu_0$, so the reluctance $\mathcal{R}_d$ of the gap is

$$\mathcal{R}_d = \frac{1}{\mu_0} \frac{d}{A} \tag{16}$$

where the gap is assumed to have the same cross sectional area A. This approximation is only valid for a gap to pole piece diameter ratio d/D much less than one. The equivalent magnetic circuit is shown in Fig. 9–1b where the mmf from the two activating coils is represented by one "mmf generator." The parallel arrangement of the two parts of the yoke $\mathcal{R}_{23}$ leads to the relation

$$\text{mmf} = \phi\,[2\mathcal{R}_1 + \mathcal{R}_d + \tfrac{1}{2}\,\mathcal{R}_{23}] \tag{17}$$

$$= \frac{B}{\mu_0} \left(\frac{2l_1 + \frac{1}{2}(l_2 + l_3)}{\mu/\mu_0} + d \right) \tag{18}$$

For a typical magnetic material

$$\mu/\mu_0 \sim 10^3 \tag{19}$$

so the reluctance of the air gap is the dominant factor in limiting the available magnetic field strength in the air gap. For a typical electromagnet

$$d << l_1 \tag{20}$$

$$2l_1 \sim l_2 \sim l_3 \tag{21}$$

and using these relations in eqs. (8) and (18), one obtains

$$B = \frac{\mu_0 n I}{l_2} \left[\frac{1}{d/l_2 + 2 \times 10^{-3}} \right] \tag{22}$$

Frequently $l_2 \sim 200$ cm and under these conditions the gap contributes half of the reluctance when

$$d = 2l_2 \times 10^{-3} = 0.4 \text{ cm} \tag{23}$$

Usually d exceeds this value in ESR applications.

The preceding calculation assumed that the cross-sectional area A of the gap is the same as that of the section l_1. For this assumption to be tenable it is necessary for the gap radius $(A/\pi)^{1/2}$ to be considerably greater than the pole piece separation d.

$$d \ll (A/\pi)^{1/2} \tag{24}$$

One may estimate the gap diameter at 30 cm, which leads to the requirement

$$d \ll 15 \text{ cm} \tag{25}$$

In practice one usually finds d between 3 and 8 cm, or in other words

$$d \sim (A/\pi)^{1/2}/3 \tag{26}$$

and as a result, a considerable amount of excess flux leaks out to the space surrounding the pole caps.

Since typical magnet gaps are close to 5 cm, one may conclude that: (1) from eq. (23) the reluctance of the magnet gap is the dominant factor in determining the intensity of the magnetic field; (2) from eq. (25) the assumption that the equivalent gap area approximates the pole piece area is not valid; (3) tapered pole caps are much less effective than the ratio $(D_1/D_2)^2$ obtained from eqs. (11) and (12). Nevertheless, the magnetic circuit concept is helpful in providing a qualitative understanding of the way magnets function, and in describing qualitatively the dependence of the magnet gap on the magnetic field strength.

C. Ferromagnetism

In paramagnetics the spins are randomly oriented in the absence of an applied magnetic field as indicated schematically on Fig. 9–3a. In the presence of an applied magnetic field to first order they align parallel or antiparallel to the field in a nonordered manner, and in accordance with a Boltzmann distribution, as shown in Fig. 9–3b. In this figure the magnetic field is directed up, and a slight excess of spins points in the direction of the field. The reader is urged to assume a g factor of two and convince himself that Fig. 9–3b corresponds to a temperature of 1.7°K in a field of 3573 G. For a paramagnetic material the interaction between neighboring spins does not have an appreciable effect on the alignment of the spins in the magnetic field.

In ferromagnetism each spin is strongly coupled to its neighbors, and to a first approximation the applied magnetic field influences the spin direction but does not uncouple it from its neighbors. The exchange coupling to neighboring spins remains the dominant interaction. As a result of this coupling the spins arrange themselves into domains about 10^{-1} or 10^{-2} mm in diameter with all of the spins parallel to each other in a given domain. In general, each domain will have its spins oriented in a different direction than its neighboring domains. The domains are separated by so-called Bloch walls $\sim$

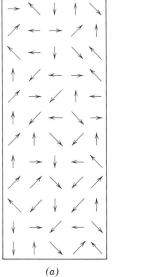 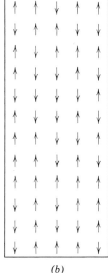

(a)   (b)

Fig. 9–3. Schematic representation of the ordering of spins in a paramagnetic material: (a) without a magnetic field; (b) in a vertical applied magnetic field.

1000 atomic spacings thick over which the spin direction gradually changes as shown schematically in Fig. 9–4a and 9–4b. The domain size corresponds to a minimum value for the energy of the spins in the domains and Bloch walls. This is because increasing the domain size from its stable equilibrium condition increases the magnetic energy to a greater extent than it decreases the Bloch wall energy, while decreasing the domain size increases the Bloch wall energy to a greater extent than it decreases the magnetic energy.

A ferromagnetic material is characterized by a permeability μ which relates the magnetic induction (flux density) B to the magnetic field strength H

$$B = \mu H \tag{1}$$

and Fig. 9–5 shows the manner in which B depends on H for a typical ferromagnet. If one starts with an unmagnetized material at $B = H = 0$ and increases the applied field H (e.g., by placing the ferromagnet in a coil carrying an electric current), the magnetic induction B will increase by following the initial magnetization curve from 0 to A. If the field strength is then decreased from its value at A to zero, the the induction B does not return to zero, but merely decreases to its

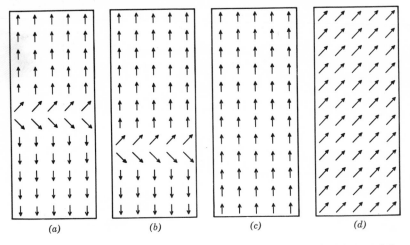

(a) (b) (c) (d)

Fig. 9–4. Spin alignment in a two-domain particle at various parts of the magnetization curve shown in Fig. 9–5. (a) Demagnetized; (b) Region I; (c) Region II; (d) Region III.

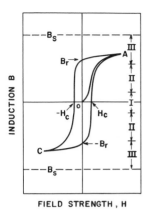

FIELD STRENGTH , H

Fig. 9–5. Magnetization curve. The initial magnetization curve is denoted by
0A and both B and H equal zero at point 0.

residual induction B_r. As a result we have a permanent magnet
characterized by the residual induction B_r. It is necessary to apply
a field strength of $- H_c$ called the coercive force to reduce the induction to zero. In like manner one may proceed around the
hysteresis loop to C, $- B_r$, H_c, and finally return to A.

The process of magnetization is characterized by the following
three regions of domain structure corresponding to the changes shown
on Fig. 9–5.

Region I: Reversible boundary displacement (dissipated energy $\ll$
stored energy). The permeability μ approximates the Rayleigh
relation

$$\mu = \mu_0 + (d\mu/dH)\, H \qquad (2)$$

$$= \mu_0 + vH \qquad (3)$$

$$B = \mu_0 H + vH^2 \qquad (4)$$

where v is a small constant.

Region II: Irreversible boundary displacement (dissipated energy
$> >$ stored energy). The permeability curve (B versus H) has an
inflection point in this region where

$$d^2B/dH^2 = 0 \qquad (5)$$

and dB/dH is very large compared to its value in Region I.   In other words

$$dB/dH \gg \mu_0 \qquad (6)$$

Region III: Domain rotation. Here the permeability approximately follows the Frölich-Kennelly relation

$$1/\mu = a + bH \qquad (7)$$

where a and b are constants, and the derivative dB/dH is sometimes close to the value of Region I.

As H is increased indefinitely, saturation sets in and the magnetic induction B approaches its saturation value B_s shown on Fig. 9–5. When this occurs the slope dB/dH approaches zero

$$\lim_{H \to \infty} (dB/dH) = 0 \qquad (8)$$

Sometimes a hysteresis loop will be entirely in Region I, such as the small loop in Fig. 9–6, while larger loops such as those in Figs. 9–5 and 9–7 extend over all three regions.

The spin system reorientations that correspond to these three regions are illustrated schematically on Fig. 9–4.   The spin system

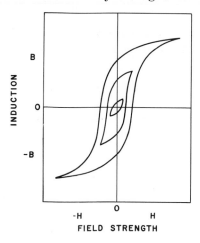

Fig. 9–6.   Three hysteresis loops corresponding to three different ranges over which the magnetic field strength is varied.

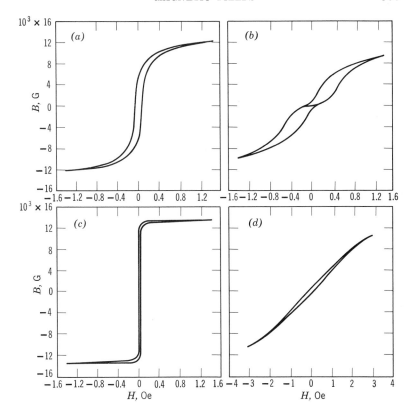

Fig. 9-7. Hysteresis loops of 65 Permalloy heat-treated in various ways: (a) annealed at 1000°C; (b) baked at 425°C for 24 hr; (c) heat-treated in a longitudinal field; (d) heat-treated in a transverse field [Bozorth (1951)].

magnetization changes occur discontinuously. This is referred to as the Barkhausen effect, and it may be observed by gradually changing the applied field strength H and measuring the rate of change of magnetic induction through the voltage induced by it in a coil. This voltage may be amplified and observed on an oscilloscope.

The normal permeability μ of any point on the magnetization curve is defined by the ratio B/H, and the incremental permeability μ_i is the ratio of a small change in B to a small change in H. More explicitly

$$\mu = B/H \tag{9}$$

and

$$\mu_i = \Delta B / \Delta H \qquad (10)$$

The incremental permeability is defined in terms of minor hysteresis loops such as the ones shown in Fig. 9–8. It is the incremental permeability that is employed when the magnetic scan of an ESR system is calibrated, since in that case the important factor is the change that occurs in B as a function of the variation in the magnet current (or the time). Such scan calibrations are useful in line width, hyperfine spacing, and g factor determinations. Care should be exercised in checking the linearity and reversibility of the scan in order to ascertain if an appreciable hysteresis effect is present. This is important when a computer is used to add the amplitudes of

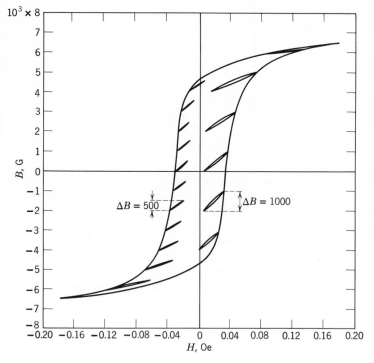

Fig. 9–8. Minor and major hysteresis loops of 4–79 Permalloy. For the minor loops ΔB is constant at 500 G (left side) or 1000 G (right side) [Bozorth, (1951)].

many successive scans in the sensitivity enhancement scheme discussed in Sec. 14-I.

The shape of the hysteresis loop depends on the range over which the magnetic field strength is varied, as Figs. 9–6 and 9–8 demonstrate. It also depends on the type of magnetic material and its pretreatment as Fig. 9–7 indicates. From this figure one sees that 65 Permalloy, heat-treated in a longitudinal field, is suitable for use as a permanent magnet because it may be magnetized in a field strength of 1 Oe $((4\pi)^{-1} \times 10^3$ At/m) and retains 12,000 G (1.2 Wb/m^2) when the field strength H is removed. The same material heat-treated in a transverse field may be employed for an electromagnet because the magnetic induction B is approximately proportional to the magnetomotive force or applied field strength H as illustrated in Fig. 9–7d.

The energy loss U_L associated with a circuit of the hysteresis loop is

$$U_L = \oint H dB \qquad (11)$$

which is numerically equal to the area enclosed by the hysteresis curve on the B–H diagram. This energy is dissipated as heat in iron core transformers, and in such ac applications it is desirable to employ a low-loss magnetic material. In selecting materials for magnets to be used in magnetic resonance spectrometers, the shape of the hysteresis curve is crucial. A linear B–H characteristic curve with a low-area hysteresis loop is best.

The magnetization curves of single crystals are strongly dependent on the orientation of the field strength H relative to the crystallographic axes. The ratio B/H is greater along easy directions of magnetization than it is along hard directions of magnetization, as Fig. 9–9 shows. It is interesting that face-centered cubic (fcc) nickel (βNi, $O_h{}^5$) and body-centered cubic (bcc) iron (αFe. $O_h{}^9$) have opposite easy and hard directions of magnetization. Hexagonal close packed (hcc) cobalt (αCo, $D_{5h}{}^4$) shows an even more startling behavior with its hard direction of magnetization located along the hexagonal or c axis below 275° C and its easy direction along the c axis above 275° C, as is shown graphically on p. 555 of Bozorth (1951).

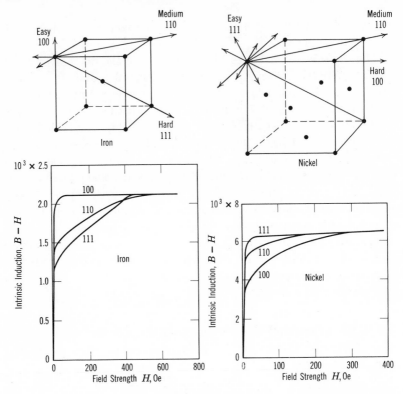

Fig. 9–9.　Magnetic properties and crystal structures of single crystals of iron and nickel [Bozorth (1951)].

D. Permanent Magnets

It was explained in the previous section that a permanent magnet is constructed from a ferromagnetic material with a large residual induction B_r such as the one shown in Fig. 9–7c [Hadfield (1962); Parker and Studders (1962)]. A large value of the permeability is also important for producing a permanent magnet that supplies a high magnetic induction B. Pertinent design data are given by Shutt and Whittemore (1951). Permanent magnets find wide application in magnetrons, isolators, relays, and other microwave electronic devices. A permanent magnet may be used in an NMR spectrometer designed for use with a single nucleus such as a proton, or in an ESR spectrometer which always operates at the same g

factor such as a vanadium analyzer [Saraceno, Fanale, and Coggeshall (1961)] or free radical detector. In these applications provision should be made for varying the magnetic field strength in the neighborhood of the resonance value (e.g., ± 10 or ± 100 G) and a current through a coil concentric with the pole pieces can provide this alignment field. Such a coil may also be employed for modulating the constant magnetic field.

The principal drawback of incorporating a permanent magnet in a magnetic resonance spectrometer is that the available magnetic field is limited to a narrow range centered at a particular g factor (e.g., $g = 2$). This prevents the study of broad resonance lines, other g factors, and the frequency dependence of ESR spectra. As a result most ESR spectrometers employ an electromagnet.

Dalman and Goodman (1957) have built a permanent magnet which produces both variable and reversible magnetic fields, but this magnet is not convenient for use in ESR spectrometers.

Several additional properties of permanent "bar" magnets are included in the next section.

E. Electromagnets

The magnetic induction in an electromagnet is usually produced by solenoids around the two pole pieces, and so this means of generating such a field will be discussed. Consider the plane circular loop of wire shown in Fig. 9–10. The magnetic field strength dH due to the current I in the element of length dl along the wire is

$$d\mathbf{H} = \frac{\mathbf{I} \times \mathbf{r}}{4\pi r^3}\, dl \tag{1}$$

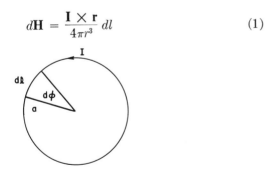

Fig. 9–10. Plane circular loop of wire carrying the current I.

where r is the distance from the current element and MKS units are employed. On the axis of the wire the current direction is perpendicular to the vector $\mathbf{r}$, and $dl = a\,d\phi$, so

$$d\mathbf{H} = \frac{Ia\,d\phi}{4\pi[a^2 + z^2]} \tag{2}$$

from Fig. 9–11. The vector $d\mathbf{H}$ may be decomposed into the component dH_z along the axis and $dH_\perp$ perpendicular to the axis. The latter cancels for current elements on opposite sides of the loop, and only the resultant H_z is nonvanishing

$$H_z = \sin \alpha \oint dH_z \tag{3}$$

$$= \frac{Ia \sin \alpha}{4\pi(a^2 + z^2)} \int_0^{2\pi} d\phi \tag{4}$$

$$= \frac{Ia^2}{2(a^2 + z^2)^{3/2}} \tag{5}$$

A solenoid may be considered as a series of loops concentric with and equispaced along the z axis, and the magnetic field strength along the axis is obtained by integrating eq. (6)

$$d\mathbf{H} = \frac{Ia^2 n}{2L(a^2 + z^2)^{3/2}}\, dz \tag{6}$$

along the solenoid, where n is the number of equispaced turns in the solenoid of length L. With the aid of Fig. 9–12 one may write

$$H = \frac{In}{2aL} \int_{L-\frac{1}{2}l}^{L+\frac{1}{2}l} \frac{dz}{[1 + (z^2/a^2)]^{3/2}} \tag{7}$$

$$= -\frac{In}{2L} \int_{\cot^{-1}[(z-\frac{1}{2}L)/a]}^{\cot^{-1}[(z+\frac{1}{2}L)/a]} \sin \theta d\theta \tag{8}$$

$$= \frac{In}{2L} (\cos \theta_2 - \cos \theta_1) \tag{9}$$

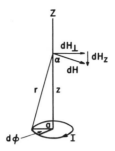

Fig. 9–11. Coordinate system for calculating the axial magnetic field strength for a loop of wire.

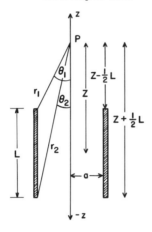

Fig. 9–12. Coordinate system for computing the magnetic field strength along the axis of a solenoid.

where θ_1 and θ_2 are defined in Fig. 9–12. At the center of the solenoid $\theta_1 + \theta_2 = \pi$ and

$$H = (In \cos \theta_1)/L \qquad (10)$$

while for a very long solenoid where $L \gg a$ and eq. (10) becomes

$$H = In/L \qquad (11)$$

At the upper end of the solenoid $\theta_1 = \pi/2$, and

$$H = (In \cos \theta_2)/2L \qquad (12)$$

which simplifies to

$$H = In/2L \tag{13}$$

for a long solenoid where $L \gg a$. Thus the field at the center of a long solenoid is twice its strength at the ends since half of the lines of force leak out the sides between the center and the end, as shown on Fig. 9–13. The magnetic field strength H inside a solenoid has exactly the same distribution as the magnetic induction B inside a uniformly magnetized bar magnet.

A large distance z from the solenoid the magnetic field strength along the axis is

$$H = \frac{In}{2L} \left[\frac{z + \tfrac{1}{2}L}{[a^2 + (z + \tfrac{1}{2}L)^2]^{1/2}} - \frac{z - \tfrac{1}{2}L}{[a^2 + (z - \tfrac{1}{2}L)^2]^{1/2}} \right] \tag{14}$$

$$= nIa^2/2z^3 \tag{15}$$

since $z \gg a$ and $z \gg L$. This is n times the result for a single turn or loop of wire when $L \ll 2a$. If one recalls that a loop of wire perpendicular to the z direction has a magnetic moment μ given by

$$\mathbf{\mu} = \mathbf{I} \times (\mathbf{Area}) = \pi a^2 I \mathbf{z}/z \tag{16}$$

one sees that

$$H = n\mu/2\pi z^3 \tag{17}$$

which is indeed n times the field strength arising from a magnetic dipole along its axis, as expected from eq. (20-I-1).

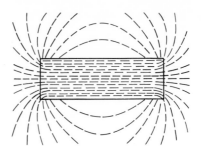

Fig. 9–13. The magnetic induction B of a uniformly magnetized bar magnet. This same figure also applies to the magnetic field strength H of a solenoid.

A torus consists of a solenoid which is bent in a circle so that its two ends are joined. More precisely, it is a doughnut-shaped solenoid with the turns of wire arranged uniformly around it. The magnetic field at any point in the torus is given by eq. (11).

$$H = In/L \qquad (11)$$

where L is the average circumference, and $L \gg a$. Thus the field everywhere in a torus is identical with that in the center of a solenoid which carries the same current and has the same number of turns per unit length.

As mentioned above, the magnetic induction B of a uniformly magnetized bar magnet is presented in Fig. 9–13. For comparison purposes, the magnetic field strength H of the same magnet is given on Fig. 9–14. The surprising thing about Fig. 9–14 is that H is "pushed out" of the magnet in the middle. In the space around the magnet, the magnetization $M = 0$ and $B = \mu_0 H$, and at its edges the normal component of B and the transverse component of H are continuous across the boundary. Inside the magnetic material H is in the opposite direction to B and the relation

$$\mathbf{B} = \mu_0 \, (\mathbf{H} + \mathbf{M}) \qquad (18)$$

is satisfied. Fig. 9–15 shows how the quantities of eq. (18) vary in a bar magnet. If a bar magnet has a discontinuity or gap whose length d is much less than the radius a (and *a fortiori* $d \ll L$) the magnetic induction will be perturbed in the manner shown in Fig.

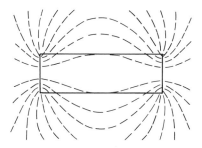

Fig. 9–14.   The magnetic field strength H of a uniformly magnetized bar magnet. The field is weakest in the center and strongest at the ends.

9–16.   If the gap d is increased, then of course the lines of force will leak out more, and the effective field strength in the gap will decrease.   In addition the increased reluctance of the magnetic circuit will decrease B both within and without the metal.   Thus when the magnet gap is increased, there are two mechanisms which cause the magnetic field in the gap to decrease in intensity.

The preceding few paragraphs have explained how a solenoid produces a magnetic field, how a magnetic field is distributed in a bar magnet, and how this field is disturbed by the presence of a gap in the bar magnet.   The reader is now prepared to construct from

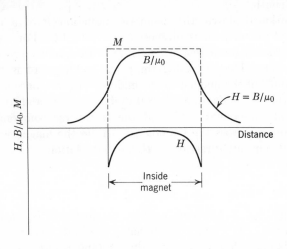

Fig. 9–15.   The relationship between the magnetization M, the magnetic induction B, and the magnetic field strength H in a uniformly magnetized (M = constant) bar magnet.   Within the magnet, B and H are oppositely directed [Sommerfeld (1948)].

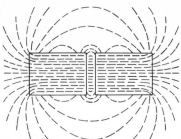

Fig. 9–16.   The magnetic induction B of a bar magnet with a gap.

these elements a magnet such as the one illustrated on Fig. 9–1. The two yokes act like a "double torus" and the magnetomotive force in the coils induces a magnetic flux which may be said to "flow" around the magnetic circuit or yokes in analogy with an electrical circuit. Since the gap is an integral part of the circuit, the flux flows across it and produces the required magnetic field for an ESR experiment.

The design of an electromagnet entails specifying the number and distribution of the turns, the selection of the proper pole pieces and yoke material, and many other details which will not be discussed here. The attainment of a very homogenous magnetic field requires the use of pole caps that are optically flat and parallel. Shims may be employed to aid in rendering the pole pieces parallel, and a lever for shimming is provided on some commercial magnets. The shim settings are somewhat field sensitive. The design of ring shims is discussed by Rose (1938), Bjorken and Bitter (1956), and Andrew and Rushworth (1952), and current shims are discussed by Golay (1958), Anderson (1961), and Zupančič (1962). In high resolution NMR, it is customary to spin the sample, and the shims are adjusted for maximum homogeneity along the axis of rotation where the averaging effect of the rotation is a minimum. Domain structures on the magnet pole faces produce microinhomogeneities at the pole faces which become negligible at the center of the gap [Brown and Bitter (1956)].

A chapter on electromagnets would not be complete without mentioning Helmholtz coils [Ruark and Peters (1926); see also Page and Adams (1949), p. 257]. These consist of two concentric and parallel circular loops of wire which have the same radii a. When the loops are placed a distance apart equal to their radius a, they produce at the midpoint between them a fairly uniform magnetic field H given by [W. T. Scott (1960)].

$$H = 8I/5^{3/2}a \qquad (19)$$

where I is the current. The field varies as $1/a$ for small distances r from the center. Double Helmholtz coils improve the magnetic field homogeneity even further [G. G. Scott (1957)]. The righthand side of eq. (19) is multiplied by n when each coil contains n turns. Sauzade and Sallé (1964) discuss the effect of the surroundings on Helmholtz coils.

One may employ NMR techniques to observe electron spin resonance. For example, solid DPPH may be detected at 34 Mc by placing the sample in the center of a Helmholtz coil and scanning the magnetic field from 9–15 G.

A number of unconventional electromagnet designs may be found in the literature. For example, Strandberg, Tinkham, Solt, and Davis (1956) built the yokeless electromagnet shown on Fig. 9–17 with the justification that for a relatively long gap the large cross section of the return path through the air supplies a reluctance which is less than the reluctance of the gap. He defines the magnet power efficiency η in terms of an equation analogous to eq. (9-B-22):

$$B = \eta \, (\mu_0 n I/d) \tag{20}$$

$$= 1.6 \times 10^{-5}\eta \, (MP)^{1/2}/ad \tag{21}$$

where M is the mass of the Cu windings in kg, P is the power input to the magnet in watts, and both the gap length d and the average

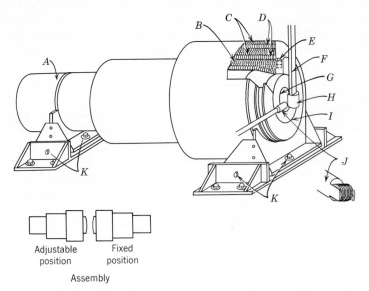

Adjustable position   Fixed position

Assembly

Fig. 9–17. Yokeless magnet: (A) core; (B) low field coils, regulated; (C) high field coils, unregulated; (D) cooling coils; (E) trimmer and modulation coils; (F) waveguide; (G) modulation feedback; (H) cavity; (I) Rose ring [cf. Rose (1938)]. (J) flip coil; (K) alignment screws [Strandberg, Tinkham, Solt, and Davis (1956)].

coil radius a are in meters. When the gap length is about one-third the pole diameter and the coils are about three times the pole diameter, the power efficiency η is about one-third up to the point of saturation. This yokeless design is low in cost and has a high power efficiency for large gaps. Disadvantages lie in the initial alignment of the pole pieces, the low power efficiency for small gaps, and the large stray fields which amount to a hundred gauss several feet away from the magnet.

An electromagnet may be constructed by circulating a large current in a superconducting coil or series of coils at liquid helium temperature. The superconductor has almost zero resistance, and so once the current is induced in the coil it will continue circulating for many hours. See Autler (1960), Adair, Squire, and Utley (1960), and Berlincourt (1963) for further details. Superconductors have also been employed for stabilizing magnets [(Foner (1963); Dunlap, Hempstead, and Kim (1963)].

Electromagnets are usually water-cooled and the water temperature may be controlled, but this is usually not necessary. A flow meter may be installed to measure the rate of flow. If the flow rate is too slow, excessive heating may occur, and if the rate is too fast, the temperature of the coil may be lowered sufficiently to cause moisture to condense on the coils and produce rusting. Slomp (1959) found that variations in the temperatures of the room air and of the magnet cooling water produced noticable drift effects on recorded NMR spectra. They alleviated the difficulty by enclosing the magnet (plywood or polystyrene foam are satisfactory) and regulating the water temperature. The resolution requirements in most ESR experiments are not sufficiently great to require such elaborate magnet control precautions. However, if the line-widths of spectra recorded from radical ions and other paramagnetic species do become much narrower, then some form of temperature regulation may become necessary. Hausser (1962, 1964) has observed ESR line-widths as low as 17 mG.

F. Magnet Power Supplies and Stabilizers

A low resistance magnet may be operated with storage batteries if it is desired to construct a spectrometer without going to the expense and trouble of buying or building a magnet power supply and stabilizer. Storage batteries have excellent short time stability, but they exhibit a gradual decrease in voltage while in use. This decrease is usually negligible for a typical ten to thirty minute scan, and can be checked by comparing the line-shape for a forward and a backward scan. It may be found possible to charge batteries while they are in use energizing the magnet, and in this capacity they serve as constant voltage sources for the battery charger which supplies constant current to the magnet coils. Such an arrangement should not be employed unless it is checked against the magnet performance when the battery charger is not operating [see Poole (1958) and Vinal (1950, 1955)].

Strandberg, Tinkham, Solt, and Davis (1956) energized their yokeless magnet shown in Fig. 9–17 with a motor generator and stabilized it with the circuit shown on Fig. 9–18. The functions of the various circuit components are as follows. The magnetic field strength in the magnet is monitored continuously by a flip coil whose output voltage is proportional to the magnetic field strength H. A reference voltage derived from a 30-cps reference generator followed by a 10-turn helipot is adjusted to be 180° out of phase with and approximately the same amplitude as the flip coil output. The two voltages are added in the 5691 (RCA red tube equivalent to a 6SL7) twin triode mixer, and the resulting error signal is amplified in a tuned amplifier. The first 6SJ7 is a 30-cps twin T amplifier which passes only frequencies close to 30 cps, and the twin T filters between the first and second, and the second and third stages reject, respectively, the fifth and second harmonics of 30 cps. Full wave synchronous detection of the amplified error voltage occurs in the Brown converter. The lower part of Fig. 9–18a shows the two-stage amplifier and phase shifter which provides the signal from the reference generator that switches the Brown converter vane between the outputs of the two 6SN7 plates. The converter output is positive if the flip coil voltage exceeds the helipot reference voltage and negative otherwise. The RC circuit at the converter output prevents unwanted oscillations from occurring. The error signal output (*) of the converter is applied to the "control" input point (*) of the 6SL7 tube of Fig. 9–18b. This tube is a cathode follower which matches the Brown converter and RC filter to the 6SF5–6L6 two-stage direct coupled dc amplifier. The amplifier output provides the grid voltage of the seven parallel 815 regulator or pass tubes, and therefore it controls the current that passes through the regulator tubes to the motor-generator.

The stabilization system works as follows. If the magnetic field deviates toward a higher field strength than the prescribed value, it causes the voltage in the flip coil to increase, and this produces an error voltage in the 5691 mixer. The Brown converter transforms the 30-cps sine wave error signal to a negative full wave rectified error signal which makes the grids of the 815 regulator tubes more negative. This increased negative grid bias decreases the plate current of the regulator tubes, which decreases the current through the motor generator and thereby lowers the magnetic field strength to its prescribed value.

The discussion of the regulated magnet power supply of Strandberg, Tinkham, Solt, and Davis is intended to illustrate the basic principles of how such circuits work. When a malfunction develops, it is particularly advantageous to understand the circuitry because such an understanding greatly facilitates troubleshooting, as discussed in Sec. 9–I. It is recommended that each ESR spectroscopist make a detailed study of all of his circuits because the time spent in so doing will be saved later in troubleshooting.

Several detailed discussions of magnet stabilizers for use in magnetic resonance spectroscopy are given in the literature. See, for example, Lawson and Tyler (1939), Sommers, Weiss, and Halpern (1951), Gilvarry and Rutland (1952), Suryan (1952), Havill and Rubin (1955), Hedgecock and Hunt (1956), Abraham, Ovenall, and Whiffin (1957), Lesaukis, Kolobkov, and Ambrasas (1962), and Kummer (1964). Current stabilizers maintain the magnet current constant, and as a result they do not properly correct for changes in the magnetic field which are not in a one to one correspondence with current changes (e.g., temperature changes). One may stabilize the magnetic field directly by means of nuclear magnetic resonance. NMR magnet stabilizers are described by Packard (1948), Vrščaj (1955), Müller-Warmuth and Servoz-Gavin (1958), Hahn (1960), Feldman (1960), Marsden (1961), Eades, Jenks and Bradbury (1961), Vincent (1960), Vincent, Kaine and King (1962), Vincent, Kaine and Titchmarsh (1964), Schwind (1962), Sasaki (1963), Denyak and Siderenko (1964), and Olsen (1964). Figure 9–19 gives a block diagram of Sasaki's NMR magnetic field stabilizer, and Fig. 9–20 gives one of the circuits from Vincent, Kaine, and King's (1962) NMR stabilizer. Maki and Volpicelli (1965) describe a magnetic field tracking NMR gaussmeter. The Hall effect may be employed

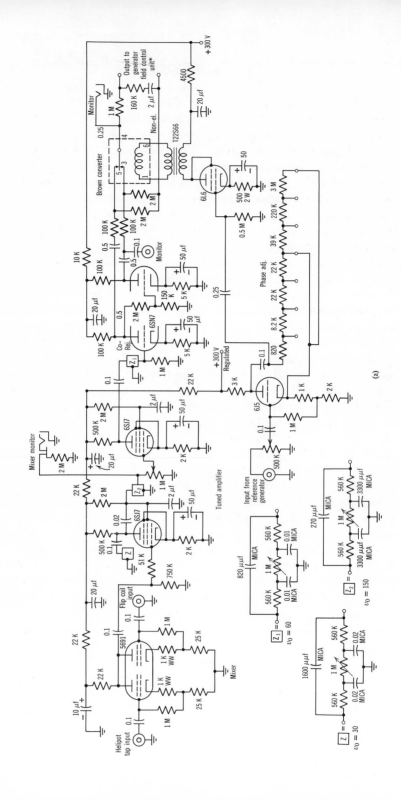

(a)

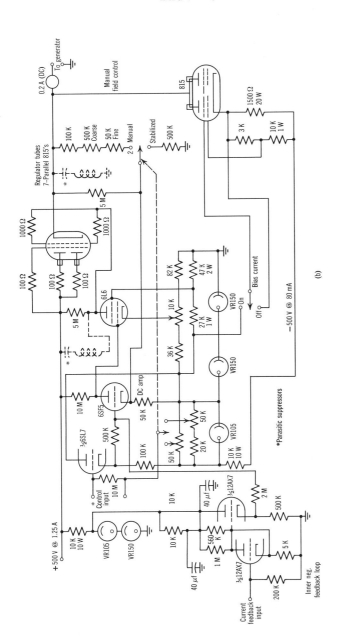

Fig. 9–18. (a) Field stabilization discriminator; (b) field stabilization dc power amplifier [Strandberg, Tinkham, Solt, and Davis (1956)].

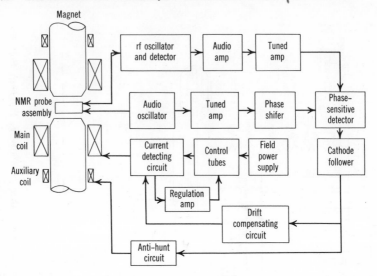

Fig. 9-19.   Block diagram of an NMR magnetic field stabilizer [Sasaki (1963)].

to stabilize the magnetic field itself rather than the current.   This is discussed in Sec. 9-H.

G. Strong Magnetic Fields

Permanent magnets are feasible up to 10,000 G and ferromagnetic core electromagnets are usually limited to field strengths below 60,000 G.   This means that electromagnets cannot be used above 170,000 Mc for ESR experiments at $g = 2$.   At higher frequencies it is necessary to produce the magnetic field in air or *in vacuo*. Pulsed magnetic fields above one MG have been produced by discharging condensers through a coil.   Information on pulsed magnetic fields may be found in the literature.   For example, see Furth and Waniek (1956) and Furth, Levine, and Waniek (1957). Air core electromagnets for continuous operation have been built for use between 100 and 125 kG, as are discussed by Giauque and Lyon (1960).   For additional information on strong magnetic fields see Kolm, Lax, Bitter, and Mills (1962), Montgomery (1963) and Karasik (1962).

Constant high magnetic fields up to and above 70 kG are best attained by superconducting magnets [Nelson and Weaver (1964);

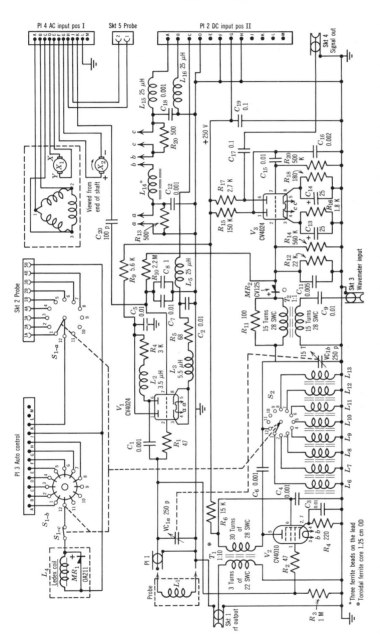

Fig. 9–20. Circuit diagram of a proton resonance magnetometer unit used in a magnetic field stabilizer. The CV4010 is equivalent to the CAK5 and the CV4024 is equivalent to a 12AT7 [Vincent, Kaine, and King (1962)].

Sauzade, Pontnau, and Girard (1964); Laverick and Lobell (1964)]. Methods of measuring the field in a superconducting solenoid up to 85 kG are described by Danilychev, Karlov, Osipov, Shirkov, and Shlippe (1964), and Maxfield and Merrill (1965). Fietz (1965) discusses a stabilizer for a superconducting solenoid.

H. Magnetometers

The strength of a magnetic field is determined by means of a magnetometer or gaussmeter. In ESR work, NMR magnetometers are ordinarily employed, but before discussing them, a brief description of other magnetometer principles will be given. An excellent review of this subject has been given by Symonds (1955), and earlier reviews were published by McKeehan (1929) and Cotton and Dupouy (1932). Since Symonds has an excellent set of references, no attempt will be made to repeat them at the end of this chapter.

The Hall Effect: When a metal of length l, width w, thickness t, and resistivity ρ, and which carries a current I, is placed in a magnetic field B directed along t perpendicular to the current direction, a potential difference V_h appears across the width w at right angles to both I and B. The magnitude of this voltage is given by the equation

$$V_h = R_H I B / t \qquad (1)$$

where R_H is the Hall coefficient in volt centimeters/ampere oersted, I is in amperes, B is in gauss, and t is in centimeters. In p-type or hole semiconductors, the Hall voltage is positive and in n-type or electon semiconductors it is negative. Second-order effects cause the Hall voltage V_h to deviate slightly from the linear dependence on the magnetic field. Hall probes covering the range from 50 to 20,000 G are available commercially, and several manufacturers incorporate them into their magnet control systems. This eliminates hysteresis effects. In addition, it allows one to set the magnet to a particular field value and scan over a predetermined interval in gauss [see Nagatomo and Iwasaki (1965); Danilychev, Karlov, Osipov, Shirkov, and Shlippe (1964); Metzger, Stampfler, Armbruste, and Taglang (1964)].

Peaking Strips: This magnetometer employs a ferromagnetic alloy with an almost rectangular hysteresis loop as described by Kelly (1951) and Symonds (1955).

Rotating and Vibrating Coils: A voltage is induced in a coil which moves (e.g., rotates or vibrates) in a magnetic field in such a manner that the total flux through the coil changes.

Forces on Conductors Carrying Currents: When a conductor carrying a current I is placed in a magnetic field B, it experiences a force proportional to both $\mathbf{I} \times \mathbf{B}$.

Miscellaneous Methods: Symonds (1955) enumerates a large number of additional physical phenomena which may be employed in the measurement of magnetic fields.

Nuclear Magnetic Resonance Magnetometers: Nuclear magnetic resonance results from the interaction of a nuclear magnetic moment $g\beta_N I$ with a magnetic field H in the same way that electron spin resonance results from the interaction of an electronic magnetic moment $g\beta S$ with a magnetic field. The magnitudes of the interactions

$$h\nu = \hbar\gamma H = g\beta_N I \cdot \mathbf{H} \qquad \text{NMR} \qquad (2a)$$

$$h\nu = g\beta \mathbf{S} \cdot \mathbf{H} \qquad \text{ESR} \qquad (2b)$$

differ by three others of magnitude since the nuclear magneton β_N incorporates the protonic mass m_p in place of the electronic mass m which enters the denominator of the expression for the Bohr magnetron β [cf. eq. (1D-6)]. The nuclei employed in magnetometers such as H^1, H^2 (D), and Li^7 have their nuclear spin $I = \frac{1}{2}$ or 1. The proton NMR signal corresponding to a typical $g = 2$ ESR X band resonance (3300 G) is about 14 Mc. More precisely, in a 1000-G field the $g = 2.000$ ESR resonances occur at 2,799.4 Mc, proton (H^1) NMR comes at 4.2577 Mc, deuteron (D) NMR appears at 0.6536 Mc, and (Li^7) NMR is detected at 1.6547 Mc. Since the principles of NMR are no doubt familiar to most ESR specialists they will not be reviewed here. For further details consult one of the books or review articles listed in the Selected Bibliography, or the review article by Symonds (1955). Specific NMR magnetometers are described by Hopkins (1949), Pound and Knight (1950), Nolle and Henneke (1957), Marcley (1961), Bonnet (1962), van Eck (1962),

Vitolin', Kirshtein, and Krumin' (1962), De Martini and Lucchini (1964); Gordienko and Antonenko (1963), Niemelä (1964), Garwin and Patlach (1965), and Muha (1965).

Two particular NMR magnetometer circuits will be discussed in detail, and then some general comments about magnetometers will be made. The first circuit by Hopkins (1949) is one of the original models, and it is shown in Fig. 9–21. The sample coil, tuning condenser, wobbling or modulaton coils and the 6AK5 regenerative detector are incorporated in the probe which is inserted into the magnet gap. The probe must be free of all ferromagnetic materials. Modulation amplitudes up to 55 G are available. The minimum usable gap was 4 cm. Four separate sample coils with 3, 9, 14, and 25 turns, respectively, were wound around water samples contained in 0.5-cm inner diameter glass tubing 1.2 cm long which was sealed with glyptal cement. The signal detected by the 6AK5 tube undergoes two stages of amplification, and is then displayed on the y axis of an oscilloscope. The lower part of Fig. 9–21 gives the magnetometer power supply.

To use the magnetometer, the regeneration control 5K potentiometer is advanced until the onset of oscillations is seen on the oscilloscope trace since the maximum sensitivity occurs when oscillations are just barely maintained. The frequency f of the magnetometer is measured by zero-beating it with a loosely coupled standard oscillator, and the magnetic field H is calculated from the relation $H = \text{const.} \times f$. The width of the resonance absorption is an indication of the magnet homogeneity since it broadens in inhomogeneous fields [Béné, (1953) and Béné, Denis, Extermann, and Bonhomme (1953)]. The magnetometer was tested from 1900 to 16,000 G but below 3000 G, the signal is difficult to locate. A more widely used circuit, devised about the same time as the Hopkins circuit, is described by Pound and Knight (1950). The noise characteristics of a marginal oscillator NMR spectrometer are described by Howling (1965) [see also Watkins (1952)]

A modern transistorized version of a marginal oscillator magnetometer is shown in Fig. 9–22. Both the 2N1744 marginal oscillator and the second 2N1744 transistor which functions as an emitter follower were located in the probe. A potentometer arrangement was used to remotely tune the frequency from 20 to 65 Mc by means of a high Q silicon voltage variable capacitor PC 117. The same

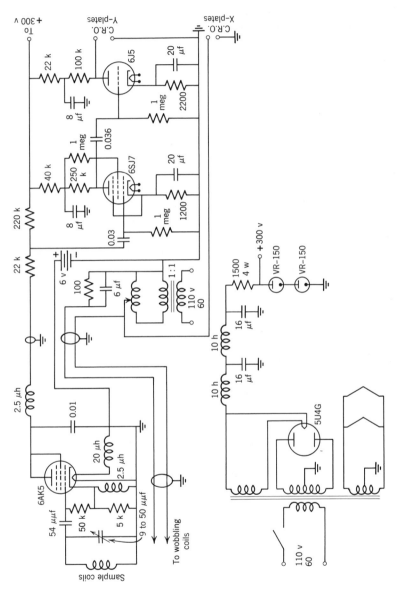

Fig. 9–21. Circuit diagram of an NMR magnetometer [Hopkins (1949)].

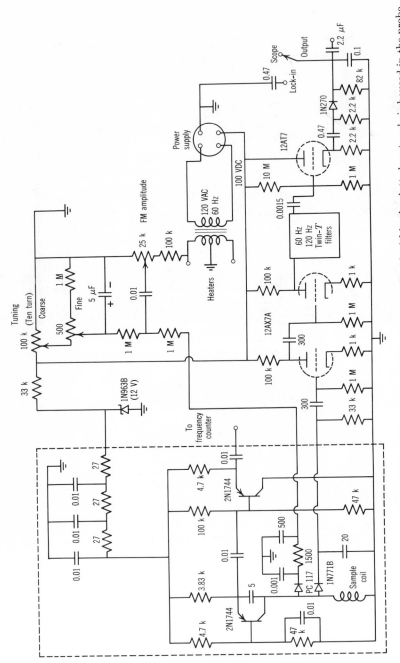

Fig. 9–22.   Circuit diagram of NMR spectrometer.   The portion enclosed within the dotted rectangle is housed in the probe. Capacitance values ≥ 1 are in μF, and those < 1 are in pF, unless otherwise specified [Pierce and Hicks (1965)].

capacitor may be used to provide 60 cps frequency modulation. No variable feedback and level controls are required. The NMR samples have a volume of 8 mm³, and the center of the NMR resonance can be determined to within one part per million.

An oscilloscope trace of the nuclear resonance signal is presented in Fig. 9–23, and the appearance of the "wiggles" shown on Fig. 9–23a is a measure of the magnetic field homogeneity. The less homogeneous the magnetic field, the less prominent are the wiggles. Water samples for proton sources are normally doped with a paramagnetic salt such as 1 N MnSO₄ to shorten the relaxation times.

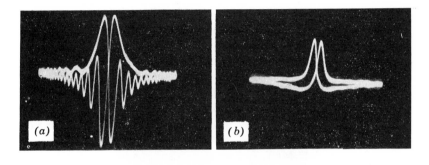

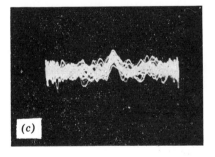

Fig. 9–23. Oscilloscopic presentation of an NMR magnetometer signal. (a) Trace on an oscilloscope of proton resonance in 0.5 cm³ of mineral oil in 6400-G field, illustrating use as a field meter. Total sweep here is about 0.5 G. The "wiggles" are very prominent owing to the good homogeneity of the field over the sample. Sweep amplitude is about 0.5 G peak-to-peak. (b) Resonance in same magnet as a, but in aqueous solution with added paramagnetic MnSO₄. Sweep amplitude is about 5 G, peak-to-peak. (c) Oscilloscope trace in field of 360 G with only about 0.5 G inhomogeneity over the sample. Sweep amplitude is about 10 G, peak-to-peak [Pound and Knight (1950)].

It is also convenient to saturate the solution with LiCl so that Li^7 NMR may be used in high magnetic fields. The Li^7 resonance is weaker due to the lower concentration of the Li^7 nuclei relative to the protons, and its presence in the solution does not effect the H^1 resonance. The magnetometer has been operated from 250 to 10,000 G (1 to 45 Mc) with protons, and if Li^7 is used, the range is extended to 25,000 G. The accuracy of the measurements is limited by the magnetic field homogeneity and the accuracy of the frequency measuring equipment. In practice, one may measure field values at points corresponding to 100 kc or 1 Mc crystal marker frequencies. For less accurate work, the capacitor dial may be calibrated against crystal markers, a frequency meter such as the BC–221, or a commercial frequency counter (plus transfer oscillator).

NMR magnetometers are convenient for use with ESR spectrometers because they are usable over a very wide range of magnetic fields, and they can easily reach an accuracy of one part in 10^5. The frequency can be measured by standard crystal-controlled oscillators, and these can be calibrated against the National Bureau of Standards (Washington, D.C.) radio station WWV which broadcasts standard frequencies at 5, 10, 15, and 20 Mc. accurate to two parts in 10^8 (2.5, 25, 30, and 35 Mc-frequencies are also broadcast at much lower power by WWV). These frequencies are modulated at one cps with a 5 msec. pulse (with an accuracy of 1 μsec.) at the start of each record. A proton magnetometer may be used to provide accurate field calibration over narrow ranges by utilizing sidebands generated by a frequency modulation technique [Mito, Okimura, and Mima (1964); Lancaster and Smallman (1965)].

An ESR magnetometer operating at typical NMR frequencies may be employed to measure weak magnetic fields [Gabillard and Germain (1955)].

I. Checking and Troubleshooting Electromagnets

It is wise for each microwave spectroscopist to learn the characteristics of his magnet. This entails keeping records of dial settings, meter readings, and magnetic field values that correspond to the field and scan positions normally used. When trouble arises, it will normally manifest itself in abnormal dial settings, meter readings, magnetic field values, or ESR spectra. Magnet drift can usually be detected by comparing a spectrum recorded with both increasing and decreasing magnetic field scans. The homogeneity of the field may be tested by observing the "wiggles" from a proton NMR magnetometer, as shown on Fig. 9–23. The wiggles vanish and the line broadens in regions of inhomogeneity, and moving the proton coil across the magnetic field allows one to map out the field homogeneity. The proton frequency indicates whether or not the actual field strength reading deviates from its customary value. A lack of stabilization may manifest itself by a proton signal which jumps around on the oscilloscope, or by fluctuations in meter readings. Sometimes it produces "spikes", excess noise, or irregular line-shapes in recorded spectra. The trouble may be isolated by disconnecting the magnet scanner and other associated equipment and ascertaining if the difficulty remains. To check for magnetometer trouble, a narrow ESR line such as DPPH may be observed visually. All test voltages should be measured and the B^+ 300 V supply should be checked on an oscilloscope for ripple (which will usually not exceed about 5 mV).

Once the characteristics of the trouble have been identified, one is ready to seek the culprit. The first thing to suspect is a bad vacuum tube or transitor, or a loose connection in a wire or cable. The transistors and tubes may be tested on a tube tester, but it is easier to stock spare ones and to replace them one by one and see if the trouble clears up after each change. The big pass tubes (e.g., 304 TL) and high voltage rectifiers (e.g., 872A) may be tested by putting a multimeter in series with the plate or cathode and measuring the plate current. Tubes with low plate currents should be replaced. *Caution: The presence of high voltages renders this test very dangerous and one should exercise extreme caution.* Sometimes one can tell bad pass tubes and high voltage rectifiers by the color of their "glow" when under load. Loose cable connections may frequently be detected by shaking or bending the cable near the junction. It is wise to have a number of test points for checking the voltages. One may check a transistor or vacuum tube by measuring its collector, emitter, and base (plate, grid, and cathode) voltages, respectively, and comparing them against the characteristics curves. Burned out resistors may frequently be spotted visually, and may be checked with a multimeter. Burned out magnet coils may be detected by measuring for continuity (resistance) at the coils.

Periodic maintenance is advisable. From time to time it will be necessary to replace vacuum tubes and transistors. Most electromagnets are water-cooled, and the filter which cleans the water should be changed periodically (e.g., every few months). If a thin film of oil is kept on the polepieces, rusting will be minimized. Reference batteries (e.g., mercury cells) should be replaced every few months. When aging occurs, their voltage drops, especially when they are tested under load (i.e., when drawing a current). Thermocouples may be mounted in the magnet coils and connected to a potentiometer to check the magnet temperature.

It is best to keep a careful record of all the trouble that occurs because the various difficulties have a tendency to recur.

J. Units

Most chemistry and some physics books employ cgs units while most engineering and some physics texts use practical or mks units. so conversion factors will be given for B and H. In cgs units $\mu_0 = 1$ and in mks units

$$\mu_0 = 4\pi \times 10^{-7} \quad \text{Wb/mA} \tag{1}$$

$$= 4\pi \times 10^{-7} \quad \text{H/m} \tag{2}$$

with the result that

$$B \; (\text{Wb/m}^2) = 4\pi \times 10^{-7} \; (\mu/\mu_0) \, H \quad \text{At/m} \tag{3}$$

$$B \; (\text{G}) = (\mu/\mu_0) \, H \quad \text{Oe} \tag{4}$$

where μ/μ_0 is the dimensionless relative permeability. The two conversion formulae are

$$H \; (\text{At/m}) = 10^3/4\pi \, H \quad \text{Oe} \tag{21}$$

and

$$B \; (\text{Wb/m}^2) = 10^{-4} \, B \quad \text{G} \tag{22}$$

Thus for a relative permeability of $\mu/\mu_0 = 1000$, a field of 10 Oe corresponds to 10,000 G $\sim$ 800 At/m and 1 Wb/m. One may make an order of magnitude estimate that for this permeability and a current of two amperes, the coils on the magnet shown on Fig. 9–1 must have at least 400 turns/m or 4 turns/cm. In practice, flux leakage at the gap, in particular, and throughout the magnetic circuit, in general, will considerably raise this requirement.

References

R. J. Abraham, D. W. Ovenall, and D. H. Whiffen, *JSI*, **34**, 269 (1957).

T. W. Adair III, C. F. Squire, and H. B. Utley, *RSI*, **31**, 416 (1960).

W. A. Anderson, *RSI*, **32**, 241 (1961).

E. R. Andrew and F. A. Rushworth, *Proc. Phys. Soc.*, **B65**, 801 (1952).

S. H. Autler, *RSI*, **31**, 369 (1960).

G. J. Béné, P. M. Denis, and R. C. Extermann, *Helv. Phys. Acta*, **26**, 267 (1953).

G. J. Béné, P. M. Denis, E. C. Extermann, and H. J. Bonhomme, *Helv. Phys. Acta*, **26**, 435 (1953).

T. G. Berlincourt, *Brit. J. Appl. Phys.*, **14**, 749 (1963).

J. D. Bjorken and F. Bitter, *RSI*, **27**, 1005 (1956).

G. Bonnet, *Ann. Geophys.*, **18**, 62, 150 (1962).

K. D. Bowers and J. Owen, *Rept. Progr. Phys.*, **18**, 304 (1955).

R. M. Bozorth, *Ferromagnetism*, van Nostrand, N. Y., 1951.

H. H. Brown and F. Bitter, *RSI*, **27**, 1009 (1956).

B. A. Coles, *Lab. Pract.*, **13**, 1073 (1964).

A. Cotton and G. Dupouy, *Congrès. Intern. Elect. III, Rept. 12*, Sec. 2E (1932).

J. A. Dalman and L. S. Goodman, *RSI*, **28**, 961 (1957).

V. A. Danilychev, N. V. Karlov, B. D. Osipov, A. V. Shirkov, and G. I. Shlippe, *PTE*, **5**, 221 (990) (1963).

F. De Martini and A. Lucchini, *Alta Frequenza*, **33**, 746 (186E) (1964).

V. M. Denyak and L. I. Siderenko, *PTE*, **6**, 176 (1181) (1963).

R. D. Dunlap, C. F. Hempstead, and Y. B. Kim, *J. Appl. Phys.*, **34**, 3147 (1963).

R. G. Eades, G. J. Jenks, and A. Bradbury, *JSI*, **38**, 210 (1961).

D. W. Feldman, *RSI*, **31**, 72 (1960).

W. A. Fietz, *RSI*, **36**, 1306 (1965).

S. Foner, *RSI*, **34**, 293 (1963).

H. P. Furth, M. A. Levine, and R. W. Waniek, *RSI*, **28**, 949 (1957).

H. P. Furth and R. W. Waniek, *RSI*, **27**, 195 (1956).

R. Gabillard and C. Germain, *Onde Élect.*, **35**, 495 (1955).

R. L. Garwin and A. M. Patlach, *RSI*, **36**, 741 (1965).

W. F. Giauque and D. N. Lyon, *RSI*, **31**, 374 (1960).

J. J. Gilvarry and D. F. Rutland, *RSI*, **23**, 111 (1952).

M. J. E. Golay, *RSI*, **29**, 313 (1958).

A. G. Gordienko and I. O. Antonenko, *PTE*, **4**, 144 (736) (1963).

D. Hadfield, *Permanent Magnets and Magnetism*, Wiley, N. Y., 1962, p. 556.

H. Hahn, *C. R. Acad. Sci.*, **250**, 2335 (1960).

K. H. Hausser, *Z. Naturforsch.*, **17A**, 158 (1962); *J. Chim. Phys.*, **61**, 1610 (1964).

K. H. Hausser, *Proc. XI Colloque Ampère*, North Holland, Amsterdam, 1963.

J. R. Havill and S. Rubin, *RSI*, **26**, 515 (1955).

F. T. Hedgecock and F. Hunt, *RSI*, **27**, 970 (1956).

N. J. Hopkins, *RSI*, **20**, 401 (1949).

D. H. Howling, *RSI*, **36**, 660 (1965).

C. A. Hutchison and R. C. Pastor, *J. Chem. Phys.*, **21**, 1959 (1953).

V. R. Karasik, *PTE*, **6**, 5 (1075) (1962).

J. M. Kelly, *RSI*, **22**, 256 (1951).

H. Kolm, B. Lax, F. Bitter, and R. Mills, *Proceedings of the International Conference on High Magnetic Fields, MIT*, Wiley, N. Y., 1962.

J. Kummer, *Z. Angew. Phys.*, **18**, 139 (1964).

G. Lancaster and A. G. Smallman, *JSI*, **42**, 341 (1965).

C. Laverick and G. Lobell, *RSI*, **36**, 825 (1965).

J. L. Lawson and A. W. Tyler, *RSI*, **10**, 304 (1939).

V. Lesauskis, V. Kolobkov, and V. Ambrasas, *Litov. Fiz. Sbornik*, **2**, 381 (1962).

L. W. McKeehan, *J. Opt. Soc. Am.*, **19**, 213 (1929).

A. H. Maki and R. J. Volpicelli, *RSI*, **36**, 325 (1965).

R. G. Marcley, *Am. J. Phys.*, **29**, 451 (1961).

K. H. Marsden, *JSI*, **38**, 471 (1961).

B. W. Maxfield and J. R. Merrill, *RSI*, **36**, 1083 (1965).

G. Metzger, A. Stampfler, R. Armbruste, and P. Taglang, *J. Phys. France, Suppl.*, **25**, 131A (1964).

S. Mito, K. Okumura, and H. Mima, *Mem. Fac. Eng. Osaka City Univ.*, **6**, 107 (1964).

D. B. Montgomery, *Rept. Progr. Phys.*, **26**, 69 (1963); see also *Brit. J. Appl. Phys.*, **14**, 741 (1963); *J. Appl. Phys.*, **36**, 893 (1965).

G. M. Muha, *RSI*, **36**, 551 (1965).

W. Müller-Warmuth and P. Servoz-Gavin, *Z. Naturforsch.*, **13A**, 194 (1958); see also W. Müller-Warmuth, *Z. Angew. Phys.*, **10**, 497 (1958).

H. Nagatomo and H. Iwasaki, *J. Radio Res. Lab.*, **12**, 39 (1965).

F. A. Nelson and H. E. Weaver, *Science*, **146**, 223 (1964).

L. Niemelä, *JSI*, **41**, 646 (1964).

A. W. Nolle and H. L. Henneke, *RSI*, **28**, 930 (1957).

W. C. Olsen, *Nucl. Instr. Methods*, **31**, 237 (1964).

J. W. Orton, *Rept. Progr. Phys.*, **22**, 204 (1959).

M. E. Packard, *RSI*, **19**, 435 (1948).

L. Page and N. L. Adams, Jr., *Principles of Electricity*, van Nostrand, N. Y., 1949, Chaps. 4, 7, 9, and 11.

R. J. Parker and R. J. Studders, *Permanent Magnets and Their Application*, Wiley, N. Y., 1962, p. 406.

W. L. Pierce and J. C. Hicks, *RSI*, **36**, 202 (1965).

C. P. Poole, Jr., Thesis, University of Maryland, 1958.

C. P. Poole, Jr., H. F. Swift, and J. F. Itzel, Jr., *J. Chem. Phys.*, **42**, 2576 (1965).

J. A. Pople, W. G. Schneider, and H. J. Bernstein, *High Resolution Nuclear Magnetic Resonance*, McGraw-Hill, N. Y., 1959.

R. V. Pound and W. D. Knight, *RSI*, **21**, 219 (1950).

M. E. Rose, *Phys. Rev.*, **53**, 715 (1938).

A. E. Ruark and M. F. Peters, *J. Opt. Soc. Am.*, **13**, 205 (1926).

A. J. Saraceno, D. T. Fanale, and N. D. Coggeshall, *Anal. Chem.*, **33**, 500 (1961).

Y. Sasaki, *Japan. J. Appl. Phys.*, **2**, 641 (1963).

M. Sauzade, J. Pontnau, and B. Girard, *C. R. Acad. Sci.*, **258**, 4458 (1964).

M. Sauzade and F. Sallé, *C. R. Acad. Sci.*, **259**, 73 (1964).

A. E. Schwind, *ETP*, **10**, 323 (1962).

G. G. Scott, *RSI*, **28**, 270 (1957).

W. T. Scott, *The Physics of Electricity and Magnetism*, Wiley, N. Y., 1960, p. 281.

R. P. Shutt and W. L. Whittemore, *RSI*, **22**, 73 (1951).

G. Slomp, *RSI*, **30**, 1024 (1959).

H. S. Sommers, Jr., P. R. Weiss, and W. Halpern, *RSI*, **22**, 612 (1951).

M. W. P. Strandberg, M. Tinkham, J. H. Solt, and C. F. Davis, Jr., *RSI*, **27**, 596 (1956).

G. Suryan, *JSI*, **29**, 335 (1952).

Y. Susaki, *Japan. J. Appl. Phys.*, **2**, 641 (1963).

J. L. Symonds, *Rept. Progr. Phys.*, **18**, 83 (1955).

J. L. Van Eck, *Rev. HF*, **5**, 143 (1962).

G. W. Vinal, *Primary Batteries*, Wiley, N. Y., 1950; *Storage Batteries*, Wiley, N. Y., 1955.

C. H. Vincent, *Nucl. Instr. Methods*, **7**, 325 (1960).

C. H. Vincent, D. Kaine, and W. G. King, *Nucl. Instr. Methods*, **16**, 163 (1962).

C. H. Vincent, D. Kaine, and R. S. Titchmarsh, *Nucl. Instr. Methods*, **27**, 156 (1964).

S. Visweswaramurthy, *Indian J. Pure Appl. Phys.*, **3**, 220 (1965).

A. Vitolin', G. Kirshtein, and Yu. Krumin', *Latvijas PSR Zinatnu Akad. Vestis*, **12**, 57 (185) (1962).

S. Vrščaj, *"J. Stefan" Inst. Rept.*, *(Ljubljana)*, **2**, 101 (1955).

G. D. Watkins, Ph.D. Thesis, Harvard University, 1952.

I. Zupančič, *JSI*, **39**, 621 (1962).

CHAPTER 10

Magnetic Field Scanning and Modulation

A. Magnet Scanning

The condition for energy absorption by the spin system is

$$h\nu \approx g\beta H \tag{1}$$

If the magnetic field H is kept constant and the frequency ν is varied, then the amount of energy absorbed will vary in accordance with the shape function $Y(\nu)$ where $Y(\nu)$ often has one of the two forms

$$Y(\nu) = y_m \exp\left[-0.693\left(\frac{\nu - \nu_0}{\tfrac{1}{2}\Delta\nu_{1/2}}\right)^2\right] \quad \text{Gaussian} \tag{2}$$

$$Y(\nu) = \frac{y_m}{1 + \left(\dfrac{\nu - \nu_0}{\tfrac{1}{2}\Delta\nu_{1/2}}\right)^2} \quad \text{Lorentzian} \tag{3}$$

In these expressions $\Delta\nu_{1/2}$ is the half amplitude full line-width in frequency units and y_m is the peak amplitude at $\nu = \nu_0$. If, on the other hand, the frequency is maintained constant and the magnetic field is varied, then one has the corresponding shape functions

$$Y(H) = y_m \exp\left[-0.693\left(\frac{H - H_0}{\tfrac{1}{2}\Delta H_{1/2}}\right)^2\right] \quad \text{Gaussian} \tag{4}$$

and

$$Y(H) = \frac{y_m}{1 + \left(\dfrac{H - H_0}{\tfrac{1}{2}\Delta H_{1/2}}\right)^2} \quad \text{Lorentzian} \tag{5}$$

387

where $\Delta H_{1/2}$ is the half amplitude full line-width in magnetic field units. These line-shapes are displayed graphically on Figs. 20-4 and 20-5. For most ESR resonances one can set

$$\Delta \nu_{1/2} = (g\beta/h) \, \Delta H_{1/2} = (\gamma/2\pi) \, \Delta H_{1/2} \tag{6}$$

where the gyromagnetic ratio γ and g factor are known from the resonance condition.

There are several reasons why it is not convenient to vary or scan the microwave frequency:

(1) The microwave generator (klystron) power output is strongly dependent on the frequency, so for best results the instrumentation would become more complex by the addition of a power stabilizer. Individual klystrons of the same model number vary in their frequency-power characteristics.

(2) The tuning of the microwave transmission line is frequency-sensitive, and it is not feasible to automatically tune the frequency-sensitive components while scanning since they have nonlinear responses. More specifically, some of the components which would have to be continuously retuned include the resonant cavity dimensions, the cavity iris, the slide screw tuner, the isolator (or attenuator), the (crystal) detector tuning stubs and plunger, the phase shifter, and the Pound stabilizer line-lengths.

(3) If the generator is a klystron, the mechanical and electronic tuning would have to be synchronized to maintain the resonant cavity pip at the top of the klystron mode during the scan.

(4) Typical klystrons can only be varied by 5 or 10% above and below their center frequency, and so very broad resonances can only be scanned in frequency over a fraction of their line-width. A carcinotron or backward wave oscillator with its lack of resonant structures, and its much wider frequency range, would be preferable in this application.

When the magnetic field is scanned, on the other hand, all of the above difficulties are automatically eliminated: (1) The microwave generator output is independent of the magnetic field strength. (2) The microwave tuning adjustments are independent of the magnetic field setting. (3) No adjustments of the microwave generator are necessary. (4) It is possible to scan from zero to several times the resonant magnetic field strength. As a result of these considerations, the magnetic field is normally scanned in ESR studies. Erickson (1966), however, describes an ESR spectrometer in which the frequency is scanned by moving the upper wall of the resonant cavity. In straight microwave spectroscopy, the frequency is usually scanned, and the resulting tuning problems often produce a drifting baseline.

A simple magnet scanner may consist of a variable resistance in series with the magnet coils, as shown on Fig. 10–1a. If the variable resistor or rheostat R is varied by a motor at a uniform rate the current through the magnet coils will also vary uniformly with time. If a second resistance R' is connected in parallel with R, then the scanning rate will become nonuniform. This type of scan is seldom employed with high voltage magnets.

An electronic magnet power supply may be scanned by varying the error voltage in the stabilization feedback loop. For example, one may employ a geared down (clock) motor to slowly rotate the ten-turn twin helical potentiometer which supplies the input to Strandberg, Tinkham, Solt, and Davis' (1956) field stabilizer shown on Fig. 9–18. This has been used to produce a linear sweep in the range from 0 to 10,000 G at any rate between 0.5 and 3000 G/min. Cook (1962), Cousins, Dupree, and Havill (1963), Jung (1964), and Blume and Williams (1964) describe electronic sweep units.

Štirand (1962) discusses the effect of the scanning rate on the recorded line-shape and position. For further details, see Sec. 14-F.

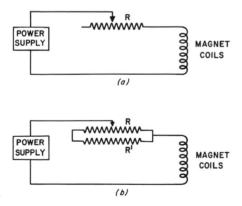

Fig. 10–1. Circuit for varying the current through the magnet coils (a) in a linear manner by the resistor R and (b) in a nonlinear manner by the resistors R and R'.

B. DC Detection

When the magnetic field is scanned through the region of resonance, the spin system in the resonant cavity absorbs a small amount of energy from the microwave (rf) magnetic field H_1, and also produces a slight change in the resonant frequency of the microwave cavity. These two factors produce a change in the amount of microwave power that is incident on the detector. For a strongly paramagnetic sample, the variation of the incident power will manifest itself by changing the detector output signal. For example, the rectified microwave power from a crystal detector may be observed by connecting a milliammeter in series with it, or the temperature change in a bolometer may be deduced from the resistance change measured by a voltmeter connected across it. These crude detection techniques could be employed with strong absorbers such as ferromagnetic samples, but with ordinary paramagnetics the absorption is excessively low.

It is possible to greatly increase the sensitivity by employing a multistage dc amplifier to enhance the signal. Feher (1957) showed that for a typical 3-cm system with the detector output proportional to the incident voltage, the fractional change in voltage $\Delta V/V$ at the detector is

$$\frac{\Delta V}{V}\bigg|_{min} \approx 2 \times 10^{-10} \tag{1}$$

for the minimum detectable signal under ideal conditions. If the detector output is proportional to the microwave power, then the relative power change $\Delta P/P$ at the detector for the same conditions is

$$\frac{\Delta P}{P}\bigg|_{min} \approx 10^{-10} \tag{2}$$

The leakage or operating current of a crystal detector is frequently about 10^{-4} A which is between the regions of linear and square law response corresponding to eqs. (11-D-4) and (11-D-5). As a result, the minimum detectable sample size will produce a current change of the order of 10^{-14} A which is very, very small. In order to achieve this sensitivity, the klystron power reflected (or transmitted) from the resonant cavity should be kept constant to within the limitations just mentioned, to insure that random power changes will not obscure the resonance absorption signal. Increased stability in the power supply voltages, plus a special power stabilization system, are both required. Unfortunately, it is not feasible to maintain the klystron power constant to this desired accuracy.

If the ESR sample is strong enough so that sensitivity is not a problem, then direct detection is capable of producing line-shapes that are free of modulation distortions. Both source and field modulation distort the line-shape when the modulation amplitude is not very small compared to the line-width ΔH expressed in gauss, or when the modulation frequency is not much less than the line-width $\Delta\nu$ expressed in frequency units, [see eq. (10-A-6)]. One instrumental shortcoming of the direct detection scheme is the fact that dc amplifiers tend to be more troublesome than ac amplifiers.

C. Source Modulation

A source-modulated spectrometer is one in which the microwave power is modulated and the ESR signal is detected and amplified at the modulation frequency. A large modulation amplitude may be obtained by switching an isolator on and off with a sawtooth voltage so that it alternately transmits first all of the microwave power, and then only a very small fraction of it. Square wave modulation of the reflector voltage shown on Fig. 6–7 can also turn the microwave power on and off [see Whitford (1961)]. A combination of frequency and amplitude modulation will result if the klystron reflector has impressed on it a sinusoidal or sawtooth waveform whose amplitude is less than the width of the klystron mode, as Fig. 6–7 indicates. Coumes and Ligeon (1964) simultaneously modulated the beam and reflector voltages to achieve a broad band-width.

Figure 10–2b shows the microwave waveform at the detector before source modulation, after source modulation, before resonance absorption, and after resonance absorption. At X band the microwave period $2\pi/\omega_0$ is about 10^{-10} sec, and a modulation frequency of 100 kc corresponds to a period of $2\pi/\omega_m = 10^{-5}$ sec. The modulation shown on this figure corresponds to the output of a sine-wave modulated isolator. It should be noticed that the amplitude of the modulation envelope before resonance is E_0, and during resonance it becomes $E_0 - \Delta E$, where

$$\Delta E/E_0 \ll 1 \qquad (1)$$

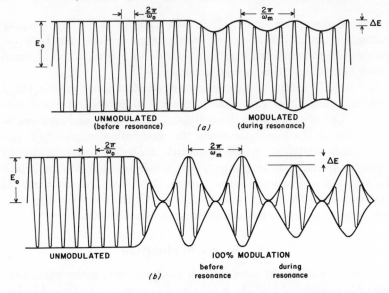

Fig. 10–2.   Microwave signal before and during resonance absorption: (a) using magnetic field modulation with the condition that the modulation amplitude E_m equals the dc absorption ΔE, and (b) using 100% source power modulation. Time increases to the right, and the microwave $(2\pi/\omega_0)$ and modulation $(2\pi/\omega_m)$ periods are indicated.

A different tuning condition could cause E_0 to increase by ΔE instead of decreasing, as assumed on Fig. 10–2.   The detector demodulates or removes the microwave carrier frequency, and only passes the signal at ω_m.   For further details one should consult a book on modulation theory [e.g., see Chap. 16 of Seely (1950)].

For optimum sensitivity, a source-modulated spectrometer requires the same precise power stability [see Munson (1950)] as the dc detection spectrometer described in the last article, and in addition, the modulating device must put out an extremely precise signal amplitude.   Physically, one may reason that random fluctuations in the modulation amplitude must be less than the change in amplitude that occurs at resonance.   Such amplitude stability would be difficult to obtain from an isolator.   In addition, unexpected low-frequency noise will appear in the source modulated spectrometer. Rinehart and Legan (1964) describe a power leveler which regulates milliwatts of K band power to within 0.5%.

Several investigators have employed source modulation for special applications, such as: (1) large line-widths [Bagguley and Griffiths (1952); Rose-Innes (1957)]; (2) low temperature work [Rose-Innes (1957)]; (3) saturation–line-shape studies [Kip, Kittel, Levy, and Portis (1953) and Portis (1953)]. These three applications will be discussed in turn.

In order to obtain maximum sensitivity when using magnetic field modulation, it is necessary to employ modulation amplitudes comparable to the line-width. In practice it is difficult to modulate at amplitudes exceeding 30 G, and so the sensitivity decreases for very broad lines. For example, if the line-width exceeds 1,000 G, the sensitivity with a 30-G modulation amplitude decreases by over a factor of 30. Source modulation does not become insensitive when broad lines are measured, and so it is sometimes applied to such a study.

The use of source modulation enables one to work at low temperatures without the inconvenience of inserting modulation coils into the Dewar. In the past, most low temperature experimental setups have either incorporated such modulation coils within the Dewar, or mounted them on the polecaps.

For accurate line shape determinations, it is necessary to use a modulation amplitude which is small relative to the line-width, which necessitates a loss of sensitivity. This is particularly important when one suspects the presence of unresolved hyperfine structure, as sometimes occurs in studies of F centers [Kip, Kittel, Levy, and Portis (1953); Portis (1953)]. Portis seems to pioneer in the use of unusual experimental setups, because more recently he continued his F center studies by microwave Faraday rotation in a bimodal cavity [Portis and Teaney (1958); Portis (1959); Teaney, Klein, and Portis (1961)]. A source modulated microwave cavity spectrometer is discussed theoretically by Weidner and Whitmer (1952) and by Hoisington, Kellner, and Pentz (1958). Several source-modulated spectrometers have been described in the literature [e.g., see Jen (1948); Artman and Tannenwald (1955); Paulevé (1955); Murina, Prokhorov, and Chayanova (1958); Dušek (1961); Hall and Schumacher (1962); Rinehart, Legan and Lin (1965)]. The undesirable effects of source modulation in an NMR spectrometer are discussed by Baker, Burd, and Root (1965).

D. Magnetic Field Modulation

Most electron spin resonance spectrometers incorporate magnetic field modulation, and therefore it will be discussed more extensively than the dc detection and source modulation schemes. When the magnetic field is modulated at the angular frequency ω_m, an alternating field $\frac{1}{2}H_m \sin \omega_m t$ is superimposed on the constant magnetic field $(H_0 + H_\delta)$. This "constant" magnetic field is ordinarily swept linearly over the range ΔH_0 from $(H_0 - \frac{1}{2}\Delta H_0)$ to $(H_0 + \frac{1}{2}\Delta H_0)$ in a time t_0, where H_0 is the magnetic field strength at the center of the scan. At any time t during the scan, the instantaneous magnetic field strength H is given by

$$H = H_0 + H_\delta + H_{\text{mod}} \tag{1}$$

$$= H_0 + \Delta H_0 \, (t/t_0 - \tfrac{1}{2}) + \tfrac{1}{2}H_m \sin \omega_m t \tag{2}$$

where

$$H_\delta = \Delta H_0 \, (t/t_0 - \tfrac{1}{2}) \tag{3}$$

It is assumed that the scan is slow enough so that there are many cycles of the modulation frequency during the passage between the peak to peak (or half amplitude) points of each resonant line, since under these conditions one may consider the magnetic field $(H_0 + H_\delta)$ as effectively constant. There are other conditions which must be satisfied for a true slow passage experiment, such as the necessity of scanning through the resonant line in a time which is long relative to the spin lattice and spin-spin relaxation times (see Sec. 18-B), but these will not concern us here.

The mechanism whereby the magnetic field modulation is transformed to microwave power modulation is shown in Fig. 10–3. The field modulated sine wave $\sin \omega_m t$ is converted by the nonlinear lineshape to a complex signal $F(H)$ which is a superposition of the fundamental modulation frequency ω_m and a large number of harmonics of ω_m:

$$F(H) = \sum_{n=0}^{\infty} [a_n(H) \cos n\omega_m t + b_n(H) \sin n\omega_n t] \tag{4}$$

The signal C at the inflection point of Fig. 10-3 is composed primarily of the fundamental $\sin \omega_m t$, while that at the center of the line A has the second harmonic $\cos 2\omega_m t$ as its principal component. Between these two points at B, the ESR signal has both the fundamental, the second harmonic, and higher harmonic terms in its Fourier series. Below the inflection point at D, the waveform resembles that at B, but is inverted and shifted by $180°$. Figure 10-2a shows the actual waveform at the detector, with the microwave carrier ω_0 modulated by the modulation fundamental ω_m at the inflection point C. The ESR signals on Figs. 10-3 and 10-4 are obtained by demodulating waveforms of the type shown in Fig. 10-2a.

If the situations depicted in Fig. 10-3 are approximated by the idealized straight line cases shown in Fig. 10-4, then the resulting ESR signals have forms which may be easily Fourier-analyzed. The

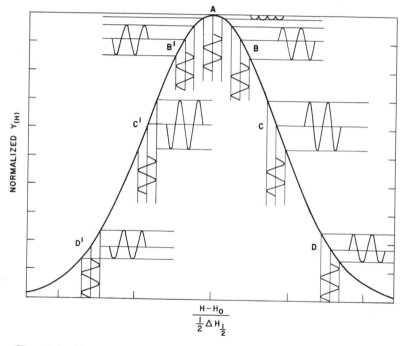

Fig. 10-3. The ESR signal produced at various points on the resonant line in a magnetic field modulated spectrometer. The vertical magnetic field modulation interacts with the bell-shaped absorption curve [χ' or $Y_{(H)}$] to produce the horizontal ESR signal.

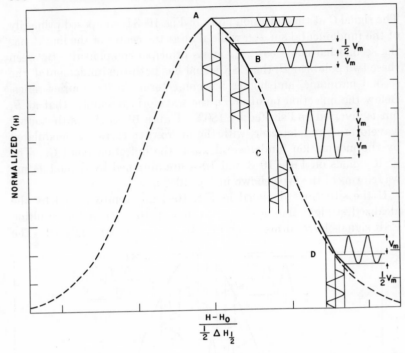

Fig. 10–4.   The ESR signal produced at various points on the resonant line using the linear approximation to the line-shape.   The wave forms for B', C', and D' are omitted for clarity.

Fourier series of two half wave and one full wave rectified signals are given on Fig. 10–5.   Using these series one may write down the expressions of the four waveforms shown on Fig. 10–4.   The first few terms of these Fourier series are:

$$A \quad V = \frac{V_m}{\pi}\left[-\frac{1}{2} + \frac{1}{3}\cos 2\omega_m t + \frac{1}{15}\cos 4\omega_m t + \dots \right] \tag{5}$$

$$B \quad V = \frac{V_m}{\pi}\left[-\frac{1}{2} + \frac{3\pi}{4}\sin \omega_m t + \frac{1}{3}\cos 2\omega_m t \right.$$

$$\left. + \frac{1}{15}\cos 4\omega_m t + \dots \right] \tag{6}$$

$$B' \quad V = \frac{V_m}{\pi} \left[-\frac{1}{2} - \frac{3\pi}{4} \sin \omega_m t + \frac{1}{3} \cos 2\omega_m t \right.$$
$$\left. + \frac{1}{15} \cos 4\omega_m t + \dots \right] \tag{7}$$

$$C \quad V = V_m \sin \omega_m t \tag{8}$$

$$C' \quad V = -V_m \sin \omega_m t \tag{9}$$

$$D \quad V = \frac{V_m}{\pi} \left[\frac{1}{2} + \frac{3\pi}{4} \sin \omega_m t - \frac{1}{3} \cos 2\omega_m t \right.$$
$$\left. - \frac{1}{15} \cos 4\omega_m t - \dots \right] \tag{10}$$

$$D' \quad V = \frac{V_m}{\pi} \left[\frac{1}{2} - \frac{3\pi}{4} \sin \omega_m t - \frac{1}{3} \cos 2\omega_m t \right.$$
$$\left. - \frac{1}{15} \cos 4\omega_m t - \dots \right] \tag{11}$$

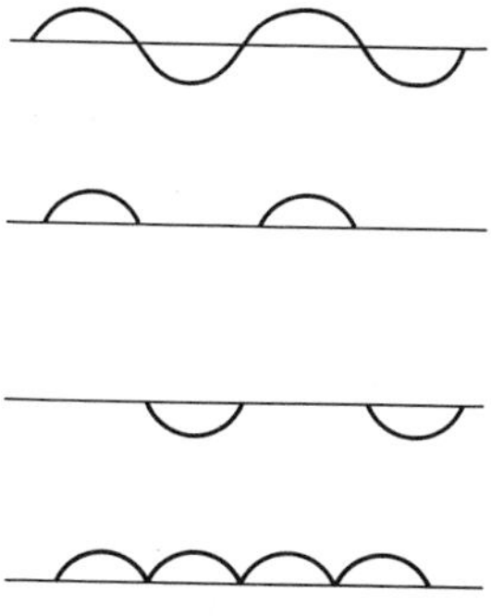

(a)

(b)

(c)

(d)

Fig. 10–5. The Fourier series corresponding to four waveforms.

(a) $V_m \sin \omega_m t$;

(b) $V_m \left[\dfrac{1}{\pi} + \dfrac{1}{2} \sin \omega_m t - \dfrac{2}{\pi} \displaystyle\sum_{k=2,4,6}^{\infty} \dfrac{\cos k\omega_m t}{(k+1)(k-1)} \right]$;

(c) $V_m \left[-\dfrac{1}{\pi} + \dfrac{1}{2} \sin \omega_m t + \dfrac{2}{\pi} \displaystyle\sum_{k=2,4,6}^{\infty} \dfrac{\cos k\omega_m t}{(k+1)(k-1)} \right]$;

(d) $V_m \left[\dfrac{2}{\pi} - \dfrac{4}{\pi} \displaystyle\sum_{k=2,4,6}^{\infty} \dfrac{\cos k\omega_m t}{(k+1)(k-1)} \right]$.

It should be emphasized that eqs. (5)–(11) merely approximate the true state of affairs, but nevertheless, they do furnish a mathematical insight into the actual physical situation, and so their form will be examined in detail. In eqs. (5)–(7), (10), and (11) the sixth harmonic has 3/7 the amplitude of the fourth, and there are no odd harmonics in the ESR signals. One should pay careful attention to the signs of these seven equations. At the same point on opposite sides of a symmetrical absorption line (e.g., B and B') the fundamental term $\sin \omega_m t$ has opposite signs, while all the harmonics plus the constant term have the same sign. The constant term and all of the harmonics have one sign for amplitudes above the inflection points C and C' and the opposite sign for amplitudes below these points, while the fundamental does not obey this relation. The fundamental is absent at the top of the resonance line A, and all the other terms are absent at the inflection points C and C'.

A careful study of the first and second derivative resonance absorption curves shown in Figs. 20–3, 20–4, and 20–5 shows that they obey the above sign rules for the fundamental and second harmonic terms, respectively, in the Fourier series. This is because to first order the amplitude of the fundamental term $\sin \omega_m t$ is a measure of the slope of the resonance absorption curve, while the second harmonic term $\cos 2\omega_m t$ measures the deviation of this slope from linearity.

An analysis similar to the one given above may be made of the dispersion mode χ' of the resonance line shown on Figs. 20–7 and 20–8, and the carrying out of this analysis is left as an *exercitatio lectori*.

Théobald et. al. (Uebersfeld and Lhote) (1960–1963) have discussed magnetic field modulation in several recent articles. Kaplan (1955), Hervé (1957), Spry (1957), Kubarev (1958), Roch (1959), Bassompierre and Pescia (1962), Doyle (1962), Goldman (1963), and Bugai (1963) discuss the effect of modulation on magnetic resonance lines.

E. Effect of Modulation Amplitude on the Resonance Line

Wahlquist (1961) studied the effect of magnetic field modulation on a Lorentzian shaped line [see also Arndt (1965)]. He combined eq. (10-A-5) with eq. (10-D-2) to obtain

$$Y(H) = \frac{y_m}{1 + (1/\tfrac{1}{2}\Delta H_{1/2})^2 [\Delta H_0(t/t_0 - \tfrac{1}{2}) + \tfrac{1}{2}H_m \sin \omega_m t]^2} \tag{1}$$

This is expanded in a Fourier series

$$Y(H) = y_m \left[a_0 + \sum_{n=1}^{\infty} a_n(\Delta H_{1/2}, H_\delta, H_m) \sin n\omega_m t \right] \tag{2}$$

where

$$H_\delta = \Delta H_0 \, (t/t_0 - \tfrac{1}{2}) \tag{3}$$

as is assumed above. The Fourier amplitudes a_n

$$a_n = \frac{\omega_m}{\pi} \int_{-\pi/\omega_m}^{\pi/\omega_m} \frac{\sin n\omega_m t}{(\tfrac{1}{2}\Delta H_{1/2})^2 + (H_\delta + \tfrac{1}{2}H_m \sin \omega_m t)^2} \tag{4}$$

were determined by contour integration, and the first three are

$$a_0 = \left(\frac{4}{H_m}\right)^2 \frac{u^{1/2}}{2(u - \gamma)\,(u - 2)^{1/2}} \tag{5}$$

$$a_1 = \pm a_0 \, (2\gamma/u - 1)^{1/2} \tag{6}$$

$$a_2 = (4/H_m)^2 + (1 + 2\gamma - 2u)\, a_0 \tag{7}$$

where

$$u = \gamma + [\gamma^2 - 16(H_\delta/H_m)^2]^{1/2} \tag{8}$$

and

$$\gamma = 1 + (2H_\delta/H_m)^2 + 3(\Delta H_{pp}/H_m)^2 \tag{9}$$

The quantity a_1 is recorded in ESR experiments when one detects at the modulation frequency ω_m, while a_2 is recorded when second harmonic detection is employed.

The properties of a_1 at the peak may be obtained by setting its derivative equal to zero

$$\frac{da_1}{dH_\delta} = -2\left(\frac{2}{H_m}\right)^3 \left(\frac{u}{u-2}\right)^{1/2} \frac{u^2 - u - 2u\gamma + 3\gamma}{(u - \gamma)^2} = 0 \tag{10}$$

which means that

$$u(1 + 2\gamma - u) = 3\gamma \tag{11}$$

From this condition one may obtain the value a_{1pp} of a_1 at the peaks of the line (inflection points of $Y(H)$):

$$a_{1pp} = \frac{\pm 2 \, (1/\Delta H_{pp})^2 \, (H_m/\Delta H_{pp})}{\{3(H_m/\Delta H_{pp})^2 + 8 + [(H_m/\Delta H_{pp})^2 + 4]^{3/2}\}^{1/2}} \quad (12)$$

and the magnetic field H_δ has the value $\pm H_{\delta pp}$ at the peaks

$$H_{\delta pp} = \pm(\Delta H_{pp}/2)\{(H_m/\Delta H_{pp})^2 + 5 - 2[4 + (H_m/\Delta H_{pp})^2]^{1/2}\}^{1/2} \quad (13)$$

The modulation amplitude broadens the resonant line by the quantity under the square root sign, and the observed modulation broadened line-width $\Delta H_{pp\,obs} = 2H_{\delta pp}$ is related to the true line-width ΔH_{pp} by the expression

$$\Delta H_{pp\,obs} = \Delta H_{pp}\{(H_m/\Delta H_{pp})^2 + 5 - 2[4 + (H_m/\Delta H_{pp})^2]^{1/2}\}^{1/2} \quad (14)$$

From the condition

$$(d/dH_m) \, a_{1pp} = 0 \quad (15)$$

one finds that the amplitude a_{1pp} reaches a maximum when $H_m = 2\Delta H_{1/2}$. Substituting this into eq. (12), one obtains

$$a_{1pp}\Big|_{max} = \pm \, 2/(\Delta H_{1/2})^2 \quad (16)$$

The maximum which occurs at $H_m = 2\Delta H_{1/2}$ is very broad; as Fig. 10–7 indicates.

Myers and Putzer (1959) considered the modulation broadening problem from a different viewpoint than Wahlquist. They Fourier-analyzed a general line-shape function Y

$$Y(H) = Y \, (H_\delta + \tfrac{1}{2}H_m \sin \omega_m t) \quad (22)$$

$$= y_m \left[a_0 + \sum_{n=1}^{\infty} (a_n \sin n\omega_m t + b_n \cos n\omega_m t) \right] \quad (23)$$

and evaluated all of the coefficients a_n and b_n explicitly for Lorentzian and Gaussian line-shapes.

The fundamental (first harmonic) results are

$$a_1 = \sum_{n=0}^{\infty} \frac{(sH_m/2)^{2n+1}}{2^{2n}(1 + sH_\delta)^{n+1}} \binom{2n + 1}{n} \sin [2(n + 1) \cot^{-1}(sH_\delta)] \quad (24)$$

subject to the condition

$$sH_m/2 < [1 + (sH_\delta)^2]^{1/2} \quad (25)$$

for a Lorentzian shape, where the quantities $\binom{2n + 1}{n}$ are the binomial coefficients $(2n + 1)!/[(n!)(n + 1)!]$, and

$$a_1 = e^{-(sH_\delta)^2} \sum_{n=0}^{\infty} \frac{(sH_m/2)^{2n+1}}{2^{2n}} \binom{2n + 1}{n}$$

$$\times \sum_{k=n+1}^{2n+1} \frac{(-1)^k}{k!} \binom{k}{2k - 2n - 1} (2sH_\delta)^{2k-2n-1} \quad (26)$$

for a Gaussian line-shape. The scaling factor s depends upon the line-shape, and has the particular forms

$$s = 2/(3^{1/2}\Delta H_{pp}) = 2/\Delta H_{1/2} \quad \text{Lorentzian} \quad (27)$$

and

$$s = 2^{1/2}/\Delta H_{pp} = 2(\ln 2)^{1/2}/\Delta H_{1/2} \quad \text{Gaussian} \quad (28)$$

for the two most important line-shapes. It may be regarded as a reciprocal line-width which normalizes the dimensionless quantities sH_m and sH_δ in eqs. (24) and (26).

The Lorentzian coefficient a_1 of eq. (26) was evaluated on a computer. The series (24) and (26) converge very slowly for high modulation amplitudes, and (24) breaks down when H_m exceeds the limits imposed by inequality (25).

The mathematical analyses of Myers and Putzer (1959) and Wahlquist (1961) which we have presented provide an insight into the manner in which the modulation amplitude broadens and distorts the resonant line. These authors and others displayed their results graphically, and we will now present some of these graphs.

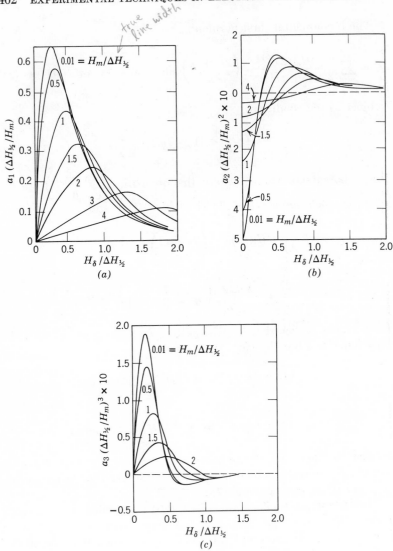

Fig. 10–6.   Modulation-broadened Lorentzian line-shape. The fundamental a_1 and the first two harmonic Fourier amplitudes a_2 and a_3 of eq. (10-E-23) are presented as a function of the normalized magnetic field $H_\delta/\Delta H_{1/2}$.   Curves are drawn for various ratios $(H_m/\Delta H_{1/2})$ of the modulation amplitude to the true line-width [Wilson (1963); Wahlquist (1959) presents a graph similar to (a)].

Wilson (1963) computed the line-shapes for the fundamental Fourier component a_1 and its second and third harmonics a_2 and a_3, respectively, defined by eq. (23) for both a Lorentzian and a Gaussian line-shape, and the results are shown on Figs. 10–6 and 10–9. The peak amplitudes of the observed signal from the first four Fourier components a_0, a_1, a_2, and a_3 vary with the modulation amplitude H_m in the manner shown on Figs. 10–7 and 10–10. The Lorentzian signals a_1, a_2, and a_3 exhibit a linear, parabolic and cubic dependence, respectively, on the modulation amplitude when $H_m \ll \Delta H_{1/2}$. The amplitudes a_1, a_2, and a_3 of the Gaussian line-shape are considerably reduced relative to the corresponding Lorentzian values.

The integrated areas A_1, A_2, and A_3 of the Fourier components a_1, a_2, and a_3 may be obtained by single, double, and triple integrations, respectively, of the suitably normalized function. The distortion of the nth Fourier component is defined in terms of the true area A by means of the expression

$$\text{Distortion} = |A - A_n|/A \tag{29}$$

Figure 10–8 shows the dependence of the distortion upon the modulation amplitude for a Lorentzian line-shape.

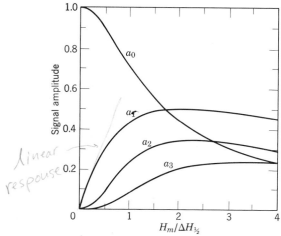

Fig. 10–7.   Dependence of the maximum Lorentzian signal amplitudes on the normalized modulation amplitude $H_m/\Delta H_{1/2}$ [Wilson (1963)].

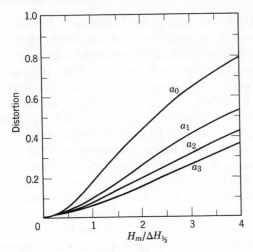

Fig. 10-8. Dependence of the distortion of the Lorentzian line-shapes on the normalized modulation amplitude $H_m/\Delta H_{1/2}$ [Wilson (1963)].

Smith (1964) examined the effect of modulation broadening on a Gaussian line-shape, and compared his results with Wahlquist's Lorentzian treatment. Figure 10-11 shows the variation of the observed modulation broadened peak-to-peak line-width $\Delta H_{pp\ obs}$ on the logarithm of the modulation amplitude H_m. Both quantities are normalized with respect to the true peak-to-peak line-width ΔH_{pp}. Experimental NMR spectra of the protons in aqueous $Cr(NO_3)_3$, shown in Fig. 10-12, with $\Delta H_{pp} = 0.19$ G agreed with the theoretical curves on Figs. 10-11 and 10-13.

Figure 10-11 is not convenient to use for comparison with experimental data because the true width ΔH_{pp} is ordinarily an unknown quantity. Figure 10-13 shows the experimentally measurable quantity $\Delta H_{pp\ obs}/H_m$ plotted against $H_m/(\Delta H_{pp})$, and one may use such a graph or the data in Table 10-1 to deduce the true line-width from an overmodulated resonant line. The graph in Fig. 10-14 is useful for determining ΔH_{pp} from a slightly overmodulated resonance, which is the case most often met in practice. For extreme over-modulation ($H_m > 2\Delta H_{pp}$), one cannot accurately determine ΔH_{pp}. The Lorentzian and Gaussian curves in Figs. 10-13 and 10-14 are so close to each other that very little error is involved in using their average to determine the true width ΔH_{pp} for a line-shape intermediate between Lorentzian and Gaussian.

The peak-to-peak amplitude varies with the modulation in the manner shown on Fig. 10–15. The curves are normalized to unity at their peaks. (Figures 10–7 and 10–10 are normalized differently.) The a_{1pp} versus $H_m/\Delta H_{pp}$ plot is much more useful for distinguishing a Gaussian from a Lorentzian line than the line-width plots.

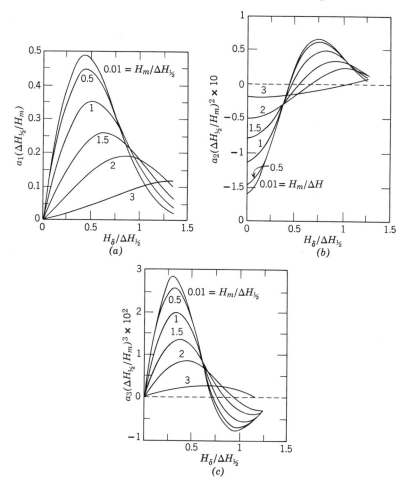

Fig. 10–9. Modulation-broadened Gaussian line-shape. The fundamental a_1 and the first two harmonic Fourier amplitudes a_2 and a_3 of eq. (10-E-23) are presented as a function of the normalized magnetic field $H_\delta/\Delta H_{1/2}$. Curves are drawn for various ratios $(H_m/\Delta H_{1/2})$ of the modulation amplitude to the true line-width [Wilson (1963)].

Chapter 20 discusses line-shapes, and Fig. 20–3 defines the inner maximum slope y_1'', the outer maximum slope y_2'', and the separation between the two outer maximum slopes H_2'' of the first derivative line-shape. Wahlquist used his equations to evaluate these quantities for a Lorentzian shape, and their dependence on the normalized

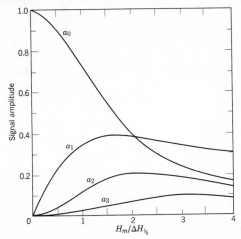

Fig. 10–10. Dependence of the maximum Gaussian signal amplitudes on the normalized modulation amplitude $H_m/\Delta H_{1/2}$ [Wilson 1963)].

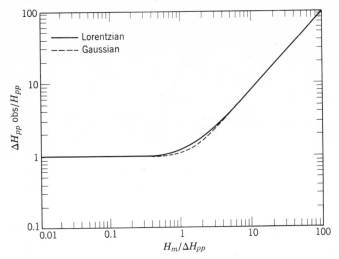

Fig. 10–11. Dependence of the amount of modulation-broadening $\Delta H_{pp\ \text{obs}}/\Delta H_{pp}$ on the normalized modulation amplitude $H_m/\Delta H_{pp}$ [adapted from Smith (1964)].

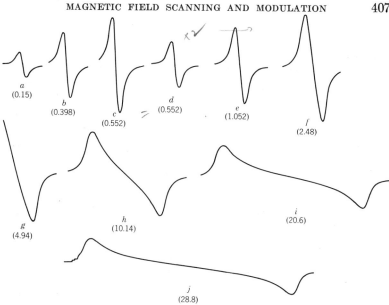

Fig. 10-12. NMR signal of protons in aqueous solution of $Cr(NO_3)_3$ ($\Delta H_{pp} = 0.19$ G) as a function of the modulation amplitude H_m. The nominal modulation frequency was 40 cps, and the field scan rate was the same in each tracing. The gain setting used for spectra (a), (b), and (c) was twice that used to record the remaining spectra. The normalized modulation amplitude $H_m/\Delta H_{pp}$ is shown in parentheses beneath each spectrum [Smith (1964)].

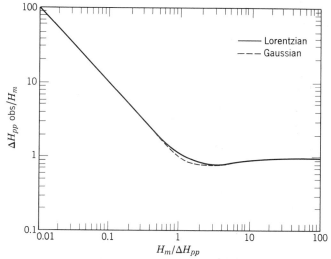

Fig. 10-13. Dependence of $(\Delta H_{pp\ obs}/H_m)$ on the normalized modulation amplitude $H_m/\Delta H_{pp}$ [adapted from Smith (1964)].

TABLE 10-1

Parameters for a Lorentzian [Wahlquist (1961)] and Gaussian [Smith (1964)]
Magnetic Resonance Lines as a Function of the Modulation Amplitude

$H_m/\Delta H_{1/2}$	$H_m/\Delta H_{pp}$	$\Delta H_{pp\ obs}/\Delta H_{pp}$	$\Delta H_{pp\ obs}/H_m$	a_{1pp} normalized
Lorentzian line				
0	0	1.000	∞	0
0.1	0.173	1.006	5.815	0.13
0.2	0.346	1.029	2.973	0.248
0.4	0.694	1.114	1.610	0.478
0.8	1.388	1.432	1.035	0.784
1.2	2.08	1.903	0.907	0.930
1.6	2.78	2.387	0.873	0.987
2.0	3.46	3.000	0.866	1.000
2.4	4.16	3.564	0.869	0.992
2.8	4.86	4.221	0.876	0.974
3.2	5.56	4.884	0.883	0.952
3.6	6.24	5.537	0.890	0.929
4.0	6.94	6.288	0.897	0.905
6.0	10.40	9.55	0.922	0.800
8.0	13.84	13.0	0.938	0.721
10.0	17.34	16.4	0.949	0.659
16.0	27.72	26.5	0.967	0.541
20.0	34.64	33.7	0.973	0.488
40.0	69.4	68.2	0.986	0.353
∞	∞	∞	1.000	0
Gaussian line				
0	0	1.00	∞	0
0.12	0.141	1.00	7.095	0.148
0.24	0.282	1.007	3.573	0.291
0.48	0.564	1.039	1.842	0.551
0.96	1.128	1.178	1.044	0.887
1.44	1.692	1.454	0.859	0.993
1.68	1.974	1.645	0.834	0.995
1.92	2.26	1.862	0.826	0.983
2.40	2.82	2.343	0.831	0.943
2.88	3.38	2.856	0.844	0.898
3.36	3.94	3.384	0.858	0.857
3.84	4.52	3.922	0.870	0.819
4.32	5.08	4.465	0.880	0.785
4.80	5.64	5.013	0.889	0.755
7.20	8.46	7.786	0.921	0.639
9.60	11.28	10.6	0.939	0.564
12.00	14.10	13.5	0.956	0.497
∞	∞	∞	1.000	0

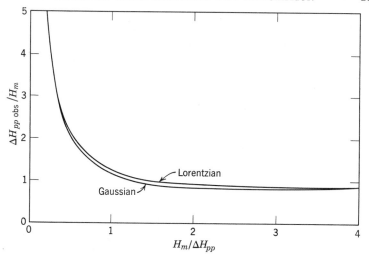

Fig. 10–14.   Linear plot of the dependence of $\Delta H_{pp\ \mathrm{obs}}/H_m$ on $H_m/\Delta H_{pp}$ in the region of moderate modulation broadening.   The data in Table 10–1 were used to construct this figure.

modulation amplitude $H_m/\Delta H_{1/2}$ is shown on Figs. 10–16 and 10–17. For comparison purposes one should recall that

$$y_1''/y_2'' = 4 \quad \text{(Lorentzian)} \tag{30}$$

$$y_1''/y_2'' = \tfrac{1}{2}e^{3/2} = 2.24 \quad \text{(Gaussian)} \tag{31}$$

so we see that modulation broadening decreases the Lorentzian ratio y_1''/y_2'' toward and eventually past the theoretical Gaussian value of 2.24.

In addition,

$$H_2'' = 3^{1/2}\Delta H_{pp} \tag{32}$$

for both a Lorentzian and a Gaussian line-shape.   It is indeed unusual to find a ratio of parameters like $H_2''/\Delta H_{pp}$ which is identical for both shapes.   In terms of the half amplitude line-width

$$H_2'' = \Delta H_{1/2} \quad \text{(Lorentzian)} \tag{33}$$

$$H_2'' = (\tfrac{3}{2}\ln 2)^{-1/2}\Delta H_{1/2} = 1.47\Delta H_{1/2} \quad \text{(Gaussian)} \tag{34}$$

The constants in eqs. (30)–(32) are listed in Table 20–5.

Berger and Günthart (1962) considered the distortion of a Lorentzian resonant line that arises in a modulation type superheterodyne spectrometer. More specifically, the magnetic field is modulated by the term $\frac{1}{2}H_m \sin \omega_m t$, and the superheterodyne detection takes place at the intermediate frequency $\omega_i \gg \omega_m$. The system which employs one lock-in detector at the frequency ω_i and another at ω_m is compared to the system which uses a square law

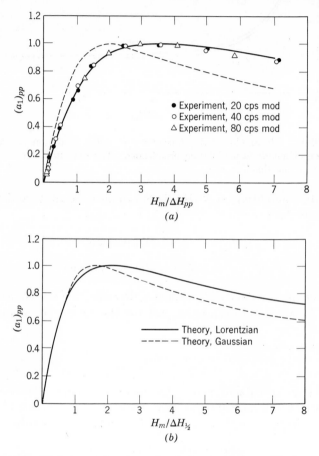

Fig. 10–15. Variation of the absorption derivative peak amplitude a_{1pp} on the modulation amplitude: (a) normalized with respect to the true peak-to-peak linewidth ΔH_{pp}, and (b) normalized with respect to the true absorption curve half amplitude line-width $\Delta H_{1/2}$ [adapted from Smith (1964)].

detector at the intermediate frequency, and only employs a lock-in detector for the magnetic field modulation frequency ω_m. When two phase-sensitive detectors are employed, the Lorentzian line-shape is reproduced sans distortion.

When the superheterodyne spectrometer employs a quadratic first detector and only one phase-sensitive detector at ω_m, then the recorded line-shape differs from a true Lorentzian. Graphs and explicit formulae for these shapes are given by Berger and Günthart (1962). Several other workers such as Halbach (1956), Bruin and van Ladesteyn (1959), Yagi (1960), and Arndt (1965) have published graphs of the type shown in Figs. 10–6 to 10–17.

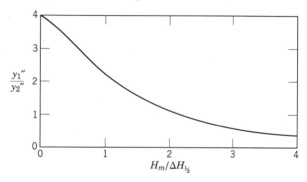

Fig. 10–16.   The dependence of the ratio y_1''/y_2'' on the normalized modulation amplitude $H_m/\Delta H_{1/2}$ for a Lorentzian-shape [adapted from Wahlquist (1961)].

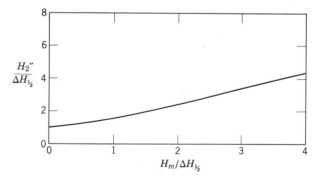

Fig. 10–17.   Variation of the quantity H_2'' on the modulation amplitude H_m for a Lorentzian shape when both are normalized relative to $\Delta H_{1/2}$ [adapted from Wahlquist (1961)].

Spry (1957) used the numerical unfolding procedure of Stokes (1948) to compute the true line-shape of an arbitrary experimental recording. The "folding function" which corrects for the modulation broadening may be either calculated mathematically, or determined experimentally.

Flynn and Seymour (1960, 1961, 1962) used a series involving the moments of a generalized broadening function to derive a general formula for correcting distorted line-shapes [see also Russell and Torchia (1962)]. Wilson (1963) developed a method for correcting line-shapes by relating the Fourier coefficients of the modulation-broadened line to those of the true integrated line-shape.

Andrew (1953) has shown that the true second moment of a resonance line $\langle H^2 \rangle$ is related to the second moment of a modulation broadened line $\langle H^2 \rangle_{obs}$ by the expression

$$\langle H^2 \rangle_{obs} = \langle H^2 \rangle + \tfrac{1}{16} H_m{}^2 \tag{35}$$

He further derived the following relation for the $2n$th moment

$$\langle H^{2n} \rangle_{obs} = \sum_{k=0}^{n} \left(\frac{H_m{}^k}{2^{2k} k!} \right)^2 \frac{(2n)! \, \langle H^{2n-2k} \rangle}{(k+1)(2n-2k)!} \tag{36}$$

which reduces to

$$\langle H^4 \rangle_{obs} = \langle H^4 \rangle + \tfrac{3}{8} \langle H^2 \rangle H_m{}^2 + \tfrac{1}{128} H_m{}^4 \tag{37}$$

for the fourth moment ($n = 2$). The odd moments vanish for a symmetrical line-shape.

Perlman and Bloom (1952) present experimental evidence in support of the dependence of the observed second moment on $(H_m)^2$. Verdier, Whipple, and Schomaker (1961) showed that the doubly integrated area or first moment of a derivative ESR absorption signal is approximately proportional to the modulation amplitude for modulations up to twice the peak-to-peak line-width. Wilson (1964) gives corrections for moments of lines detected at any harmonic of the modulation frequency. Rädler (1961) discusses the influence of the modulation amplitude on the Overhauser effect [see also Visweswaramurthy (1965)].

Halbach (1960) generalized the above expressions by taking into account the effect of both the modulation amplitude H_m and the modulation frequency ω_m on the line-shape. It is assumed that there is no phase shift between the field modulation and the lock-in detector reference signal. His formulae are in terms of frequency moments $\langle \omega^n \rangle$, and using the transformation $\langle \omega^n \rangle = \gamma^n \langle H^n \rangle$, we obtain

$$\langle H^2 \rangle_{\text{obs}} = \langle H^2 \rangle + \tfrac{1}{3}(\omega_m/\gamma)^2 + \tfrac{1}{16} H_m^2 \tag{38}$$

$$\langle H^4 \rangle_{\text{obs}} = \langle H^4 \rangle + \langle H^2 \rangle[2(\omega_m/\gamma)^2 + \tfrac{3}{8} H_m^2] + \tfrac{1}{5}(\omega_m/\gamma)^4$$
$$+ \tfrac{3}{16}(\omega_m/\gamma)^2 H_m^2 + \tfrac{1}{128} H_m^4 \tag{39}$$

These expressions are valid in the absence of saturation when the line-width, the modulation frequency, and γH_m are small compared to the resonant frequency. They are derived under the assumption that frequency and field modulation are equivalent, and this assumption is justified by Halbach (1960).

In this book we have defined the modulation magnetic field by $\tfrac{1}{2}H_m \sin \omega_m t$. This means that H_m is the peak-to-peak modulation amplitude, so that the magnetic field strength ranges between $(H_0 + H_\delta - \tfrac{1}{2}H_m)$, and $(H_0 + H_\delta + \tfrac{1}{2}H_m)$ during one modulation cycle. Some authors work in terms of the definition $H_m \sin \omega_m t$, so their expressions will differ from ours by a factor of two. In addition, some authors express their results in terms of half of the line-width, instead of the full line-width. These divergent definitions can lead to considerable confusion when comparing the results reported by various workers.

F. Effect of the Modulation Frequency on the Resonance Line

In practice, the frequency $\omega_m = 2\pi f_m$ of the magnetic field modulation ordinarily satisfies the inequality

$$\omega_m/\gamma \ll \Delta H \tag{1}$$

where $\gamma = g\beta/\hbar$. When the modulation frequency ω_m exceeds the line-width $\gamma \Delta H$, then sideband resonances develop which are separated by the intervals of ω_m/γ G. These sidebands are centered at the resonant field H_0 and extend over a range of H_m G, where H_m is the peak-to-peak modulation amplitude. When n, defined by

$$n = \gamma H_m/2\omega_m \tag{2}$$

is close to an integer, it gives the number of prominent sidebands on each side of the center line, and for certain values of n, the center line itself disappears. Burgess and Brown (1952) extended the work of Smaller (1951) and Karplus (1948) to obtain the following mathematical expressions for the real and imaginary parts of the rf susceptibility χ:

$$\chi' = A \cos \omega_m t + B \sin \omega_m t \tag{3}$$

$$\chi'' = C \cos \omega_m t + D \sin \omega_m t \tag{4}$$

where

$$A = \frac{1}{2}\chi_0\omega_0 \sum_{k=-\infty}^{\infty} \frac{4\omega_m k J_k^2(n)}{\gamma H_m} \frac{[\gamma(H - H_0) + k\omega_m]}{[\gamma(H - H_0) + k\omega_m]^2 + 1/T_2^2} \tag{5}$$

$$B = \frac{1}{2}\chi_0\omega_0 \sum_{k=-\infty}^{\infty} \frac{J_k(n)\,[J_{k+1}(n) - J_{k-1}(n)]}{T_2}$$
$$\times \frac{1}{[\gamma(H - H_0) + k\omega_m]^2 + 1/T_2^2} \tag{6}$$

$$C = -\frac{1}{2}\chi_0\omega_0 \sum_{k=-\infty}^{\infty} \frac{4\omega_m k J_k^2(n)}{\gamma H_m T_2} \frac{1}{[\gamma(H - H_0) + k\omega_m]^2 + 1/T_2^2} \tag{7}$$

$$D = \frac{1}{2}\chi_0\omega_0 \sum_{k=-\infty}^{\infty} J_k(n)[J_{k+1}(n) - J_{k-1}(n)]$$
$$\times \frac{[\gamma(H - H_0) + k\omega_m]}{[\gamma(H - H_0) + k\omega_m]^2 + 1/T_2^2} \tag{8}$$

and $J_k(n)$ is the kth order Bessel function. The function χ' is symmetric and χ'' is antisymmetric about the point $H = H_0$. When $\omega_m > \gamma \Delta H$, the spectrum of both χ' and χ'' consists of a series of components which resemble absorption curves, dispersion curves, or a mixture of both, depending on the setting of the lock-in detector phase (i.e., on whether $\cos \omega_m t$, $\sin \omega_m t$, or a mixture is detected). The functions A and D are dispersion types, while B and C are absorption types.

Burgess and Brown (1952) studied the NMR of protons in water, and confirmed these equations experimentally for $n = 1$, 2, and 4 using $f_m = 100$ cps and $H_m = 0.048$, 0.096, and 0.192 G, as shown on Figs. 10–18 to 10–20. When f_m is reduced by a factor of four to

25 cps, the sidebands overlap, and a broadened line is observed, as shown in Fig. 10–21.   A further reduction in f_m leads to $\omega_m \ll \gamma H_m$, and the modulation effect disappears.   Gabillard and Ponchel (1962) observed sidebands in the ESR of DPPH for n in the range from 1 to 3.6 [see also Garif'yanov (1957)].   Hyde and Brown (1962) observed sidebands with the tetracene positive ion.   Macomber and Waugh (1965) generalized Karplus' (1948) theory.

Modulation frequency effects become negligible when f_m becomes much less than the line-width ΔH expressed in frequency units

$$f_m \ll (\gamma/2\pi)\,\Delta H \qquad (9)$$

For $g = 2$, the conversion factor $\gamma/2\pi$ has the value

$$f/H = \gamma/2\pi = 2.8 \times 10^6 \text{ cps/G} \qquad (10)$$

where f is in cps and H is in gauss.

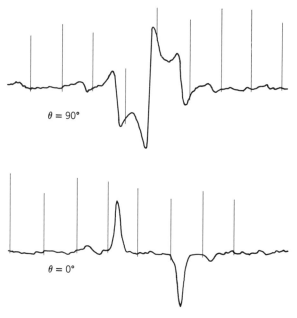

Fig. 10–18.   Lock-in amplifier output versus radio frequency at a modulation frequency of 100 cps and $(\gamma H_m/2\omega_m) = 1$ using two different phases θ of the lock-in amplifier.   Vertical lines indicate 100-cps frequency intervals [Burgess and Brown (1952)].

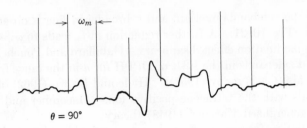

$\theta = 90°$

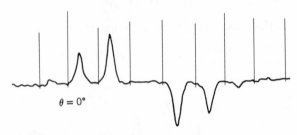

$\theta = 0°$

Fig. 10–19.   Same conditions as shown in Fig. 10–18 except $(\gamma H_m/2\omega_m) = 2$
[Burgess and Brown (1951)].

Therefore, we obtain the explicit condition

$$f_m/\Delta H \ll 2.8 \times 10^6 \text{ cps/G} \tag{11}$$

which must be satisfied if modulation effects are to be neglected. A resonance line $1/10$ G wide with $g = 2$ observed with a 100-kc modulation frequency corresponds to

$$f_m/\Delta H = 10^6 \text{ cps/G} \tag{12}$$

Therefore, it is not advisable to employ 100 kc modulation to record lines that are narrower than about a hundred milligauss. More explicitly, we may say that a 100-kc modulation frequency corresponds to 36 mG in magnetic field units. Since lower modulation frequencies reduce the spectrometer sensitivity because of the $1/f$ crystal noise, it is recommended that a superheterodyne spectrometer be employed for such narrow lines. Hyde and Brown (1962) found that a line-width of 100 mG recorded with a superheterodyne spectrometer broadens by about 15% with 100 kc modulation, and their data indicate that a 25 mG line-width will double in going from superheterodyne to 100 kc operation. When they adjusted the lock-in detector phase away from its proper value, they found significant narrowing, in addition to the expected decrease in amplitude of a modulation broadened resonance. Hausser (1962) has observed line-widths of 17 mG in the 1,3-bisdiphenylene allyl radical.

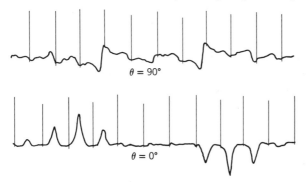

Fig. 10–20.   Same conditions as in Fig. 10–18 except $(\gamma H_m/2\omega_m) = 4$ [Burgess and Brown (1952)].

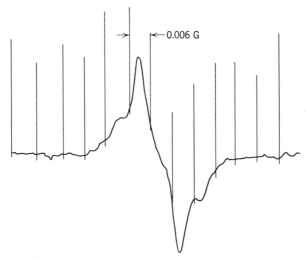

Fig. 10–21.   Lock-in amplifier output at a modulation frequency of 25 cps. Frequency intervals are 25 cps (0.006 G) apart [Burgess and Brown (1952)].

Rinehart, Kleen, and Lin (1960) discuss the effect of frequency modulation on the line-shape in a microwave spectrometer, and Acrivos (1962) and Parikh (1965) describe modulation frequency effects in NMR. Glarum's (1965) field modulation techniques for resolution enhancement are discussed in Sec. 14-I.

G. Experimental Details of Magnetic Field Modulation Apparatus

To produce audio frequency modulation of the magnetic field, one usually mounts Helmholtz coils either on the resonant cavity itself, or on the magnet pole pieces. When they are mounted on the pole pieces, they modulate the field throughout the gap, and can interfere with the use of a proton magnetometer. When mounted on the resonant cavity, they require a much lower power input for a given modulation amplitude H_m. Pole piece mounting is not feasible for frequencies above the audio range (e.g., for 100 kc). As discussed in Sec. 9-E, the two Helmholtz coils have a radius a, and they are separated by a distance equal to this radius a. The amplitude of the magnetic field at the center between the coils with n turns on each is easily deduced from eq. (9-E-5), and has the form

$$H = B/\mu = 8nI/5^{3/2}a \qquad \text{At/m} \qquad (1)$$

where a is in meters, and I is in amperes. Using the free space permeability $\mu = 4\pi \times 10^{-7}$ H/m, expressing a in centimeters, and converting to gauss one obtains

$$B = 0.64\pi nI/5^{1/2}a \approx 0.9\, nI/a \qquad \text{G} \qquad (2)$$

with I still in amperes. These expressions assume that the radius of the coil is much greater than the length of the two individual coils (i.e., $a \gg L$ on Fig. 9–12). The sample in the resonant cavity should be located at the center of the coils, as the modulating field is most homogeneous there. See Sec. 9-E for further details.

The inductance L of a circular loop of wire is given by

$$L \approx \mu a[\ln (8a/t) - 2] \qquad \text{H} \qquad (3)$$

where a is the radius of the loop, t is the radius of the wire that forms the loop, and it is assumed that $a \gg t$. A coil of n turns whose thickness and length both equal $2t \ll a$ has an inductance L given by

$$L \approx \mu a n^2 [\ln (8a/t) - 2] \qquad \text{H} \qquad (4)$$

The quantity t may be considered as the radius of the cross section of the group of wires that form the coil. The resistance R of a piece of wire of length l and cross-sectional area A may be computed from the relationship

$$R = \rho l / A \qquad (5)$$

where ρ is the resistivity. A loop of wire of radius a has a length $l = 2\pi a$, and therefore n turns in series have the resistance R

$$R = 2\pi n a \rho / A \qquad (6)$$

The impedance Z is

$$Z = R + j\omega L \qquad (7)$$

$$= (R^2 + \omega^2 L^2)^{1/2} e^{j\phi} \qquad (8)$$

where

$$\phi = \tan^{-1} (\omega L / R) \qquad (9)$$

Usually $\omega L \gg R$, and the impedance of the coil is almost entirely inductive

$$Z \approx j\omega L \qquad (10)$$

Equations (4) and (6)–(8) for the inductance, resistance, and impedance, respectively, apply to one side of a Helmholtz coil. They should be halved or doubled depending on whether or not the two sides are connected together in parallel or in series.

For Helmholtz coils to be effective, it is necessary for the modulating magnetic field to penetrate through the resonant cavity walls. An X band waveguide has a wall thickness of 0.13 cm (0.05 in.), and a glance at Fig. 3–4 indicates that this is about the skin depth δ of copper at about 3 kc. Therefore, modulation frequencies above ~ 1

kc should not be used with this waveguide. A frequency of 100 kc has a skin depth in copper of 0.02 cm, and the microwave frequency of 9000 Mc has $\delta = 7 \times 10^{-5}$ cm, so if one makes a cylindrical resonant cavity out of glass and plates it inside with copper to a thickness of about 0.002 cm (0.005 in.), then it may be used with 100 kc modulation. The requirement is that the metallic wall thickness be much greater than the skin depth at the microwave resonant frequency, and much less than the skin depth at the modulation frequency. The first requirement is of somewhat greater importance than the second.

There are a number of other methods for introducing the high frequency modulation into the resonant cavity. Several of these are: (1) One may cut a slot in the side of the cavity parallel to lines of microwave current flow [see Sec. 13-H; Buckmaster and Scovil (1956)]. (2) A loop of wire may be located within the resonant cavity and oriented parallel to the magnetic lines of force [see Sec. 13-L; Llewellyn (1957)]. (3) The wall of the resonant cavity adjacent to the modulation coil may be made a thickness intermediate between the skin depths of the microwave and modulation frequencies [see Sec. 13-L; Llewellyn (1957), Bennett, Hoell, and Schwenker, (1958)]. (4) The magnetic field modulation may be excited by two vertical posts symmetrically placed on the base plate of a TE_{011} mode cylindrical cavity [Sec. 13-K; Bowers, Kamper, and Knight (1957)].

An example of a simple modulation coil amplifier is shown in Fig. 10-22. The audio signal from an oscillator is impressed on the grids of a push-pull amplifier, and the modulation coils are connected to the plates. The coils act like a load of impedance Z

$$Z \approx j\omega_m L \tag{11}$$

in the ac equivalent circuit, while they act like the resistance R of eq. (6) for the dc current. The two push-pull tubes are balanced by the 75-Ω cathode potentiometer, and the B^+ voltage is supplied by a full wave rectifier and π-filter. The modulation amplitude is adjusted by varying the ac input, and the output is monitored at the banana jacks connected across a 2.7-Ω plate resistor.

Fitzky (1958) describes modulation circuits, and Cook (1962) presents a slow sweep generator circuit.

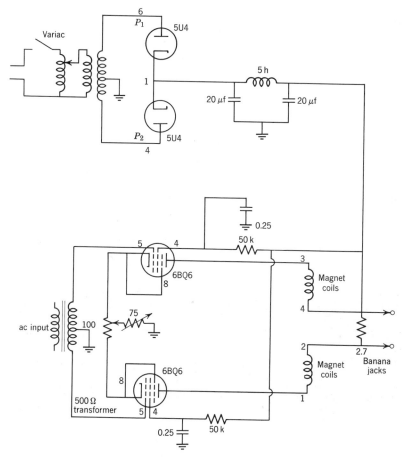

Fig. 10–22. Modulation coil circuit. The resistors are in ohms and the capacitors are in μf [Poole (1958)].

H. Double Modulation

Some spectrometers employ a high frequency field modulation for use with narrow band detection, and also a simultaneous audio frequency modulation for use with video observation of the absorption line. The oscilloscope which is synchronized at the audio frequency displays the modulus of the derivative line-shape, as shown on Fig. 10–23 [see Secs. 13-H; 13-L; Buckmaster and Scovil (1956); Llewellyn

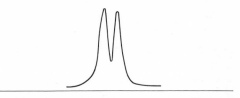

Fig. 10–23. Modulus of absorption line-shape obtained with solid DPPH at modulation frequencies of 60 cps plus 462 kc [Buckmaster and Scovil (1956)].

(1957)]. The audio frequency modulation is turned off when spectra are recorded after narrow band, high frequency detection.

Unterberger, Quevedo, and Stoddard (1957) described a double modulation method which entails both amplitude modulating the magnetic field, and frequency modulating the klystron. As a result, the resonance observed with the klystron mode that is displayed on an oscilloscope appears much narrower than it does in the absence of the klystron frequency modulation, as illustrated on Fig. 10–24. The authors derived an equation which relates the apparent line-

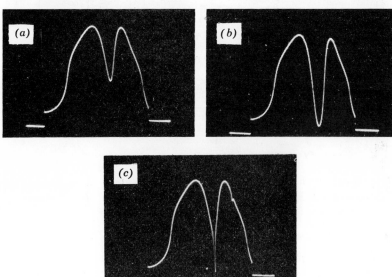

Fig. 10–24. Oscilloscopic presentation of a klystron mode and resonant cavity pip: (a) off resonance, (b) on resonance, and (c) on resonance plus magnetic field modulation. The cavity contains solid DPPH [Unterberger, Quevedo, and Stoddard (1957)].

width using double modulation to the true line width obtained with a single (field) modulation, and they easily obtained a reduction in width by a factor of 17. The technique may be found useful in searching for new resonances with a sillyscope.

Muromtsev, Piskunov, and Verein (1957) discuss the use of triple modulation for recording the second derivative of the resonance line. See also Rinehart and Lin (1961).

References

J. V. Acrivos, J. Chem. Phys., 36, 1097 (1962).
E. R. Andrew, Phys. Rev., 91, 425 (1953).
R. Arndt, J. Appl. Phys., 36, 2522 (1965).
J. O. Artman and P. E. Tannenwald, J. Appl. Phys., 26, 1124 (1955).
D. M. S. Bagguley and J. H. E. Griffiths, Proc. Phys. Soc., A65, 594 (1952).
E. B. Baker, L. W. Burd, and G. N. Root, RSI, 36, 1495 (1965).
A. Bassompierre and J. Pescia, C. R. Acad. Sci., 254, 4439 (1962).
R. G. Bennett, P. C. Hoell, and R. P. Schwenker, RSI, 29, 659 (1958).
P. A. Berger and H. H. Günthart, Z. Angew. Math. Phys., 13, 310 (1962).
R. J. Blume and W. L. Williams, RSI, 35, 1498 (1964).
K. D. Bowers, R. A. Kamper, and R. B. D. Knight, JSI, 34, 49 (1957).
F. Bruin and D. van Ladesteyn, Appl. Sci. Res., 7B, 270 (1959).
H. A. Buckmaster and H. E. D. Scovil, Can. J. Phys., 34, 711 (1956).
A. A. Bugai, Fiz. Tverd. Tela, 4, 3027 (2218) (1963).
J. H. Burgess and R. M. Brown, RSI, 23, 334 (1952).
P. D. Cook, Electron. Eng., 34, 320 (1962).
A. Coumes and M. Ligeon, J. Phys., 25, Suppl. No. 3, 45A (1964).
J. E. Cousins, R. Dupree, and R. L. Havill, JSI, 40, 407 (1963) [see Brit. J. Appl. Phys., 16, 1687 (1965)].
W. T. Doyle, RSI, 33, 118 (1962).
J. Dušek, Czech. J. Phys., 11, 528 (1961).
L. E. Erickson, Phys. Rev., 143, 295 (1966).
G. Feher, Bell System, Tech. J., 36, 449 (1957).
H. G. Fitzky, Z. Angew. Phys., 10, 489 (1958).
C. P. Flynn and E. F. W. Seymour, Proc. Phys. Soc., 75, 337 (1960); JSI, 39, 352 (1962); C. P. Flynn, Proc. Phys. Soc., 78, 1546 (1961).
R. Gabillard and B. Ponchel, C. R. Acad. Sci., 254, 2727 (1962).
N. S. Garif'yanov, Zhur. Eksper. Teor. Fiz., 32, 609 (503) (1957).
S. H. Glarum, RSI, 36, 771 (1965).
M. Goldman, C. R. Acad. Sci., 256, 3643 (1963).
K. Halbach, Helv. Phys. Acta, 29, 37 (1956); Phys. Rev., 119, 1230 (1960).
J. L. Hall and R. T. Schumacher, Phys. Rev., 127, 1892 (1962).
K. H. Hausser, Z. Naturforsch., 17A, 158 (1962); 11th Colloque Ampère, Eindhoven, 1962, p. 420.
J. Hervé, C. R. Acad. Sci., 244, 1182 (1957).
J. S. Hyde and H. W. Brown, J. Chem. Phys., 37, 368 (1962).

R. W. R. Hoisington, L. Kellner, and M. J. Pentz, *Proc. Phys. Soc.*, **72**, 537 (1958).

C. K. Jen, *Phys. Rev.*, **74**, 1396 (1948); **76**, 1494 (1949).

P. Jung, *12th Colloque Ampère*, Bordeaux, 1963, p. 564.

J. I. Kaplan, *Am. J. Phys.*, **23**, 585 (1955).

R. Karplus, *Phys. Rev.*, **73**, 1027 (1948).

A. F. Kip, C. Kittel, R. A. Levy, and A. M. Portis, *Phys. Rev.*, **91**, 1066 (1953).

A. V. Kubarev, *PTE*, **3**, 68 (393) (1958).

P. M. Llewellyn, *JSI*, **34**, 236 (1957).

J. D. Macomber and J. S. Waugh, *Phys. Rev.*, **140**, A1494 (1965).

I. K. Munson, *RSI*, **21**, 622 (1950).

T. M. Murina, A. M. Prokhorov, and E. A. Chayanova, *Radiotekhn. i Electron.*, **3**, 1402 (1958).

V. Muromtsev, A. K. Piskunov, and N. V. Verein, *Radiotekhn. i Electron.*, **7**, 1206 (1129) (1962).

O. E. Myers and E. J. Putzer, *J. Appl. Phys.*, **30**, 1987 (1959).

P. Parikh, *Indian J. Pure Appl. Phys.*, **3**, 34 (1965).

J. Paulevé, *Onde Élect.*, **35**, 494 (1955).

M. M. Perlman and M. Bloom, *Phys. Rev.*, **88**, 1290 (1952).

C. P. Poole, Jr., Ph.D. thesis, University of Maryland, 1958.

A. M. Portis, *Phys. Rev.*, **91**, 1071 (1953).

A. M. Portis, *J. Phys. Chem. Solids*, **8**, 326 (1959).

A. M. Portis, and D. T. Teaney, *J. Appl. Phys.*, **29**, 1692 (1958).

K. H. Rädler, *Ann. Phys.*, **7**, 45 (1961).

E. A. Rinehart, R. H. Kleen, and C. C. Lin, *J. Mol. Spect.*, **5**, 458 (1960).

E. A. Rinehart and R. L. Legan, *RSI*, **35**, 103 (1964).

E. A. Rinehart, R. L. Legan, and C. C. Lin, *RSI*, **36**, 511 (1965).

E. A. Rinehart and C. C. Lin, *RSI*, **32**, 562 (1961).

J. Roch, *C. R. Acad. Sci.*, **248**, 663 (1959).

A. C. Rose-Innes, *JSI*, **34**, 276 (1957).

A. M. Russell and D. A. Torchia, *RSI*, **33**, 442 (1962).

S. Seeley, *Electron Tube Circuits*, 2nd Ed., McGraw-Hill, N. Y., 1958.

B. Smaller, *Phys. Rev.*, **83**, 812 (1951); B. Smaller and E. L. Yasaitis, *RSI*, **24**, 991 (1953).

G. W. Smith, *J. Appl. Phys.*, **35**, 1217 (1964).

W. J. Spry, *J. Appl. Phys.*, **28**, 660 (1957).

O. Štirand, *ETP*, **10**, 313 (1962).

A. R. Stokes, *Proc. Phys. Soc.*, **61**, 382 (1948).

M. W. P. Strandberg, M. Tinkham, I. H. Solt, and C. F. Davis, Jr., *RSI*, **27**, 596 (1956).

D. T. Teaney, W. E. Blumberg, and A. M. Portis, *Phys. Rev.*, **119**, 1851 (1960).

D. T. Teaney, M. P. Klein, and A. M. Portis, *RSI*, **32**, 721 (1961).

J. G. Théobald, *Arch. Sci.*, **14**, Spec. No., 128 (1961); J. G. Théobald and J. Uebersfeld, *Arch. Sci.*, **13**, *Fasc. Spec.*, 347 (1960); *J. Phys. Radium*, **21**, 676 (1960); *C. R. Acad. Sci.*, **252**, 3030 (1961); **254**, 255 (1962); *11th Ampère Colloquium*, Eindhoven, 1962, p. 445; G. Lhote and J. G. Théobald, *C. R. Acad. Sci.*, **256**, 1248 (1963).

R. R. Unterberger, J. L. Garcia de Quevedo, and A. E. Stoddard, *RSI*, **28**, 616 (1957).

P. H. Verdier, E. B. Whipple, and V. Schomaker, *J. Chem. Phys.*, **34**, 118 (1961).

S. Visweswaramurthy, *Indian J. Pure Appl. Phys.*, **3**, 261 (1965).

H. Wahlquist, *J. Chem. Phys.*. **35**, 1708 (1961).

R. T. Weidner and C. A. Whitmer, *RSI*, **23**, 75 (1952).

B. G. Whitford, *RSI*, **32**, 919 (1961).

G. V. H. Wilson, *J. Appl. Phys.*, **34**, 3276 (1963).

G. V. H. Wilson, *JSI*, **41**, 98 (1964).

M. Yagi, *Sci. Rep. Tohoku Univ. First Ser. (Japan)*, **44**, 5 (1960).

CHAPTER 11

Detectors

Electronic components cannot pass microwave frequencies, and so a detector is employed to convert microwave energy to a lower frequency (e.g., dc, af, or rf). The present chapter describes several detectors and detector circuits. The ultimate sensitivity that may be achieved with both bolometers and crystal detectors is discussed in Sec. 14-C. Other types of detectors are discussed by Dicke (1946), Goodwin and Jones (1961), and Taylor and Herskovitz (1961).

A. Calorimetric Detection

When microwave energy is absorbed in a matched load, it is converted to heat and the temperature of the load rises. In the absence of a mechanism for heat removal the increase in temperature ΔT in degrees centigrade is related to the incident power P in watts and the time t in seconds by the relation

$$\int_0^t P dt = 4.186 \, CM \Delta T \tag{1}$$

where C is the heat capacity in calories per gram degree and M is the mass of the load in grams. Heating effects are unimportant at typical ESR power levels (e.g., 100 mW). The high power loads ordinarily employed with magnetrons, on the other hand, are equipped with cooling fins to dissipate excess power.

High microwave power levels may be measured by means of a water load with circulating water. The power in watts is computed from the rate of flow of the water (dV/dt cm³/sec) and the temperature difference ΔT between the input and output water from the relation

$$P = 4.186 \, (dV/dt) \, \Delta T \tag{2}$$

This equation follows from (1) since 1 cm³ of water weighs one gram, and the heat capacity C of water is 1 cal/g deg. Water loads are discussed at the end of the third chapter in *RLS*-11.

The bolometers and the thermistors discussed in the next two sections, respectively, are the most common types of calorimetric or thermal detectors.

B. Bolometers (Barretters)

A bolometer (or barretter) consists of a thin piece of wire which is heated by the incident microwave radiation. As a result of its positive temperature coefficient, the bolometer exhibits an increase in electrical resistance which may be detected by a Wheatstone bridge circuit such as the one shown in Fig. 11–1. From a knowledge of the increase in resistance, the thermal coefficient of resistance, and the heat capacity, one may deduce the microwave power. Commercial power meters which employ bolometer detectors incorporate more sophisticated circuits than the one shown on Fig. 11–1. Platinum is frequently employed as the thermoelectric element in the bolometer. When in use, a bolometer is ordinarily biased by passing about 8 mA of direct current through it, and thus provides it with an operating resistance R of 100 or 200 Ω. The resistance R of a bolometer with the microwave power P incident on it is related to its resistance R_0 at zero power by the expression

$$R = R_0 + kP^n \tag{1}$$

where k is a constant and n is close to unity.

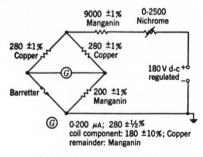

Fig. 11–1. Wheatstone bridge for use with a bolometer (*RLS*-11, p. 170).

A bolometer may be employed to detect the ESR signal in a spectrometer. In this application it is most sensitive when about 20 mW of microwave power are incident upon it, and for a simple detection scheme the sensitivity decreases when the power falls below this value, as shown in Fig. 11–2. A balanced mixer detection scheme such as the one discussed in Sec. 11–F may be employed to render the sensitivity independent of power. Every bolometer has a burnout power, and if the incident microwave radiation exceeds this power the bolometer melts and "burns out".

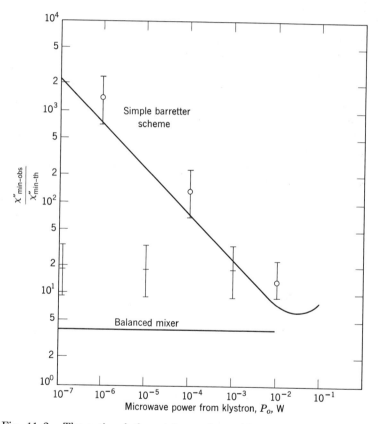

Fig. 11–2. The ratio of the minimum detectable rf susceptibility to the minimum theoretical value vs. microwave power for two different bolometer (barretter) schemes. The curves correspond to the predicted sensitivity, and the vertical lines bracket the experimental values [Feher (1957)].

A bolometer is ordinarily operated with a modulation frequency in the audio range of tens or hundreds of cycles per second because its response time is slow. It is advisable to keep the modulation frequency below 1 kc. The slow response of bolometers will also distort signals which are swept through in less than a millisecond, and this severely limits their adaptability to the signal enhancement scheme of Sec. 14-I.

In theory, bolometer detection can be as sensitive as crystal detection, but in practice, it is less versatile to use. A bolometer's noise temperature is unity since it produces only Johnson noise $dN = kT\Delta f$. Several highly sensitive spectrometers which incorporate bolometers have been described in the literature (e.g., see Sec. 13-B).

Some authors use the word bolometer interchangeably with barretter, and others use bolometer to mean thermal detectors with both positive and negative temperature coefficients. The first usage is adapted in this book. An extensive treatment of bolometers may be found in RLS–11, Chap. 3, Feher (1957), and Long (1960). Urano (1955) gives a bolometer equivalent circuit. Lalevic (1962) discusses the use of carbon resistors as bolometers at low rf powers. Byrne and Cook (1963) describe a bolometer for submillimetric wavelengths (see Sec. 11-E).

C. Thermistors

A thermistor is a thermal detector which consists of a semiconducting bead with a negative temperature coefficient of resistance. The resistance of thermistors may be varied over a much wider range than that of bolometers, and thermistors have excellent overload and burnout characteristics. They are less reproduceable and more sluggish than bolometers [Beck (1956)], and therefore are seldom employed as ESR detectors. An extensive discussion of thermistors is found in RLS–11, Chap. 3.

D. Crystals

The most commonly used detector in electron spin resonance is the crystal rectifier or diode. A common crystal conversion element consists of a "crystal" of silicon in contact with a tungsten cat whisker. The silicon contains a trace of impurity which renders it

semiconducting. A typical current-voltage characteristic is shown
in Fig. 11–3. A ceramic cartridge crystal is shown in Fig. 11–4 and
a shielded cartridge crystal is illustrated in Fig. 11–5.

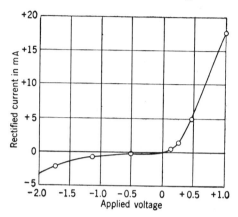

Fig. 11–3. Typical characteristic curve of a silicon rectifier (*RLS*–15, p. 20).

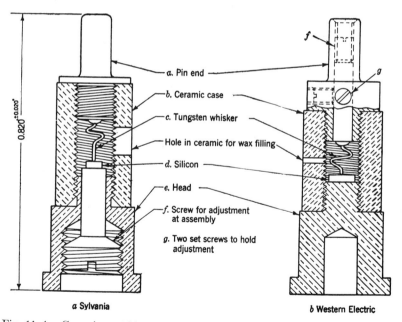

Fig. 11–4. Ceramic cartridge crystals [*RLS*-11, p. 5 and also *RLS*–15, p. 16).

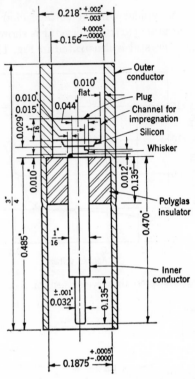

Fig. 11–5.   Coaxial cartridge crystal (RLS–11, p. 6; RLS–15, p. 327).

To understand crystal detection one must become familiar with the concepts of dc resistance R_{dc}, i-f impendance, noise power, dN, noise temperature t, conversion loss L, current sensitivity β, and figure of merit M.   These quantities are tabulated in crystal detector catalogs, and one must know their definitions in order to evaluate the relative merits of different crystals.   More information on crystal detectors may be found in RLS–11, RLS–15, RLS–16, and Long (1960).

The rectification properties of a silicon crystal are defined in terms of the equivalent circuit shown in Fig. 11–6.   The incident microwave power induces the voltage drop V across the crystal and causes the current I to flow through the variable resistor R.   If the resistance R is changed by a small amount, ΔR, then the voltage V and current I

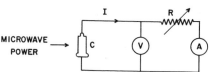

Fig. 11–6. Ammeter I and voltmeter V used for measuring the rectified current I and the rectified voltage V at the crystal C. The resistor R can be adjusted between open circuit $(R \sim \infty)$ and closed circuit $(R \sim 0)$ conditions.

will change by the increments ΔV and ΔI, respectively. The dynamic output impedance R_{dc} defined by

$$R_{dc} = \Delta V / \Delta I \qquad (1)$$

is called the "dc" impedance" or the "video resistance". The dc impedance of a typical crystal varies with the microwave power in the manner shown on Fig. 11–7. The same figure shows the power dependences of the short circuit current obtained when $R = 0$ and the open circuit voltage obtained when $R = \infty$. At microwatt powers, the dc impedance is fairly constant and the rectified current is proportional to the rf power. As a result, we say that the crystal is a square law detector. In the milliwatt region, the rectified crystal current becomes proportional to the square root of the microwave power, and the crystal is said to be a linear detector. The transition from square law to linear behavior is very gradual, and the crossover point between the two regions is typically near the power range 10^{-5} to 10^{-4} W. Crystal detectors of ESR spectrometers often operate in this transition region.

When the magnetic field is modulated at an intermediate frequency (i.f.) denoted by f_{mod}, the microwaves become amplitude modulated at f_{mod} during the passage through resonance. At the crystal the microwave signal is demodulated, and the ESR signal enters the receiver or preamplifier as an i.f. signal. The i.f. impedance "seen" at the input terminals of the receiver is the ratio of the i.f. current to the i.f. voltage at these terminals. The theory of frequency conversion (RLS–15, Chap. 5) predicts that the i.f. impedance and dc resistance are identical for crystal mixers used with low Q microwave systems. (RLS–15, p. 40f). An electron spin resonance spectrometer ordinarily employs a high-Q resonant cavity, so in this case the two may not be equal.

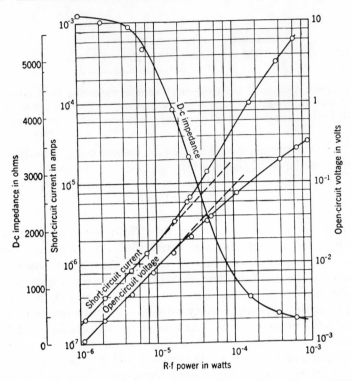

Fig. 11–7. Rectification properties of a silicon crystal rectifier at 3300 Mc
(*RLS*–11, p. 498; *RLS*–15, p. 334).

The available noise power or Johnson noise dN arising from a resistor radiating into a "cold" or noiseless load at the temperature T is

$$dN = kT\Delta f \tag{2}$$

where Δf is the band-width. A crystal rectifier generates more noise than a resistor, and its noise power dN is given by

$$dN = tkT\Delta f \tag{3}$$

where the dimensionless quantity $t > 1$ is the so called "noise temperature" or output noise ratio. Physically, t is the amount by which a resistor has to be raised in temperature to make it equivalent in noise power to a crystal maintained at room temperature. The excess noise is inversely proportional to the modulation frequency f_{mod}, and for the square law region ($P_c < 10^{-6}$ W) one may write

$$dN = (\gamma P_c{}^2/f_{\mathrm{mod}} + 1)\, kT\Delta P \tag{4}$$

while in the linear region

$$dN = (\gamma' P_c/f_{\mathrm{mod}} + 1)\, kT\Delta P \tag{5}$$

Feher (1957) quotes for an X band crystal

$$\gamma \approx 5 \times 10^{14}\ \mathrm{W}^{-2}\ \mathrm{sec}^{-1} \tag{6}$$

$$\gamma' \approx 10^{11}\ \mathrm{W}^{-1}\ \mathrm{sec}^{-1} \tag{7}$$

For further details, see RLS-15, Miller (1947) and Nicoll (1954). Andrews and Bazydlo (1959) found that the noise figure in decibels from a IN23E crystal decreased linearly with increasing frequency below 100kc, and remained constant above this value. Bosch, Gambling, and Wilmshurst (1961) found a $1/f_{\mathrm{mod}}$ law obeyed from 25 cps to 300 kc, with excess noise still present at higher frequencies. They used SIM2 and SIM5 crystals.

The conversion loss L of a crystal is the ratio of the available ESR signal power in the microwaves incident on the crystal, to the available output power at the frequency f_{mod} after detection. The conversion gain G is the reciprocal of L. From Feher (1957)

$$L = S'/P_c \tag{8}$$

in the square law region, and

$$L = C' \tag{9}$$

in the linear region where S' and C' are constants. For a 1N23C crystal $S' = 0.002$ W and $C' \approx 3.3$.

It is desirable to have both a low conversion loss L and a low noise temperature t. As Fig. 11–8 indicates, the conversion loss becomes very great at low crystal currents and the noise temperature becomes

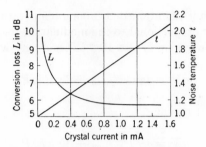

Fig. 11–8. Conversion loss L and noise temperature t as a function of the rectified current for a typical 1N23B crystal rectifier (RLS–15, p. 34).

excessive at high crystal currents. The best operating point is at an intermediate current which corresponds to an intermediate power level. The leakage or amount of microwave power incident on the crystal should be adjusted to this value, but the setting is not critical since the range of power which provides a maximum signal-to-noise ratio is fairly broad. Setting the leakage in this manner is called rf bucking (see Fig. 11–10). Sometimes a dc bias is employed to improve the crystal noise figure, as explained in RLS–16, Secs. 5–7 and 5–8. Long (1960) gives specific data on seven crystal diodes. His measurements on the minimum detectable relative power are shown on Fig. 11–9.

The current sensitivity β of a crystal is the number of microamperes of rectified current per microwatt of available rf power. The figure of merit M is defined by

$$M = \beta R/(R_{dc} + R_A)^{1/2} \qquad (10)$$

where R_{dc} is the dc or video resistance, and R_A is the equivalent noise resistance of a video amplifier (see RLS–15, Sec. 11–5). The JAN specifications have set R_A equal to 1200 Ω. It is desirable to have a high value of M.

There are two principal types of crystals. A *mixer crystal* is designed to convert a microwave frequency to an intermediate frequency, and is ideally suited for superheterodyne detection. It is usually characterized by its conversion loss L, output noise ratio (noise temperature) t, receiver noise figure (see Sec. 14-C), i.f. impedance, and burnout rating. Mixer crystals are discussed by Strum (1953) and Pritchard (1955). A *video crystal* is designed for the detection of very low power microwave energy, and is often used in spectrometers that do not employ superheterodyne detection. It is frequently characterized by its figure of merit M, its current sensitivity β, its video or dc impedance R_{dc}, and its burnout rating. A video crystal is also characterized by its minimum detectable signal, which is a signal voltage about equal to the RMS noise, and by its tangential signal (minimum sensitivity) which is the pulse power which raises the noise by its own width. The latter is of

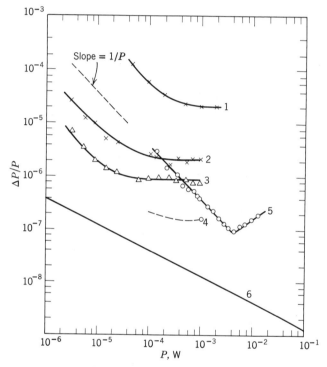

Fig. 11–9. Minimum detectable $\Delta P/P$ vs. P normalized for a 1-cps bandwidth. Curve 1 was computed from data on a 1N26 diode. Curve 2 is for a 1N23E diode, and is typical of 1N23 crystals. Curve 3 is for a 1N23B diode, and is the most sensitive of diode data measured by Long (1960). Curve 4 is for a 1N23E diode; the circle indicates computed sensitivity, and the result was confirmed by $CFCl_3$ measurements. Curve 5 is typical of 610B bolometer data. Curve 6 represents calculated sensitivity. The signal frequency for curve 1 was 24,000 Mc; the signal frequency for curves 2, 3, 4, and 5 was 10,000 Mc. The modulation frequency for curves 1, 2, 3, and 5 was 1 kc; the modulation frequency for curve 4 was 85 kc (Long (1960)].

interest in pulsed radar applications and is defined elsewhere (*RLS–15*, p. 347).

Crystals perform very well as detectors in ESR spectrometers, as Fig. 11–10 indicates, but their conversion characteristics are not uniform enough to render them suitable for accurate power measurements. Very high powers can damage crystals. A crystal may be checked for burnout by means of an ohmmeter. For this test the positive terminal of the ohmmeter is connected to the pointed or pin end of the crystal to measure the low resistance in the forward direction. The resistance in the forward direction should be about a thousand times that in the backward direction. For typical crystals

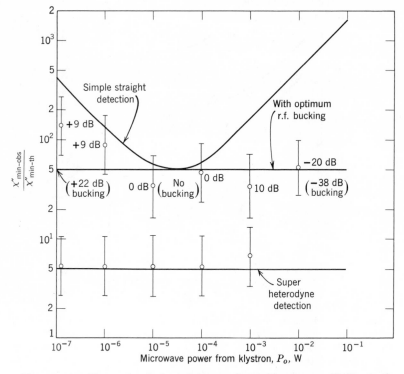

Fig. 11–10. The ratio of the minimum observable rf susceptibility to the minimum theoretical value vs. the microwave power for three crystal detection schemes. The straight detection and rf bucking schemes employed a modulation frequency of 1 kc. The curves correspond to the predicted sensitivity, and the vertical lines bracket the experimental values [Feher (1957)].

the limiting back current obtained with a potential difference of 1 V across the crystal is between 0.1 and 0.4 mA. A simple crystal test circuit and limiting back current data for specific crystals are found in *RLS*–16, Secs. 2–19 to 2–21.

The use of crystals as frequency multipliers at microwave frequencies is discussed in Sec. 6-F.

E. Submillimeter Detectors

The microwave-infrared gap [Coleman (1962)] can be spanned by thermal detectors [DeWaard and Wormser (1959); Petritz (1959); Goodwin and Jones (1961); Long and Rivers (1961); Byrne and Cook (1963)], and by an InSb photodetector [Putley (1960, 1961)]. Other detectors are operative in the submillimeter region, but will not cover as wide a wavelength band.

In Table 11–1 are listed eight detectors suitable for use at submillimetric wavelengths [Coleman (1963)]. The detectors are rated in terms of their detectivity D

$$D = (S/N)(\Delta f/A)^{1/2} \, (1/P) \, (\text{cps})^{1/2} \, \text{cm}^{-1} \, \text{W}^{-1} \qquad (1)$$

where S/N is the signal-to-noise ratio, Δf is the band-width, A is the area in square centimeters, and P is the power in watts. It is evident from the second column of the table that the InSb and germanium cyclotron resonance detectors are the most sensitive.

TABLE 11–1

Submillimeter Detectors [Coleman (1963)]

Detector	Detectivity $D \times 10^{-9}$	Response time τ, sec
Carbon resistor, 4°K	3	$< 10^{-3}$
Thermistor bolometer	0.2	$< 10^{-3}$
Superconductor bolometer		
Golay cell	1	$< 10^{-2}$
Ge-Zn photodetector 38 μ, 4°K	15	$\sim 10^{-3}$
InSb (Putley) photodetector $H \sim 5$ kG, 77°K	200	$\sim 10^{-6}$
Ge cyclotron resonance detector, 4°K	100	$\sim 10^{-6}$
Crystal diode, 0.7 mm		$< 10^{-2}$

It is believed that these detectors absorb microwave energy by means of their free or conduction electrons, and this leads to a change in the electrons' mobility and the material's conductivity [Rollin (1961)]. These detectors also have short enough response times for use with a 100-kc modulation frequency.

Crystal detectors are useful at low millimetric wavelengths. A dc bias may be used to increase the gain and sensitivity, and to decrease the noise of a IN53 crystal diode [Ishii and Brault (1962)]. Gallium arsenide is superior to either silicon or germanium in the low-milli-meter wavelength band [Sharpless (1961)]. A tunnel diode balanced near oscillation is a sensitive detector [Montgomery (1961)]. Burrus (1963) and DeLoach (1964) discuss several other millimeter wave detectors such as varactors, tunnel diodes, backward diodes, and Eski diodes. Erickson (1966) used a backward diode detector with his ESR spectrometer. Hot carrier diodes are discussed by Crane (1965) and Sorensen (1965). They consist of a metal semiconductor junction, and have response times less than 10^{-10} sec.

F. Balanced Mixers

A balanced mixer employs two detectors arranged in such a manner that the ESR signal arrives at each of them in the same phase while the power coming directly from the klystron arrives out of phase (*RLS*-16, Chap. 6). The i.f. output at the modulation frequently f_{mod} is the sum of the signals that appear at the two crystals, and so the phase relations cause the ESR signals to add and the klystron noise to cancel. Only half of the ESR signal appears at each crystal, but the two signals add so that the overall conversion loss of a balanced mixer is the same as that of a single crystal.

A balanced mixer is often constructed from a magic T in accordance with Fig. 11–11. As discussed in Sec. G, the wave amplitudes B_1 and B_2 produced in the crystal arms 1 and 2 are related to the incident amplitudes A_E and A_H in the E and H arms, respectively, by the relations [eq. (7F-2)]

$$B_1 = [j/2^{1/2}) \, (A_H + A_E) \tag{1}$$

$$B_2 = (j/2^{1/2}) \, (A_H - A_E) \tag{2}$$

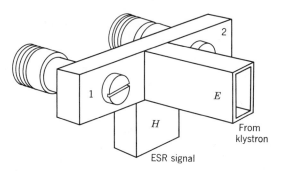

Fig. 11–11. X band magic T balanced mixer (RLS–16, p. 270).

Thus the magic T automatically causes the ESR signal to add and the klystron noise to cancel. If the klystron arm has the internal admittance Y_E and power P_E and the ESR cavity arm has the admittance Y_H and power P_H, then the power P_1 delivered to the crystal arm 1 is (RLS–16, p. 266)

$$P_1 = \frac{8g_1[g_H P_H (1 + Y_2 Y_E)^2 + g_E P_E (1 + Y_2 Y_H)^2]}{[(1 + Y_1 Y_H)(1 + Y_2 Y_E) + (1 + Y_1 Y_E)(1 + Y_2 Y_H)]^2} \quad (3)$$

where all the admittances are normalized relative to the characteristic admittance Y_0. A similar expression may be obtained for the power P_2 in arm 2 by interchanging the subscripts 1 and 2. The quantities g_i are the conductances in the various arms of the bridge (real part of Y_i).

To estimate the liability that results from unbalanced crystals ($Y_1 \neq Y_2$; $g_1 \neq g_2$), one may simplify eq. (3) by letting

$$Y_E = Y_H = g_E = g_H = g \quad (4)$$

As a result, one obtains the power ratio in the two arms

$$\frac{P_1}{P_2} = \frac{g_1}{g_2}\left(\frac{1 + gY_2}{1 + gY_1}\right)^2 \quad (5)$$

When $gY_1 \ll 1$ and $gY_2 \ll 1$, the power splits at the crystals in the ratio of the if conductances, or in other words, in the inverse ratio of the rf resistances. In general, the noise suppression in a magic T balanced mixer is a complicated function of the rf resistances of the two crystals, and a simplified relation such as eq. (5) cannot be used.

To estimate the extent to which the klystron noise suppression is dependent upon the closeness of their conversion losses to each other, let each crystal have the same incident rf power from both the ESR signal and the local oscillator. If L_1 and L_2 are the two conversion losses, then the ESR signal power is proportional to $(L_1^{1/2} + L_2^{1/2})^2$ and the klystron noise power is proportional to $(L_1^{1/2} - L_2^{1/2})^2$. The factor by which the klystron noise is suppressed relative to the signal is $(L_1^{1/2} + L_2^{1/2})^2/(L_1^{1/2} - L_2^{1/2})^2$. For a 3-dB difference in conversion loss, $L_1 = 2L_2$, and therefore

$$\left(\frac{L_1^{1/2} + L_2^{1/2}}{L_1^{1/2} - L_2^{1/2}}\right)^2 = 34 \tag{8}$$

so even this small unbalance suppresses the klystron noise by 15.3 dB.

In Sec. 11–B it was mentioned that at low powers the conversion gain of a bolometer is low. A balanced mixer such as the one shown in Fig. 11–11 may feed a large amount of power P_2 to mixer bolometers or barretters. This improves the conversion gain without increasing the noise because the bolometer noise should not be

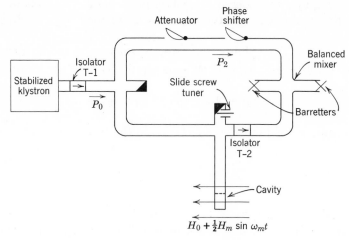

Fig. 11–12.   Bolometer (barretter) system with balanced mixer [Feher (1957)].

power-dependent, and much of the noise from the bypassed power P_2 in Fig. 11–12 cancels in the balanced mixer. A phase shifter is provided for the bypassed power since an incorrect phase will reduce the ESR sensitivity and also produce an admixture of χ' and χ''. This system is somewhat inconvenient to operate because the phase must be reset every time either the bypassed power level P_2 is adjusted by the attenuator, or the slide screw tuner setting is changed.

G. Superheterodyne Detectors

A superheterodyne receiver employs the frequency converter shown diagrammatically on Fig. 11–13 to convert the microwave ESR signal to an intermediate frequency (i.f.) signal $\Delta\omega$ that is two or three orders of magnitude lower in frequency. In a typical case a local oscillator klystron supplies a frequency $(1/2\pi)\,\omega_L = 9030$ Mc and the ESR absorption experiment is carried out at $(1/2\pi)\,\omega_0 = 9000$ Mc. The two frequencies ω_L and ω_0 mix in the frequency converter and produce the sum and difference frequencies $\omega_L \pm \omega_0$. The difference or i.f. frequency is detected by the mixer and later demodulated to provide the ESR resonance signal which is either seen visually, or recorded in the usual way. The magic T mixer shown in Fig. 11–11 is often employed in superheterodyne detection, and it provides for the usual cancellation of the klystron noise. Seidel (1962) and Llewellyn, Whittlestone, and Williams (1962) modulate the klystron and use a sideband as the local oscillator frequency. This simplifies the superheterodyne instrumentation by eliminating the necessity of a second klystron.

The big advantage of a superheterodyne detector is that it operates at a frequency which is sufficiently high so that the $1/f$ noise in the crystal is negligible. The 30 or 60-Mc i.f. frequency of typical superheterodyne spectrometers considerably exceeds the modulation frequency of almost every field modulation system that has been

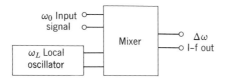

Fig. 11–13.   Block diagram of a converter or mixer (RLS–16, p. 26).

described in the literature. In addition, it resolves very narrow resonant lines (e.g., tens of milligauss wide) which are beyond the limits of resolution with very high frequency (e.g., 100 kc) field modulation systems.

In a superheterodyne spectrometer it is necessary to stabilize the frequency of the signal klystron, and at the same time to stabilize the frequency of the local oscillator klystron in such a manner that the difference frequency remains constant. This entails either the use of two independent AFC circuits, or the addition of a system which maintains the constant difference $\Delta\omega$ between the two klystrons. The latter is preferable.

England and Schneider (1950) describe the first superheterodyne spectrometer mentioned in the literature. Table 13–1 lists a number of such spectrometers, and several are described in Chap. 13. The basic principles of superheterodyne receivers are discussed in *RLS*–16 and *RLS* 23, while associated i.f. amplifiers are covered in *RLS*–18.

H. Detector Holders

Bolometer holders are described in *RLS*–11, Sec. 3–27. Crystal holders are discussed in *RLS*–11, Sec. 1–3, and at several places in *RLS*–15 and *RLS*–16. A tunable *X* band crystal mount is shown in

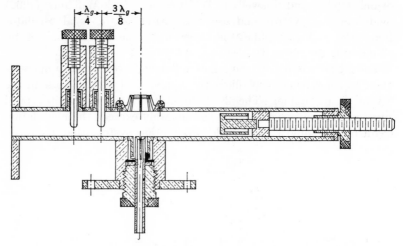

Fig. 11–14.   Tunable *X* band crystal mount (*RLS*–16, p. 132).

Fig. 11–14. Blomfield (1964) describes a detector in oversized waveguide for use at millimetric wavelengths.

References

G. B. Andrews and H. A. Bazydlo, *Proc. IRE*, **47**, 2018 (1959).

A. Beck, *JSI*, **33**, 16 (1956).

D. L. H. Blomfield, *JSI*, **41**, 517 (1964).

B. G. Bosch, W. A. Gambling, and T. H. Wilmshurst, *Proc. IRE*, **49**, 1226 (1961).

C. A. Burrus, Jr., *IEEE Trans.*, **MTT-11**, 357 (1963).

J. F. Byrne and C. F. Cook, *IEEE Trans.*, **MTT-11**, 379 (1963).

P. D. Coleman, *Proc. IRE*, **50**, 1219 (1962).

P. D. Coleman, *IEEE Trans.*, **MTT-11**, 271 (1963).

M. Crane, *Hewlett Packard J.*, **17**, 6 (1965).

B. C. DeLoach, *IEEE Trans.*, **MTT-12**, 15 (1964).

R. DeWaard and E. M. Wormser, *Proc. IRE*, **47**, 1508 (1959).

R. H. Dicke, *RSI*, **17**, 268 (1946).

T. S. England and E. E. Schneider, *Nature*, **166**, 437 (1950).

L. E. Erickson, *Phys. Rev.*, **143**, 295 (1966).

G. Feher, *Bell System Tech. J.*, **36**, 449 (1957).

D. W. Goodwin and R. H. Jones, *J. Appl. Phys.*, **32**, 2056 (1961).

K. Ishii and A. L. Brault, *IRE Trans.*, **MTT-10**, 258 (1962).

B. Lavelic, *RSI*, **33**, 103 (1962).

P. M. Llewellyn, P. R. Whittlestone, and J. M. Williams, *JSI*, **39**, 586 (1962).

M. W. Long, *RSI*, **31**, 1286 (1960).

M. W. Long and W. K. Rivers, *Proc. IRE*, **49**, 1024 (1961).

P. H. Miller, *Proc. IRE*, **35**, 252 (1947).

M. D. Montgomery, *Proc. IRE (Corresp.)*, **49**, 826 (1961).

G. R. Nicoll, *Proc. IEE*, **101**, 317 (1954).

R. L. Petritz, *Proc. IRE*, **47**, 1458 (1959).

W. L. Pritchard, *Trans. IRE*, **MTT-3**, 37 (1955).

E. H. Putley, *J. Phys. Chem. Solids*, **22**, 241 (1961).

E. H. Putley, *Proc. Phys. Soc.*, **76**, 802 (1960).

RLS–11.

RLS–15.

RLS–16.

RLS–18.

RLS–23.

B. V. Rollin, *Proc. Phys. Soc.*, **77**, 1102 (1961).

H. Seidel, *Z. Angew. Phys.*, **14**, 21 (1962).

W. M. Sharpless, *IRE Trans.*, **MTT-9**, 6 (1961).

H. O. Sorensen, *Hewlett Packard J.*, **17**, 1 (1965).

P. D. Strum, *Proc. IRE*, **41**, 875 (1953).

R. L. Taylor and S. B. Herskovitz, *Proc. IRE*, **49**, 1901 (1961).

Y. Urano, *J. Phys. Soc. Japan*, **10**, 864 (1955).

CHAPTER 12

Electronic Circuitry

An electron spin resonance spectrometer consists of electronic circuits which supply power to the microwave generator and magnet, amplify and record the ESR absorption signal, modulate the magnetic field, etc. Indeed most of the parts that enter into the construction of an ESR spectrometer are transistors, vacuum tubes, resistors, capacitors, inductances, transformers, and other electronic components. It will be assumed that the reader has a knowledge of basic electronics, and in this chapter we will emphasize circuits which are frequently incorporated into ESR spectrometers. Well known circuits such as a cathode follower (emitter follower) and a push-pull amplifier will only be discussed in sufficient detail to enable the reader to understand their functions in the spectrometer. More specialized circuits such as a twin T amplifier and a lock-in detector will be elaborated upon in order to explicate their principles of operation, in addition to presenting their function in the spectrometer.

During the discussion of the various electronic components, the reader should refer to the circuit diagrams found throughout the book. These circuits show the components in actual use, and a perusal of this chapter in conjunction with a careful examination of these circuits will prepare the spectroscopist for isolating and repairing malfunctions of the electronic instrumentation.

Most recently designed electronic circuits are transistorized, but space does not permit an extensive discussion of transistor circuitry.

A. Preamplifiers

The preamplifier is the first stage of amplification following the detection of the ESR absorption (or dispersion) signal. The signal which enters the preamplifier consists of a combination of the ESR signal itself and noise (cf. Secs. 14-B and 14-C). The noise may arise from one or more sources such as the klystron, the detector, microphonics, etc. The function of the preamplifier is to amplify this incident signal without adding significant noise to it. Thus the principal attribute of a good preamplifier is its low noise characteristic.

It is shown in Sec. 14-C that the overall noise figure F of n successive stages of amplification is

$$F = F_1 + \frac{F_2 - 1}{G_1} + \frac{F_3 - 1}{G_1 G_2} + \cdots + \frac{F_n - 1}{G_1 G_2 \ldots G_{n-1}} \qquad (1)$$

where F_i and G_i are the individual noise figure and gain, respectively, of the ith stage of amplification. Since in practice it is usually true that

$$G_i \gg 1 \qquad (2)$$

and F_i is the same order of magnitude for all the stages, it follows that only the first stage will contribute appreciably to the overall noise figure, with the result that

$$F \approx F_1 \qquad (3)$$

It should be emphasized that the function of a preamplifier is to amplify both the signal and the noise that are impressed on its input terminals (e.g., its emitter or grid) without introducing an appreciable amount of additional noise. Successive stages such as narrow band amplifiers and the lock-in detector preferentially remove noise without apprecially decreasing the signal. Sometimes, the narrow band function is combined with the low noise feature in the preamplifier.

It is helpful to precede the preamplifier with a step-up transformer which provides a voltage gain before the introduction of transistor or vacuum tube noise [Strandberg, Tinkham, Solt, and Davis (1956)]. Some of the preamplifier tubes that have been employed in ESR spectrometers include: the 6AU6, 6SJ7, 12AU7, 12AY7, 6112, 2N2189 and the nuvistor [see Brophy (1955)].

Preamplifiers may be employed in other parts of the spectrometer, such as in the NMR magnetometer, and in the magnet power supply error signal loop.

B. Push-Pull Amplifiers

A push-pull amplifier such as the one shown on Fig. 10–22 has its cathodes joined together and its plates connected through a load resistance or inductance. On this figure the magnet coils form an inductive load. The input signal drives one grid positive while the other is negative, and vice versa. The amplified signals from the two tubes add in the load connected between the plates, and there they produce an output signal that is free of even harmonics of the input frequency. The push-pull amplifier accepts a balanced input signal and produces a balanced output. The input and output signals are often transformer-coupled to and from the amplifier.

C. Cathode and Emitter Followers

A cathode follower such as the 6J5 (V18) on Fig. 6–17 is a triode which has its input signal applied from the grid to B⁻, and provides an output signal between the cathode and B⁻. (This entire circuit is "upside down" with grounded plates.) The grid is usually connected to ground through a resistor, and the plate is ordinarily connected through a resistor to the B⁺ power supply. The transistor analog of a cathode follower is the emitter follower or common collector transistor such as the 2N1744 shown on Fig. 9–22 [Pierce and Hicks (1965)].

Both the cathode follower and the emitter follower have a high input impedance and low output impedance, so they find frequent use as impedance matching devices. Other follower characteristics include a low effective input capacitance, low nonlinear distortion, and a gain somewhat less than unity.

The reader is advised to look for cathode and emitter followers in other figures of this book in order to develop his facility in recognizing them. Sometimes a cathode follower serves as a dual purpose tube, e.g., by amplifying the main signal in the plate circuit while at the same time acting as a cathode follower for a reference signal.

D. Tuned Amplifiers

When an amplifier incorporates a narrow band filter so that it only passes signals near a particular frequency then it eliminates noise at other frequencies. The narrow band 100-kc amplifier desribed on p. 61 of *Microwave Spectroscopy*, by Gordy, Smith, and Trumbarulo (1953) employs parallel tuned LC circuits connected to the grids and plates of several series amplifiers.

E. Twin T Amplifiers

The twin T shown in Fig. 12-1 is a three-terminal nonplanar network which has bilateral symmetry so that two of the terminals are equivalent. It is convenient to consider it as a two-terminal pair network with two of its terminals grounded together. This circuit is discussed by Tuttle (1940) and Terman (1943).

For very high frequencies where

$$\omega \gg 1/RC \tag{1}$$

one has

$$|X_c| \ll R \tag{2}$$

and the capacitive reactance may be considered negligible relative to the resistance. As a result, the equivalent circuit has the form shown in Fig. 12-2a, and a voltage V_i impressed at the input terminals produces an open circuit voltage $V_0 = V_i$ across the output terminals. A dc voltage impressed at the input terminals corresponds to $X_c = \infty$, and leads to the equivalent circuit shown in Fig. 12-2b. Again the application of an input voltage V_i produces the open circuit output voltage $V_0 = V_i$. Thus we see that for frequencies much greater and much less than the resonant frequency $\omega_0 = 1/RC$, the twin T does

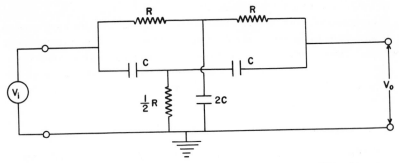

Fig. 12-1. Twin T with angular resonant frequency $\omega_0 = 1/RC$ rad/sec.

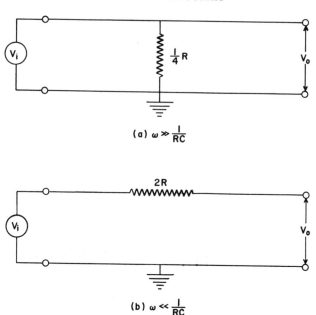

Fig. 12-2. The equivalent circuit of a twin T for frequencies (a) $\omega \gg 1/RC$; (b) $\omega \ll 1/RC$.

not directly attenuate the input voltage, but merely adds a resistance in parallel or in series with the input voltage V_i. This resistance will of course lead to a loss of power, but an appreciable loss of this kind would be the result of a poor impedance match to the output or load that is connected at the output terminals.

A twin T may be looked upon as a low pass T filter connected in parallel to a high pass T filter. Its reactances are chosen in such a way that the two cutoff frequencies effectively coincide, and as a result the resonant frequency $\omega_0 = 1/RC$ is attenuated, while higher and lower frequencies are transmitted. This makes the twin T a band-stop filter which passes all frequencies except those near ω_0. The band-stop filters Z_1 and Z_2 in the tuned amplifier shown on Fig. 9-18 are twin T's.

A twin T band stop filter may be incorporated into an amplifier to produce a band pass twin T amplifier. This is accomplished by providing a degenerative feedback path through the twin T so that the frequencies above and below ω_0 act to nullify the input signal, and thereby prevent it from appearing at the output (cf. Sec. 12-G). Since the resonant frequency ω_0 is stopped by the twin T, the degenerative feedback is absent at this frequency, and amplification results. The first 6SJ7 amplification stage on Fig. 9–18 is a twin T amplifier. Gheorghiu and Valeriu (1962) discuss the signal-to-noise ratio obtained with a twin T bridge in NMR applications.

Occasionally, twin T amplifiers have a tendency to oscillate. This is usually the result of regenerative feedback, and it should not depend on the input signal. The unwanted oscillations will be detected as a large signal which appears on the plate of the twin T amplifier even when the input is short-circuited. It may be necessary to replace the tube or some circuit components such as resistors or capacitors to suppress these oscillations.

F. Lock-In Detectors

Other sections of this chapter discuss electronic components such as narrow band (e.g., twin T) amplifiers and long-time constant filters which preferentially suppress noise without appreciably attenuating the signal. These components perform their function as a result of their frequency selectivity since they reject undesired frequencies. A lock-in detector is more efficient than these other components because it is both frequency-sensitive and phase-sensitive. In other words, it only passes signals which have the proper frequency, and in addition, which arrive in phase with a reference signal. Thus a lock-in detector only accepts signals which "lock in" to the reference signal. Sometimes a lock-in detector is given one of the more descriptive titles "phase-sensitive detector", or "coherent detector".

The Schuster lock-in detector circuit [Schuster (1951)] shown in Fig. 12–3 consists of the pentode V_2 whose plate load is switched between the resistors R_1 and R_2 by means of the reference signal which is applied to the grids of the double triode switching tube V_1. This reference voltage alternately cuts off one side of V_2 and causes the other side to conduct.

The equivalent circuit of this lock-in detector is shown in Fig. 12–4. The signal input is represented by the voltage μV_g where μ is the tube amplification factor. If the input signal has the same frequency and phase as the reference signal, then the positive half of it will always

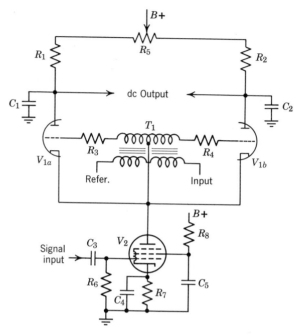

Fig. 12–3.   Lock-in-detector circuit [Schuster (1951)].

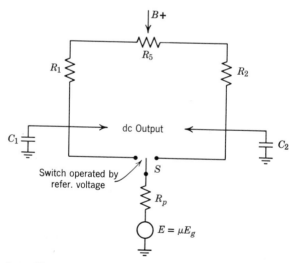

Fig. 12–4.   Equivalent circuit of a lock-in-detector [Schuster (1951)].

go through V_{1a}, and the negative half will be passed by V_{1b}, which means that the two plates will have half-wave rectified signals of opposite polarity. The dc components of these two signals will be added in the following long time constant filter to produce a net output signal which is twice the magnitude of either dc component alone. If the input signal is 90° out of phase with the reference signal then the average dc component on each plate will be zero, as shown in Fig. 12–5. Of course intermediate phase settings produce intermediate output signals.

If the input signal frequency ω_i is slightly different from the reference frequency ω_r, then it will act like an input signal of gradu-

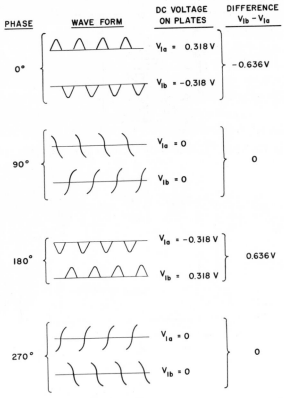

Fig. 12–5. Waveform and dc voltage on the lock-in detector plates for four values of the phase of the input signal V. The half amplitude of the waveform on the plate is V, and the applied frequency ω_i equals the reference frequency ω_r.

ally changing phase, and the voltages on the plates will oscillate back and forth at the difference frequency $|\omega_i - \omega_r|$. The amplitude of this signal at $|\omega_i - \omega_r|$ becomes smaller as $|\omega_i - \omega_r|$ becomes greater. If one assumes that the input noise spectrum is independent of frequency in the neighborhood of ω_r, then the output noise will peak near ω_r and decrease with $|\omega_i - \omega_r|$ for frequencies both above and below ω_r. In addition, most of the noise at the frequency $|\omega_i - \omega_r|$ will itself be rejected because it will be out of phase with the reference signal. Fig. 12-6 shows the waveforms on the lock-in detector plates for $\omega_i = 2\omega_r$ and $\omega_i = \frac{1}{2}\omega_r$. This figure is drawn to the same scale as Fig. 12-5 to facilitate a comparison with the analogous zero phase (i.e., properly phased) signal for $\omega_i = \omega_r$.

To insure phase coherence, the reference signal for the lock-in detector must be obtained from the same oscillator that produces the magnetic field (or source) modulation. Ordinarily an adjustable phase shifter is provided to insure that the modulation and reference signals arrive in phase at the lock-in detector. A second phase shifter may be employed to synchronize the oscilloscope x axis sweep with the lock-in detector output for visual observation of the latter. These two phases should be adjusted, respectively, to (1) maximum signal amplitude and (2) a symmetrical scope pattern.

The lock-in detector of Strandberg, Tinkham, Solt, and Davis (1956) employs a mechanical switch or Brown converter instead of a vacuum tube for the switch S shown in the equivalent circuit of Fig. 12-4. One may also employ two diodes, since a diode acts like a short circuit for a positive polarity and an open circuit for a negative polarity. Strandberg, Tinkham, Solt, and Davis also incorporated a Brown converter in their magnet stabilizer (Fig. 9-18).

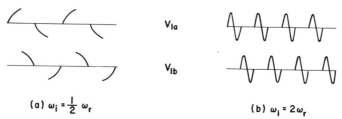

(a) $\omega_i = \frac{1}{2}\omega_r$

(b) $\omega_i = 2\omega_r$

Fig. 12-6. Waveforms on the lock-in-detector plates V_{1a} and V_{1b} for an input angular frequency ω_i which is (a) half and (b) twice the reference frequency ω_r. The dc voltages of both V_{1a} and V_{1b} are zero in each case.

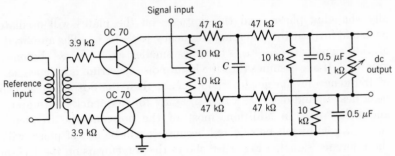

Fig. 12-7.   Transistorized, drift-free, phase-sensitive detector [Faulkner (1959)].

Faulkner (1959) designed the transistorized lock-in detector shown in Fig. 12-7. The reference signal is transformer coupled to the bases of the OC70 transistors, and the ESR signal is applied to the collectors. In the two halves of the switching cycle the transistor impedance alternates between a value very small and very large relative to the 10-kΩ load. A band-width of 0.2 cps is obtained when a 100 μf capacitance is used for the integrating capacitor C. The dc drift is less than 5 μV.

The lock-in detector is essentially a narrow band filter which is phase-sensitive, and as such, it is characterized by an effective band-width Δf and quality factor Q. This will be discussed in Secs. 14-C, 14-D, and 14-F.

Lock-in detector circuits are also discussed in *RLS*-19, and by Cox (1953), Nuckolls and Rueger (1953), Baker (1954), Bösnecker (1960), (1961), and Dereppe Memory (1964). The Popov (1960) circuit operates up to 12 Mc. Van Gerven, Van Itterbeek, and Stals (1963) used a wattmeter as the active element in their coherent detector. Raether and Bitzer (1964) built a polarity coincidence detector. Blentzinger, Garscadden, Alexeff, and Jones (1965) show how an oscilloscope may be used as a lock-in detector. Beers (1965) describes a lock-in detector mode of operation which removes spurious coherent signals. Arnal and Beuchot (1964) and Williams (1965) describe transistorized phase-sensitive detectors.

G. Oscillators

An ordinary amplifier is a transistor or vacuum tube which accepts an ac input voltage V_i at the control grid, increases its amplitude by the factor K, and produces the output voltage $V_0 = KV_i$ at the plate. As discussed earlier in this chapter, the voltage gain K is dependent on the frequency, and in addition, it is also dependent on other factors such as the circuit impedance. Suppose that a fraction βV_0 of the output voltage is fed back to the grid. When this is the case, then the effective input signal becomes $V_i + \beta V_0$, and the output voltage has the form

$$V_0 = K(V_i + \beta V_0) \tag{1}$$

The voltage gain G in the presence of feedback is defined by the ratio V_0/V_i, and therefore,

$$\text{gain} = V_0/V_i \tag{2}$$

$$= K/(1 - \beta K) \tag{3}$$

If the feedback voltage βV_0 is in phase with the externally applied input signal V_i, then the product βK is positive, and for $0 < \beta K < 1$, the gain is increased over its value in the absence of feedback. This is referred to as positive or regenerative feedback. If, on the other hand, the feedback voltage βV_0 is out of phase with the applied input voltage, then βK is negative, and the gain is decreased as the result of negative or degenerative feedback. The twin T amplifier discussed in Sec. 12-E operates on the principle of degenerative feedback. In general, both β and K can assume any phase angle relative to each other, and accordingly the product βK may be complex.

It may be seen from eq. (3) that as βK approaches unity for regenerative feedback, the gain becomes arbitrarily large. When $\beta K = 1$, the gain becomes infinite and oscillations result. In other words, the applied input voltage V_i may be removed and the feedback voltage βV_0 itself sustains the oscillation.

Another characteristic of an oscillator is the presence of a tuned circuit to limit the oscillations to a single frequency. For example, the CV4024 NMR oscillator that is incorporated in the super regenerative circuit shown in Fig. 9–20 employs an LC parallel-tuned circuit [Vincent, Kaine, and King (1962)]. The coil of this circuit holds the NMR sample while the capacitance is variable so that the frequency f

$$f = \omega/2\pi = [2\pi(LC)^{1/2}]^{-1} \tag{4}$$

may be tuned.   An RC Wien bridge oscillator does not employ an
LC-tuned circuit, and it may be recognized by the tungsten filament
in the cathode circuit, as explained by Seely (1950).   Some circuits
employ external oscillators, or generate frequencies that are crystal-
controlled.

H. Modulation

A high frequency signal is said to be modulated if either its amplitude V or its angular frequency $\omega = 2\pi f$ is varied in a regular manner.

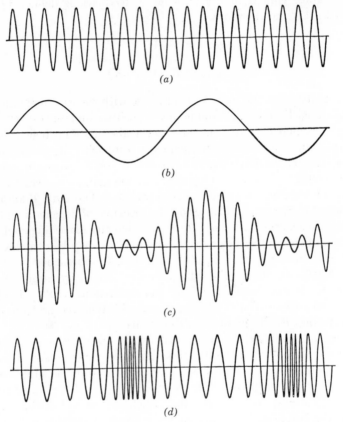

Fig. 12–8.   Amplitude and frequency modulation of a high frequency carrier
by a sine wave signal: (*a*) unmodulated carrier; (*b*) modulating waveform;
(*c*) amplitude-modulated wave; (*d*) frequency-modulated wave [Black (1953)].

Figure 12–8 shows an unmodulated, an amplitude-modulated, and a frequency-modulated rf carrier. The present section will open with a discussion of amplitude modulation. This will be followed by a treatment of frequency modulation, and finally the theory of modulation will be applied to magnetic resonance. For simplicity in the remainder of this section, the high frequency or carrier signal $V_0 \cos \omega_0 t$ will be referred to as the radio frequency (rf) and the modulating signal $V_m \cos \omega_m t$ will be designated the audio frequency (af). In practice, one sometimes actually uses modulation frequencies as high as 60 Mc, which is actually in the rf region.

Amplitude Modulation (AM): If an rf wave $V_0 \cos \omega_0 t$ is amplitude-modulated by an af wave $V_m \cos \omega_m t$, the resulting wave form V is

$$V = V_0(1 + m \cos \omega_m t) \cos \omega_0 t \tag{1}$$

where m is the modulation index and $100m$ is the percentage modulation. A trigonometric identity may be employed to rearrange eq. (1) to the form

$$V = V_0 \cos \omega_0 t + \tfrac{1}{2} m V_0 \cos (\omega_0 + \omega_m)t$$
$$+ \tfrac{1}{2} m V_0 \cos (\omega_0 - \omega_m)t \tag{2}$$

The first term in eq. (2) is the carrier frequency, while the second and third terms are the upper and lower sidebands, respectively. These three frequencies may actually be separated by means of narrow band filters.

Demodulation is the process of recovering the modulation signal $V_m \cos \omega_m t$ from the sidebands. It may be looked upon as a frequency-shifting procedure. Diodes are often employed for demodulation purposes. In ESR, the modulation is removed from the microwave carrier by the crystal detector, or bolometer as discussed in Chap. 11.

Frequency Modulation (FM): The carrier waveform $V_0 \sin \omega t$ is frequency-modulated when its angular frequency ω varies in a regular manner. For example, in sinusoidal frequency modulation one has

$$V = V_0 \sin (\omega_0 t + \delta \sin \omega_m t) \tag{3}$$

where δ is the deviation ratio which is defined in terms of the maximum instantaneous FM frequency ω_{max} and the minimum frequency ω_{min} defined by

$$\omega_{max} = \omega_0 + \omega_m\delta \tag{4}$$

$$\omega_{min} = \omega_0 - \omega_m\delta \tag{5}$$

The maximum variation of the angular frequency from its mean value ω_0 is referred to as the frequency deviation ω_d

$$\omega_d = \omega_m\delta = \begin{cases} \omega_0 - \omega_{min} \\ \omega_{max} - \omega_0 \end{cases} \tag{6}$$

The modulation index m is defined by

$$m = \omega_d/\omega_0 \tag{7}$$

The frequency modulation waveform of eq. (3) may be expanded by the use of a trigonometric identity to

$$V = V_0[\sin \omega_0 t \cos (\delta \sin \omega_m t) + \cos \omega_m t \sin (\delta \sin \omega_m t)] \tag{8}$$

If one makes use of the two expressions

$$\cos (\delta \sin \omega_m t) = J_0(\delta) + 2 \sum_{n=1}^{\infty} J_{2n}(\delta) \cos 2n\omega_m t \tag{9}$$

$$\sin (\delta \sin \omega_m t) = 2 \sum_{n=0}^{\infty} J_{2n+1}(\delta) \sin (2n + 1)\omega_m t \tag{10}$$

where $J_n (\delta)$ is the nth order Bessel function of the first kind, then the frequency-modulated waveform may be written [Seely (1950)]

$$V = J_0(\delta) V_0 \sin \omega_0 t + J_1(\delta) V_0 [\sin (\omega_0 + \omega_m)t - \sin (\omega_0$$
$$- \omega_m)t] + J_2(\delta) V_0 [\sin (\omega_0 + 2\omega_m)t + \sin (\omega_0 - 2\omega_m)t]$$
$$+ J_3(\delta) V_0 [\sin (\omega_0 + 3\omega_m)t - \sin (\omega_0 - 3\omega_m)t] \tag{11}$$
$$+ \ \cdot \ \cdot \ \cdot \ \cdot \ \cdot \ \cdot$$

This result means that the spectrum of an *FM* wave consists of a carrier plus an infinite number of side bands whose amplitudes are the Bessel functions $J_n(\delta)$ E_0. The side band distributions for several *FM* waves are shown in Figs. 12–9 and 12–10.

Modulation in ESR Spectrometers: The most important modulation in ESR is the magnetic field (or source) modulation. At resonance the paramagnetic sample absorbs microwave energy, and as a result the microwave carrier ω_0 is amplitude-modulated at the modulation frequency ω_m and higher harmonics of ω_m, as discussed in Sec. 10-D. The crystal diode removes the carrier ω_0 and passes the ESR signals at ω_m and its harmonics to the preamplifier. When either the amplitude or the frequency of the magnetic field modulation becomes too high, the result is the generation of many large amplitude harmonics of ω_m and considerable distortion of the detected line shape, as discussed in Secs. 10-E and 10-F.

Some Pound stabilizer (Sec. 6-H) and superheterodyne (Sec. 11-G) arrangements beat two klystrons together to produce an inter-

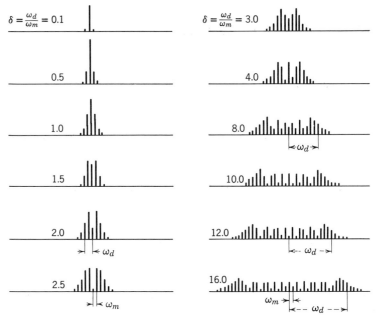

Fig. 12–9. The spectral distribution of an *FM* wave for a fixed value of ω_m and several different values of δ and ω_d [Seely (1950)].

mediate frequency (i.f.).   For example, the beat between two klystrons at 9000 and 9030 Mc, respectively produces the i.f. of 30 Mc
which is detected by the crystal.   This i.f. is said to amplitude
modulate the microwave carrier.

The reflector modulation klystron stabilizer discussed in Sec. 6-H,
modulates the klystron reflector with a very small modulation index

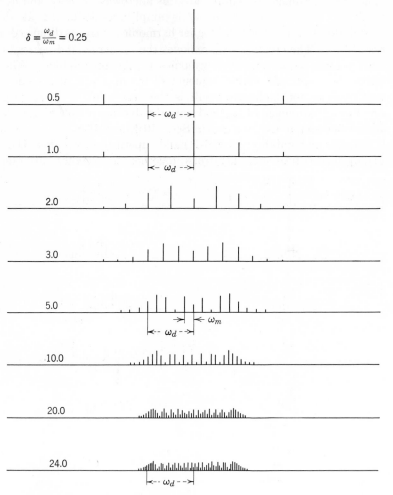

Fig. 12–10.   The spectral distribution of an FM wave for a fixed value of ω_d and
several different values of δ and ω_m [Seely (1950)].

m. The result is actually a combination of frequency modulation and amplitude modulation (cf. Fig. 6–7), but the klystron stabilizer only makes use of the fundamental AM component. It is the high Q of the resonant cavity that is responsible for the AM of the klystron's output power.

Sometimes vibrations or other microphonics in the microwave system modulate the microwave carrier, and produce a large contribution to the noise incident on the detector.

I. Oscilloscopic Presentation of the ESR Signal

For tuning purposes and rapid searching for unknown resonances, it is convenient to display the resonant absorption on an oscilloscope. For example, a strong absorber like α,α'-diphenyl-β-picryl hydrazyl (DPPH) may be observed visually to set the magnetic field strength dial, adjust the modulation phase, check the magnet homogeneity and modulation amplitude, etc. A proton NMR magnetometer may be employed to calibrate the oscilloscope screen for the purpose of visually determining the line-width, hyperfine spacings, and g factor. Oscilloscope presentation of ESR data was widely used before Whitmer, Weidner, Hsiang, and Weiss (1948), and Weidner and Whitmer (1952) demonstrated the utility of recorders.

If the modulation amplitude is made several times the line-width and the signal is impressed on the oscilloscope before it reaches the narrow band amplifiers, then the 'scope will present the actual absorption (or dispersion) line-shape. When one employs a high frequency plus a low frequency modulation and narrow band detection, the oscilloscope display is the modulus of the absorption line-shape as shown in Figs. 10–23 and 13–9. These patterns differ from the first (or second) derivative signals that result from phase-sensitive detection with a lock-in detector.

For oscilloscopic presentation of the magnetic resonance signal, it is best to obtain the oscilloscope sweep frequency from the same oscillator that modulates the magnetic field. A phase shifter may be employed to center the pattern on the oscilloscope. When the double frequency modulation technique is employed the low or audio frequency is used for the oscilloscope sweep. (e.g., see Sec. 13–H).

J. Recorder Presentation and Response Time

When the electron spin resonance signal emerges from the lock-in detector, it still contains a considerable amount of noise. A great deal of this noise may be removed by passing the signal through a low pass filter. The filter has associated with it a time constant or response time τ_0 which is a measure of the cutoff frequency of the filter. In other words, the filter fails to pass frequencies that are much greater than the reciprocal of the time constant $1/\tau_0$; it attenuates, distorts, and retards (in phase) those waveforms which have frequencies which are in the neighborhood of τ_0, and it transmits, undisturbed, those frequencies which are considerably below $1/\tau_0$.

The waveform that is impressed on the ESR response filter may be considered as the derivative of the absorption (or dispersion) line, and for comparison with the above criteria, its effective frequency may be taken as the inverse of the time that it takes to scan through the resonance from one peak to the next. In other words, if the time that it takes to scan through the magnetic field range ΔH_{pp} is very short compared to the time constant τ_0, then no signal will appear on the recorder; if this time equals the time constant, then a distorted signal will result; while if one waits many time constants to complete the scan, then the recorder will faithfully reproduce the true line-shape. Of course, other criteria such as the absence of both over-modulation and saturation effects must also be met to produce an undistorted line-shape. Sometimes one encounters a drifting recorder base line which must be recentered during a scan. Torgeson and Rhinehart (1963) have designed an automatic recorder recentering circuit.

It will be helpful to give a more quantitive treatment of the distortion that occurs at intermediate scanning rates. The time constant of a resistor R in series with a capacitor C is RC sec (ohm $\times$ farad = second). Strandberg, Johnson, and Eshbach (1954) studied the distortion of an absorption signal in terms of the parameter α

$$\alpha = RC/\tau_{1/2} = \tau_0/\tau_{1/2} \tag{1}$$

where $\tau_{1/2}$ is half the time that it takes to scan through the signal between the half amplitude points. They define the parameter ρ which depends on the time t as follows:

$$\rho = (t - t_0)/\tau_{1/2} \tag{2}$$

where t_0 is the time at the peak of the filter's input signal. Their Lorentzian curve illustrated on Fig. 12–11 exhibits the following three distortions at $\alpha = 1$: (1) the peak amplitude decreases, (2) the peak appears at a later time than it would for zero time constant, and (3) the resonance appears broader on the right than on the left, but it continues to have the same integrated area. The peak of the actual output signal always occurs where this curve intercepts the undisturbed $\alpha = 0$ curve.

If accurate line-width and g factor measurements are to be made, one must be careful not to employ a response time τ_0 which is too long. One can recognize response time distortion by scanning both forward and backward through the resonance, and observing whether or not the asymmetry reverses phase since true g factor asymmetry will always be more pronounced on the same side of the line, while response time distortion will always broaden more on the side which appears last on the recorder. For g factor measurements one may average the values obtained with forward and backward scans when it is not feasible to reduce α.

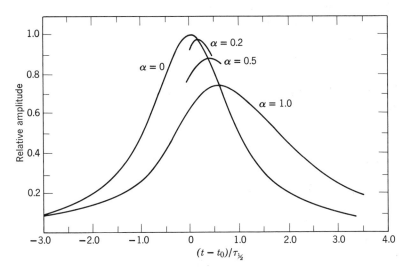

Fig. 12–11. The distortion that results from scanning too quickly through a magnetic resonance absorption line. The abscissa gives the time t relative to the time t_0 at the center of the resonance normalized with respect to the time $\tau_{1/2}$ that it takes to scan through the width $\frac{1}{2}\Delta H_{1/2}$. The parameter α is defined by eq. (12-J-1) [Strandberg, Johnson, and Eshbach (1954)].

In theory, one may always increase the signal-to-noise ratio by increasing the response time and decreasing the rate of scan, but this always prolongs the time required to obtain data.   If one carries this process too far by using scans of several hours' duration then one encounters long time drift and stability problems which can produce a drifting baseline and other deleterious effects (e.g., room temperature variations may change the magnetic field value).

It is recommended that inexperienced ESR spectroscopists practice recording the spectrum of a well known sample like solid DPPH under a variety of scanning rates and response times.   When a spectrum is being recorded to obtain quantitative data such as the g factor and line-shape, it is recommended that one employ a response time that is less than $1/10$ of the time τ_{pp} required to scan through the two peaks of the line.

The time constant may be measured by setting the magnetic field considerably off resonance, starting the recorder, and then suddenly and rapidly turning the magnet control knob to near the peak of the resonance.   When this is done, the recorder will plot an exponential increase in the ESR signal I to its maximum value I_0 in accordance with the relation ($t_0 = 0$)

$$I = I_0(1 - e^{-t/RC}) = I_0(1 - e^{-t/\tau_0}) \tag{3}$$

A time-constant criterion may be established by observing that at the time

$$t = 0.693\tau_0 \tag{4}$$

one obtains

$$I = \tfrac{1}{2}I_0 \tag{5}$$

and at the time

$$t = \tau_0 \tag{6}$$

one has

$$I = 0.632I_0 \tag{7}$$

Either point may be employed to compute τ_0.   The experimental technique requires that one use a strongly absorbing sample, that the resonance be set near its peak value in a time short compared to τ_0, and that the magnetic field and ESR frequency be maintained constant during the measurement. Further details are given in Sec. 14-F.

K. Integrators

Narrow band detection at the fundamental of the modulation frequency produces a recorder plot which is the first derivative of the absorption line shape. Schwenker (1959) described the electromechanical analog integrator shown on Fig. 12–12 which converts the first derivative recorder pattern shown in Fig. 12–13a to the absorption curve shown in Fig. 12–13b. This integrator is useful in applications where integrating times exceed one minute. Kramer and Müller-Warmuth (1963) also designed an electronic integrator, and Collins (1959) and Randolph (1960) describe analog computers for use in integrating ESR spectra. See also Camponovo, (1956). Van Der Lugt and Van Overbeek (1964) obtained a direct absorption signal on an x-y recorder by driving the x-axis with a voltage proportional to the instantaneous modulation amplitude.

When one desires to obtain the number of unpaired spins that contributes to the recorded spectrum, it is considerably easier and quicker to perform a graphical integration of Fig. 12–13b than it is to carry out a double integration of 12–13a. This advantage is offset by the fact that the individual hyperfine lines are much better resolved in the derivative spectrum, and so derivative presentation is preferable to use for obtaining hyperfine splittings and amplitude ratios. This improvement in resolution forms the basis for the resolution enhancement of spectra, as described in Sec. 14-I.

L. Power Supplies

The alternating (ac) input voltage is converted to a direct (dc) voltage by means of a full wave vacuum tube rectifier (e.g., 5R4 of Fig. 6–17 or 5U4 of Fig. 10–22) or crystal rectifier. The dc voltage is then filtered by a π or T section to remove ripple. In a B^+ or other regulated power supply, all of the current goes through regulator or pass tubes (e.g., the 807 and of Fig. 6–17). Voltage regulation is achieved by selecting an error signal from across the load (e.g., 100K potentiometer of Fig. 6–17), amplifying it in a dc amplifier and impressing the resultant voltage on the grid of the regulator tube.

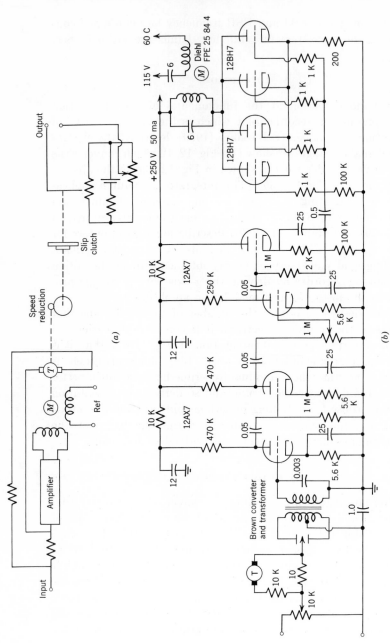

Fig. 12–12. Analog integrator for ESR spectra: (a) diagram showing the servomotor M which is mechanically connected to the tachometer generator T that supplies the feedback to the Brown converter and (b) details of the "amplifier" circuits. The capacitors are in microfarads [Schwenker (1959)].

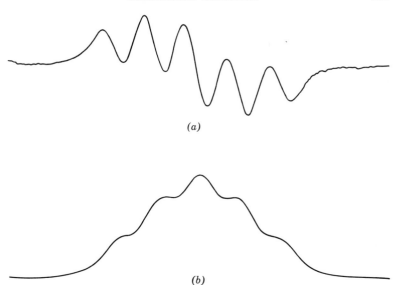

(a)

(b)

Fig. 12–13. The ESR spectrum of DPPH in benzene: (a) the derivative curve and (b) the same curve after passage through an integrator [Schwenker (1959)].

The potential change impressed on this grid changes the conductivity of the regulator tube, returns it to the value required for a zero error signal, and regulation results. Further details on power supplies may be found in Secs. 6-G and 9-F.

For troubleshooting purposes, it is convenient to know the appearance of the waveforms obtained after rectification (on the cathode of the rectifier tube), after filtering (just past the coil or choke), and after regulation (the output voltage). Typical waveforms and exemplary peak-to-peak voltages for these three waveforms are given in Fig. 12–14. If one-half of the rectifier tube fails to work then the result will be half wave rectification, with the appearance on the rectifier cathode of the waveform shown on Fig. 12–14b. The ripple that results from a full wave rectifier appears at twice the ac frequency. For example, a 60-cps input voltage produces ripple at 120 cps. Note the unsymmetrical appearance of the ripple in Fig. 12–14d and 12–14e.

If the waveforms shown on Fig. 12–14 are Fourier-analyzed (cf. Secs. 10-D and 10-E), they will be found to have a dc component

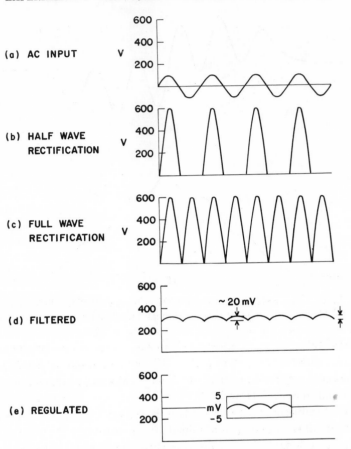

Fig. 12–14. Waveforms at several points of a regulated power supply. An expanded ordinate sacle is presented on the insert of (e).

V_{dc} plus a series of ac components V_{ac} at harmonics of 60 cps. The root mean square or rms value of a voltage V is defined by

$$V_{rms} = \left(\frac{1}{2\pi} \int_0^{2\pi} V^2 d\theta \right)^{1/2} \tag{1}$$

$$= \left(V_{dc}^2 + \frac{1}{2\pi} \int_0^{2\pi} V_{ac}^2 d\theta \right)^{1/2} \tag{2}$$

where θ is the phase angle which goes from 0 to 2π radians. The ripple factor r is

$$r = \frac{\text{rms value of ac components}}{\text{dc component}} \tag{3}$$

$$= [(V_{\text{rms}}/V_{\text{ac}})^2 - 1]^{1/2} \tag{4}$$

$$= \begin{cases} 1.21 & \text{half wave rectifier} \\ 0.482 & \text{full wave rectifier} \end{cases} \tag{5}$$

Note from eq. (2) that V_{rms} includes both V_{ac} and V_{dc}. The object of a filter and regulated power supply is to reduce the ripple factor to a very small value.

M. Troubleshooting

This section will contain several miscellaneous suggestions for troubleshooting electronic circuits. When trouble occurs, it is best to check the dc and ac components of all power supply voltages. If the difficulty is not in the power supplies, then the input and output voltages to all suspected circuits should be examined. In particular, the cables should be checked for loose connections (e.g., by shaking them while monitoring the next input signal). When the trouble appears at the output but not at the input of a particular circuit, then it probably arises within the circuit. In this case the tubes and other removable parts may be removed successively one by one from the input to the output end until the trouble vanishes at the output. In other words, the first basic principle of troubleshooting is to isolate the trouble. This is frequently much easier than eliminating the trouble. A corollary to this is that a knowledge of the proper input and output voltages is essential for troubleshooting. The ac voltages may be measured with the oscilloscope, and the dc voltages with a vacuum tube voltmeter or multimeter.

Once the trouble has been isolated, one may either check the vacuum tubes on a tube tester, or replace them one by one until an improvement is observed. The latter procedure seems somewhat preferable from the viewpoint of both time and effectiveness. The plate, grid, and cathode dc voltages of the vacuum tubes (collector, emitter and base voltages of transistors) may be measured and compared to values given in the manual to ascertain if they have satisfactory operating points. The currents through the tube or transistor via the various electrodes (plate, collector, etc.) may be determined by measuring the dc voltages across resistors connected in series with the electrodes, and then they may be compared with the manual values. It will sometimes be necessary to replace capacitors. Resistors may be checked on the multimeter resistance scales, and replaced if necessary. One should always check for loose solder joints before replacing resistors and capacitors.

References

R. Arnal and G. Beuchot, *Nucl. Instr. Methods*, **28**, 277 (1964).

E. B. Baker, *RSI*, **25**, 390 (1954).

Y. Beers, *RSI*, **36**, 696 (1965).

H. S. Black, *Modulation Theory*, Van Nostrand, N. Y., 1953, p. 25.

P. Bletzinger, A. Garscadden, I. Alexeff, and W. D. Jones, *JSI*, **42**, 358 (1965).

D. Bosnecker, *Z. Angew. Phys.*, **12**, 306 (1960).

J. J. Brophy, *RSI*, **26**, 1076 (1955).

X. Camponovo, *Arch. Sci.*, **11**, *Spec. No.*, 203 (1956).

R. L. Collins, *RSI*, **30**, 492 (1959).

H. L. Cox, Jr., *RSI*, **24**, 307 (1953).

J. M. Dereppe, *RSI*, **32**, 979 (1961).

E. A. Faulkner, *JSI*, **36**, 321 (1959).

D. Gheorghiu and A. Valeriu, *Nucl. Distr. Methods*, **16**, 313 (1962).

W. Gordy, W. V. Smith, and R. F. Trambarulo, *Microwave Spectroscopy*, Wiley, N. Y., 1953.

K. D. Kramer and W. Müller-Warmuth, *Z. Angew. Phys.*, **16**, 281 (1963).

J. D. Memory, *Am. J. Phys.*, **32**, 83 (1964).

R. G. Nucholls and L. J. Rueger, *Phys. Rev.*, **85**, 731 (1952).

W. L. Pierce and J. C. Hicks, *RSI*, **36**, 202 (1965).

Yu. V. Popov, *PTE*, **3**, 77 (433) (1960).

M. Raether and D. Bitzer, *RSI*, **35**, 837 (1964).

M. L. Randolph, *RSI*, **31**, 949 (1960).

RLS–19, Chap. 14.

N. A. Schuster, *RSI*, **22**, 254 (1951).

R. P. Schwenker, *RSI*, **30**, 1012 (1959).

S. Seely, *Electron Tube Circuits*, McGraw-Hill, N. Y., 1950.

M. W. P. Strandberg, H. R. Johnson, and J. R. Eshbach, *RSI*, **25**, 776 (1954).

M. W. P. Strandberg, M. Tinkham, I. H. Solt, Jr., and C. F. Davis, Jr., *RSI*, **27**, 596 (1956).

F. E. Terman, *Radio Engineer's Handbook*, McGraw-Hill, N. Y., 1943.

D. R. Torgeson and W. A. Rhinehart, *RSI*, **34**, 1447 (1963).

W. N. Tuttle, *Proc. IRE*, **28**, 23 (1940).

W. Van Der Lugt and J. Van Overbeeke, *JSI*, **41**, 702 (1964).

L. Van Gerven, A. Van Itterbeek, and L. Stals, *Paramagnetic Resonance*, **2**, 684 (1963); see also *Appl. Sci. Res.*, **B10**, 243 (1963).

C. H. Vincent, D. Kaine, and W. G. King, *Nucl. Instr. Methods*, **16**, 163 (1962).

R. T. Weidner and C. A. Whitmer, *RSI*, **23**, 75 (1952).

C. A. Whitmer, R. T. Weidner, J. S. Hsiang, and P. R. Weiss, *Phys. Rev.*, **74**, 1478 (1948).

P. Williams, *JSI*, **42**, 474 (1965).

CHAPTER 13

Overall Spectrometer Systems

The preceding chapters have discussed in detail the various components that enter into electron spin resonance spectrometers, and at the beginning of Chap. 7, a spectrometer block diagram was presented to show the location of the principal components in the overall system. A great deal may be learned from studying some of the principal spectrometers that have been discussed in the literature. The following sections contain block diagrams and brief discussions of several spectrometers. The discussions tend to emphasize the novel features of the various spectrometers. It is recommended that the original articles be consulted for further details, as they contain a great deal of information which cannot be included here due to the lack of space.

The spectrometer block diagrams are presented as the original authors drew them so that the reader may become familiar with the various conventions that are in use for signifying the components. The reader may find it helpful to redraw several in a more conventional manner.

Table 13–1 presents a summary of the characteristics of several score ESR spectrometers. Reviews of spectrometers have been given by Al'tshuler and Kozyrev (1964), Gordy, Smith, and Trumbarulo (1953), Ingram (1955, 1958), Jeffries (1961), the NMR–EPR staff of Varian (1960), Semenov (1962), and Townes and Schawlow (1955). Some descriptions of spectrometers [e.g., del Rosal, Zorn, and Pinkel (1965); Low (1965)] were too brief to enter in Table 13–1.

A. Jen, 1948

Jen studied the Zeeman effect in the microwave spectroscopy of gases by means of the apparatus shown in Fig. 13–1. Strictly speaking, this apparatus was not designed for electron spin resonance,

TABLE

Characteristics of Spectrometers

Author	Year	Sec.	Figure no.	Frequency generator[b]	Frequency band[c]	Cavity or other sample chamber[d]
Jen	1948	13-A	13–1	2K33	K	Cy, Rf, large
Beringer and Castle	1950	13-B	13–2	723A/B (P-dc)	X	Cy, T, TM_{011}
Bagguley and Griffiths	1952	13-C	13–3	CV 223	X	Two TE_{111}
Mackey and Hershberger	1953			723A/B	X	Cy, T, TE_{011}
Maxwell and McGuire	1953			Klystron	X	Rt
Beringer and Heald	1954	13-D	13–4	723A/B (P-dc)	X	Cy, T, TE_{101}
Collier	1954	13-E	13–5 13–6	707A (P-dc)	S	Cx, TEM_2
Berthet	1955			723A/B (P)	X	Rt, Rf
Artman and Tannenwald	1955			Klystron	X	Cy, Rf, TE_{111} (Rt TE_{011})
Feher and Kip	1955	13-G	13–8	UHF generator	300 Mc	Cx, T, TEM
Hirshon and Fraenkel	1955	13-F	13–7	2K25 (P-i-f)	X	Rt, Rf, TE_{101} or TE_{102}
Paulevé	1955			2K25	X	Rt, Rf
Ryter, Lacroix, and Extermann	1955			723A/B(P)	X	Rf
Uebersfeld	1955			723A/B	X	Cy, T, TE_{011}
Buckmaster and Scovil	1956	13-H	13–9	2K33A	K	Cy, T, TE_{111}
Charru	1956				S	Cy, T, TE_{112}
Hoisington, Kellner, and Pentz	1956				S, 35 Gc	Absorption cell
Lutze	1956			723A/B	X	Cy, T, TE_{011}
Manenkov and Prokhorov	1956	13-J	13–12, 13–13	Klystron	X	Rt, Rf, TE_{101}
Strandberg, Johnson, and Eshbach (1954); Strandberg, Tinkham, Solt and Davis (1956)	1956	13-I	13–10, 13–11	707B, 2K25,2K50 (P-i-f)	S,X,K	Rf, Rt, TE_{10n}, Cy, TE_{011}
Uebersfeld	1956			2K25, KL2T1	X, 36 Gc	Cy, Rf, TE_{011}

13–1

Described in the Literature[a]

Detector[e]	Modulation frequency[f]	Temperature, °K	Sensitivity, moles DPPH[g]	Comments[h]
C	S, 100 kc	300		Gas sample
Bo	F, 30 cps	≥300	10^{-10}	Gas sample
C, BM	S, 1 Mc	170–670		
C	F, 32 cps	300		
C	S	300		
Bo	F, 30 cps	≥300		Gas sample, NMR field stabilization, 1 ppm resolution
Bo	F, 30 cps	300		Gas sample, no magnet
C	F, 1 kc, 50 cps	300	10^{-7}	
C	S	300		Circular polarization
Grid leak	F, 6 kc	4–300	2×10^{-8}	Solenoidal magnet
C, SH	F, 38 cps, SH 30 Mc	Low to 625	2×10^{-11}	
C	S, 300 cps	300		
C, SH	F, 25 cps	300		
C	F, 50 cps		10^{-8}	
C	F, 60 cps and 460 kc	4–300	10^{-11}	
	F, 50 cps	300		Polarized microwaves give sign of g
C, SH	25 cps, 100 kc	170–300		Gas sample, NMR field stab.
C	8 Mc and 10 Mc SH			
	30 to 60 cps S			
C, BM, SH	50 cps, 75 Mc SH		4×10^{-10}	
C, BM, SH	50 cps, 30 Mc SH	Variable		Yokeless electromagnet
C	F, 50 cps, or 1.3 kc	300	10^{-10}	

(continued)

TABLE 13-1

Author	Year	Sec.	Figure no.	Frequency generator[b]	Frequency band[c]	Cavity or other sample chamber[d]
Albold, Eischner, and Wenzel	1957			723A/B (N)	X	Rt, Rf, TE_{102}
Bowers, Kamper, and Knight	1957	13-K	13-14, 13-15	CV129 (P)	X	Cy, T, TE_{011}
Bresler, Saminskii, and Kazbekov	1957			Klystron (P)	X	Cy, T, TE_{011}
Feher	1957	13-M	13-18	Klystron	X	Rf
Frait	1957			2K25 (P)	X	Cy, Rf, TE_{011}
Llewellyn	1957	13-L	13-16, 13-17	CV 129	X	Rt, T, TE_{101}
Rose-Innes	1957	13-N	13-19, 13-20	CV 129	X	Rf
Abraham, Ovenall, and Whiffin	1958			723A/B, R2222 (RM)	X	Cy, TE_{112}, Rt TE_{102}
Galkin and Kichigin	1958			12S3S triode	<500 Mc	Condenser
Misra	1958			V-23 (dual cavity)	X	Rt
Stieler	1958			2K25 (P)	X	Rt, Rf, TE_{106}
Akhmanov, Gvozdover, Konstantinov, and Trofimenko	1959			BWO	X	Cavity, T
Gravlin and Cowen	1959			723A/B (N)	X	T (horns)
Shamfarov	1959			51-I; K-19 (P)	X	Rf
Unterberger	1959			Klystron (P)	X	Rt, T, TE_{102}
Bösnecker	1960			723A/B	X	Cy, Rf, TE_{011}
El'sting	1960			12SZS	230–400Mc	Loop
Mock	1960	13-P	13-26 to 13-29	BWO (N)	50–150 Gc	T, waveguide
Pescia	1960			Carcinotron	X	T
Scoffa and Ristau	1960			20SR51 (P)	X	Cy TE_{111} and TE_{011}, Rt TE_{014}
Bogle, Symmons, Burgess, and Sierins	1961			X-13 and HO-4B BWO	8–18 Gc	T or Rf, waveguide cell

(*Continued*)

Detector[e]	Modulation frequency[f]	Temperature, °K	Sensitivity, moles DPPH[g]	Comments[h]
C	F, 50 cps, 115 cps	300	2×10^{-9}	
C	F, 115 kc	300	2×10^{-11}	NMR field stab.; gas sample
Bo, (C)	F, 30 cps, 400 cps (1.6 Mc)	300	2×10^{-13}	
C, BM, SH	100–1000 cps, 30–60 Mc, SH	Variable	2×10^{-12}	
C	F, 50 cps		10^{-9}	
C	F, 115 kc	14–300	10^{-11}	Modulus displayed
C, SH	S, SH, 50 cps, 45 Mc	4–300		Good for broad lines
C	F, 490 cps			
C, BM, SH	F, SH, 30 Mc	90–300 300	10^{-14}	Dual channel, uses klystron amplifier (V-27)
C	F, 73 cps	300–500	10^{-10}	
	F, 50 cps	300	10^{-8}	TWT feedback circuit discussed
C	F, 60 cps	300	10^{-5}	Simple, inexpensive
C, BM, SH	F, 125 cps; SH 30 Mc		10^{-8}	Similar to Hirshon and Fraenkel (1955)
C	F, 100 cps	300		
C	F or S, 50 cps, 500 kc, 81 cps	>90	3×10^{-11}	
	F, 6 kc	300	10^{-8}	
Wafer [cf. Sharpless (1956)]	F, 400 cps	1.2–300		Suitable for zero field studies
C	F, 50 cps, S 1 to 10 Mc	300	10^{-7}	15 W microwave power
C, BM, SH	50, 123 cps	90–300	5×10^{-10}	
C, Bo	F, 3000 cps	4.2–300		No magnet, for zero field studies

(*continued*)

TABLE 13-1

Author	Year	Sec.	Figure no.	Frequency generator[b]	Frequency band[c]	Cavity or other sample chamber[d]
Dusek	1961			723A/B (RM)	X	Rt, T, TE_{103}
Henning	1961			723A/B (RM)	X	Rt, Rf, TE_{102}
Kipling, Smith, Vanier, and Woonton	1961			2K39 (P)	X	Rf
La Force	1961			Acorn tube (955)	100–300 Mc	Sample is near shorted end of grid line
Marcley	1961			GAF4A	315 Mc	$\frac{1}{4}\lambda_g$ coax, line
Pascaru and Valeriu	1961				X	
Portis and Teaney (1958); Teaney, Klein, and Portis (1961)	1961	13-Q	13–30 to 13–33	Klystron	X	Cy, T, TE_{111} (bi-modal)
Zverev	1961			Klystron	X	Rf, toroidal cavity
Atsarkin, Zhabotinskii, and Frantsesson	1962			Klystron, (RM, phase stab.)	X	
Benoit and Ruby	1962			Klystron	X	Cy, Rf, TE_{111}
Bolef, deKlerk, and Gosser	1962			Acoustic	10–1000 Mc	T
Hall and Schumacher	1962			203B (RM, P-i-f)	X, K (harmonic)	Rt, Rf
Holton and Blum	1962			V-58 (P)	X	Rt, Rf, TE_{101}
Kaplan	1962			Pulsed magnetron	X	Rt, Rf, TE_{102}
Kolbasov, Mukhina and Nazarov	1962			51-I	X	Rt, T, TE_{101}, tunable
Laffon, Servoz-Gavin, and Uchida	1962			Klystron (P)	X	Rf, TE_{112}
Lecar and Okaya	1962			X-13 (QK-306 pump)	X, K	Rt, TE_{102}
Llewellyn, Whittlestone, and Williams	1962	13-R	13–34	V153	X	Cy, T, TE_{011}
Mehlkopf and Smidt	1962			X-13 (P)	X	Two Wonderstone cavities, T
Théobald	1962			2K25, V63 (two cavities)	X	Cy, Rf, TE_{011}

(*Continued*)

Detector[e]	Modulation frequency [f]	Temperature, °K	Sensitivity, moles DPPH[g]	Comments[h]
C		300		
C, BM	F, 30 cps	300	3×10^{-11}	Battery-powered magnet dual channel
	F, 200 cps	300		
Synchronous	30 cps	300		No magnet
Same GAF4A	F, 60 cps	300		Simple, inexpensive
CSH	SH, 450 cps	1.5–300	2×10^{-9}	
C, BM, SH	SH 30 cps, 30 Mc	4–300	6×10^{-11}	Microwave induction spectrometer; sign of g factor
SH	60 Mc	2–300		
C, BM, SH	F, 50 cps, 420 cps, 30 Mc		2×10^{-12}	
BM, SH		0.3–1.5		Meas. relaxation times
C	20–200 cps	1.5–300		
BM, C, SH	S 63 Mc	≤300		
C, SH		1.3–300	2×10^{-11}	Endor cavity
SH		1.6–300	2×10^{-11}	See Kaplan, Browne, and Cowen (1961)
C	F, 50 cps, 465 Kc	77 or 300	10^{-11}	
C, BM, SH	SH	300	2×10^{-12}	
C	F, audio	4		Uses a ruby maser
C, SH	S, 10 Mc	1–300		Pulsed, meas. relax. time
C, SH	SH, 30 Mc	300	10^{-13}	Dual channel
C, SH	F, 50 cps, 0.1–14 Mc	300		

(*continued*)

TABLE 13-1

Author	Year	Sec.	Figure no.	Frequency generator[b]	Frequency band[c]	Cavity or other sample chamber[d]
Anderegg, Cornax, and Borel	1963			Tunnel diode	2000 Mc	Cx, TEM
Battaglia, Iannuzzi, and Polacco	1963			2K33	K	Rf, TE_{111}
Brodwin and Burgess	1963			V-290, 723A/B, (P-dc)	X	H plane T junction
Elliston, Troup, and Hutton	1963			Harmonic of R5146	64 Gc	Rf, no cavity
Fedorov	1963			Autodyne	42 Mc	Coil of LC circuit
Gambling and Wilmshurst	1963			Klystron and tripler	K	Rf
Glauche and Voigt	1963			2K25 (RM)	X	Rt, T, TE_{102}
Ghosh, Bagchi, and Pal	1963			2K33	K	Cy, T, TE_{111}
Ingram	1963					
Kolbasov and Mukhina	1963			51-1	X	Rt, Rf, TE_{101}
Kramer and Müller-Warmuth	1963			2K28	S	Rt, Rf, TE_{105}
Lebedev	1963			51-1 (RM)	X	Cy, Rf, TE_{011}
Lenzo	1963			955 (Marginal 200–1000 osc.)	Mc	Loop
Lichtenstein, Gallagher, and Cupp	1963			OKI	150–217Gc	FPI
Müller-Warmuth	1963				10–100 Mc (30–60 kc)	Coil
Tuong Tai-chian	1963			Klystron	X	Cy, Rf, TE_{011}
Assenheim	1964					
Goldsborough and Koehler	1964			Klystron	X	Rt, Rf
Haupt, Müller-Warmuth, and Schultz	1964			Autodyne; pulsed	15, 30 Mc	Coil

(*Continued*)

Detector[e]	Modulation frequency[f]	Temperature, °K	Sensitivity, moles DPPH[g]	Comments[h]
		300	3×10^{-6}	
C		300		Gives polarization of lines and sign of g factors
C	F, 30 Mc SH	300	$\sim 10^{-10}$	
C, BM	F, 630 cps		10^{-8}	Shorted waveguide holds sample
	F, 0.5 cps	0.15–4.2	10^{-5}	Helmholtz coils
SH	F, 130 cps, 465 Kc	300	10^{-11}	
	Faraday modulator, 9 kc	Variable		Contains single crystal rotator; designed for ferromagnetic resonance
C	F, 33 cps			
C	F, 50 cps, 465 Kc	300	3×10^{-12}	Circuits given
C	F, 400 and 4000 cps	110–500	10^{-5}	
C		300	10^{-10}	
Regeneration	F, 60 cps	300		
C (run-in)		300		This is a microwave spectrometer.
	F	300	10^{-6}	Double resonance
C	F, 50 cps; S 100 kc	300	5×10^{-9}	
C, SH, BM	F, 400 cps, 30 Mc	5–300		Condensed rf discharge
	F, 30–300 cps	300		

(*continued*)

TABLE 13-1

Author	Year	Sec.	Figure no.	Frequency generator[b]	Frequency band[c]	Cavity or other sample chamber[d]
Pascaru	1964			Klystron	X	Rt, Rf, TE_{102} tunable
Payne	1964			TWT	X	T, TE_{111}
Richards and White	1964			8FK1	K	T, TE_{01n}
Zakrevskii and Toma-shevskii	1964				36 Gs	
Brown, Mason, and Thorp	1965			Klystron	35 Gs	Cavity
Buckmaster and Dering	1965			VA-232	X	Rt, Rf, TE_{101}
Duncan and Schneider	1965			Tuned anode-tuned grid	250–1000 Mc	Cx, Rf, 1/4 λ
Grützediek, Kramer, and Müller-Warmuth	1965				493 Mc	Cx, 1/4 λ
Jefferts and Jones	1965			Super reg.	200–1000 Mc	1/2 λ Transmission line Osc.
Kenworthy and Richards	1965			K350, K336	X	Helix or Cy, TE_{011}
Mergerian, Stombler, and Harrup	1965			DX-237	115–148 Gc	Cy, Rf
Tsung-tang, Wen-chia, Lien-fong, and Tin-fong	1965			DX-247 (RM)		
Erickson	1966			TWT	1–4.6 Gc	reentrant, T

[a] The data in this table were compiled with the assistance of O. F. Griffith III.

[b] All generators are klystrons unless otherwise specified; (BWO) backward wave oscillator; (N) sans stabilization; (osc.) oscillator. (P), (Pif), and (Pdc) Pound stzbilization; (RM) reflector modulation, (TWT) traveling wave tube; (uhf) ultrahigh frequency.

[c] $(K) \sim 24$ Gc (1.2 cm); $(S) \sim 3$ Gc (10 cm); $(X) \sim 10$ Gc (3 cm).

(Continued)

Detector[e]	Modulation frequency[f]	Temperature, °K	Sensitivity, moles DPPH[g]	Comments[h]
C	F, 430 cps or 171 Kc	77, 300	2×10^{-13}	
C	F, 100 Kc	300	2×10^{-11}	Uses generalized feedback microwave oscillator
C	F, 50 cps, 5 Kc	300		Double resonance; rf coil inside cavity
	F	300	3×10^{-13}	
C, SH	F, 45 Mc, 160 Kc	300		
C, BM	F, ~1 kc, ~100 kc	300	$\sim 10^{-12}$	No AFC is required
SH	F, 175 cps, 10.7 Mc	4–300	$\sim 10^{-10}$	
Q-meter	F, 5 cps, 50 cps	300		Double resonance (706–760 kc NMR)
		2–300		
C, SH		300		Double resonance
C	F, 100 cps	2–300		Uses oversize waveguide and cavity
			3×10^{-12}	
Backward diode	F 10 kc, S 160 kc (phase)	4–300		

[d] (Cx) coaxial; (Cy) cylindrical; (Rf) reflection; (Rt) rectangular; (T) transmission; TE_{mnp} and TM_{mnp} = modes; (FPI) Fabry-Perot interferometer.

[e] (BM) Balanced mixer; (Bo) bolometer; (C) crystal; (SH) superheterodyne.

[f] (F) Field modulation; (S) source modulation.

[g] For DPPH, 472 g = 1M = 6×10^{23} spins (assuming one benzene molecule of "hydration").

[h] (ppm) Parts per million.

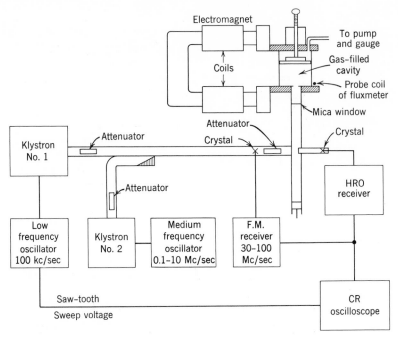

Fig. 13-1.   A schematic diagram of a spectrometer used for measurements of microwave Zeeman spectra [Jen (1948)].

but it may be considered as a sort of prototype of an ESR spectrometer. Whitmer, Weidner, Hsiang, and Weiss (1948) give a block diagram of an early ESR spectrometer.

B. Beringer and Castle, 1950

As shown on Fig. 13-2, Beringer and Castle employed a 723 A/B klystron, a dc Pound stabilizer and a TM_{01} mode cylindrical transmission cavity isolated by vacuum tight mica windows.   The loaded and unloaded Q's are 3500 and 8400, respectively.   The bolometer detector forms one arm of a high impedance dc bridge which is balanced by the bolometer's 200-Ω resistance.   In place of the usual balance meter found on a Wheatstone bridge, there was connected an audio amplifier, with a gain of over two million and a 2 cps bandwidth centered at 30 cps.   The lock-in mixer output deflects a critically damped galvanometer of 0.04-cps band-width.   The modu-

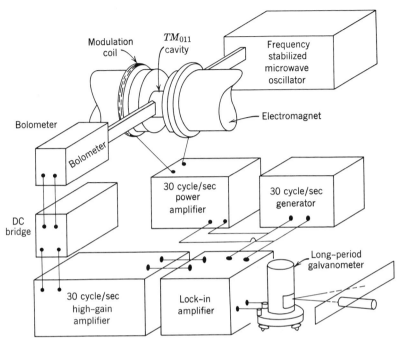

Fig. 13-2. Schematic diagram of a microwave magnetic resonance absorption apparatus [Beringer and Castle (1950)].

lation coils mounted on the pole pieces produce a modulating field amplitude between 1 and 200 G. More modern spectrometers make use of a recorder in lieu of the galvanometer.

C. Bagguley and Griffiths, 1952

The dual channel spectrometer built by Bagguley and Griffiths is shown in Fig. 13-3. The reflector voltage of the C.V. 223 klystron was modulated with a frequency of 1 Mc and an amplitude of 40 V from a quartz-controlled oscillator. The klystron power output was split between the two resonant cavities R_1 and R_2. The sample cavity R_1 was coupled to the waveguide by a coaxial line and probe, while the reference cavity R_2 was iris-coupled. Each had a Q of 5000 at 3.1 cm. The 2-Mc second harmonic of the modulation frequency was detected by a pair of silicon tungsten crystals D_1 and D_2, and the two resulting signals were fed out of phase to the mutually

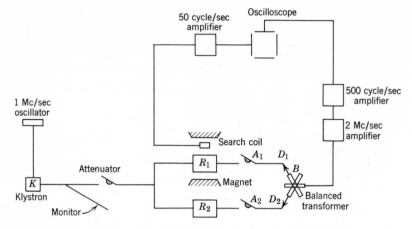

Fig. 13–3.   Block diagram of ESR apparatus [Bagguley and Griffiths (1952)].

perpendicular windings of the balanced transformer B. The transformer output undergoes narrow band amplification at 2 Mc, and then, after conversion to 500 cps, it is again amplified. The two attenuators A_1 and A_2 were employed for initially balancing the system. The output of the balanced transformer is proportional to the absorption in the sample cavity at resonance since the antiphase arrangement in B balances out the carrier. This system employs source modulation instead of field modulation. It provides high sensitivity and actual absorption line-shapes for broad absorption lines. See Sec. 10-C for further information on source modulation.

D. Beringer and Heald, 1954

The block diagram for the spectrometer of Beringer and Heald is similar to some of the others in this chapter, and may be found in the original article. The spectrometer was employed to study atoms generated in a gas discharge and pumped through the cavity as shown on Fig. 13–4. The TE_{011} mode cylindrical cavity contained a quartz tube which was coated with fused metaphosphoric acid above the cavity to prevent atom recombination. Very accurate ESR and NMR frequency measurements were made, and the ratio of the ESR to NMR g factors for hydrogen atoms was measured to better than 1 ppm.

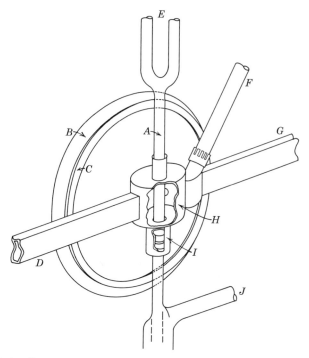

Fig. 13–4. Cutaway view of atom cavity in magnet gap. The wave guide to the bolometer is offset to permit centering of the proton coil in the magnet gap. (A) Pyrex-to-quartz graded seal; (B) 8-in. magnet pole; (C) Rose shim [Rose (1938)]; (D) waveguide-to-generator; (E) discharge tube; (F) proton regulator probe; (G) waveguide-to-bolometer; (H) TE_{011} cavity; (I) O ring demountable vacuum joint; (J) to pumps [Beringer and Heald (1954)].

E. Collier, 1954

Most spectrometers in microwave spectroscopy employ gas absorption cells and Stark modulation to study the frequency dependence of gas absorption lines in the absence of a magnetic field. Collier built a 10-cm microwave spectrometer with a TEM_{012} mode coaxial transmission cavity. The frequency is stabilized on the resonant cavity by means of a dc Pound stabilizer. The frequency is swept by gradually varying the cavity length through a gear chain and moveable plunger in such a way that the Pound discriminator maintains the klystron stabilized on the instantaneous cavity fre-

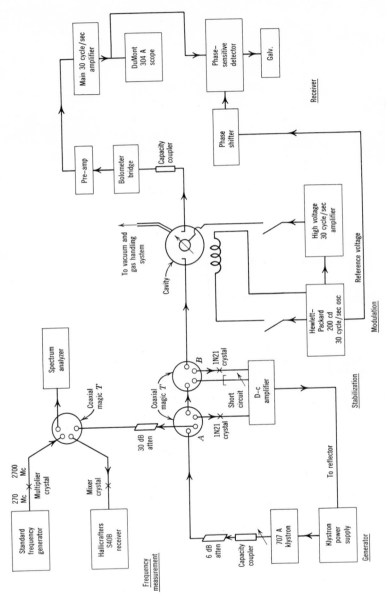

Fig. 13-5.   A block diagram of a 10-cm microwave spectrometer [Collier (1954)].

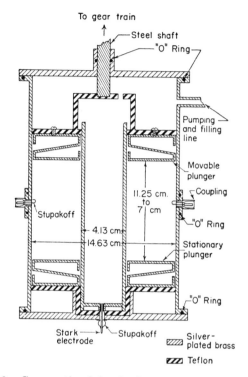

Fig. 13–6.   Cross sectional sketch of a coaxial cavity [Collier (1954)].

quency.   Even though this is a microwave spectrometer rather than an electron spin resonance spectrometer, its design incorporates many features of interest in ESR, and its details are presented in Figs. 13–5 and 13–6.

F. Hirshon and Fraenkel, 1955

The superheterodyne spectrometer of Hirshon and Fraenkel shown in Fig. 13–7 is somewhat more complicated than the ones previously discussed.   This spectrometer employs four magic T's, five attenuators (A_1 to A_5), two klystrons, a wavemeter (λ), two directional couplers (D_1 and D_2) and three crystals (X).   The signal klystron frequency ν_0 and the local oscillator klystron frequency $\nu_0 + 30$ Mc are mixed in the "beat T" to produce the intermediate frequency i-f $= 30$ Mc.   The signal klystron frequency ν_0

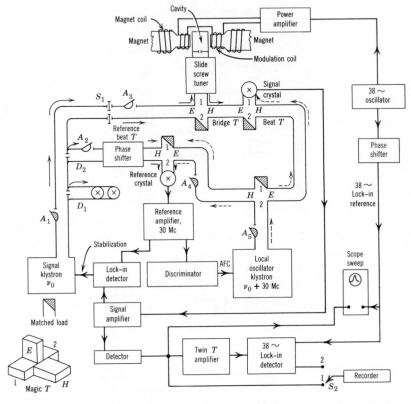

Fig. 13-7.　Block diagram of ESR spectrometer [Hirshon and Fraenkel (1955)].

is stabilized on the sample cavity, and at the same time the local oscillator klystron is stabilized to remain 30 Mc above ν_0. The two AFC error signals are obtained from the signal crystal and the reference crystal, respectively. The magnetic field is modulated at 38 cps, and this audio frequency is separated from the 30-Mc carrier in the detector (second detector) that is placed between the signal amplifier and the twin T amplifier. This ESR spectrometer achieved a higher sensitivity than most of the earlier ones as Table 13–1 indicates.

G. Feher and Kip, 1955

An ESR spectrometer designed to operate at 300 Mc between liquid helium temperature (4°K) and room temperature (300°K) was built by Feher and Kip, and is shown in Fig. 13–8. The coaxial resonant cavity is a half wavelength long with a Q between 1000 and 2000. It is a transmission cavity with two identical coupling loops which may be adjusted to achieve the proper coupling conditions. Line stretchers and a voltage standing wave ratio (VSWR) meter are used to achieve the proper match. The cavity output is rectified by a grid leak detector and fed to a 6-Kc narrow band amplifier with a Q of 85, a 120-dB maximum gain, and an equivalent noise input of 0.05 μV. The magnetic field is supplied by a water-cooled solenoid, and measured by a standard resistor and potentiometer to an accuracy of one part in 10^5.

Temperatures between 77 and 300°K are obtained by adjusting a heater placed in thermal contact with the cavity while the surrounding Dewar is filled with liquid nitrogen. Temperatures between 4 and 77°K are covered by mounting a brass rod at the lower end of the cavity and immersing it in a liquid helium bath. The level of the liquid helium determines the temperature. Parts of the brass rod are thermally short-circuited by copper which has a thermal conductivity two orders of magnitude greater than that of brass at 4°K. The liquid helium evaporates at the rate of 30 ml/hr. An

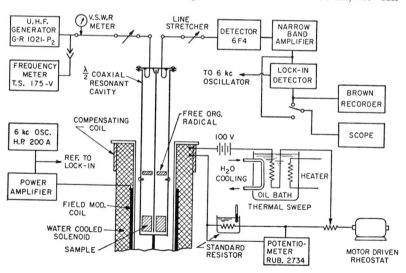

Fig. 13–8. Experimental setup for electron spin resonance absorption at 300 Mc [Feher and Kip (1955)].

AgAu–AuCo thermocouple is employed for determining the temperature down to 4°K. When the resonant cavity was filled with liquid helium, a great deal of noise was produced, and this was eliminated by filling the cavity with styrofoam, a low loss material with a relative dielectric constant of 1.0.

This spectrometer was employed by Feher and Kip for studying the electron spin resonance of metals. The organic free radical DPPH was utilized for calibration purposes.

H. Buckmaster and Scovil, 1956

The K band (1.25 cm) double magnetic field modulation spectrometer developed by Buckmaster and Scovil for use at liquid helium temperatures (4°K) is shown on Fig. 13–9. The 2K33A klystron supplies the microwave power, and a TE_{111} cylindrical resonant cavity supports the sample on its end plate. The magnetic field is modulated at $f_1 = 60$ cps and $f_2 = 462.5$ kc, and the frequency $f_2 \pm f_1$ is passed by the 1N26 crystal and rf amplifier. For broad band detection, either the 462.5 kc carrier may be sent through a 462.5 kc lock-in detector and then displayed on an oscilloscope, or the audio frequency f_1 may be removed from the f_2 carrier and then amplified and displayed on an oscilloscope. The former gives the modulus of the absorption line while the latter gives the first derivative of the resonance, as sketched on Fig. 13–9. For narrow band

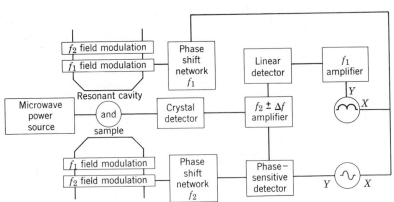

Fig. 13–9.   Block diagram of a double field modulation paramagnetic resonance spectrometer [Buckmaster and Scovil (1956)].

(high sensitivity) operation, the output of the phase-sensitive detector is fed through a long time-constant network to a recorder, and the audio frequency modulation f_1 is not required.

The skin depth effect prevents the 462.5-kc signal from penetrating the resonant cavity walls, although the 60-cps modulation gets through easily. To gain entrance for the f_2 modulation, a narrow slot was cut in the cavity walls along lines of rf current flow, so that the cavity Q is only slightly disturbed. The f_2 modulation current of up to 75 A flows around the slot, and some penetrates it and sets up the high frequency magnetic field modulation inside the cavity at the sample site.

For liquid helium temperature operation, the waveguide to and from the cavity is constructed from silver-plated German silver waveguide (0.32 × 0.63 cm ID, and 0.01 cm wall thickness) which is filled with Teflon. Taper sections match this to the standard K band waveguide (0.432 × 1.016 cm ID). The Teflon permits the waveguide size to be reduced. The Teflon filled waveguides terminate on coupling slots at the cavity top. Mica windows and Lucite screws electrically insulate the cavity from the remaining waveguide components.

I. Strandberg, Tinkham, Solt, and Davis, 1956

Strandberg, Tinkham, Solt, and Davis designed the spectrometer presented in Fig. 13-10. It is shown with a 2K25 3-cm klystron, but the author also obtained satisfactory performance with a type 707B tube at 10 cm, and a type 2K50 tube at 1.25 cm. More modern klystrons would certainly also perform satisfactorily. The klystron is stabilized by the i.f. Pound system as modified by Tuller, Galloway, and Zaffarano (1948). The first magic T contains the sample cavity in one arm and the 30-Mc modulator crystal in the other. Half of the incident microwave power goes to the sample cavity and half to the modulation crystal. The two reflected waves mix in the first magic T and proceed to the second magic T. Here half of the signal is detected in the signal crystal after which it undergoes narrow band amplification followed by second detection in the demodulator to remove the 50-cps ESR signal from the 30-Mc carrier. Finally, it is displayed on the chart recorder. The other half of the signal goes to the Pound mixer crystal to provide the

AFC error voltage.   For making asbolute power measurements a
bolometer is used as the detector.

For most work a rectangular TE_{10n} mode cavity was found to be
very convenient.   Interchangeable fixed coupling irides are employed, which is less convenient than the present custom of installing
a variable coupling iris.   The cavity is gold-plated to maximize the
Q and minimize possible spurious signals from the presence of paramagnetic impurities in the cavity walls.   For low temperature work
the cylindrical TE_{011} mode cavity shown in Fig. 13–11 is used.   The

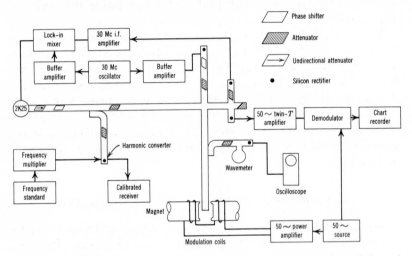

Fig. 13–10.   ESR spectrometer block diagram [Strandberg, Tinkham, Solt, and
Davis (1956)].

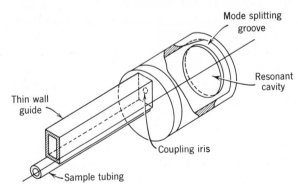

Fig. 13–11.   Resonant cavity [Strandberg, Tinkham, Solt, and Davis (1956)].

mode splitting groove in this cavity suppresses the degenerate TM_{111} mode. Special cavities for circular polarization were designed by Tinkham and Strandberg (1955). A calibrated wavemeter measures the frequency with an ultimate accuracy of about one part in 10^4, and for more accurate g factor measurements, the microwave frequency is beat against the known harmonic of a standard crystal. The resulting beat frequency is measured by a calibrated frequency standard [see, e.g., Beers (1959); Townes and Schawlow, Chap. 17 (1955)]. The accuracy is limited only by the stability of the receiver and the accuracy of the crystal standard.

J. Manenkov and Prokhorov, 1956

The superheterodyne spectrometer of Manenkov and Prokhrov is shown in Fig. 13–12. It makes use of a hybrid ring, a balanced

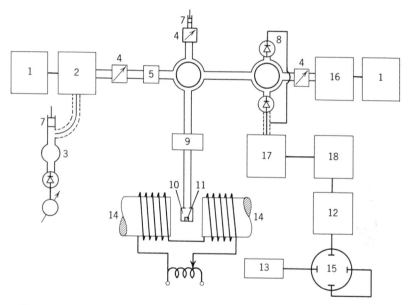

Fig. 13–12. Block diagram of superheterodyne spectrometer. (1) Stabilized voltage source; (2) klystron generator; (3) bolometer; (4) attenuator; (5) phase shifter; (6) lost; (7) plunger; (8) crystal detector; (9) tuner; (10) resonator; (11) sample; (12) low-frequency amplifier; (13) sweep; (14) electromagnet with 50 cps modulation coils; (15) oscilloscope; (16) klystron generator; (17) intermediate frequency amplifier; (18) second detector [Manenkov and Prokhorov (1956)].

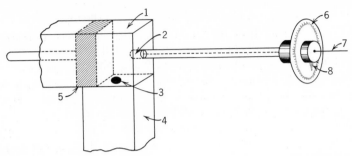

Fig. 13–13. Sketch of a resonant cavity. *(1)* resonator; *(2)* sample; *(3)* coupling hole; *(4)* waveguide; *(5)* plunger; *(6)* goniometer dial; *(7)* pivot; *(8)* pointer [Manenkov and Prokhorov (1956)].

mixer, and narrow band amplification. The hybrid ring is unusual because three of the angles between the arms are 100°, with the remaining angle equal to 60°. The rectangular resonant cavity shown on Fig. 13–13 is designed for studies of the orientation dependence of single crystals. The frequency of the cavity is tuned by means of the plunger.

K. Bowers, Kamper, and Knight, 1957

The high-precision spectrometer of Bowers, Kamper, and Knight is shown outlined on Fig. 13–14. It provides a precision of 3 ppm. The TE_{011} mode cylindrical resonator is made of tellurium copper which is completely free of ferromagnetic impurities. It is constructed in a number of sections. Two vertical posts inside the cavity are fed with a current of up to 2 A rms to modulate the magnetic field at 115 kc with amplitudes up to 2 G. The magnetic field is stabilized to within 20 ppm by the scheme shown in Fig. 13–15, and additional stabilization to better than 1 ppm is provided by the proton resonance technique. The strength of the magnetic field is determined by the proton NMR of an 0.163 molar solution of nickel sulfate, since in this solution the bulk diamagnetism of the water is exactly cancelled [Dickinson (1951)].

L. Llewellyn, 1957

The spectrometer block diagram of Llewellyn shown in Fig. 13–16 is similar to some of the others, and so will not be elaborated upon.

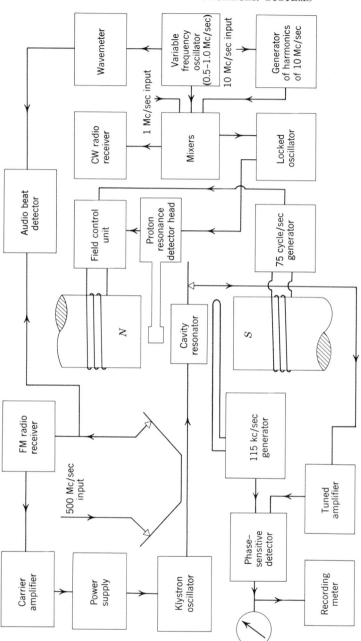

Fig. 13-14. Block diagram of ESR apparatus; the upper lefthand side shows the microwave frequency stabilizer, the lower lefthand side, the detection system, and the righthand side the proton resonance field stabilizer [Bowers, Kamper, and Knight (1957)].

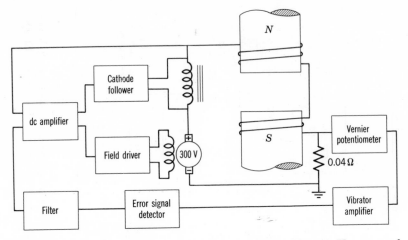

Fig. 13–15.   Block diagram of magnet current stabilizer [Bowers, Kamper, and Knight (1957)].

In one of the resonant cavities used with this spectrometer, the modulating magnetic field of several amperes is supplied to a loop of wire located inside the cavity, parallel to the microwave magnetic field lines of force. Another design shown on Fig. 13–17 incorporates a modulation coil above the sample with an intervening cavity wall whose thickness is intermediate between the skin depths at the 10-Gc microwave frequency and that at the 115-kc modulation frequency. The wall is made of German silver which has an almost constant resistance down to the lowest spectrometer operating temperature at the triple point of hydrogen (14°K). The cavity is connected to both the input and the output coaxial lines by microwave coupling probes. The resonant cavity itself is made of brass, and is split in the middle where no rf currents flow. The cavity supports are of German silver which has a low thermal conductivity. The spectrometer gives a visual presentation of the modulus of the differential absorption line-shape, or a recording of the absorption first derivative itself.

M. Feher, 1957

Feher found the superheterodyne spectrometer to be the most sensitive of the ones that he analyzed, and the block diagram of his design is shown in Fig. 13–18. The power from the signal klystron I is fed to the resonant cavity, and the signal reflected therefrom

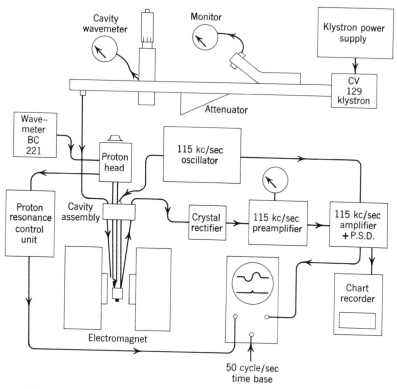

Fig. 13–16.   Block diagram of ESR spectrometer [Llewellyn (1957)].

enters the balanced mixer magic T to be mixed with the output of the reference klystron II. The resulting intermediate frequency $(\Omega_1 - \Omega_2)$ is detected, amplified, and demodulated to remove the magnetic field modulation frequency ω_M. It is then sent through a lock-in detector, and finally recorded. The microwave frequency is measured by means of a frequency meter, and when a more precise frequency determination is required, a transfer oscillator and high speed counter are employed. The signal from an NMR magnetometer is recorded on the same trace as the ESR signal.

N. Rose-Innes, 1957

The spectrometer of Rose-Innes shown in Fig. 13–19 employs frequency modulation by applying a 50 cps voltage to the klystron

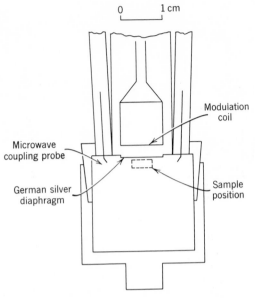

Fig. 13-17.   Resonant cavity and modulation coil detail [Llewellyn (1957)].

reflector.   The signal is the cavity pip, and a portion of the klystron mode is shown in Fig. 13-20.   At resonance the height of the cavity pip from the baseline changes, so one must detect a very small change in a large signal.   This is accomplished by the use of an i-f amplifier operating as an inverted "class C" or saturated amplifier. This frequency modulation technique is useful for the study of broad resonance lines.   The spectrometer may be adapted for low temperature (e.g., 4°K) investigations without the necessity of incorporating field modulation coils with their eddy current heating effect.   Lutze (1956) has also described a frequency modulation spectrometer.

O. McWhorter and Mayer, 1958

Masers have been employed as preamplifiers to increase the sensitivity of ESR spectrometers [Townes (1963); Gambling and Wilmshurst (1963); Lecar and Okaya (1963); cf. Sec. 14-H].   Strictly speaking, the description of a maser is not germane to the subject matter of this chapter.   Nevertheless, we will discuss the solid state

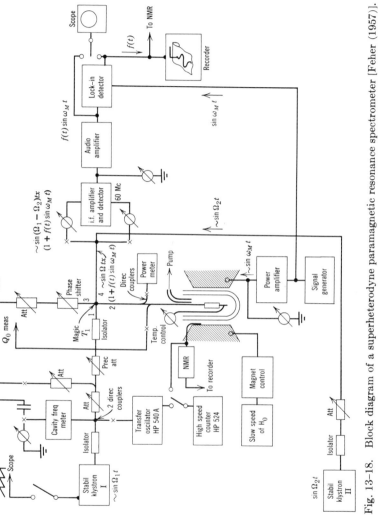

Fig. 13–18. Block diagram of a superheterodyne paramagnetic resonance spectrometer [Feher (1957)].

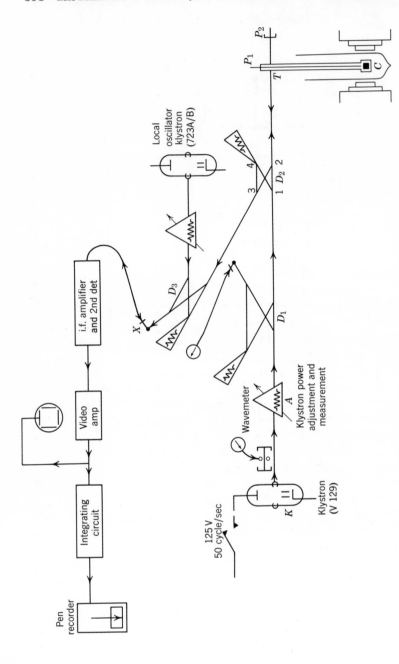

Fig. 13-19. 3-cm band ESR apparatus [Rose-Innes (1957)].

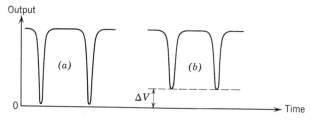

Fig. 13–20. Time dependence of the output signal. (a) Without electron resonance absorption; (b) during electron resonance absorption. The ESR signal ΔV is shown [Rose-Innes (1957)].

maser of McWhorter and Mayer (1958) in terms of its block diagram shown in Fig. 13–21, and the dual mode cavity of Fig. 13–22. Masers have been reviewed by Wittke (1957), Singer (1959), and Weber (1959).

The working substance of the maser was a single crystal of $K_3Cr(CN)_6$ oriented in the bottom of the cavity with the c axis parallel to the steady magnetic field. With this orientation the two zero field levels split in the manner shown on Fig. 13–23. The maser operates between the energy level pairs characterized by the spin quantum numbers $-1/2 \to 3/2$ and $3/2 \to 1/2$, which correspond to 9400 Mc and 2800 Mc, respectively, as shown on Fig. 13–23. The bimodal coaxial cavity operates simultaneously in the TEM mode at 2800 Mc and the TE_{113} mode at 9400 Mc. The 9400-Mc saturating or pump power between 0.3 and 30 mW traverses an isolator and two attenuators before reaching the cavity. The 2800-Mc signal power passes through a variable attenuator, a 20-dB directional coupler, and finally a 30-dB directional coupler before it arrives at the bimodal cavity. In the cavity, the pump power equalizes the spin populations between the $-1/2$ and $3/2$ levels, and the signal power induces transitions from $3/2$ to $1/2$, becoming amplified in the process. The maser amplifier output proceeds through the low-pass filter, isolator, and variable attenuator before it arrives at the spectrum analyzer where its amplitude is monitored. The amplifier gain G, band-width B, output power, and efficiency are shown on Figs. 13–24 and 13–25 as a function of the 9400 Mc pump power. The product of the square root of the gain times the band-width $G^{1/2}B$ was constant, as predicted by Strandberg (1957). The band-width is the spread between the positive and negative deviations from the midband frequency that lower the amplifier power output by a factor of two.

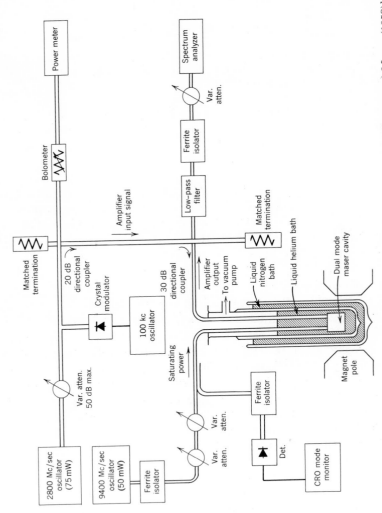

Fig. 13-21. Block diagram of microwave instrumentation for a maser [McWhorter and Meyer (1958)].

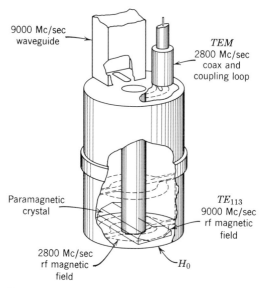

9000 Mc/sec
waveguide

TEM
2800 Mc/sec
coax and
coupling loop

Paramagnetic
crystal

TE_{113}
9000 Mc/sec
rf magnetic
field

2800 Mc/sec
rf magnetic
field

H_0

Fig. 13–22. Dual frequency maser cavity [McWhorter and Meyer (1958)].

It should be emphasized that Fig. 13–21 depicts a maser amplifier and not an ESR spectrometer. The reader is referred to the original article for further details.

P. Mock, 1960

A block diagram of Mock's basic 50 to 150-Gc spectrometer is shown in Fig. 13–26. It employs a backward wave oscillator (BWO) of the type TE67 and TE68. The power supply was stable to one part in 10^5, so no automatic frequency control (AFC) was needed. The frequency was measured relative to a known harmonic of a 200-Mc transfer oscillator with the aid of a frequency (HP) counter. A waferlike detector designed by Sharpless (1956) was used. The sample was placed directly in the waveguide, as is illustrated in the diagram of the zero field system shown in Fig. 13–27. By placing the sample in one side of the waveguide in accordance with Fig. 13–28, a microwave magnetic field of circular polarization predominated. As a result, positive and negative applied magnetic fields gave different resonant frequencies, corresponding to the ruby data shown in Fig. 13–29. If measurements were

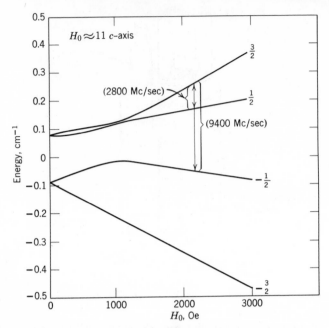

Fig. 13–23. Energy level diagram of $K_3Cr(CN)_6$ showing point of maser operation with the pump power inducing $-1/2 \rightarrow 3/2$ transitions, and the signal power operating between the $3/2 \rightarrow 1/2$ levels [McWhorter and Meyer (1958)].

carried out with the opposite circular polarization, it would reflect Fig. 13–29 about the $H = 0$ axis [cf. Sec. 8-M].

The advantage of Mock's system is that it permits measurements to be carried out over a wide range of frequencies, as is required for a determination of zero field splittings. Bogle, Symmons, Burgess, and Sierins (1961) describe two broad band spectrometers which cover the frequency range from 7.2 to 18 Gc, and which are also useful for determining zero field splittings.

Q. Teaney, Klein, and Portis, 1961

The block diagram of the bimodal cavity superheterodyne induction spectrometer designed by Teaney, Klein, and Portis (1961) is shown on Fig. 13–30. It differs from an ordinary heterodyne spectrometer by the incorporation of the bimodal cavity shown in

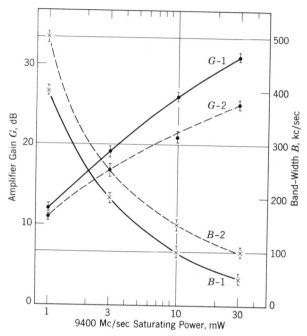

Fig. 13-24. (*G*) Gain and (*B*) band-width curves of a maser amplifier for two degrees of coupling (*1*) and (*2*) [McWhorter and Meyer (1958)].

Fig. 13-31 in place of the regular (monomodal) cavity. As described by Portis and Teaney (1958), the bimodal cavity is a TE_{111} mode cylindrical resonator with the two waveguides coupled to the cavity in such a way that each corresponds to a degenerate TE_{111} mode polarized at right angles to the other. One can picture the two mode configurations by rotating the TE_{112} mode diagram shown on Fig. 8-11 through 90°. The equivalent circuit is shown in Fig. 13-32. Since the modes are orthogonal or uncoupled, it follows that the power which is incident through one iris does not escape out through the other, but is either dissipated in the cavity or reflected back to the klystron. At resonance, an isolation as high as 60 dB is easily maintained.

When microwaves traverse a paramagnetic sample at resonance, their plane of polarization undergoes a Faraday rotation through an angle θ. If the sample is in a resonant cavity, then on the average, the microwaves bounce back and forth from the walls and through

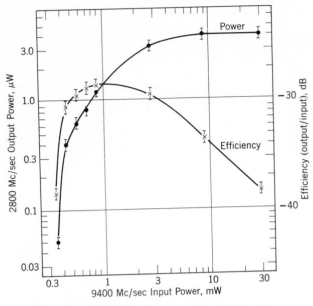

Fig. 13–25. Power output and efficiency characteristics of maser oscillator [McWhorter and Meyer (1958)].

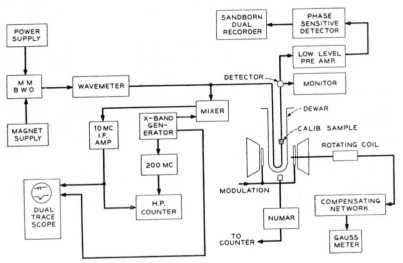

Fig. 13–26.   Broad band ESR spectrometer for use between 50 and 150 Gc [Mock (1960)].

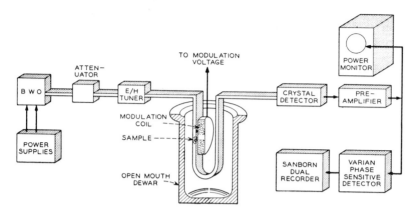

Fig. 13-27. Zero field ESR spectrometer [Mock (1960)].

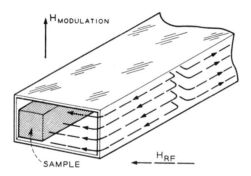

Fig. 13-28. Sample placement in waveguide [Mock (1960)].

the sample about Q times before they are finally dissipated, so the angle of rotation θ in the cavity is Q times what it would be in a waveguide. This rotation is additive for each passage of radiation through the sample since the sense of the Faraday rotation depends only on the magnetic field direction, and not on the direction of propagation. As a result of this Faraday rotation the cavity mode excited by the microwave generator is coupled at resonance to the output iris of the perpendicular mode, and so the signal that traverses the cavity at resonance is proportional to the paramagnetic resonance signal.

The scheme discussed in the preceding paragraph is essentially a zero leakage scheme which produces an output which is a combination

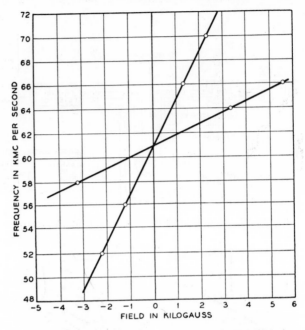

Fig. 13–29. Transitions in positive and negative magnetic fields for ruby subjected to circularly polarized microwaves [Mock (1960)].

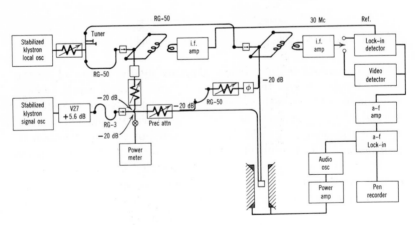

Fig. 13–30. Bimodal cavity induction spectrometer [Teaney, Klein, and Portis (1961)].

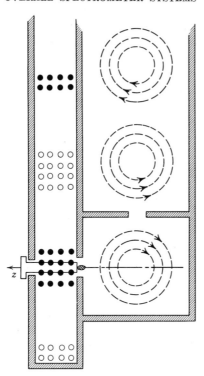

Fig. 13-31. The bimodal cavity, showing the crossed input and output wave-guides. The sample is mounted on the end wall, which is removable [Teaney, Klein, and Portis (1961)].

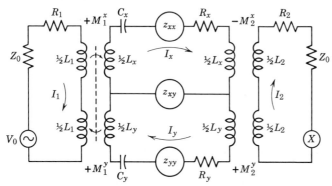

Fig. 13-32. Equivalent circuit for the bimodal cavity [Teaney, Klein, and Portis (1961)].

of absorption χ'' and dispersion χ'. The cavity may be provided with the series of metal plugs, resistive plugs, and a dielectric vane shown in Fig. 13–33 to produce a resistive or reactive unbalance between the two degenerate modes. As a result of such an unbalance, one will obtain absorption or dispersion, respectively.

This arrangement is the microwave analog of the nuclear induction NMR spectrometer of Bloch, Hansen, and Packard (1946). This NMR system consisted of two perpendicular coils surrounding the sample, and at balance, the rf energy did not couple from the transmitter coil to the receiver coil. When in use, a deliberate resistive or reactive unbalance is set up by means of a carbon or copper paddle, respectively, and one obtains absorption or dispersion. As a result of this analogy Teaney, Portis, and Klein call their instrument a microwave induction spectrometer. ESR induction spectrometers were also built by Brodwin and Burgess (1963) and Raoult, Chandezon, Chenon, Duclaux, and Perrin (1963). Brodwin and Burgess used an H-plane microwave junction to achieve the "induction" operation.

The heterodyne microwave induction spectrometer was found to maintain its very high sensitivity up to 1 W of incident power, while an ordinary superheterodyne spectrometer begins to lose sensitivity one or two orders of magnitude below this. Teaney, Klein, and

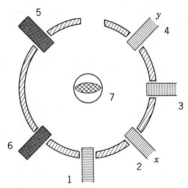

Fig. 13–33.   Cross section of the bimodal cavity showing the arrangement of the tuning plugs and dielectric vane.   Metal plugs *1* and *3* decouple the x and y normal modes; metal plugs *2* and *4* adjust the frequencies of the two modes; resistive plugs *5* and *6* adjust the losses of the two modes.   The dielectric vane, *7*, is rotated in the iris to differentially adjust the coupling to the two modes [Teaney, Klein, and Portis (1961)].

Portis (1961) attribute this improvement to the removal of the extreme frequency dependence in the bridge balance at high powers where almost complete isolation is required [see Sec. 14–C; Misra (1958)]. The bimodal cavity automatically provides this isolation. This cavity is suitable for use at low temperatures. It has been employed for the study of F centers in NaCl [Teaney, Blumberg, and Portis (1960)]. One particularly useful feature is the fact that the sign of the g factor can be obtained because the direction of the Faraday rotation depends on this sign [cf. Sec. 8–M].

R. Llewellyn, Whittlestone, and Williams, 1962

Llewellyn, Whittlestone, and Williams describe the superheterodyne pulse spectrometer shown on Fig. 13–34. It was designed to measure relaxation times from 1 μsec to 100 msec at temperatures between 1 and 20°K.

The system employs one V153 klystron [see Seidel (1962)]. It is frequency modulated at 10 Mc (30 Mc is preferable*) with a deviation ratio adjusted to put 4% of the power ($\sim$4mW) in each of the first two sidebands at $f \pm 10$ Mc, and a negligible amount of power in the second and third sidebands [cf. Sec. 12–H]. The tunable cavity C_1 transmits only the local oscillator frequency $f + 10$ Mc to the lower right waveguide, while all three frequencies f and $f \pm 10$ Mc are carried by the waveguide directly to the right of C_1. The sample cavity C_2 which contains the sample is tuned to transmit only the carrier f. The carrier and LO signals are brought together in the magic T where the microwave silicon–tungsten mixer diode (CS 10B or CS 3B) detects the 10 Mc intermediate frequency. The ESR signal traverses a 10 Mc i.f. amplifier, second detector, video amplifier, and limiter before reaching the oscilloscope.

The microwave switching diode permits power levels with zero and 29-dB attenuation to be incident on the sample cavity. In operation, the switch generates high power pulses with a rise time of 0.1 μsec or less, and the remainder of the time the saturated spin system is monitored at lower power. The pulse generator provides a signal to synchronize the oscilloscope, and another called the "paralysis" signal to control the i.f. amplifier gain during the pulse. Time delay networks are associated with the pulse generator.

* J. M. Williams, private communication.

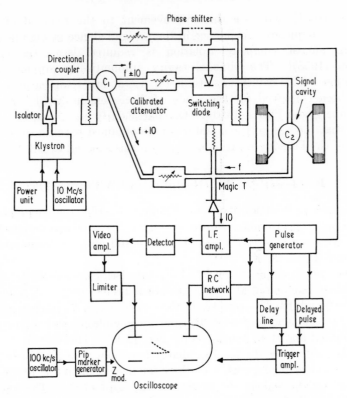

Fig. 13–34.   Superheterodyne pulse spectrometer [Llewellyn, Whittlestone, and Williams (1962)].

The sensitivity is limited by the large band-width that is required to reproduce the change in the ESR absorption close to the pulses. It is very difficult to reach times as short as 10^{-7} sec [see Kaplan, Browne, and Cowen (1961)]. This spectrometer detects as few as 10^{16} spins/cm^3 at liquid helium temperatures. It is not suited for use in ordinary ESR studies at powers exceeding 100 μW. Pulse measurements are also described by Davis, Strandberg, and Kyhl (1958).

S. Candela and Mundy, 1965

Candela and Mundy designed a spectrometer for measuring the static dc susceptibility χ_0 as a function of the microwave power

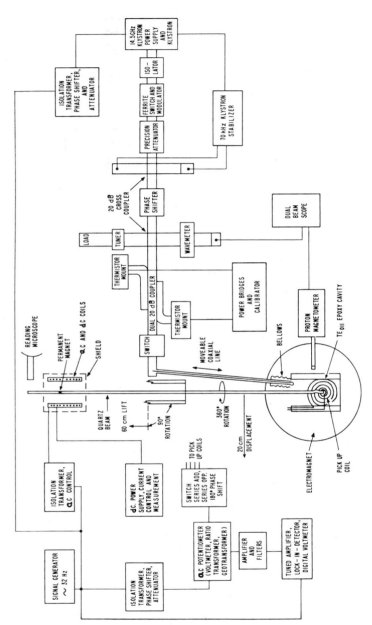

Fig. 13-35. Spectrometer for measuring magnetic susceptibilities [Candela and Mundy (1965)].

absorbed at resonance. The spin lattice relaxation time T_1 is related to the difference between the static susceptibility χ_0 at zero microwave power and the susceptibility χ_p when the sample is absorbing the microwave power P

$$T_1 = [(\chi_0 - \chi_p)/P\Gamma_M] M_s H_0^2$$

where M_s is the sample weight, H_0 is the applied magnetic field, and Γ_M is a constant [Candela (1965)].

The spectrometer shown on Fig. 13–35 permits one to measure the quantities in this equation. The susceptibilities χ_0 and χ_p were determined by means of an electromagnetically controlled beam balance [Thorpe and Senftle (1959); Candela and Mundy (1961, 1962); Frederick (1960)]. This consists of a quartz beam, permanent magnet, ac and dc cores, and reading microscope. The microwave power P was determined by the power bridges and calibrator which received their input signals from thermistors mounted on directional couplers. This arrangement permits the measurement of both the incident and the reflected microwave power. A proton magnetometer determined the magnetic field H_0. The original article should be consulted for further details.

References

R. J. Abraham, D. W. Ovenall, and D. H. Whiffin, *Trans. Faraday Soc.*, **54**, 1128 (1958).

S. A. Akhmanov, S. D. Gvozdover, Yu. S. Konstantinov, and I. T. Trofimenko, *PTE*, **2**, 38 (1959).

E. Albold, B. Eischner, and P. Wenzel, *ETP*, **5**, 254 (1957).

S. A. Al'tshuler and B. M. Kozyrev, *Electron Paramagnetic Resonance*, translated by Scripta Technica and edited by C. P. Poole, Jr., Academic Press, N. Y., 1964.

S. A. Al'tshuler and B. T. Kozyrev, *Uspekhi Fiz. Nauk.*, **63**, 533 (1957); review of spectrometers.

M. Anderegg, P. Cornaz, and J. P. Borel, *Z. Angew. Math. Phys.*, **14**, 201 (1963).

J. O. Artman and P. E. Tannenwald, *J. Appl. Phys.*, **26**, 1124 (1955); Cy-TE_{11n} and Rt-TE_{01n} cavity theory for circular polarization discussed.

H. M. Assenheim, *Lab. Pract.*, **13**, 1079 (1964).

V. A. Atsarkin, M. E. Zhabotinskii, and A. V. Frantsesson, *Radiotekh. i Electron. Phys.*, **7**, 866 (820) (1962); sensitivity theory discussed.

D. M. S. Bagguley and F. H. E. Griffiths, *Proc. Phys. Soc.*, **A65**, 594 (1952).

M. J. A. Bakker and J. Smidt, *Appl. Sci. Res.*, **B9**, 199 (1961).

A. Battaglia, M. Iannuzzi, and E. Polacco, *Ric. Sci. 11A*, **3**, 119 (1963).

Y. Beers *RSI*, **30**, 9 (1959).

H. Benoit and R. H. Ruby, *Paramagnetic Resonance*, **2**, 414 (1963).

R. Beringer and J. G. Castle, *Phys. Rev.*, **78**, 581 (1950).

R. Beringer and M. A. Heald, *Phys. Rev.*, **95**, 1474 (1954).

G. Berthet, *Onde Élect.*, **35**, 489, 490 (1955); *C. R. Acad. Sci.*, **241**, 1730 (1955).

F. Bloch, W. W. Hansen, and M. Packard, *Phys. Rev.*, **70**, 474 (1946).

G. S. Bogle, H. F. Symmons, V. R. Burgess, and J. V. Sierins, *Proc. Phys. Soc.*, **77**, 561 (1961).

D. I. Bolef, J. de Klerk, and R. B. Gosser, *RSI*, **33**, 631 (1962).

D. Bösnecker, *Z. Angew. Phys.*, **12**, 306 (1960); theory of phase-sensitive detector discussed.

K. D. Bowers, R. A. Kamper, and R. B. D. Knight, *JSI*, **34**, 49 (1957).

S. E. Bresler, E. M. Saminskii, and E. N. Kazbekov, *Zh. Tekh. Fiz.*, **27**, 2535 (2357) (1957); sensitivity theory discussed.

M. E. Brodwin and T. J. Burgess, *IEEE Trans. Instr. Meas.*, **IM-12**, 7 (1963).

G. Brown, D. R. Mason, and J. S. Thorp, *JSI*, **42**, 648 (1965).

H. A. Buckmaster and J. C. Dering, *Can. J. Phys.*, **43**, 1088 (1965).

H. A. Buckmaster and H. E. D. Scovil, *Can. J. Phys.*, **34**, 711 (1956).

G. A. Candela, *J. Chem. Phys.*, **42**, 113 (1965).

G. A. Candela and R. E. Mundy, *RSI*, **32**, 1056 (1961); **36**, 338 (1965); *IRE Trans. Instr.*, **I-2**, 106 (1962).

A. Charru, *C. R. Acad. Sci.*, **243**, 652 (1956); see also M. Chenot, *J. Phys. Radium*, **16**, 101 (1955).

R. J. Collier, *RSI*, **25**, 1205 (1954).

J. Combrisson and J. Uebersfeld, *J. Phys. Radium*, **14**, 104, 724 (1953).

C. F. Davis, M. W. P. Strandberg, and R. L. Kyhl, *Phys. Rev.*, **111**, 1268 (1958).

E. del Rosal, J. C. Zorn, and D. Pinkel, *Rev. Mexican Fis.*, **14**, 175 (1965).

W. C. Dickinson, *Phys. Rev.*, **81**, 717 (1951).

G. F. Dionne, *Phys. Rev.*, **139**, A1648 (1965).

W. Duncan and E. E. Schneider, *JSI*, **42**, 395 (1965).

J. Dušek, *Czech. J. Phys.*, **11**, 528 (1961).

P. R. Elliston, G. J. Troup, and D. R. Hutton, *JSI*, **40**, 586 (1963).

O. G. El'sting, *PTE*, **5**, 64 (753) (1960).

L. E. Erickson, *Phys. Rev.*, **143**, 295 (1966).

B. V. Fedorov, *PTE*, **4**, 98 (686) (1963).

G. Feher, *Bell System Tech. J.*, **36**, 449 (1957); sensitivity theory discussed.

G. Feher and A. F. Kip, *Phys. Rev.*, **98**, 337 (1955).

Z. Frait, *Czech. J. Phys.*, **7**, 222, 577 (1957).

N. V. Frederick, *IRE Trans. Intsr.*, **I-9**, 194 (1960).

A. A. Galkin and D. A. Kichigin, *PTE*, **3**, 71 (396) (1958); modifies Zavoiskii's method.

W. A. Gambling and T. H. Wilmshurst, *Phys. Letters*, **5**, 228 (1963); *Proc. XII Colloque Ampere*, Bordeaux, 1963, p. 171.

U. S. Ghosh, R. N. Bagchi, and A. K. Pal, *Indian J. Phys.*, **37**, 555 (1963).

E. Glauche and F. Voigt, *ETP*, **11**, 196 (1963).

J. P. Goldsborough and T. R. Koehler, *Phys. Rev.*, **133**, A135 (1964).

W. Gordy, W. V. Smith, and R. F. Trambarulo, *Microwave Spectroscopy*, Wiley, N. Y., 1953.

E. S. Gravlin and J. A. Cowen, *Am. J. Phys.*, **27**, 566 (1959).

H. Grützediek, K. D. Kramer, and W. Müller-Warmuth, *RSI*, **36**, 1418 (1965).

J. L. Hall and R. T. Schumacher, *Phys. Rev.*, **127**, 1892 (1962).

J. Haupt, W. Müller-Warmuth, and G. Schultz, *Z. Angew. Phys.*, **18**, 132 (1964).

J. C. M. Henning, *RSI*, **32**, 35 (1961); good diagram.

J. Hervé, J. Pescia, and M. Sauzade, *C. R. Acad. Sci.*, **249**, 1486 (1959).

J. M. Hirshon and G. K. Fraenkel, *RSI*, **26**, 34 (1955).

R. W. R. Hoisington, L. Kellner, and M. J. Pentz, *Nature*, **178**, 1111 (1956); *Proc. Phys. Soc.*, **72**, 537 (1958).

W. C. Holton and H. Blum, *Phys. Rev.*, **125**, 89 (1962).

D. J. E. Ingram, *Free Radicals as Studied by Electron Spin Resonance*, Butterworths, London, 1958.

D. J. E. Ingram, *Lab. Pract.*, **12**, 518 (1963); review.

D. J. E. Ingram, *Spectroscopy at Radio and Microwave Frequencies*, 2nd Ed., Butterworths, London, 1955.

K. B. Jefferts and E. D. Jones, *RSI*, **36**, 983 (1965).

C. D. Jeffries, *Progr. Cryogenics*, **3**, 129 (1961).

C. K. Jen, *Phys. Rev.*, **74**, 1396 (1948); *ibid.*, **76**, 1494 (1949).

D. E. Kaplan, *J. Phys. Radium*, **23**, Suppl. No. 3, 21A (1962).

D. E. Kaplan, M. E. Browne, and J. A. Cowen, *RSI*, **32**, 1182 (1961).

J. G. Kenworthy and R. E. Richards, *JSI*, **42**, 675 (1965).

A. L. Kipling, P. W. Smith, J. Vanier, and G. A. Woonton, *Can. J. Phys.*, **39**, 1859 (1961); see Dionne (1965).

V. A. Kolbasov and M. M. Mukhina, *PTE*, **1**, 84 (77) (1963).

V. A. Kolbasov, M. M. Mukhina, and V. P. Nazarov, *PTE*, **2**, 107 (328) (1962).

K. D. Kramer and W. Müller-Warmuth, *Z. Angew. Phys.*, **16**, 281 (1963).

J. L. Laffon, P. Servoz-Gavin, and T. Uchida, *J. Phys. Radium*, **23**, 951 (1962).

R. C. La Force, *RSI*, **32**, 1387 (1961).

V. B. Lebedev, *Izv. Akad. Nauk SSSR, Ser. Fiz.*, **27**, 69 (73) (1963).

H. Lecar and A. Okaya, *Paramagnetic Resonance*, **2**, 675 (1962).

P. V. Lenzo, *RSI*, **34**, 1374 (1963).

M. Lichtenstein, J. J. Gallagher, and R. E. Cupp, *RSI*, **34**, 843 (1963).

P. M. Llewellyn, *JSI*, **34**, 236 (1957).

P. M. Llewellyn, P. R. Whittlestone, and J. M. Williams, *JSI*, **39**, 586 (1962).

W. Low, *Proc. Intern. Conf. Magnetism*, Inst. Phys. and Phys. Soc., London, 1965, p. 462.

E. Lutze, *Z. Angew. Phys.*, **8**, 61 (1956).

R. C. Mackey and W. D. Hershberger, *Trans. Inst. Radio Engr. Prof. Group on Microwave Theory and Tech.*, **MTT-1**, 3 (1953).

A. L. McWhorter and J. W. Meyer, *Phys. Rev.*, **109**, 312 (1958).

A. A. Manenkov and A. M. Prokhorov, *Radiotekh. i Elektron.*, **1**, 469 (1956).

R. G. Marcley, *Am. J. Phys.*, **29**, 492 (1961).

L. R. Maxwell and T. R. McGuire, *Rev. Mod. Phys.*, **25**, 279 (1953).

A. F. Mehlkopf and J. Smidt, *Ampere Colloquium Eindhoven*, North Holland, Amsterdam, 1962, p. 758; see also *RSI*, **32**, 1421 (1961); see Bakker and Smidt (1961) for cavity details.

D. Mergerian, M. P. Stombler, and I. H. Harrop, *Bull. Am. Phys. Soc.*, **10**, 1109 (1965).

H. Misra, *RSI*, **29**, 590 (1958); second cavity reduces *FM* noise by 10×.

J. B. Mock, *RSI*, **31**, 551 (1960).

W. Müller-Warmuth, *Z. Naturforsch.*, **19A**, 1309 (1964).

The NMR-EPR Staff of Varian Associates, *NMR and EPR Spectroscopy*, Pergamon, N. Y., 1960.

I. Pascaru, *Nuclear Instr. Methods*, **26**, 333 (1964).

I. Pascaru and A. Valeriu, *Stud. Cercetari Fiz.* (*Roumania*), **12**, 165 (1961).

J. Paulevé, *Onde Élect.*, **35**, 494 (1955).

J. B. Payne, III, *IEEE Trans.*, **MTT-12**, 48 (1964).

J. Pescia, *Arch. Sci. Fasic. Spec.*, **13**, 350 (1960); see Hervé, Pescia, and Sauzade (1959) for frequency stabilization.

A. M. Portis and D. T. Teaney, *J. Appl. Phys.*, **29**, 1692 (1958).

G. Raoult, J. Chandezon, M. T. Chenon, A. M. Duclaux, and M. Perrin, *Proc. 12th Colloque Ampère*, Bordeaux, 1963, p. 167.

R. E. Richards and J. W. White, *Proc. Roy. Soc.*, **A279**, 474 (1964).

M. E. Rose, *Phys. Rev.*, **53**, 715 (1938).

A. C. Rose-Innes, *JSI*, **34**, 276 (1957).

Ch. Ryter, R. Lacroix, and R. Extermann, *Onde Élect.*, **35**, 490 (1955).

G. Schoffa and O. Ristau, *ETP*, **8**, 217 (1960).

H. Seidel, *Z. Angew. Phys.*, **14**, 21 (1962).

A. G. Semenov, *PTE*, **5**, 5 (1962); review of commercial spectrometers.

Ya. L. Shamfarov, *PTE*, **6**, 57 (916) (1959).

W. M. Sharpless, *Bell System. Tech. J.*, **35**, 1385 (1956).

J. R. Singer, *Masers*, Wiley, N. Y., 1959.

W. Stieler, *Z. Angew Phys.*, **10**, 89 (1958).

M. W. P. Strandberg, *Phys. Rev.*, **106**, 617 (1957).

M. W. P. Strandberg, H. R. Johnson, and J. R. Eshbach, *RSI*, **25**, 776 (1954).

M. W. P. Strandberg, M. Tinkham, I. H. Solt, and C. F. Davis, *RSI*, **27**, 596 (1956).

Sun Tsung-tang, Chaing Wen-chia, Shun Lien-fong, and Mao Tin-fong, *Acta Phys. Sinica*, **21**, 866 (1965).

D. T. Teaney, W. E. Blumberg, and A. M. Portis, *Phys. Rev.*, **119**, 1851 (1960).

D. Teaney, M. P. Klein, and A. M. Portis, *RSI*, **32**, 721 (1961); sensitivity theory discussed.

J. G. Théobald, *Ann. Phys.* (*Paris*), **7**, 585 (1962).

A. Thorpe and F. E. Senftle, *RSI*, **30**, 1006 (1959).

M. Tinkham and M. W. P. Strandberg, *Proc. IRE*, **43**, 734 (1955).

C. H. Townes, *Phys. Rev. Letters*, **5**, 428 (1960).

C. H. Townes and A. L. Schawlow, *Microwave Spectroscopy*, McGraw-Hill, N. Y., 1955.

W. G. Tuller, W. C. Galloway, and F. P. Zaffarano, *Proc. IRE*, **36**, 794 (1948).

Tuong Tai-chian, *Acta. Phys. Sinica*, **19**, 407, 816 (1963).

J. Uebersfeld, *Onde Élect.* **35**, 492 (1955); *Ann. Phys.*, **1**, 395 (1956).

J. Uebersfeld and E. Erb, *J. Phys. Radium*, **17**, 90A (1956); see Combrisson and Uebersfeld (1953).

R. R. Unterberger, *Electronics*, **32**, 142 (1959).

J. Weber, *Rev. Mod. Phys.*, **31**, 681 (1959).

C. A. Whitmer, R. T. Weidner, H. C. Hsiang, and P. R. Weiss, *Phys. Rev.*, **74**, 1478 (1984).

J. P. Wittke, *Proc. IRE*, **45**, 291 (1957).

V. A. Zakrevskii and E. E. Tomashevskii, *PTE*, **4**, 102 (821) (1964).

G. M. Zverev, *PTE*, **5**, 109 (930) (1961).

CHAPTER 14

Sensitivity

This chapter will begin by presenting Feher's (1957) classical analysis of the sensitivity of electron spin resonance spectrometers [see also Ingram (1958)] and will then discuss several other approaches to the same subject. The latter part of the chapter will elaborate upon the manner in which various instrumental parameters and experimental conditions affect the sensitivity, and will recommend ways of selecting optimum conditions. We assume throughout that allowed transitions are being observed with the microwave magnetic field H_1 perpendicular to the constant applied field. Forbidden transitions with lower intensity are observed with these fields parallel to each other, and Brogden and Butterworth (1965) even reported the detection of doubly forbidden satellites. Chapter 21 may be referred to for specific details on tuning ESR spectrometers.

A. Q and Frequency Changes at Resonance

When a paramagnetic sample in a resonant cavity is tuned through the resonance condition $\hbar\omega = g\beta H$, the unpaired spins interact with the rf field H_1 at the sample. This interaction manifests itself as a frequency change (dispersion) or a Q change (absorption) in the resonant cavity. The absorption mode will be discussed in detail, and then a few words will be said about dispersion. Most ESR spectrometers detect only absorption, but some [e.g., see Ryter, Lacroix, and Extermann (1955) and Faulkner (1962)] operate in both modes.

A paramagnetic sample in a resonant cavity of frequency $\omega_0 = 2\pi\nu_0$ will absorb incident microwave energy at the resonant magnetic field H_0 given by

$$\hbar\omega_0 = g\beta H_0 \tag{1}$$

where $\hbar$ is Planck's constant divided by 2π, β is the Bohr magneton, and g is the dimensionless g factor which is often close to two. The average power absorbed per unit volume is given by

$$P = \tfrac{1}{2}\omega_0 H_1{}^2 \chi'' \tag{2}$$

where H_1 is the amplitude of the microwave magnetic field at the sample and χ'' is the microwave or rf susceptibility. The power absorbed at resonance will manifest itself as a change in the quality factor or Q of the cavity

$$1/Q = 1/Q_u + 1/Q_x \tag{3}$$

where Q_u is the unloaded Q of the cavity in the absence of resonant absorption and Q_x is the contribution of the resonant absorption to the Q. This quantity Q_u includes cavity losses plus the dielectric and conductivity losses in the sample. At resonance, the Q changes by an amount ΔQ

$$\Delta Q = -Q^2 \Delta(1/Q) = -Q_u{}^2/Q_x \tag{4}$$

where we assume

$$Q_x \gg Q_u \tag{5}$$

The loaded Q is defined in Sec. 8-B and Q_x has the form

$$Q_x = \frac{\dfrac{\mu_0}{2}\displaystyle\int_{\text{cavity}} H_1^2 dV}{\dfrac{\mu_0}{2}\displaystyle\int_{\text{sample}} H_1^2 \chi'' dV} \tag{6}$$

If χ'' is homogeneous over the sample volume, then one has

$$Q_x = \frac{\displaystyle\int_{\text{cavity}} H_1^2 dV}{\chi'' \displaystyle\int_{\text{sample}} H_1^2 dV} = \frac{1}{\chi'' \eta} \tag{7}$$

where η is the filling factor discussed in Sec. 8-H and χ'' is considered a constant for each sample. The filling factor is a measure of the fraction of the microwave energy that interacts with the sample, and explicit values of η are given in Sec. 8-H for several commonly used sample arrangements. Equations (4) and (7) furnish the change in Q

$$\Delta Q = \chi'' \eta Q_u^2 \tag{8}$$

where the negative sign is omitted for simplicity. To convert this equation from MKS to cgs units, multiply the righthand side by 4π.

The equivalent circuits for reflection and transmission cavities are shown on Figs. 8–21 and 8–22, respectively. The coupling coefficients to the waveguide are discussed in Sec. 8-F, and the same terminology will be used here.

Reflection Cavity and Square Law Detector: The power P_c into a resonant cavity is given by [Feher (1957)]

$$P_c = \frac{\frac{1}{2}(nE)^2 R_c}{(R_c + R_g n^2)^2} = \frac{2P_w(R_c/R_g n^2)}{(1 + R_c/R_g n^2)^2} \tag{9}$$

and the maximum power P_w available from the source is

$$P_w = \frac{1}{4}(E^2/R_g) \tag{10}$$

where R_g is the generator's internal resistance, R_c is the resonant cavity resistance and n is the turns ratio of the equivalent circuit transformer.

At match $R_c = R_g n^2$. At resonance, the change in reflected power ΔP_r equals the change in the power ΔP_c absorbed by the sample in the cavity as a result of the change ΔR_c in the equivalent cavity resistance R_c

$$\frac{\Delta P_c}{P_w} = \frac{1}{P_w} \frac{\partial P_c}{\partial R_c} \Delta R_c = \frac{2\Delta R_c}{R_g n^2} \frac{1 - (R_c/R_g n^2)}{(1 + R_c/R_g n^2)^3} \tag{11}$$

For a square law detector whose output is proportional to the incident power (e.g., crystals in the microwatt region, or bolometers), we optimize ΔP_c with respect to the coupling parameter $R_g n^2$ by setting

$$\frac{\partial \Delta P_c}{\partial (R_g n^2)} = 0 \tag{12}$$

with the result that

$$\frac{R_g n^2}{R_c} = 2 \pm 3^{1/2} = \begin{cases} \text{VSWR} & R_g n^2 \geqslant R_c \\ 1/\text{VSWR} & R_g n^2 \leqslant R_c \end{cases} \quad (13)$$

The positive sign is for an overcoupled cavity and the negative sign for an undercoupled cavity. Each case gives a VSWR of $2 + 3^{1/2}$, and from eq. (11), we have for the two cases

$$\Delta P_c / P_w = \pm 0.193 \ \Delta R_c / R_c = \mp 0.193 \ \Delta Q / Q = \mp 0.193 \ \chi'' \eta Q_u \quad (14)$$

for the maximum ESR signal. An overcoupled cavity produces less noise, as will be shown below. Equation (11) is plotted in Fig. 14–1, and the symmetry of the graph shows that for a given VSWR,

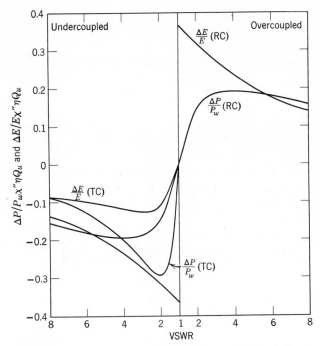

Fig. 14–1. The ESR signal $\Delta P / P_w$ and $\Delta E / E$ normalized relative to $\chi'' \eta Q_u$ as a function of VSWR for square law ($\Delta P / P_w$) and linear ($\Delta E / E$) detectors used with a reflection (RC) and transmission (TC) cavity [Feher (1957)].

the same sensitivity is obtained with both the overcoupled and the undercoupled cases.

Transmission Cavity with Square Law Detector: The power into the load P_l is

$$P_l = \frac{E^2 n_1^2 n_2^2 R_g}{[R_g n_1^2 + R_c + R_l n_2^2]^2} \tag{15}$$

The change in power ΔP_l at resonance is related to the maximum available power $P_w = E^2/(4R_g)$ by the expression

$$\frac{\Delta P_l}{P_w} = \frac{1}{P_w} \frac{\partial P_l}{\partial R_c} \Delta R_c = \frac{8 n_1^2 n_2^2 R_g^2 \Delta R_c}{(R_g n_1^2 + R_c + R_l n_2^2)^3} \tag{16}$$

and at match $R_g = R_l$. If we maximize ΔP_l with respect to both $R_g n_1^2$ and $R_l n_2^2$, we obtain

$$R_g n_1^2 = R_l n_2^2 = R_g n^2 = R_c \tag{17}$$

Since the cavity input impedance equals the sum of R_c and $R_l n_2^2$, it follows that the cavity is overcoupled, and the VSWR has the form

$$\text{VSWR} = (R_l n_2^2 + R_c)/R_g n_1^2 \tag{18}$$

It is not possible to undercouple a transmission cavity with equal input and output coupling constants. Using condition (17) and setting $n_1 = n_2$ we obtain

$$\frac{\Delta P_l}{P_w} = \frac{1}{P_w} \frac{\partial P_l}{\partial R_c} \Delta R_c = \frac{8}{27} \frac{\Delta R_c}{R_c} = -\frac{8}{27} \frac{\Delta Q}{Q} = -\frac{8}{27} \chi'' \eta Q_u \tag{19}$$

Reflection Cavity and Linear Detector: In this case, one detects the reflected voltage E_r which is related to the incident voltage E by

$$E_r = E\Gamma = -E \left(1 - \frac{2\,\text{VSWR}}{1 + \text{VSWR}} \right) \tag{20}$$

where the reflection coefficient Γ is defined by eq. (2-B–20). The VSWR for a reflection cavity is given by

$$\text{VSWR} = (R_g n^2/R_c)^{\pm 1} \tag{21}$$

where we shall adopt the convention that the upper sign is for the overcoupled case and the lower sign for the undercoupled case. At resonance, the change in the reflected voltage ΔE_r arises from a change ΔR_c in the equivalent cavity resistance R_c

$$\frac{\Delta E_r}{E} = \frac{1}{E}\frac{\partial E_r}{\partial R_c}\Delta R_c = \pm 2\Delta R_c \frac{R_g n^2}{(R_g n^2 + R_c)^2} \qquad (22)$$

using the same sign convention. For a linear detector whose output is proportional to the input voltage (e.g., crystals at milliwatt or watt power levels), the optimum coupling occurs when

$$\frac{\partial \Delta E_r}{\partial R_g n^2} = 0 \qquad (23)$$

which corresponds to the condition of match

$$R_g n^2 = R_c \qquad (24)$$

As a result, eq. (22) gives

$$\Delta E_r/E = \pm \Delta R_c/2R_c = \mp \Delta Q/2Q = \mp \chi''\eta Q_u/2 \qquad (25)$$

Thus we should work near match for maximum sensitivity, but to avoid distortion, it is best to detune the cavity sufficiently so that it will remain on one side of match while sweeping through the resonant line. The observed sign of the signal will indicate the type of coupling, since during resonance absorption the reflected voltage E_r will increase for an undercoupled cavity and decrease for an over-coupled cavity.

Transmission Cavity and Linear Detector: The voltage E_l observed at a linear detector after passing through a transmission cavity is

$$E_l = \frac{E n_1 n_2 R_g}{R_g n_1^2 + r + R_l n_2^2} \qquad (26)$$

where again for maximum sensitivity both couplings are the same $(R_g n_1^2 = R_l n_2^2 = R_g n^2)$. At resonance, one obtains

$$\frac{\Delta E_l}{E} = \frac{1}{E}\frac{\partial E_l}{\partial R_c}\Delta R_c = -\frac{\Delta R_c}{R_c}\frac{R_c R_g n^2}{(R_c + 2R_g n^2)^2} \qquad (27)$$

When

$$\frac{\partial E_l}{\partial R_g n^2} = 0 \quad \text{then} \quad R_g n^2 = \frac{1}{2} R_c \tag{28}$$

and we arrive at the condition

$$\Delta E_l / E = -\frac{1}{8} \chi'' \eta Q_u \tag{29}$$

Figure 14–1 shows $\Delta P/P_w$ and $\Delta E/E$ from eqs. (11), (16), (22), and (27) plotted as a function of the VSWR. Crystal detectors used with reflection cavities are ordinarily operated somewhere between their linear and square law regions, and so in this case one may work at an intermediate VSWR, perhaps at a value near two. When noise is taken into account (see Sec. 11-D), then we see that in the milliwatt and watt range it is advisable to operate crystal detectors with a constant amount of incident power or "leakage" P_d that is independent of the power P_c that enters the resonant cavity. At high powers, $P_c \gg P_d$, this corresponds to tuning the cavity close to match.

This section has discussed the change in Q that results from the behavior of the absorption or the imaginary part of the magnetic susceptibility χ'' at resonance. During resonance there will also be a dispersion mode which corresponds to a change in the frequency of the resonant cavity as a result of the real part of the rf magnetic susceptibility χ'. The reason for this frequency change may be deduced by considering the velocity v of electromagnetic radiation in a dielectric medium

$$v = 1/(\mu\epsilon)^{1/2} = \lambda f \tag{30}$$

with a dielectric constant ϵ and a permeability $\mu = \mu_0 (1 + \chi)$, where ϵ and μ are considered real. In a resonant cavity the wavelength λ (or the guide wavelength λ_g) is fixed by the dimensions of the resonator. As a result, if the susceptibility or dielectric const is changed by the amount $\Delta\chi$ and losses are neglected (i.e., $\chi'' = 0$), then the frequency will change by

$$\Delta f = \frac{1}{\lambda(\mu_0\epsilon)^{1/2}} \left[\frac{1}{(\chi')^{1/2}} - \frac{1}{(\chi' + \Delta\chi)^{1/2}} \right] \tag{31}$$

At resonance, $\chi = \chi' + j\chi''$ changes both its real and imaginary parts in conformity with the Kramers-Kronig relations [Kronig (1926); Kramers (1927); Gorter and Kronig (1936); Pake and Purcell (1948); RLS-13, Chap. 8; Abragam (1961); Bolton, Troup, and Wilson (1964); Scott (1964); Sharnoff (1964); Troup and Walter (1965)]

$$\chi'(\omega) = \chi'(\infty) + \frac{2}{\pi} \int_0^\infty \frac{\omega' \chi''(\omega')}{\omega'^2 - \omega^2} d\omega' \tag{32}$$

$$\chi''(\omega) = -\frac{2\omega}{\pi} \int_0^\infty \frac{\chi'(\omega') - \chi'(\infty)}{\omega'^2 - \omega^2} d\omega' \tag{33}$$

These relations are very important physically because they ensure that the amplitude of the observed signal from χ' will be comparable to that observed from χ'' [Rajan (1962)]. If a phase shifter or slide screw tuner is employed to vary the effective length of line in front of the resonant cavity [cf. Ellerbruch (1965) and Sec. 7-R], then the shape of the observed first derivative signal will change with the phase in the manner shown on Fig. 14–2. If the klystron is stabilized

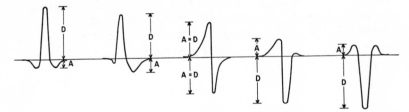

Fig. 14–2. Change in shape of a spectrum from solid DPPH when the bridge is tuned from dispersion to absorption and then back to dispersion.

on the sample resonant cavity, then it will "follow" the frequency variations, and the dispersion mode χ' will be stabilized out. This is why most ESR spectrometers record only the absorption mode χ''.

If a mixed mode is recorded, then the percentage of absorption $\%\chi''$ may be approximated from the expression

$$\%\chi'' = 100\chi''/(\chi' + \chi'') \tag{34}$$

$$\approx 100 \left[\frac{\dfrac{2A}{A+D} - \left(\dfrac{2A}{A+D}\right)_{\chi'}}{1 - \left(\dfrac{2A}{A+D}\right)_{\chi'}} \right] \tag{35}$$

where the parameters A and D are defined on Fig. 14–2. For pure absorption, $D = A$, and for pure dispersion, D/A has the values [Sec. 20-G; Table 20-5; Pake and Purcell (1948)]

$$\frac{D}{A} = \begin{cases} 8 & \text{Lorentzian} \\ 3.5 & \text{Gaussian} \end{cases} \tag{36}$$

which lead to

$$\left(\frac{2A}{A+D}\right)_{\chi'} = \begin{cases} 2/9 & \text{Lorentzian} \\ 4/9 & \text{Gaussian} \end{cases} \tag{37}$$

Peter, Shaltiel, Wernick, Williams, Mock, and Sherwood (1962) also discuss a technique for obtaining the ratio of χ'' to χ'.

If the klystron is stabilized at the frequency f_k on a reference cavity, and recordings are made of a DPPH sample in a second resonant cavity at the frequency f_c, then the $\%\chi''$ was found experimentally to vary with the frequency deviation $\Delta f = f_k - f_c$ in the manner shown on Fig. 14–3.

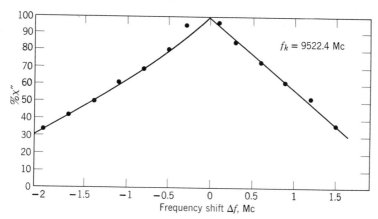

Fig. 14–3. Per cent absorption ($\%\chi''$) as a function of the frequency deviation Δf of the resonant cavity frequency f_c from the klystron frequency f_k where $\Delta f = f_k - f_c$. The measurements were made using $f_c = 9522.4$ Mc. The data were obtained by Mr. J. F. Itzel, Jr.

B. Noise Sources

In the previous section, the magnitude of the ESR signal detected on the crystal (or bolometer) was discussed for several experimental arrangements. The factor which determines the sensitivity of a spectrometer is the signal-to-noise ratio, and so the present section will discuss the various types of noise that are capable of effecting this ratio (see RLS-24). Obvious noise sources such as the lack of voltage regulation and mechanical transients will not be mentioned. The next section will discuss the signal-to-noise ratio itself.

Johnson Noise: The available noise power or Johnson noise dN arising from a resistor radiating into a "cold" or noiseless load at a temperature T is (RLS-16, p. 11)

$$dN = kT\Delta f \tag{1}$$

where k is Boltzmann's constant and Δf is the band-width in cps. A crystal rectifier generates more noise than a resistor, and so its noise power is characterized by the noise temperature t as discussed in Sec. 11-D.

Vacuum Tube Noise: Shot effect noise arises in vacuum tubes as a result of randomness in the emission of electrons by the filament. Partition noise results from randomness in the partition of the total current among the electrodes. Other noise sources include the flicker effect, induced grid noise, and positive ion fluctuations, as discussed in RLS-24, Chap. 4.

Detector Noise: A bolometer detector produces Johnson noise $dN = kT\Delta f$ while a crystal detector produces the noise power $dN = tkT\Delta f$, where the dimensionless "noise temperature" t exceeds one. The excess noise in a crystal is inversely proportional to the modulation frequency f_{mod} [Miller (1947)], and this may be expressed analytically by writing

$$t - 1 = F(P)/f_{\mathrm{mod}} \tag{2}$$

The term $F(P)$ is a quadratic function of the power in the microwatt region and a linear function of the power in the milliwatt and watt region, as discussed in Sec. 11-D [e.g., eqs. (11-D-3), (11-D-4), and (11-D-5)]. In a superheterodyne spectrometer the second detector sometimes introduces appreciable noise. Klystron noise suppression in a balanced mixer is discussed in Sec. 11-E. A comparison of crystals and bolometers is given by Long (1960).

Klystron Noise: The noise figure F of a klystron is related to noise power dN in the frequency interval Δf by [*RLS*-7, p. 472; *RLS*-24, p. 113; Feher (1957)]

$$dN = FkT\Delta f \tag{3}$$

and this may be rearranged to

$$\tfrac{1}{2}F = \tfrac{1}{2}(dN/P_w)(P_w/kT\Delta f) = sP_w \tag{4}$$

in terms of the klystron power output P_w. Feher (1957) quotes the values of s shown in Table 14–1 corresponding to the side band noise for three klystrons at an intermediate frequency of 60 Mc. Note that the relative klystron noise decreases in going to higher modes. FM klystron noise is considerably more troublesome than AM noise. Kuper and Waltz (1945) found that a 3-cm klystron produced between 10^{-12} and 10^{-11} W of noise within a 2.5-Mc band-width located 30 Mc away from the klystron frequency. There is a considerable decrease in the klystron noise output in going from an intermediate frequency of 30 Mc to one of 90 Mc. At 90 Mc, the klystron noise was sufficiently low so as not to increase the effective crystal noise temperature, while the reverse was true at 30 Mc (*RLS*-24, p. 113). There are very few data of this type available on modern klystrons (see *RLS*-11, p. 276).

TABLE 14–1

Ratio s of the Noise Figure $(dN/2kT\Delta f)$ to the Incident Klystron Power P_w for Several Klystrons

Klystron	Klystron mode	Parameter s, W^{-1}
723A[a]	—	5000
V-153[b]	Higher	1000
V-153[b]	Lower	3000
X-13[b]	Higher	200
X-13[b]	Lower	400

[a] From *RSL*-7, p. 475.
[b] From Feher (1957).

A microwave generator such as a klystron will produce a great deal of noise if its supply voltages are not maintained at constant values. The klystron output is most sensitive to fluctuations in the reflector voltage, and least sensitive to variations in the filament supply, with variations of the beam or accelerator voltage in an intermediate category. Sections 6-G and 6-H discuss klystron power supplies and stabilization schemes.

Feher (1957) points out that, for some common operating conditions, noise voltages which result from frequency instabilities enter as a first order effect when one is tuned to the dispersion mode χ', and as a second order effect when one is tuned to the absorption mode χ''. An overcoupled cavity is less sensitive than an undercoupled one to this source of noise. The original article should be consulted for further details.

Amplifier Noise: An amplifier will amplify the impressed signal plus its accompanying noise, and in addition it will add some noise of its own. Sometimes noise is generated in the i.f. receiver. This will be discussed in the next section.

Cavity Vibrations: One should be sure of having a sufficiently rigid mounting of the resonant cavity to avoid vibrations which will increase the noise level. It is particularly important to make sure that all of the screws are tight, etc. Another noise source arises from eddy currents generated in the cavity walls by a high frequency modulation signal. Mechanical vibrations can be produced by an interaction of these currents with the applied magnetic field. The amplitude of this interaction is approximately proportional to the applied field strength, and the frequency of vibration is the modulation frequency or a harmonic thereof. It will effect the recorder trace by producing a continuous shift of the baseline. Amplitude and phase shifts may also occur. This interference may be minimized in a rectangular cavity by properly orienting it relative to the magnetic field, or by using a glass cavity coated with silver to a thickness which is much greater than the microwave skin depth but much less than the modulation skin depth, as suggested by Feher (1957). Vibrations in unsupported thin cavity walls may be damped out by a thick coat of cement or other dielectric material.

At high modulation amplitudes, the eddy currents in the cavity walls will heat the cavity and shift its frequency. Sometimes, it is necessary to await the establishment of thermal equilibrium at the high modulation amplitude to obviate a sloping background signal. In low temperature experiments, this heat dissipation effect may boil off refrigerant excessively.

Spin Noise: Bonnet (1961) suggested that statistical fluctuations in the magnetization may give rise to noise peaked near the resonant frequency.

C. Signal-to-Noise Ratio

The sensitivity of an ESR spectrometer is proportional to the ratio of the signal amplitude to the noise amplitude on a recorder or oscilloscope. The results of the last section will be applied toward a determination of the minimum detectable rf susceptibility with various types of detecting systems. This will provide us with the tools needed for deriving a general formula for computing the number of spins in a sample. The derivation itself will be postponed until the next section. In this section and the remainder of the chapter, we will assume that the resonant cavity is properly matched to the transmission line.

As the noise and the signal proceed from the generator through various networks, the ratio of the incremental noise power dN to the signal power S increases because of the extra noise generated by the networks themselves. The noise power is written as a differential dN because it corresponds to noise in the band-width Δf centered at the signal frequency f_m, while the signal S is ordinarily at only one frequency (e.g., the modulation frequency). The ratio of dN to S at the output of a network dN_1/S_1 is related to the corresponding ratio dN_0/S_0 at the input by (RLS-16, Sec. 1.4)

$$dN_1/S_1 = F_1 \, (dN_0/S_0) \tag{1}$$

where $F_1 \geqslant 1$ is the noise figure of the network. For a network without any internal sources of noise, $F_1 = 1$ since both the noise and the signal undergo equal amplification at the gain G_1

$$G_1 = S_1/S_0 \tag{2}$$

As a result, at a detection and amplification temperature T_d,

$$dN_1 = F_1 G_1 dN_0 = F_1 G_1 k T_d \Delta f \tag{3}$$

$$= G_1 k T_d \Delta f + (F_1 - 1) \, G_1 k T_d \Delta f \tag{4}$$

where we equated the input noise power dN_0 to the Johnson noise $kT_d\Delta f$. This equation means that the network amplifies the input noise $kT_d\Delta f$ by its gain G_1, and in addition it adds the noise $(F_1 - 1) G_1kT_d\Delta f$ to the signal.

The overall or integrated noise figure N_1 of the network is obtained by integrating over all frequencies

$$N_1 = \int_0^\infty F_1 G_1 kT_d df \tag{5}$$

The noise power that would have appeared at the output of an ideal or noiseless network is

$$\int_0^\infty G_1 kT_d df$$

so we write

$$\langle F_1 \rangle = \frac{\displaystyle\int_0^\infty F G_1 kT_d df}{\displaystyle\int_0^\infty G_1 kT_d df} \tag{6}$$

The effective noise band-width B is defined by

$$B = \frac{1}{G_{\max}} \int_0^\infty G df \tag{7}$$

For two networks in series, the second network with the noise figure F_2 and gain G_2 will amplify its input noise dN_1 by the gain G_2, and in addition, it will add the noise $(F_2 - 1) G_2 kT_d df$ to the signal. As a result, the output noise power dN_2 from the second network has the form

$$dN_2 = G_2 dN_1 + (F_2 - 1) G_2 kT_d\Delta f \tag{8}$$

and using eq. (3) we may write

$$dN_2 = [F_1 + (F_2 - 1)/G_1] G_1 G_2 kT_d\Delta f \tag{9}$$

$$= F_{12} G_1 G_2 kT_d\Delta f \tag{10}$$

where F_{12} is the overall noise figure

$$F_{12} = F_1 + (F_2 - 1)/G_1 \qquad (11)$$

For n cascaded sections

$$dN_n = F_{12,\ldots,n} G_1 G_2 \ldots G_n k T_d \Delta f \qquad (12)$$

and eq. (11) can be generalized to

$$F_{12,\ldots,n} = F_1 + (F_2 - 1)/G_1 + (F_3 - 1)/G_1 G_2$$
$$+ \ldots + (F_n - 1)/G_1 G_2 \ldots G_{n-1} \qquad (13)$$

Thus after any high gain network, the overall noise figure is not appreciably influenced by additional networks, even though their individual noise figures are relatively high. We can immediately see the advantage of using a maser preamplifier because it introduces a gain G_1 with a noise figure F_1 close to one.

In an ordinary spectrometer random fluctuations in the source and microwave components result in an input noise figure $F_K > 1$ before the signal reaches the detector. Hence the noise power dN_K incident on the detector is given by $(F_1 = F_K; G_1 = G_K \cong 1)$

$$dN_K = F_K k T_d \Delta f \qquad (14)$$

from eq. (3) since the gain G_K before reaching the detector is assumed to be close to unity. The output noise power from the detector dN_d depends upon the detector noise figure F_d and upon the detector gain G_d. These quantities may be used to replace F_2 and G_2 in eq. (10), but it is more customary to characterize detectors by their noise temperature t defined by

$$t = G_d F_d = G_2 F_2 \qquad (15)$$

and the insertion loss L which is the reciprocal of the conversion gain G_d

$$L = 1/G_d \qquad (16)$$

Upon placing these relations in eq. (9), we obtain for the noise power at the output of the detector

$$dN_d = (F_K/L + t - 1/L) \, kT_d\Delta f \tag{17}$$

From eqs. (12) and (13) we obtain for the noise power dN_{amp} at the output of the preamplifier ($F_{amp} = F_3$; $G_{amp} = G_3$)

$$dN_{amp} = (F_K/L + t - 1/L + F_{amp} - 1) \, G_{amp} \, kT_d\Delta f \tag{18}$$

Now that the noise output from the preamplifier has been evaluated, we will consider the ESR signal under ideal conditions. For the linear detector with the reflection cavity, we have the magnitude

$$\Delta E_r = \tfrac{1}{2} \chi'' \eta Q_u E \tag{19}$$

where the incident power is

$$P_w = E^2/4R_0 \tag{20}$$

For the limit of detectability χ''_{min}, we equate the ESR signal ΔE_r with the RMS voltage across a terminating resistance R_0 on a transmission line of characteristic impedance R_0

$$\Delta E_r = (4R_0 kT_d\Delta f)^{1/2} \tag{21}$$

with the result that

$$\chi''_{min} = (2/\eta Q_u) \, (kT_d\Delta f/P_w)^{1/2} = \chi''_{min\,TH} \tag{22}$$

One should bear in mind that χ'' is in MKS units, and the right hand side of eq. (22) must be divided by 4π to convert it to the usual cgs units. Feher's expression for eq. (22) has the factor $2^{1/2}$ in the numerator. Throughout this chapter we will freely quote Feher's results without bothering to correct for this factor. We shall see in the next section that it is more convenient to replace P_w in eq. (22) and the subsequent ones by an expression containing the energy density $(1/2\mu) \langle H_1{}^2 \rangle_w$ immediately outside the cavity iris. At X band we have the typical values $Q_u = 5000$, $\Delta f = 0.1$ cps, $P_w = 10^{-2}$W, $V_c \approx 10$ cm^3, and $\eta = 2V_s/V_c$ [eq. (8-H-20)]. Hence [Feher (1957)]

$$\chi''_{min} \, V_s \approx \frac{8\pi \times 10^{-15}}{P_w{}^{1/2}} \tag{23}$$

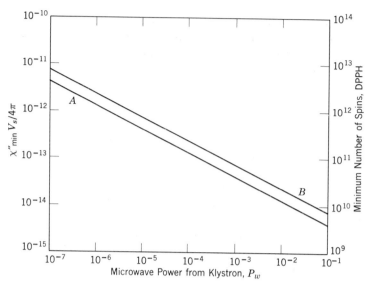

Fig. 14–4. (A) The minimum detectable number of DPPH spins; (B) the minimum detectable rf susceptibility $\chi''_{min} V_s/4$ as a function of the applied microwave power P_w in watts. The curves correspond to the conditions $Q_u = 5000$, $\Delta f = 0.1$ sec,$^{-1}$ $T = 300°$K, $\omega/\Delta\omega = 1500$, and no saturation [Feher (1957)].

This expression is plotted in Fig. 14–4 as a function of the microwave power P_w in watts. Similar expressions are obtained for the other cavity arrangements.

The minimum voltage ΔE_R will become $(G_{amp}/L)\ \Delta E_R$ at the output of the preamplifier, and so we may take into account the noise introduced by the detector and preamplifier by replacing (G_{amp}/L) ΔE_R from eq. (22) by dN_{amp} of eq. (18) to obtain

$$\chi''_{min\ OB} = \frac{2}{Q_u\eta} \left[(F_k - 1 + (t + F_{amp} - 1)\ L)\ \frac{kT_d\Delta f}{P_w} \right]^{1/2} \quad (24)$$

We denote χ''_{min} defined by eq. (22) as $\chi''_{min\ TH}$ and χ''_{min} defined by eq. (24) as $\chi''_{min\ OB}$, and consider the ratio $\chi''_{min\ OB}/\chi''_{min\ TH}$

$$\chi''_{min\ OB}/\chi''_{min\ TH} = [F_k - 1 + (t + F_{amp} - 1)L]^{1/2} \geqslant 1 \quad (25)$$

as a measure of the extent to which a spectrometer approaches the ideal sensitivity where

$$L = F_k = F_{amp} = t = 1 \text{ and } \chi''_{min\ OB} = \chi''_{min\ TH}$$

The response laws and noise temperature relations found in Secs. 11-B and 11-D may be used to evaluate these last two expressions, and this was done by Feher (1957). For bolometer detection employing a balanced mixer

$$\chi''_{\min \text{ OB}}/\chi''_{\min \text{ TH}} \sim 4 \tag{26}$$

as may be seen by consulting Fig. 11–2. A complicated expression is required for the simple bolometer curve on this figure.

Figure 11–10 shows the ratio of the observed to the theoretical minimum susceptibility for three arrangements of the crystal detector. In the simple straight detection scheme, the bridge is adjusted so that the microwave power P_d that is incident on the crystal equals 10% of the microwave power P_w that is incident on the cavity. We assume $F_{\text{amp}} \sim 1$ which approximates a step-up transformer. For this arrangement at a modulation frequency of 1000 cps we obtain [Feher (1957)]

$$\frac{\chi''_{\min \text{ OB}}}{\chi''_{\min \text{ TH}}} = \begin{cases} \left(\dfrac{1 + 5 \times 10^9 P_w^2}{50 P_w}\right)^{1/2} & \text{quadratic} \\ (3 \times 10^7 P_w)^{1/2} & \text{linear} \end{cases} \tag{27}$$

for the square law (quadratic) and linear regions respectively of the IN23C crystalline response. If optimum bucking is employed, then the actual power level at the crystal is maintained equal to the minimum value in the simple detection scheme of Fig. 11–10, and this entails biasing the crystal with a power $P_B \sim 1.4 \times 10^{-6}$ W. Using the relations of Sec. 11-D, one may show that

$$\frac{\chi''_{\min \text{ OB}}}{\chi''_{\min \text{ TH}}} = \left[2S'\left(\frac{\gamma F_{\text{amp}}}{f}\right)^{1/2}\right]^{1/2} \approx \frac{300}{f^{1/4}} = 55 \tag{28}$$

for the typical modulation frequency of 1 kc. The optimum bucking power is proportional to the square root of the modulation frequency. Negative bucking or the reduction of the power ratio P_d/P_w when $P_w > P_B$ is easily accomplished by using the slide screw turner to bring the bridge closer to balance. When $P_B > P_w$, then it is necessary to employ an arrangement like that shown in Fig. 11–12 to obtain the necessary power at the crystal. When making saturation curve measurements at very low powers (e.g., $P_w < P_B$) in order to determine the relaxation times T_1 and T_2, it is often more convenient to work with $P_d < P_B$ on an ordinary ESR spectrometer, and thereby sacrifice some sensitivity. This avoids the necessity of setting up an arrangement such as that shown in Fig. 11–12. An examination of Fig. 11–10 reveals that when $P_d = 0.1 \, P_B$, the sensitivity $\chi''_{min \, OB}/\chi''_{min \, TH}$ decreases by less than a factor of two, but this allows the power measurements to be conveniently made an order of magnitude lower than is possible with the optimum leakage condition $P_d = P_B$. Indeed, by sacrificing a factor of ten in sensitivity one can work conveniently at a power level 1/200th of the value that can be reached with the setting $P_d = P_B$.

A superheterodyne spectrometer ordinarily operates at 30 or 60 Mc, and thereby renders negligible the generation of crystal noise. For this case, Feher estimates for a balanced mixer operating in the linear region of the crystal

$$\chi''_{min \, OB}/\chi''_{min \, TH} \sim [L(t + F_{i.f.} - 1)]^{1/2} \sim 5 \qquad (29)$$

which is independent of the microwave power, where $F_{i.f.}$ is the noise figure of the 30- or 60-Mc receiver. The klystron noise tends to cancel and the ESR signal adds in the balanced mixer. Note that the sensitivity obtained with superheterodyne detection is comparable to that obtained by using a 100-kc field modulation scheme. Bolometer detection also gives about the same sensitivity. The 100-kc field modulation arrangement is easier to set up and operate than the superheterodyne one, but it is not useful for detecting resonant lines that are much less than 100 mG wide. Hausser (1962) has observed lines as narrow as 17 mG.

Frater (1965) designed a synchronous demodulator which subtracts a modulated microwave signal from a calibrated microwave source and thereby increases the signal-to-noise ratio. A balanced mixer produces the same result and is more useful in ESR applications.

Teaney, Klein, and Portis (1961) compared the sensitivity of a superheterodyne spectrometer to that of the bimodal spectrometer discussed in Sec. 13-Q. They studied several superheterodyne receivers and found the noise figures shown on Fig. 14–5 for video

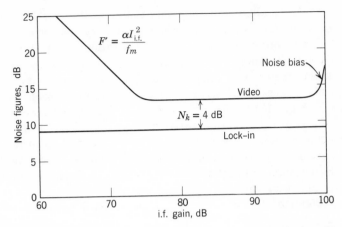

Fig. 14–5.   Noise figures for superheterodyne receivers employing video and homodyne (phase-sensitive) detection of the intermediate frequency. The improved noise figure of the lock-in scheme results from the suppression of carrier noise.   In the video system, the excess noise F at low i.f. gain results from flicker noise generated by the i.f. current in the mixer diodes, while that at high i.f. gain arises from the audio frequency beat between noise components at the second detector [Teaney, Klein, and Portis (1961)].

(homodyne) and lock-in detection.   At low powers the conventional superheterodyne spectrometer produced a signal-to-noise ratio proportional to the square root of the microwave power, as expected, but the sensitivity fell off above a klystron power of 10 mW in accordance with Fig. 14–6.   The decrease in sensitivity at high power levels is the result of random frequency modulation which disturbs the bridge balance.   This source of noise is more troublesome when detecting dispersion than it is with absorption.   It increases with the microwave power because of the bridge being brought closer to match when it is tuned to maintain the optimum power P_d at the detector.   The bimodal spectrometer employs a bimodal cavity [Portis and Teaney (1958)] whose balance is completely independent of the frequency.   As a result, this source of noise is minimized, and the bimodal spectrometer maintains its expected sensitivity at high powers, as shown in Fig. 14–7.   Brodwin and Burgess (1963) discuss an induction spectrometer which uses an H plane microwave junction in lieu of a bimodal cavity.

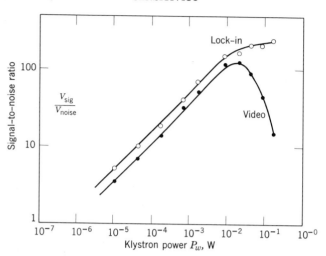

Fig. 14–6. Signal-to-noise ratios for a bridge spectrometer. The linear parts of the curves correspond to a noise figure of 9 dB for lock-in detection and 13 dB for video detection [Teaney, Klein, and Portis (1961)].

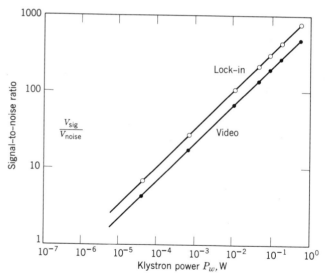

Fig. 14–7. Signal-to-noise ratios for a bimodal cavity spectrometer. The noise figures are the same as those noted on Fig. 14–6 for the bridge spectrometer [Teaney, Klein, and Portis (1961)].

Gozzini and Iannuzzi (1960) proposed the use of sixteen microwave spectrometer systems connected in parallel and fed by the same source in order to achieve a factor of four gain in sensitivity. They reason that the sensitivity is proportional to the square root of the number of systems. It is interesting to note that this sedecuple arrangement did not burgeon forth from an opulent American laboratory. For the ESR case, it seems to the author that in the absence of saturation one could achieve the same factor of four gain in sensitivity by sending all of the microwave power down only one channel instead of scattering it among sixteen. Mahendru and Parshad (1964) discuss the merit of using several parallel crystal detectors when operating at high microwave power levels.

Hedvig (1959) used a dielectric slab in a rectangular resonant cavity to appreciably increase the filling factor η and thereby enhance the sensitivity. Section 8-I gives the theory behind this technique. An enormous increase in sensitivity is obtained by making a properly shaped single crystal into a dielectric resonant cavity as discussed by Okaya (1963) (cf. Sec. 8-L).

Several detailed theoretical discussions of the sensitivity of ESR spectrometers have appeared recently [e.g., see Bresler, Saminskii, and Kazbekov (1958); Goldsborough and Mandel (1960); Smidt (1960); Müller (1960); Atsarkin, Zhabotinskii, and Frantsesson (1962); Muromtsev, Piskunov, and Verein (1962); Wilmshurst, Gambling, and Ingram (1962); Misra (1963); Schneider (1963); Valeriu and Pascaru (1963); Payne (1964); Buckmaster and Dering (1965); Tsung-tang, Wen-chia, Lien-fong, and Tin-fong (1965)]. Various spectrometer arrangements are discussed and their sensitivities are compared by Faulkner (1964).

D. Number of Spins

The results of the last section may be combined with the Curie law to provide a general formula for the number of spins in the sample. The dependence of the minimum detectable number of spins on various parameters such as the instrumental conditions (e.g., frequency), the spin system's environment (e.g., temperature), and its characteristics (e.g., line-width) will now be discussed in detail.

In the previous section we derived the expression [eq. (14-C–24)]

$$\chi_{\min} = \frac{2}{Q_u \eta} \left[\frac{F_k - 1 + (t + F_{\mathrm{amp}} - 1) L}{P_w} (kT_d \Delta f) \right]^{1/2} \tag{1}$$

for the minimum detectable rf susceptibility. The rf susceptibility $\chi''(\omega)$ is related to the static susceptibility χ_0 by the Bloch equation

$$\chi''(\omega) = \frac{\frac{1}{2}\chi_0\omega_0 T_2}{1 + (\omega - \omega_0)^2 T_2^2} \tag{2}$$

This expression reaches its maximum value at $\omega = \omega_0$

$$\chi''(\omega_0) = \frac{\chi_0\omega_0}{3^{1/2}\Delta\omega_{pp}} \tag{3}$$

where we have replaced the spin-spin relaxation time T_2 by its equivalent reciprocal line-width $\Delta\omega$

$$T_2 = \frac{2}{\Delta\omega_{1/2}} = \frac{2}{3^{1/2}\Delta\omega_{pp}} \tag{4}$$

The static susceptibility χ_0 is related to the g factor, spin S, and sample temperature T_s by the Curie-Weiss law*

$$\chi_0 = \frac{Ng^2\beta^2 S(S + 1)}{3V_sk(T_s + \Delta)} \tag{5}$$

where N is the number of spins in the sample of volume V_s. When the Weiss constant Δ vanishes, we have the Curie law*

$$\chi_0 = \frac{Ng^2\beta^2 S(S + 1)}{3V_skT_s} \tag{6}$$

From eqs. (1), (3), and (6), the minimum detectable number of spins for systems obeying the Bloch equations and Curie law is [Poole (1958)]

$$N_{\min} = \frac{6V_skT_s}{Q_u\eta g^2\beta^2 S(S+1)} \left(\frac{\Delta\omega_{pp}}{\omega_0}\right)$$

$$\times \left[\frac{F_k - 1 + (t + F_{\text{amp}} - 1)\,L}{P_w} (3kT_d\Delta f)\right]^{1/2} \tag{7}$$

To work in magnetic field units one merely replaces the ratio $\Delta\omega_{pp}/\omega_0$ by $\Delta H_{pp}/H_0$. If all of the constants are combined into one

* This is for free radicals and the first transition series. For rare earths, replace S by J.

constant K, and P_w is replaced by $P_w \omega_0^2$ for reasons discussed below, then eq. (7) simplifies to

$$N_{\min} = \frac{V_s T_s K}{Q_u \eta g^2 S(S+1)\omega_0} \left(\frac{\Delta H_{pp}}{H_0}\right)$$

$$\times \left[\frac{T_d \Delta f}{P_w} [F_k - 1 + (t + F_{\text{amp}} - 1) L]\right]^{1/2} \quad (8)$$

One wishes to make $N_{\min}$ as small as possible for maximum sensitivity. The number of spins in the sample N_{spin} is given by

$$N_{\text{spin}} = y_m' N_{\min} \quad (9)$$

where y_m' is the signal-to-noise ratio.

For the three typical detection schemes discussed in Sec. 14-C we have

$$F_k - 1 + (t + F_{\text{amp}} - 1) L$$

$$\begin{aligned} &= 16 && \text{bolometer} \\ &= \left(\frac{1}{500\, P_d} + 10^9 P_d\right) && \text{square law} \quad \left.\begin{aligned}&\\&\end{aligned}\right\}\text{IN23C} \quad (10) \\ &= 3 \times 10^8 P_d && \text{linear} \qquad\qquad \text{crystal} \end{aligned}$$

where P_d is the "leakage" power incident on the crystal. In Sec. 8-H we found that

$$V_s/\eta = (\text{const}) \; V_c \quad (11)$$

where the dimensionless constant is of the order of unity. The factor $g^2 S(S+1)$ must be taken into account when one compares spectra from two spin systems which differ in their g factors and spins. Decreasing the sample temperature T_s increases the Q so that there are two reasons why the sensitivity increases with decreasing temperature. Decreasing the temperature of the detector also increases the sensitivity, but this is not ordinarily done in practice. Decreasing the detection–amplification band-width Δf by means of a narrow band amplifier and a lock-in detector can produce a pronounced improvement in sensitivity. This is elaborated upon in Secs. 14-F and 14-I. For unsaturated lines, $N_{\min}$ is inversely proportional to the square root of the microwave power while above saturation N_{min} increases with increasing power. Thus oversaturation decreases the sensitivity.

The dependence of the sensitivity upon the frequency can be clarified by grouping into a constant K all of the terms in eq. (7) which are independent of the frequency. It is assumed that the detection and amplification stages are in this category. In addition, the resonant cavity has its dimensions scaled in proportion to the wavelength, and the same sample is in the same relative position in the cavity. As a result eq. (8) with $\Delta\omega_{pp}/\omega_0$ simplifies to

$$N_{min} = \frac{KV_s}{Q_u\eta\omega_0^2(P_w)^{1/2}} \tag{12}$$

This expression has the extra ω_0 which we added to eq. (8) in order to take into account the dependence of the energy density (i.e., $\langle H^2 \rangle_w$) in the waveguide outside the cavity iris on the total microwave power P_w. Before proceeding further, we shall justify this modification of Feher's results.

It is the average value of H_1^2 at the sample $\langle H_1^2 \rangle_s$ which produces ESR absorption, and this is related to the root mean square value of H_1^2 in the cavity $\langle H_1^2 \rangle_c$ through the filling factor η. Equation (8-H-74) relates $\langle H_1^2 \rangle_c$ to the rms rf magnetic field outside the cavity $\langle H^2 \rangle_w$ that results from Poynting's vector $\frac{1}{2}\mathbf{E} \times \mathbf{H}$

$$\langle H_1^2 \rangle_c = Q_L(V_w/V_c) \langle H^2 \rangle_w \tag{13}$$

We will of course maintain the ratio V_w/V_c constant when we vary the frequency. For a rectangular waveguide with the large dimension $a = \frac{1}{2}\lambda_g$ ($2a = d$) and small dimension b we obtain from eqs. (8-H-66) and (8-H-70) the following expression for the microwave power P_w incident on the cavity

$$P_w = abZ_0 \langle H^2 \rangle_w \tag{14}$$

Since the waveguide dimensions a and b are each inversely proportional to the frequency it follows that

$$\langle H^2 \rangle_w \propto \omega_0^2 P_w \tag{15}$$

which justifies the extra ω_0 that we inserted into eq. (8).

The physical significance of eq. (15) may be illustrated from another point of view. The total power incident on the cavity per cycle is given by $(2\pi/\omega_0) P_w$

$$(2\pi/\omega_0) P_w = 2\pi(ab/\omega_0) Z_0 \langle H^2 \rangle_w \quad \text{J/cycle} \tag{16}$$

and at match it all enters and is dissipated in the cavity. Since Q is defined as 2π times the ratio of the total stored energy U to the total energy dissipated per cycle [eq. (8-A-13)], we have

$$U = (Q_L/\omega_0) P_w \tag{17}$$

By definition

$$U = \frac{1}{2} \mu \int_{\text{cavity}} H_1^2 dV = \frac{1}{2} \mu V_c \langle H_1^2 \rangle_c \tag{18}$$

and therefore

$$\langle H_1^2 \rangle_c = \frac{2Q_L}{\mu V_c \omega_0} P_w \tag{19}$$

in agreement with a similar expression of Zverov (1961). The use of eq. (13) allows us to write

$$\langle H^2 \rangle_w = \frac{2}{\mu V_w \omega_0} P_w \tag{20}$$

which has the same frequency dependence as eq. (14) since both ab and $V_w \omega_0$ are inversely proportional to ω_0^2.

Another way to arrive at this proportionality is to say that $\langle H^2 \rangle_w$ is proportional to Poynting's vector $\frac{1}{2}\mathbf{E} \times \mathbf{H}$, and that P_w is proportional to Poynting's vector times the waveguide cross sectional area.

Constant Incident Power P_w: Now we return to the discussion of the frequency dependence of $N_{\min}$ in accordance with eq. (12). If the sample size is scaled to the same extent as the sample dimensions, then the filling factor η remains constant. We saw in Secs. 8-C and 8-D that Q_u equals a geometric factor times λ/δ. Scaling the cavity dimensions produces a Q_u proportional to λ/δ which is inversely proportional to $\omega_0^{1/2}$, so we obtain for the minimum detectable spin concentration N_{min}/V_s (spins/cm^3 or moles/l) at a constant micro-wave power P_w

$$N_{min}/V_s \propto 1/\omega_0^{3/2} \tag{21}$$

Therefore for a constant filling factor η and microwave power level P_w, a factor of two increase in frequency produces about a factor of three increase [i.e., $2(2^{1/2})$] in sensitivity. This case corresponds to the usual experimental situation in which there is plenty of sample available, and the limiting factor is the amount that can be put into the cavity without appreciably lowering the Q. In a practical case, the sample dielectric loss may be frequency-sensitive, and the same filling factor may not be optimum at both frequencies.

If the sample is small and cannot conveniently be varied in size (e.g., a small single crystal), then we assume that the filling factor η is proportional to V_s/V_c independent of the frequency, which gives

$$N_{min} = KV_c/Q_u\omega_0^2 \tag{22}$$

Since the cavity volume V_c is proportional to ω_0^{-3} we obtain

$$N_{min} \propto 1/\omega_0^{9/2} \tag{23}$$

Thus for a constant sample size and a constant microwave power, it is very advantageous to go to higher frequencies. The physical reason for this is that at the higher frequency the energy density in the cavity increases and in addition the sample fills a much greater percentage of the cavity volume, which results in a greatly enhanced filling factor. A factor of two increase in frequency provides a factor of twenty-two increase in sensitivity.

Constant rf Field at Sample; It was shown in Sec. 18-C that there is an optimum value of $\langle H_1^2 \rangle_s$ at the onset of saturation which produces the greatest signal-to-noise ratio. If there is enough power available to saturate the spin system at two microwave frequencies, then the maximum sensitivity for each frequency will correspond to the same $\langle H_1^2 \rangle_s$ value. To attain this condition, each microwave generator or klystron will be set at the appropriate power level P_w. This may be deduced by noting that for the same sample–cavity relationship (except for a scaling factor) the ratio $\langle H_1^2 \rangle_s/ \langle H_1^2 \rangle_c$ will be independent of frequency.   From eq. (19), we see that it is necessary to maintain a constant ratio $(Q_l P_w / V_c \omega_0)$ in order to preserve the same $\langle H_1{}^2 \rangle_s$ at the sample.   As a result, eq. (12) gives

$$N_{\min} = \frac{KV_s}{\eta \omega_0{}^2 (V_c Q_u \omega_0)^{1/2}}$$ (24)

and for the two cases of a constant ratio of V_s / V_c and a constant V_s we obtain

$$N_{\min}/V_s \propto 1/\omega_0{}^{3/4}$$ (25)

$$N_{\min} \propto 1/\omega_0{}^{15/4}$$ (26)

Constant Incident Poynting Vector: Feher (1957) compared sensitivities for the case in which $\langle H^2 \rangle_w$ is kept constant, and he obtained the resulting equations for $V_s / V_c = \text{const}$ and $V_s = \text{const}$, respectively [see eq. (15)]

$$N_{\min}/V_s \propto 1/\omega_0{}^{1/2}$$ (27)

$$N_{\min} \propto 1/\omega_0{}^{7/2}$$ (28)

The results obtained for these six cases are summarized in Table 14–2.

The effect of modulating the magnetic field at an amplitude $H_{\mod}$ much less than the line-width ΔH_{pp} is to produce a resonant line whose amplitude is proportional to $H_{\mod}$.   When $H_{\mod}$ greatly exceeds ΔH_{pp}, then further increases produce a weaker ESR line. One may approximate the effects of $H_{\mod}$ on the sensitivity by multiplying eq. (7) or (8) by $(\Delta H_{pp}/H_{\mod})$ when $H_{\mod} \ll \Delta H_{pp}$ as is done explicitly in eq. (31).   Section 10-E gives further details on this effect.

The area A of an ESR resonance absorption is given by (Table 20–5)

$$A = \begin{cases} 1.06 \; y_m \Delta H_{1/2} & \text{Gaussian} & (28a) \\ 1.57 \; y_m \Delta H_{1/2} & \text{Lorentzian} & (28b) \\ \Lambda y_m \Delta H_{1/2} & \text{general} & (28c) \end{cases}$$

TABLE 14-2
Dependence of the Minimum Detectable Concentration (N_{min}/V_s) and the
Minimum Detectable Number of Spins (N_{min}) on the Microwave Frequency ω_0

Spectrometer conditions	N_{min}/V_s (η = const)	N_{min} (V_s = const)
Constant microwave power P_w	$1/\omega_0^{3/2}$	$1/\omega_0^{9/2}$
Constant energy density at sample ($<H_1^2>_s$ = const) ($<H_1^2>_c$ = const)	$1/\omega_0^{3/4}$	$1/\omega_0^{15/4}$
Constant energy density in waveguide outside sample ($\frac{1}{2}\,\mathbf{E} \times \mathbf{H}$ = const) ($<H_w^2>$ = const)	$1/\omega_0^{1/2}$	$1/\omega_0^{7/2}$

where y_m is the peak amplitude, and Λ is a general shape factor.
For a first derivative spectrum, Table 20-4 gives

$$\Lambda = \begin{cases} 1.03\ y_m'(\Delta H_{pp})^2 & \text{Gaussian} & (29a) \\ 3.63\ y_m'(\Delta H_{pp})^2 & \text{Lorentzian} & (29b) \\ \Lambda' y_m'(\Delta H_{pp})^2 & \text{general} & (29c) \end{cases}$$

where y_m' is the derivative amplitude and Λ' is a function characteristic of the line-shape. The sensitivity relations such as eq. (8) developed earlier in this section were for a Lorentzian line-shape. They may be generalized by multiplying the righthand side by $\Lambda/1.57$ for absorption lines and $\Lambda'/3.64$ for first derivative lines as is done in eq. (31). This is important when comparing two resonances with different line-shapes.

When the resonance consists of several hyperfine components, we may take this into account by a summing over the signal-to-noise ratios y_i of the component lines $\Sigma y_i'$. Let

$$D_m = \frac{1}{y_m'} \sum y_i' \qquad (30)$$

where y_m' is the signal-to-noise ratio of the strongest line, and D_m is the corresponding multiplicity factor. The parameter D is the amount by which the signal-to-noise ratio of the strongest hyperfine component must be multiplied to give the equivalent amplitude of the singlet which would result if all of the hfs collapsed to a single line of the same width. For n equally coupled protons or other spin $\frac{1}{2}$ nuclei, we have the multiplicity factors shown in Table 14–3. These data assume fully resolved hyperfine components with a binomial intensity ratio.

TABLE 14–3

Multiplicity Factors D_m for n Fully Resolved Equally Coupled Nuclei with Nuclear Spin $I = \frac{1}{2}$ [Poole (1958)]

n	D_m	n	D_n
1	2.00	5	3.20
2	2.00	6	3.20
3	2.67	7	3.66
4	2.67	8	3.66

Hydrazyl (DPPH) in benzene solution has two equally coupled nitrogen nuclei with spin $I = 1$, and an intensity ratio $1:2:3:2:1$. Therefore its D_m value is 3. However, the first derivative lines overlap so that the minimum of one line is near the maximum of the next, and as a result all but the two outside components are considerably decreased in intensity. Consequently the measured D_m value is much greater than the calculated value. To circumvent this difficulty, one may use the outermost peak (line number 1) of the hfs since its amplitude is not effected by the overlap of the components. Its multiplicity factor D_1 is 9, which means that the amplitude of this first component is $1/9$ of the singlet amplitude that would result if I equaled zero for nitrogen. Knowing this enables the outside DPPH line to be used in checking ESR spectrometer sensitivity, as shown on Fig. 14–8.

The appropriate D value may be placed in the numerator of the righthand side of the sensitivity relations (χ''_{min} and N_{min}) to deduce N_{min} in the presence of hfs.

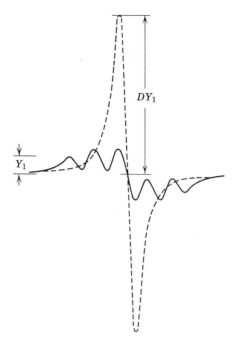

Fig. 14–8. Spectrum of DPPH showing the hypothetical singlet which would be obtained if $I = 0$ for N^{14}. The figure was prepared by O. F. Griffith III.

If the modulation amplitude, line-shape, and hyperfine structure (multiplicity factor) are taken into account, then eq. (8) will have the form

$$N_{\min} = \frac{V_s T_s DK}{Q_u \eta g^2 S(S+1)\,\omega_0}\left(\frac{\Delta H_{pp}}{H_0}\right)\left(\frac{\Delta H_{pp}}{H_{\mathrm{mod}}}\right)$$

$$\left(\frac{\Lambda'}{3.64}\right)\left[\frac{T_d \Delta f}{P_w}\,[F_k - 1 + (t + F_{\mathrm{amp}} - 1)\,L]\right]^{1/2} \quad (31)$$

for first derivative lines. If the sample is lossy, then Q_u in a sensitivity formula such as this should be replaced by Q_u' defined in Sec. 14-J. The number of spins in a sample N_{spin} is related to the minimum detectable number $N_{\min}$ by the signal-to-noise ratio y_m'

$$N_{\mathrm{spin}} = N_{\min} y_m' \quad (32)$$

In practice, the number of spins in a sample is often determined by comparing the sample under study with a standard sample. It is customary to carry out this comparison with the same spectrometer, so most of the terms in eq. (31) will be identical for both samples. Therefore one may write

$$
\frac{N_{\text{spin}}^A}{N_{\text{spin}}^B} = \frac{\dfrac{V_s^A D^A}{Q_u^A \eta^A (g^A)^2 S^A (S^A + 1)\,(P_w^A)^{1/2}}}{\dfrac{V_s^B D^B}{Q_u^B \eta^B (g^B)^2 S^B (S^B + 1)\,(P_w^B)^{1/2}}}
$$

$$
\times \frac{\left(\dfrac{\Delta H_{pp}^A}{H_0}\right)\left(\dfrac{\Delta H_{pp}^A}{H_{\text{mod}}^A}\right)\left(\dfrac{\Lambda'^A}{3.64}\right) y_m'^A}{\left(\dfrac{\Delta H_{pp}^B}{H_0}\right)\left(\dfrac{\Delta H_{pp}^B}{H_{\text{mod}}^B}\right)\left(\dfrac{\Lambda'^B}{3.64}\right) y_m'^B} \tag{33}
$$

where the subscripts A and B refer to the two types of spins. A comparison of this type is ordinarily carried out in the same sample tube ($\eta = $ const, $V_s = $ const), with a negligible change in Q ($Q_l = $ const), and at the same power level ($P_w = $ const) and modulation amplitude ($H_{\text{mod}} = $ const), so that one may simplify eq. (33) to

$$
\frac{N_{\text{spin}}^A}{N_{\text{spin}}^B} = \left(\frac{D^A}{D^B}\right)\left(\frac{g^B}{g^A}\right)^2 \left[\frac{S^B(S^B + 1)}{S^A(S^A + 1)}\right]
$$

$$
\times \left(\frac{\Delta H_{pp}^A}{\Delta H_{pp}^B}\right)^2 \left(\frac{\Lambda'^A}{\Lambda'^B}\right)\left(\frac{H_{\text{mod}}^B}{H_{\text{mod}}^A}\right)\left(\frac{y_m'^A}{y_m'^B}\right) \tag{34}
$$

This expression is simplified even further when both types of spins have the same spin S and g factor (e.g., when both are free radicals). The ratio ($y_m'^A / y_m'^B$) may be looked upon as the ratio of the amplitudes on the recorder.

E. Temperature

When a spin system is studied at a series of temperatures and microwave frequencies, it is often desirable to compare the resulting data with each other. In this section the ordinary ESR doublet is discussed in terms of its Boltzmann populations, and two graphs are presented to assist in comparing experimental data. The less common triplet state is treated from the same viewpoint, and the results are compared graphically to those obtained with the doublet.

Doublet State: For a spin system with $S = \frac{1}{2}$ the population of spins in the upper energy level n_2 will be related to the number in the lower energy level n_1 by the Boltzmann distribution

$$n_2 = n_1 \exp\left(-\Delta E/kT_2\right) \tag{1}$$

where the energy separation ΔE for the Zeeman term in the Hamiltonian for $g = 2$ has the value

$$\Delta E = \hbar\omega = g\beta H \sim \frac{1}{3} \text{ cm}^{-1} \sim 6.3 \times 10^{-24} \text{ J} \tag{2}$$

at X band (9.6 Gc). Since $k = 1.38 \times 10^{-23}$ J/deg, we obtain

$$n_2 = n_1 \exp\left(-0.46/T\right) \sim n_1\left(1 - 0.46/T\right) \tag{3}$$

where the binomial expansion is valid above liquid helium temperature. The ESR signal Y_D is proportional to the population difference $n_1 - n_2$, and this has the form

$$Y_D = Y_0\left(\frac{n_1 - n_2}{n_1 + n_2}\right) = Y_0\left[\frac{1 - \exp\left(-\hbar\omega/kT\right)}{1 + \exp\left(-\hbar\omega/kT\right)}\right] \tag{4}$$

where Y_0 is the signal amplitude at $T \to 0$. The temperature dependence of the ESR signal Y_D is shown in Figs. 14–9 and 14–10 for several typical microwave frequencies and for several typical magnetic field strengths (assuming $g = 2.0$ in the latter case). Note that at X band (10^4 Mc), it is necessary to lower the temperature to the liquid helium range to appreciably populate the lower Zeeman level and render the ratio Y_D/Y_0 greater than 10%.

At high temperatures ($\hbar\omega \ll kT$), the exponential term may be expanded in a power series, and the sensitivity becomes inversely proportional to the temperature. At low temperature ($\hbar\omega \gg kT$), the exponentials may be neglected, and the sensitivity becomes

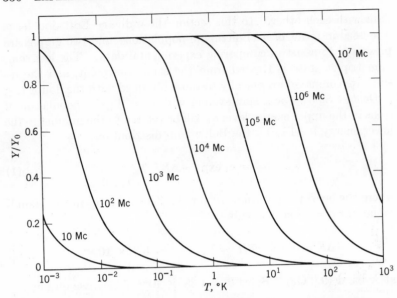

Fig. 14–9. Temperature dependence of the ESR amplitude $Y = Y_D$ relative to its value Y_0 at $T = 0$ for several microwave frequencies.

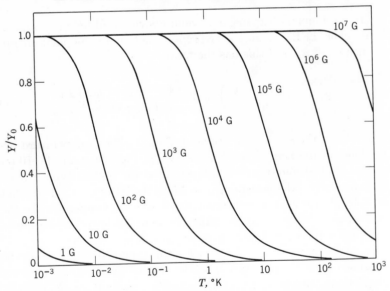

Fig. 14–10. Temperature dependence of the ESR amplitude $Y = Y_D$ relative to its value Y_0 at $T = 0$ at several magnetic field strengths for a g factor of 2.0.

independent of temperature. These limiting cases may be summarized by the relations

$$Y_D = (\hbar\omega/2kT)\, Y_0 = (g\beta H/2kT)\, Y_0 \qquad \hbar\omega \ll kT \qquad (5)$$

$$Y_D = Y_0 \qquad \hbar\omega \gg kT \qquad (6)$$

Equation (5) corresponds to almost every case discussed elsewhere in this book. In particular, the discussion in the last section is based entirely upon the Curie law (14-D-6) which assumes eq. (5).

Variations in the temperature will result in other more complicated effects which influence the sensitivity. As the temperature is lowered, the Q of the cavity will increase to render the system more sensitive. For liquid helium studies the spin lattice relaxation time of solids often becomes very long in accordance with eq. (18-E-1) or (18-E-2). This produces resonant lines which saturate at relatively low (e.g., microwatt) power levels [cf. eqs. (18-C-3) and (18-C-4)].

Triplet State: The paramagnetic absorption associated with a triplet state has been discussed by Bijl, Kainer, and Rose-Innes (1959). It corresponds to the energy level diagram (*b*) or (*c*) of Fig. 14–11. In the case of a *low lying triplet* (Fig. 14–11*b*), the ESR

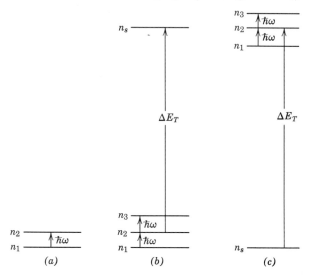

Fig. 14–11. Energy level diagrams for (*a*) a doublet, (*b*) a low lying triplet plus a singlet, and (*c*) a singlet plus a high lying triplet state. The symbol n_i refers to the population of the *i*th energy level.

signal arises from the two transitions $1 \to 2$ and $2 \to 3$, and its amplitude Y_{LT} is determined by the average populations as follows

$$Y_{LT} = Y_0 \left[\frac{n_1 - n_2}{n_1 + n_2 + n_3 + n_s} + \frac{n_2 - n_3}{n_1 + n_2 + n_3 + n_s} \right] \qquad (7)$$

$$\approx \frac{1 - \exp(-2\hbar\omega/kT}{1 + \exp(-\hbar\omega/kT) + \exp(-2\hbar\omega/kT + \exp(-\Delta E_T/kT)} Y_0 \qquad (8)$$

where the singlet population $n_s \ll n_1$ is neglected since $\Delta E_T \gg \hbar\omega$. Above the liquid helium temperature range $\hbar\omega \ll kT$ and

$$Y_{LT} \approx \frac{2\hbar\omega Y_0}{kT} \frac{1}{[3 + \exp(-\Delta E_T/kT)]} \qquad (9)$$

For a *high lying triplet* such as the one shown in Fig. 14–11c, one has from eq. (7)

$$Y_{HT} \approx \frac{[1 - \exp(-2\hbar\omega/kT)]}{1 + [1 + \exp(-\hbar\omega/kT) + \exp(-2\hbar\omega/kT)]}$$

$$\times \frac{\exp[(\hbar\omega - \Delta E_T)/kT]}{\exp[(\hbar\omega - \Delta E_T)/kT]} Y_0 \qquad (10)$$

$$\approx \frac{2\hbar\omega Y_0}{kT} \frac{1}{[3 + \exp(\Delta E_T/kT)]} \qquad (11)$$

since we assume $\Delta E_T \gg \hbar\omega$.

The ratio of the sensitivity (i.e., amplitude ratio) for each triplet case relative to the doublet one for $\hbar\omega \ll kT$ is given by

$$\frac{Y_{LT}}{Y_D} = \frac{4}{3 + \exp(-\Delta E_T/kT)} \qquad (12)$$

$$\frac{Y_{HT}}{Y_D} = \frac{4}{3 + \exp(\Delta E_T/kT)} \qquad (13)$$

The temperature dependence of these ratios is shown graphically on Fig. 14–12. The low lying triplet provides greater ESR sensitivity than an ordinary doublet at all temperatures, while the ESR signal

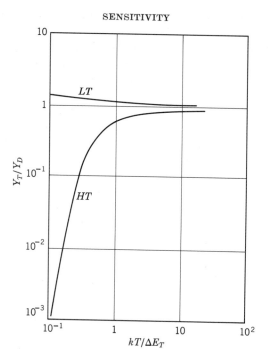

Fig. 14–12. Ratio of the ESR amplitude for a triplet state Y_T relative to a doublet state Y_D for a low lying triplet LT and a high lying triplet HT. The abscissa kT is normalized relative to the triplet energy ΔE_T [adapted from Bijl, Kainer, and Rose-Innes (1959)].

from the high lying triplet is relatively strong only for temperatures which correspond to $kT \gg \Delta E_T$. The ratios Y_{LT}/Y_0 and Y_{HT}/Y_0 may be obtained by comparing Figs. 14–9, 14–10, and 14–12. In this section we did not take into account the $S(S + 1)$ term in eqs. (14-D-7) and (14-D-31) which will also effect the sensitivity ratio of triplet to doublet spin states. Kottis and Lefebvre (1963, 1964) discuss the line-shapes obtained in triplet state ESR spectra.

F. Narrow Band Amplification and Detection

The ESR signal appears at a single frequency (e.g., 100 kc or 30 Mc) while the noise that accompanies the signal has components extending over the entire spectrum of frequencies that can be passed by the detector and preamplifier. The signal-to-noise ratio is considerably increased by narrow band amplification and detection using the electronic components discussed in Secs 12-D, 12-E, 12-F, 12-H, and 12-J. The narrow band amplifiers remove noise components that lie outside of their passband of width Δf centered at the modulation frequency f_m.

The lock-in detector (synchronous detector or coherent detector) is more efficient because it removes noise components that differ from the signal in either frequency or phase. The time constant network between the lock-in detector and the recorder removes the noise whose frequency exceeds the reciprocal of the time constant. The enhancement scheme discussed below in Sec. 14-I removes noise at frequencies both above and below the reciprocal of the effective time constant. Since the Johnson noise power discussed earlier in this chapter is proportional to the band-width, the noise-reducing circuits under discussion may be looked upon as decreasing the effective band-width of the system. Figure 14–13 shows schematically the relationship between the effective band-width Δf_2, of the tuned amplifier and that of the lock-in detector RC filter combination. A 100-kc narrow band amplifier might have a Q of 20 to give it a band-width of 5 kc while a 100-kc coherent detecter followed by a 10-sec time constant might have an effective band-width of 0.1 cps.

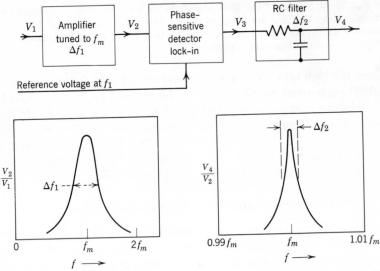

Fig. 14–13. The decrease in the effective band-width Δf when the voltage V_2 traverses the phase-sensitive detector and RC filter [adapted from Feher (1957)].

Štirand (1962) studied the effects of a linear network of time constant τ on the position and shape of a first derivative signal. He assumed a Gaussian line-shape

$$Y'(H) = 1.65 y'_m \left(\frac{H - H_0}{\frac{1}{2}\Delta H_{pp}} \right) \exp\left[-\tfrac{1}{2} \left(\frac{H - H_0}{\frac{1}{2}\Delta H_{pp}} \right)^2 \right] \quad (1)$$

with a linear scan

$$(H - H_0)/\Delta H_{pp} = t/b_0 \quad (2)$$

where b_0 is the peak-to-peak line-width ($b_0 = \Delta t_{pp}$) of the undistorted line in temporal units. The undistorted line-shape $Y'(t)$ considered as a function of time t is

$$Y'(t) = 1.65 y'_m \left(\frac{t}{b_0/2} \right) \exp\left[-\tfrac{1}{2} \left(\frac{t}{b_0/2} \right)^2 \right] \quad (3)$$

When the first derivative signal (3) emerges from the lock-in detector, it frequently traverses a time constant (τ) network which converts it to a new distorted shape function $U(t)$. When $\tau \ll b_0$, we have no distortion, and so

$$\lim_{\tau/b_0 \to 0} U(t) = Y'(t) \quad (4)$$

When the time constant τ is not negligible relative to the undistorted temporal linewidth b_0, then the distorted line-shape $U(t)$ has the form shown on Fig. 14-14. Note that for increasing values of the t/b_0, the following three changes take place in $U(t)$: (1) the amplitude decreases, (2) the line-width b broadens ($b = \Delta t_{pp}$ OB increases), and (3) it takes longer to reach the crossover point in the center of the line where $U(t) = 0$. The normalized increase in the peak-to-peak line-width b/b_0 is shown on Fig. 14-15, and the time delay $\delta t/b$ in reaching the crossover point is depicted in Fig. 14-16 as a function of the normalized time constant τ/b_0.

These figures show that when $\tau \ll b_0$, the time delay effect is much greater than the increase in width or distortion in shape. Fortunately we are ordinarily not bothered by the time delay, while the amplitude–width–shape errors can be serious. One should note that the line-shape of the first half of the spectrum (the part which traverses

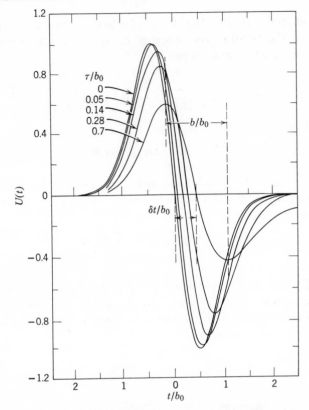

Fig. 14–14. Variation in the shape and position of the ESR line $U(t)$ after it emerges from a filter of time constant τ. Values of b/b_0 and $\delta t/b_0$ are shown for the broadest line where $\tau/b_0 = 0.7$ [adapted from Štirand (1962)].

the filter first) corresponding to $t/b_0 < 0$ is much more distorted than the second half where $t/b_0 > 0$. Figure 12–11 exhibits the same characteristics as the above figures. For best reproducibility one should work with $\tau \ll b_0$, while for best sensitivity it is advantageous to use $\tau \sim b_0$. A useful *lex pollicis* is to select τ equal to one tenth b_0.

G. Resonant Cavities and Helices

Wilmshurst, Gambling, and Ingram (1962) analyzed the sensitivity of various ESR spectrometers in terms of their optimum

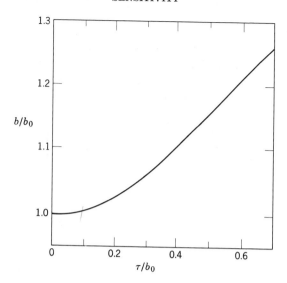

Fig. 14–15. The variation in the line-width b/b_0 as a function of the normalized filter time constant τ/b_0 [adapted from Štirand (1962)].

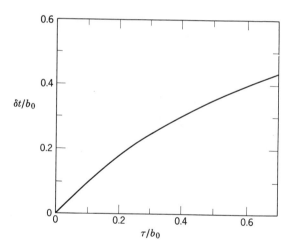

Fig. 14–16. The variation of the shift in position $\delta t/b_0$ of the ESR line as a result of the passage through the filter of normalized time constant τ/b_0 [adapted from Štirand (1962)].

operating points on a Smith chart (Sec. 2-C). They examined the transmission cavity, absorption cavity, and reflection cavity schemes shown on Fig. 14–17 and found the corresponding relative sensitivities Y_{min} to vary with the tuning conditions in the manner shown on Fig. 14–18. The data on these three figures fit the equations

$$Y_{min} = \begin{cases} \dfrac{4(\alpha - 1)}{\alpha^2} & \begin{cases} \text{transmission } (Y_T) \\ \text{absorption } (Y_A) \end{cases} \\ \dfrac{1 + \Gamma}{1 - \Gamma} & \text{reflection } (Y_R) \end{cases} \tag{1}$$

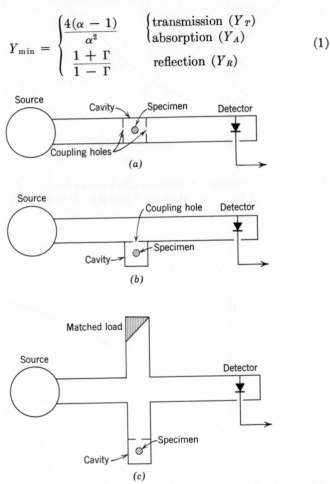

Fig. 14–17. Schematic representation of (a) transmission, (b) absorption, and (c) reflection cavity spectrometers [Wilmshurst, Gambling, and Ingram (1962)].

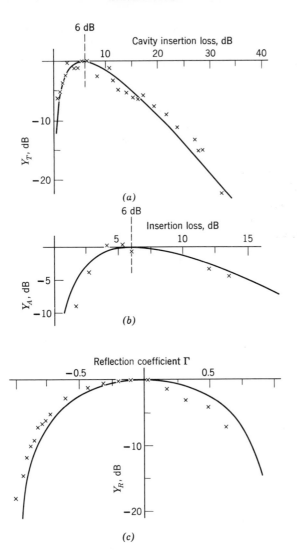

Fig. 14–18. Variation of the relative sensitivity Y with (a) the insertion loss of a transmission cavity, (b) the insertion loss of an absorption cavity, and (c) the reflection coefficient of a reflection cavity. The calculated solid curves are fitted to the data at their respective maxima [Wilmshurst, Gambling, and Ingram (1962)].

where α is the voltage insertion ratio, Γ is the voltage reflection coefficient, and of course, $Y_R = $ VSWR for the reflection cavity. In terms of Q, the optimum coupling in each case corresponds to a loaded Q equal to one half of the unloaded Q.

Under the conditions of maximum sensitivity the dispersion mode χ' is repressed with the transmission and absorption cavity arrangements. The reflection cavity is considerably more flexible since it may be conveniently tuned to provide either absorption χ'' or dispersion χ' under optimum coupling conditions. The absorption cavity is useful for generating circular polarization to determine the sign of the g factor (see Sec. 8-M).

The diagram of a reflection helix or traveling wave tube spectrometer is given in Fig. 14–19, and the equivalent circuits of three helix spectrometers are shown in Fig. 14–20. Wilmshurst, Gambling, and Ingram (1962) showed that for the transmission case the rate of change of the detected voltage E_l with the resistivity of the helix r is given by

$$\frac{1}{E_g} \frac{\partial E_l}{\partial r} = -\tfrac{1}{2} j\omega c x \frac{2 \sinh \gamma x + (n^2 + 1/n^2) \cosh \gamma x}{[2 \cosh \gamma x + (n^2 + 1/n^2) \sinh \gamma x]^2} \tag{2}$$

where γ is the propagation constant in the helix

$$\gamma = \alpha + j\beta = [j\omega c(r + j\omega l)]^{1/2} \tag{2-D-13}$$

and normally $r \ll \omega l$. In these relations E_g is the generator voltage, n is the transformer ratio, and x is the length of the helix. Equation (2) has a maximum with respect to n^2 when

$$n^2 = 1 \qquad \text{traveling waves} \tag{3}$$

$$n^2 + \frac{1}{n^2} = \frac{2(1 - \sinh^2 \gamma x)}{\sinh \gamma x \cosh \gamma x} \qquad \text{standing waves} \tag{4}$$

The traveling wave mode leads to the expression

$$\frac{1}{E_g} \frac{\partial E_l}{\partial r} = -\frac{j\omega c x}{4\gamma} \exp(-\gamma x) \tag{5}$$

and its solution

$$E_l = \tfrac{1}{2} E_g \exp(-\gamma x) \tag{6}$$

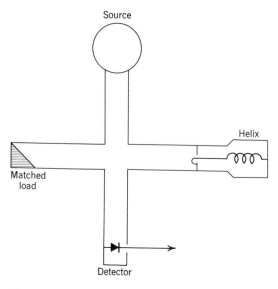

Fig. 14–19. The essential elements of a reflection helical spectrometer [Wilmshurst, Gambling and Ingram (1962)].

The sensitivity for absorption $(2r/E_g)(\partial E_l/\partial r)$ is a maximum when $x = 1/\alpha$, and varies with the length of the helix, as shown in Fig. 14–21. At the point of maximum sensitivity we have

$$\frac{2r}{E_g}\frac{\partial E_l}{\partial r} = \frac{1}{e} \tag{7}$$

where e is the natural logarithm base (cf. Table 20–5). The standing wave mode leads to maximum sensitivity when x is an integral number of half wavelengths $(\beta x = m\pi)$ in the range $0 < \alpha x < (1/2) \ln 3$, with the explicit values at its endpoints

$$\frac{2}{E_g}\frac{\partial E_l}{\partial r} = \begin{cases} -j\omega c/8\gamma\alpha & \alpha x = 0 \\ -0.63j\omega c/8\gamma\alpha & \alpha x = \tfrac{1}{2}\ln 3 \end{cases} \tag{8}$$

It is best to keep x as small as possible to maximize the sensitivity $(2/E_g)(\partial E_l/\partial r)$. From eq. (8) with $\alpha x = 0$ and with the aid of eqs. (2-D-15) and (2-D-16a) (with $G = 0$) we obtain

$$\frac{2r}{E_g}\frac{\partial E_l}{\partial r} = -\frac{1}{4} \tag{9}$$

The sensitivities of the two modes are compared in Fig. 14–21 as function of αx. Equation (9) leads to the same result for the minimum detectable signal as (14-C-19). Wilmshurst made a similar analysis of the absorption and reflection traveling wave spectrometers and found that they all produce about the same sensitivity as the cavity spectrometers, provided the cavities are no more than a few half wavelengths long.

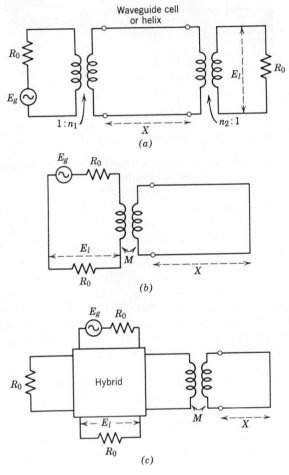

Fig. 14–20. The equivalent circuits for (a) transmission, (b) absorption, and (c) reflection helical spectrometers [Wilmshurst, Gambling, and Ingram (1962)].

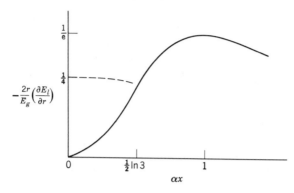

Fig. 14–21.   Variation in the relative sensitivity of the helix with length x when operating in (—) the traveling wave mode and (- -) the standing wave mode [Wilmshurst, Gambling, and Ingram (1962)].

The advantages of a slow wave structure or traveling wave tube are that the effective length is increased by the slowing factor S defined by

$$S = \frac{\text{velocity of light } \textit{in vacuo}}{\text{effective axial velocity of microwave energy}} \tag{10}$$

This is another way of saying that the microwave energy is concentrated by the factor S.   Modulating coils and optical irradiation may easily be introduced into the helix, and in double resonance experiments, the helix can also serve as the NMR coil.   Since the helix is broadbanded, it is not necessary to stabilize the source as precisely as in the cavity case, and frequency modulation noise [Bosch and Gambling (1961, 1962)] becomes unimportant.   The helix can be used over a wide range of frequencies.   It may be matched at room temperature and then immersed in liquid nitrogen or helium without appreciably changing its properties [Webb (1962)].   A slight disadvantage is the fact that the axis of polarization varies periodically along the helix.   Slowing factors of 100 can be achieved by helices, and other types of slow wave structures are able to produce $S \sim 1000$ with smaller band-widths.   [DeGrasse, Schulz-Du Bois, and Searl (1959)].   The effective Q of a slow wave structure of length x is given by

$$Q = 4\pi S(x/\lambda) \tag{11}$$

where λ is the free space wavelength. Mittra (1963) discusses wave propagation on helices.

Webb (1962) discusses the matching of a helix to a transmission line, and three of his arrangements are presented in Fig. 14–22. In this figure, screw A compensates for the frequency dependence of the match and screw B adjusts for different sample loadings. Screw A may be adjusted to provide either absorption or dispersion modes. A complete double resonance spectrometer incorporating a helix is shown on Fig. 14–23. Hausser and Reinhold (1961) used a helical waveguide for an Overhauser effect experiment. ESR double resonance spectrometers which employ helices were designed by Werner (1964) and Kenworthy and Richards (1965). Helices may also be used for antennae [e.g., see Blume, Habermehl, and Walter (1965)].

Before concluding this section a few words of practical importance will be added about resonators. It is very important to keep clean the inside surface of the resonant cavity and everything that enters it such as sample tubes and Dewars. After a spectrum is recorded, it is always wise to repeat the scan with an empty sample tube. Sometimes quartz produces a weak "blank" absorption near $g = 2$, but it is much superior to Pyrex in this respect. The inner surface of a resonant cavity is often gold-plated to minimize spurious resonances [Strandberg, Tinkham, Solt, and Davis (1956)]. A resonant

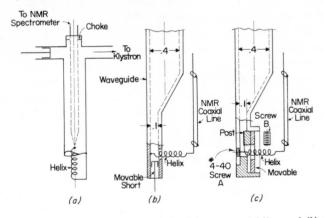

Fig. 14–22. Methods of matching a helix (a) to a coaxial line and (b) and (c) to a waveguide. The latter two cases show the NMR input for double resonance studies [Webb (1962)].

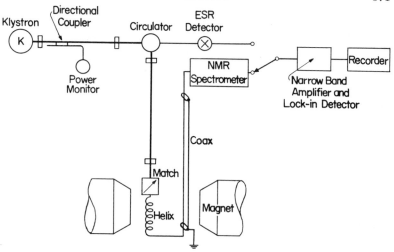

Fig. 14–23. A double resonance spectrometer employing a helix [Webb (1962)].

cavity may be effectively cleaned with dilute nitric acid, and phene (benzene) or dimethylketone (acetone) may be employed to remove organic deposits.

During low temperature studies, the condensation of moisture within the resonant cavity can be troublesome due to its high dielectric loss. The losses due to water vapor and oxygen are discussed in *RLS-23*, p. 663.

H. Masers and Parametric Amplifiers

It was shown in Secs. 14-B and 14-C that the detector and preamplifier not only amplify the incoming signal with its accompanying noise, but in addition, they introduce additional noise of their own. It is possible to minimize the introduction of such additional noise by the use of a maser, parametric amplifier, or traveling wave amplifier. The first two will be discussed here. A maser is described in Sec. 13-O, and Sec. 6-D treats traveling wave tubes.

Masers or microwave amplifiers for stimulated emission of radiation are reviewed by Wittke (1957), Weber (1959), J. R. Singer (1959), Townes (1960), and Schulz-Du Bois (1961). The generation and amplification of millimeter waves have been reviewed by Willshaw (1961). A mechanical analog of maser action is presented by

Karbowiak (1963). A detailed discussion of masers as such is beyond the scope of this book, so we will limit ourselves to their application to ESR spectrometers. The advantage of employing a maser for a preamplifier is its very low noise figure [Shimoda, Takahasi, and Townes (1957); Strandberg (1957); Weber (1957);

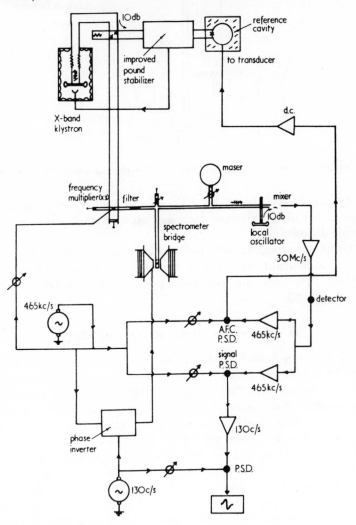

Fig. 14-24. Block diagram of an ESR spectrometer incorporating an ammonia maser preamplifier [Gambling and Wilmshurst (1963)].

McWhorter and Arams (1958)]. This arrangement gives us one stage of amplification before detector and vacuum tube noise enters to obscure the signal.

Shimoda (1959), Shimoda and Wang (1955), Townes (1960), and Thaddeus and Krisher (1961) discuss the use of maser techniques to improve the sensitivity of microwave spectrometers. Krupnov and Skvortsov (1964) described a beam microwave spectroscope which incorporates a maser. Beers (1961) compared cavity microwave spectrometers to maser microwave spectrometers, and found that under some experimental conditions the maser spectrometer is superior.

Gambling and Wilmshurst (1963) describe the superheterodyne K band ESR spectrometer shown on Fig. 14–24 which incorporates an ammonia maser with a 30 cps band-width as a preamplifier. It employs a Pound-stabilized X band klystron and a frequency tripler to obtain 23 kMc. In order to avoid saturating the maser at powers in excess of 10^{-12} W, the magnetic field is modulated at 465 kc and the maser is tuned to one of the microwave sidebands at $f + 465$ kc. The high power carrier f is outside the 30-cps maser band-width, and so it is suppressed. The 465-kc AFC signal is introduced at the doubler. The resulting error signal undergoes dc amplification and is employed to feed a piezoelectric transducer which corrects for thermal drift by deforming the wall of the reference cavity. The AFC and ESR signals are separated by inverting the 465-kc field modulating signal at 130 cps and employing separate phase-sensitive detectors (P.S.D.) at 465 kc. In addition, the ESR signal traverses a 130 cps phase-sensitive detector before being displayed on the recorder. Figure 14–25 shows the ESR signal with and sans the

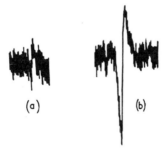

(a)   (b)

Fig. 14–25. An ESR signal recorded (a) sans maser and (b) after maser amplification [Gambling and Wilmshurst (1963)].

maser.   The maser provides up to a 17-dB improvement in signal-to-noise ratio and operates at liquid nitrogen temperature.   Using a 30-μW power generator and a 1-sec time constant, the sensitivity for a signal-to-noise ratio of 1 is 3×10^{12} ΔH spins.

A three-level solid state maser has a larger band-width ($\sim$10 Mc) and higher saturation power ($\sim$$10^{-5}$ W), so its use obviates some of the electronic problems intrinsic to an ammonia maser.   It has the disadvantage of requiring liquid helium refrigeration techniques. Lecar and Okaya (1963) describe an ESR spectrometer which uses a ruby maser.

One of the principal competitors of the maser for low noise, high frequency applications is the parametric amplifier.   This device also goes under the name of junction diode, mavar (modulation amplification through variable reactance), reactance amplifier, varactor (variable reactor), and variable resistance amplifier.   The principle of operation is illustrated by the LC-tuned circuit with the applied sinusoidal voltage V shown on Fig. 14–26a.   The capacitance is varied in the manner shown in Fig. 14–26b, and this causes the voltage across the capacitor $V = Q/C$ to increase as indicated.   The energy for the voltage buildup is supplied by the work done in changing the capacitor spacing.   At low frequencies the capacitance

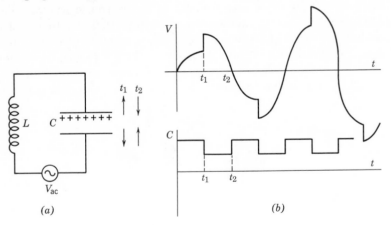

Fig. 14–26.   (a) The equivalent circuit of a parametric amplifier and (b) the change in capacitance and voltage during its operation [Hemenway, Henry, and Caulton (1962)].

can be varied mechanically, while for high frequency applications, one may employ an electronically variable reactance such as the junction capacitance of a silicon diode. Further details on the principle of operation are given by Uhlir (1959), Stevens (1960), and Hemenway, Henry, and Caulton (1962).

Parametric amplifiers are much smaller and much less complex than masers, and they may be operated at room temperature, while masers usually require refrigeration techniques (e.g., 77 or 4.2°K). The effective noise temperature or relative noisiness [Mortenson (1960)] of parametric amplifiers (junction diodes) is compared with that of other types of amplifiers in Fig. 14–27. Suhl (1957) discusses the theory of ferrite parametric amplifiers. Berteaud and LeGall (1963) describe a 4700-Mc parametric amplifier.

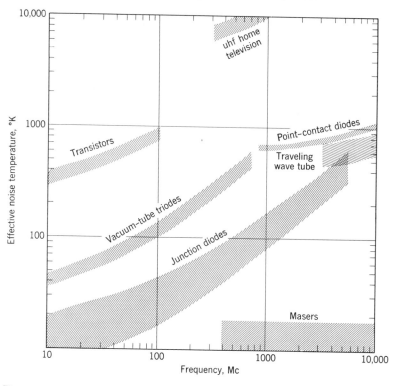

Fig. 14–27. The frequency dependence of the effective noise temperature as a function of the type of detector [Uhlir (1959)].

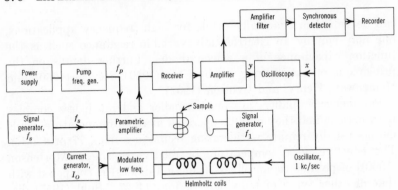

Fig. 14–28.   Block diagram of a spectrometer employing a parametric amplifier [Jelenski (1962)].

Jelenski (1962) designed a parametric ESR spectrometer which employed a pump frequency f_p of ~700 Mc and a signal frequency f_s of ~220 Mc.   The block diagram of the spectrometer presented in Fig. 14–28 shows the sample located in the coil of the parametric amplifier.   The 1-kc oscillator is employed for recorder presentation after passage through the amplifier, filter, and synchronous detector, while 100 cps is used for visual presentation.   From Fig. 14–27 we see that in this application parametric amplifiers are still low enough in frequency to eliminate noise effectively, while at X band, masers are theoretically much superior.   Hollocher, From, and Bromberg (1964) employed a commercial varactor diode parametric amplifier to reduce the noise figure of their ESR spectrometer from 15 to 4.1 dB.   Deloach (1963) described a 54-Gc parametric amplifier. Electron spin oscillator spectrometers employing a regenerative microwave feedback loop are described by Payne (1964) and Sloan, Ganssen, and La Vier (1964).

I. Enhancement of Spectra

The earlier sections in this chapter discussed the sensitivity attainable using standard electronic components, including a long time constant filter preceding the recorder.   This filter is very efficient in removing high frequency noise, but it does not affect the low frequency noise.   An enhancement technique of continuous averaging may be employed to remove both low and high frequency noise, and thereby increase the signal-to-noise ratio. The theory and application of this technique are presented in this section. The section concludes with another type of enhancement technique designed to increase the resolution of an ESR spectrum.

Signal-to-Noise Enhancement: Klein and Barton (1963, 1963) decribe a digital computer technique which makes use of a multichannel pulse height analyzer [Schumann and McMahon (1956)] to enhance the signal-to-noise ratio of ESR spectra by continuous averaging. These pulse height analyzers have been used previously in neutron time of flight measurements [Schumann (1956)], mass spectrometry [Barton, Gibson, and Tolman (1960)], the Mössbauer effect [Ruby, Epstein, and Sun (1960)], and bioelectric experiments [Clark, Brown, Goldstein, Molnar, O'Brien, and Zieman (1961); Clynes and Kohn (1961)]. Analog computers have also been employed [Dawson (1954)], but they have a limited dynamic range and are not as stable.

In conventional lock-in detector techniques, the ESR signal is sent through a long time-constant filter and then recorded. The signal-to-noise ratio is enhanced by increasing the time constant τ and the time T required for the scan, while keeping the ratio τ/T constant. The continuous average or time domain filtering technique [Klein and Barton (1963)] requires the same overall time T for the measurement, but divides this time into T/n intervals and makes a total of n scans while using a time constant of τ/n. The n scans are summed, and this causes the signals to add and produce a resultant with n times the amplitude of a single scan. The noise components, on the other hand, will add randomly and give a resultant which is $n^{1/2}$ times the noise of a single traverse. As a result the signal-to-noise ratio increases as the square root of the time constant τ (or total scanning time T). This is the same result that is obtained for the high frequency components of noise when a single long scan is used. However, the long scan does not filter out very low frequency noise, and it tends to be upset by very strong noise impulses or spikes. The prominent low frequency noise arises from the crystal $1/f$ noise power and other sources. The continuous averaging technique achieves its remarkable enhancement by its efficient removal of both high and low frequency noise.

The multichannel pulse height analyzer and its associated equipment are shown on Fig. 14–29. It employs a voltage to frequency converter [Anderson and Schulteis (1959) ; Stejskal (1963)] to con-

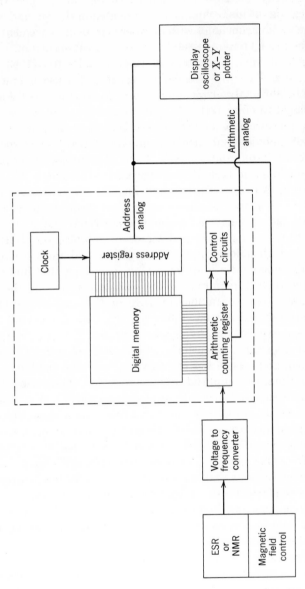

Fig. 14–29. Multichannel pulse–height analyzer (within dotted line) and associated electronic equipment. The system is arranged to operate as an average response computer [Klein and Barton (1963)].

vert the output voltage of the lock-in detector to a form that is suitable for storage in the memory of the analyzer. This unit produces a pulse train whose rate is proportional to its instantaneous input voltage. The magnetic field H is driven from the address in order to set up a one-to-one correspondence between the channel number and H. A field sweeping regulator [Barton, Tolman, and Roulette (1960)] is employed to insure that the field rather than the current follows the address analog. To avoid magnet time constant effects, the address advance is programed in a triangular manner. The data are displayed on either a recorder or a sillyscope.

The apparatus shown in Fig. 14–29 is arranged to operate as an average response computer. The ferrite core memory unit consists of 400 channels, and each has a capacity of 10^6 counts. The clock which advances the address by one channel for each pulse is continuously adjustable from a rate of 1 msec/channel upward. The arithmetic counting register and control circuits constitute the logic units which add (or subtract) the pulses entering the input circuit to (or from) the count stored in the memory.

Figure 14–30 shows the enhancement that has been obtained with ESR spectra. Signal-to-noise ratios have been enhanced by one to two orders of magnitude without sacrifice of band-width. When hyperfine structure is present, there should be enough channels to allow over 25 for each hfs component. Sampling techniques can be used with transient signals [Robinson and Yogi (1965)]. Pulse height analyzers are available with 10^{-8} sec rise times and 13 Mc maximum input repetition rates [Welter (1965)]. Sampling techniques applied to magnetic resonance are also discussed by Crosnier and Gabillard (1963), Aubrun, Veillet, and Van Hiep (1963), Mayo and Goldstein (1964), Coles and Bruce (1965), Ernst (1965), Ernst and Anderson (1965, 1966), Kent and Mallard (1965), and Visweswaramurthy (1965). Sigmond (1965) describes a simple pulse height averager [see also Gabillard (1959) and Aubrun (1965)]. This enhancement technique should become routine in the near future.

Resolution Enhancement: Many ESR spectra containing partially resolved hyperfine structure are composed of individual resonant lines whose width and shape are either known or may be approximated. In this case the spectrum may be sharpened by the method [Allen, Gladney, and Glarum (1964)] shown in Fig. 14–31. The second derivative of the line-shape $(d^2/dt^2) f(t)$ shown in the center is multiplied by a constant C and then subtracted from the upper line-shape $f(t)$ [denoted by $Y'(t)$ or $U(t)$ in Sec. 14-F] to produce the narrowed lower line-shape. A Gaussian line narrowed by sub-tracting some of its second derivative and adding some of its fourth derivative is shown in Fig. 14–32, and the effect of varying the mixing coefficients is shown in Fig. 14–33. The success of this method depends upon the fact that the even derivatives of absorption lines are narrower in the center than the original line-shape, and

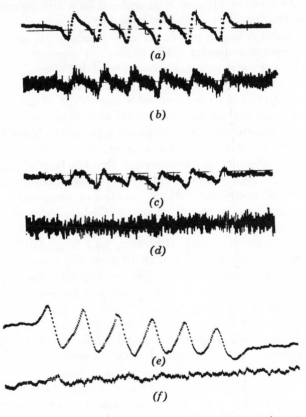

Fig. 14–30.   First derivative ESR spectra of Mn^{+4} in H_2O at the output of the pulse height analyzer. The time constant was 10^{-2} sec and each traverse lasted for 5 sec.   (a) 100 traverses, 5×10^{14} spins; (b) 1 traverse, 5×10^{14} spins; (c) 500 traverses, 5×10^{13} spins; (d) 1 traverse, 5×10^{13} spins; (e) 5000 traverses, 5×10^{13} spins; (f) 1 traverse, 5×10^{13} spins [Klein and Barton (1963)].

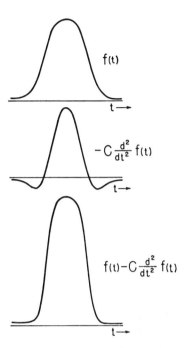

Fig. 14–31. Qualitative representation of the principle of resolution enhancement. $f(t)$ = the line-shape function; C = a constant dependent on line-width [Allen, Gladney, and Glarum (1964)].

similarly higher order odd derivatives are narrower than the first one (cf. Sec. 14-K and Fig. 14–38). Allen, Gladney, and Glarum (1964) discuss filters that may be employed to perform the differentiations, additions, and subtractions. They made use of both digital and analog computers in their experimental arrangements. Filtered and unfiltered ESR spectra are presented in Fig. 14–34.

The digital equipment required for the above resolution enhancement scheme is rather expensive, and the substitution of analog techniques introduces noise and makes sharpening adjustments critically dependent on the rate of scan. Glarum (1965) presented an alternative technique which avoids these difficulties. He showed that modulating the magnetic field with a complex (nonsinusoidal) waveform and using phase-sensitive detection can reduce the observed width of the spectral lines. This resolving technique has

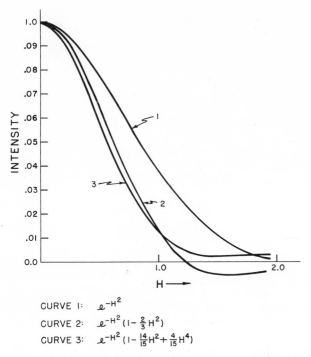

CURVE 1: e^{-H^2}

CURVE 2: $e^{-H^2}(1-\frac{2}{3}H^2)$

CURVE 3: $e^{-H^2}(1-\frac{14}{15}H^2+\frac{4}{15}H^4)$

Fig. 14–32.   Gaussian absorption line: (1) undistorted, (2) sharpened to its second derivative, (3) sharpened to its fourth derivative [Allen, Gladney, and Glarum (1964)].

several advantages: (1) the sharpening is independent of the rate of scan; (2) the sharpened spectrum is obtained directly on the recorder; (3) distortion due to ringing is eliminated; (4) derivatives higher than the third can be included; and (5) the required equipment is inexpensive and readily integrated into existing spectrometer systems.

In the Glarum technique, the magnetic field is modulated at several frequencies f_{mod}, $f_{mod}/3$, $f_{mod}/5$, . . . , etc, while retaining a single receiver and detector at f_{mod}. For small amplitude modulation ($H_{mod} \ll \Delta H_{pp}$ for all frequencies), this method is mathematically equivalent to using detector circuits at f_{mod}, $f_{mod}/3$, $f_{mod}/5$, etc., and recombining terms later, as suggested by Russell and Torchia (1962).

Figure 14–35 shows a transistorized line sharpening field modulator. The 100-kc reference signal from a conventional modulation circuit

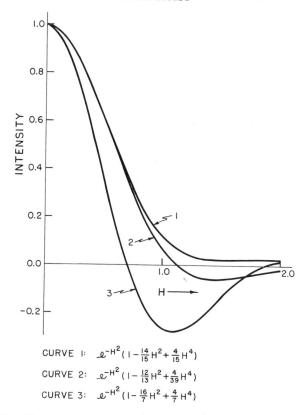

CURVE 1: $e^{-H^2}(1 - \frac{14}{15}H^2 + \frac{4}{15}H^4)$

CURVE 2: $e^{-H^2}(1 - \frac{12}{13}H^2 + \frac{4}{39}H^4)$

CURVE 3: $e^{-H^2}(1 - \frac{16}{7}H^2 + \frac{4}{7}H^4)$

Fig. 14–33. The effect on a Gaussian line-shape of modifying the derivative mixing coefficients [Allen, Gladney, and Glarum (1964)].

triggers two multivibrators to produce the 33-kc and 20-kc sharpening frequencies. Each frequency is filtered, adjusted in phase and amplitude, and then impressed on the modulation coils. Figure 14–36 shows a spectrum of DPPH in benzene after sharpening with one (33 kc) and two (33 kc plus 20 kc) modulation subharmonics.

It is believed that resolution enhancement or line sharpening techniques will be widely used in the future.

J. Choice of Sample Size

The discussion of Sec. 8-H and the calculations of the type that are summarized in Table 8–2 show that, in general, the ESR signal

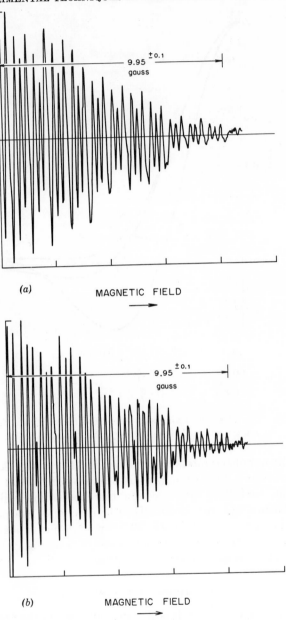

Fig. 14-34. ESR patterns of K$^+$(benzophenone)$^-$ (a) before and (b) after filtering by the analog circuit [Allen, Gladney, and Glarum (1964)].

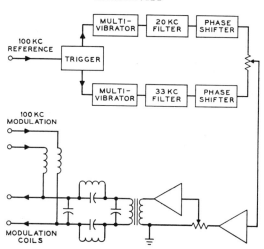

Fig. 14–35. Block diagram of field modulation line sharpener [Glarum (1965)].

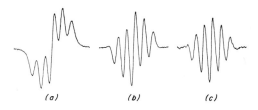

Fig. 14–36. First derivative spectrum of DPPH in benzene with (a) no, (b) one, and (c) two sharpening terms [Glarum (1965)].

increases with an increase in the size of the paramagnetic sample, and also with an increase in Q. If a sample is lossy, then an increase in its size will (a) increase the number of paramagnetic centers and (b) will decrease Q, and these two factors will have opposite effects on the sensitivity. Feher (1957) distinguishes two limiting cases: (a) insulators and semiconductors which exhibit a dielectric loss proportional to E^2 arising from the imaginary part ϵ'' of the dielectric constant ϵ

$$\epsilon/\epsilon_0 = \epsilon' + j\epsilon'' \tag{1}$$

and (b) low resistivity samples which produce losses that are proportional to H^2 and which e.g., may arise from surface currents. Each will be considered in turn.

We showed in Sec. 14-D that the ESR signal y_m' is proportional to the product ηQ_u

$$\eta Q_u \propto V_s Q_u \tag{2}$$

where the filling factor η, which is proportional to the sample volume V_s, has been evaluated explictly for several experimental arrangements in Sec. 8-H.   In the presence of a lossy sample, the factor Q_u in the sensitivity formulae [e.g., (14-D-1) to (14-D-34)] should be replaced by Q_u' defined by

$$\eta Q_{u'} = \frac{\eta}{1/Q_u + 1/Q_\chi + 1/Q_\epsilon + 1/Q_\mu} \tag{3}$$

where Q_ϵ and Q_μ, respectively, arise from the dielectric and H^2 losses mentioned above.   These are defined by

$$\frac{1}{Q_\epsilon} = \frac{\displaystyle\int_{\text{sample}} \epsilon_0 \epsilon'' |E|^2 dV}{\displaystyle\int_{\text{cavity}} \mu H_1^2 dV} = \frac{\epsilon_0}{\mu_0 V_c \langle H_1^2 \rangle_c} \int_{\text{sample}} \epsilon'' |E|^2 dV \tag{4}$$

$$\frac{1}{Q_\mu} = \frac{\displaystyle\int_{\text{sample}} \mu_0 \mu'' H_1^2 dV}{\displaystyle\int_{\text{cavity}} \mu H_1^2 dV} = \frac{1}{V_c \langle H_1^2 \rangle_c} \int_{\text{sample}} \mu'' H_1^2 dV \tag{5}$$

where ϵ'' and μ'' are the losses under consideration where $\mu/\mu_0 = \mu' + j\mu''$.   We shall consider the optimum sample size V_s for two specific sample shapes and orientations.

First let us consider a sample of the type shown in Fig. 8–5 placed in a "square" TE_{102} mode with $2a = d$.   From eq.(8-H-31) we have

$$\eta = V_s/V_c = (\pi d/V_c)\, r^2 \tag{6}$$

for a sample tube of radius r.   Using eqs. (8-H-8) to (8-H-10), eq. (8-H-18), and the coordinate system of Fig. 8–24 in eq. (4), we obtain

$$\frac{1}{Q_\epsilon} = \frac{1}{abd} \left(4\epsilon'' \right) \int_0^a \sin^2 \frac{\pi x}{a} \, dx \int_0^r \sin^2 \frac{2\pi z}{d} \, dz \int_{r \sin \varphi}^{r \sin \varphi} dy \tag{7}$$

$$= \frac{4r\epsilon''}{bd} \int_0^r \left[1 - \left(\frac{z}{r} \right)^2 \right]^{1/2} \sin^2 \frac{2\pi z}{d} \, dz \tag{8}$$

Ordinarily the tube radius r is sufficiently small relative to the cavity dimension a, so that we may approximate $\sin 2\pi z/d$ by its argument, and ergo, we obtain

$$\frac{1}{Q_\epsilon} = \frac{4\pi^2 r^4}{a^2 bd} \, \epsilon'' \int_0^1 \left[1 - \left(\frac{z}{r}\right)^2\right]^{1/2} \left(\frac{z}{r}\right)^2 d\left(\frac{z}{r}\right) \qquad (9)$$

$$= \frac{\pi^3 r^4}{4a^2 bd} \, \epsilon'' = \frac{\pi^3 r^4}{2V_c d} \, \epsilon'' \qquad (10)$$

where ϵ'' is the ratio of the imaginary part of the dielectric constant of the sample to that of free space. [More properly, E^2 should be replaced by a value closer to $\epsilon' E^2$ (cf. Sec. 8-D)]. For the dielectric loss case, $1/Q_\mu = 0$, and we neglect the resonance absorption $1/Q_x$, which gives

$$\eta Q_{u'} = \frac{(\pi d/V_c)\, r^2}{\dfrac{1}{Q_u} + \dfrac{\pi^3}{2V_c d} \epsilon'' r^4} \qquad (11)$$

This has a maximum when

$$\frac{\partial(\eta Q_{u'})}{\partial r} = 0 \qquad (12)$$

which leads to the condition

$$\frac{\pi^3}{2V_c} \epsilon'' r^4 = \frac{1}{Q_u} = \frac{1}{Q_\epsilon} \qquad (13)$$

or in other words

$$(Q_{u'} \text{ with sample}) = \tfrac{1}{2}(Q_u \text{ sans sample}) \qquad (14)$$

This result is only valid for $r \ll a$. Thus to obtain the highest sensitivity, one should use a sample which reduces the loaded Q of the cavity to one-half of its initial value.

For the case of magnetic losses

$$\frac{1}{Q_\mu} = \frac{\displaystyle\int_{\text{sample}} \mu'' H_1^2 dV}{V_c \langle H_1{}^2 \rangle_c} = \frac{\tfrac{1}{4}(\pi r^2 d) H_0^2}{V_c \langle H_1{}^2 \rangle_c} \, \mu'' \qquad (15)$$

$$= \mu'' \frac{\pi r^2}{ab} \qquad (16)$$

where the integration is similar to eq. (8-H-27)ff.   As a result

$$\eta Q_{u'} = \frac{(\pi d/V_c)\, r^2}{\dfrac{1}{Q_u} + \left(\mu'' \dfrac{\pi}{ab} \right) r^2} \tag{17}$$

which has no maximum, so the larger the sample tube, the higher the sensitivity.

These calculations were presented in detail to illustrate the method.   Feher (1957) considered the case of a planar sample of dimensions $a \times b \times \delta$ with $\delta \ll d$ placed at the bottom of a rectangular TE_{102} mode cavity.   He obtained the condition

$$(Q_{u'} \text{ with sample}) = \tfrac{2}{3}(Q_u \text{ sans sample}) \tag{18}$$

for dielectric losses and found that the larger the sample size the greater the sensitivity for $H_1{}^2$ losses.

The physical reason why an optimum sample size exists for the two cases with dielectric loss is as follows.   When the size increases by an increment Δr or Δz, the additional sample is located in a position of lower $H_1{}^2$ and higher E^2, and so it contributes less to the signal and more to the losses than the rest of the sample.   This process becomes more pronounced as the size increases until a point is reached where the loss term predominates, and a further increase in size lowers the sensitivity.   When the losses are proportional to $H_1{}^2$ on the other hand, both the signal and the losses increase at the same rate, and the constant term $1/Q_u$ which is in the denominator of eq. (3) prevents an optimum size from being reached.

One of the most frequently employed lossy sample materials is water (aqueous solutions).   Several authors [Cook and Mallard (1963); Stoodley (1963, 1963); Wilmshurst (1963)] have discussed the feasibility of employing long cavities to increase the sensitivity with such samples.   For the reasons advanced by Stoodley and Wilmshurst and from arguments similar to those presented in Sec. 8-H, one may conclude that it is best to keep the resonant cavity as short as possible.   Lossy samples may be analyzed in capillary tubes, and their cylindrical shape is most adaptable for use with cylindrical resonators.   The most efficient arrangement for a rectangular TE_{102} cavity is a thin flat quartz sample cell located at the region of maximum magnetic field strength and minimum electric field strength, and oriented parallel to the smallest cross section of the cavity (i.e., parallel to the iris). Electrolytic or polarographic studies (cf. Sec. 15-F) are often carried out with such a cell. Lagercrantz and Persson (1964) used two flat cells in a dual cavity. A thin flat cell also works well in the center of a TE_{011} mode cylindrical cavity. Dielectric losses may be reduced by operating at S band (3000 Mc) or lower in frequency. Kent and Mallard (1965) describe a vhf (80 Mc) spectrometer designed for use with wet biological tissue samples.

Roberts and Derbyshire (1961) describe a universal crystal mount designed for use with a rectangular TE_{102} resonant cavity. It provides for rotation of a crystal about two orthogonal axes, and gives a reproducibility of 2°. Similar crystal mounts are described by Bil'dyukevich (1963, 1964, 1965), Engel (1964), and Danilyuk, Pokhol'chik, and Koleda (1965).

K. Standard Samples and Number of Spins

To obtain quantitative spin concentrations and g factors by electron spin resonance, it is necessary to compare an "unknown" sample to a known one. The calibration sample may be "run" before and after the unknown, or it may be placed in the cavity simultaneously and recorded superimposed on the unknown. A dual cavity (cf. Sec. 8-K) provides the best features of both methods. Several standard samples useful for calibration purposes are discussed in this section.

One of the most frequently used calibration samples is α,α'-diphenyl-β-picryl hydrazyl (DPPH) [Holden, Kittel, Merritt, and Yager (1950); Townes and Turkevitch (1950); Pake, Weissman, and Townsend (1955); Livingston and Zeldes (1956)]. Goldschmidt and Renn (1922) describe its preparation, and it is available commercially. It has been used in the solid state as a g factor standard ($g = 2.0036 \pm 0.0003$), and in benzene solution, its hyperfine structure has been used to calibrate the number of gauss per recorder division. It may be employed in both phases as an intensity standard, and it does not saturate easily [Lloyd and Pake (1953); Bloembergen and Wang (1954); Berthet (1955)]. A series of standard solutions diluted successively by factors of $10^{1/2}$ or 10 can be very useful.

Solid DPPH exhibits a g factor anisotropy [Cohen, Kikuchi, and Turkevich (1952); Kikuchi and Cohen (1954)] which is more pronounced at low temperatures [Singer and Kikuchi (1955)]. The narrow Lorentzian-like singlet line-width of solid DPPH is due to exchange narrowing, and the Lorentzian-shaped quintet observed in dilute solutions arises from the Brownian motion or molecular tumbling.   If one could remove the exchange interaction in the solid, then one would observe a dipolar broadened Gaussian resonance. The line-width in solid DPPH varies from 1.5 to 4.7 G depending on the solvent from which it is crystallized [Lothe and Eia (1958); Arbuzov, Valitova, Garif'yanov, and Kozyrev (1959); Bodi and Goara (1964); see Table 7.1 of Al'tschuler and Kozyrev (1964)]. Mattuck and Strandberg (1958) employed DPPH in a micromodulator technique to determine intensities in a microwave Stark spectrometer.

Despite its advantages, DPPH also has certain undesirable features [e.g., see Feher (1957) and Uebersfeld (1959)].   As a result, several other standards have been proposed.   L. S. Singer (1959) and Singer, Smith, and Wagoner (1961) suggested the use of a small single crystal of ruby (0.5% Cr/Al_2O_3) as a secondary standard because it is chemically stable, and has an ESR signal which is strongly orientation-dependent.   The crystal may be permanently situated at the edge of the resonator and oriented to produce a signal at a g factor which will not interfere with the spectra under study. (e.g., $g = 1.5$ or 2.5 is often convenient).   The ruby spectrum may be recorded under the same instrumental conditions immediately before or after the unknown, and since both are in the same resonator, there will be an automatic compensation for such effects as the cavity Q and the modulation amplitude.   Figure 16–3 shows Singer's experimental arrangement.   Thompson and Waugh (1965) describe an adjustable ruby standard in which the amplitude and effective g factor may be varied at will.

Tinkham and Strandberg (1955), Krongelb and Strandberg (1959), Westenberg and DeHaas (1964), and Evenson and Burch (1966) used a molecular oxygen standard.   Filipovich and Sanders (1959) proposed the use of gaseous $O^{16}O^{18}$ as an intensity standard, while Westenberg and DeHaas (1965) used gaseous NO.   Hoskins and Pastor (1960) recommend the use of charred dextrose as a frequency marker because the line-width (10.6 G), g value, and spin lattice relaxation time are constant between liquid helium and room temperature.   This material is easily prepared and is stable when stored in a sealed container.   The Varian standard is $3.3 \times 10^{-4}\%$ pitch on KCl.

It contains 10^{13} spins per centimeter of length and has $g = 2.0028$, $\Delta H_{pp} = 1.7$ G, and $A/(y_m'\Delta H_{pp}^2) = 5.46$ (Hyde; cf. Sec. 20-B).

Fremy's salt or peroxylamine disulfonate dissolved in saturated sodium carbonate forms the $NO(SO_3)_3^=$ ion with three hyperfine components separated by 13.00 ± 0.07 G, and has $\Delta H_{pp} = 0.26 \pm 0.02$ G, and $g = 2.0057 \pm 0.0001$ [Wartz, Reitz, and Dravnieks (1961)]. The solution may be stored in a refrigerator for several months, but decays if stored at room temperature [see Lloyd and Pake (1954); Burgess (1958); Cram and Reeves (1958)]. These may be used for calibrating the magnet scan. McBrierty and Cook (1965) recommend a nitric oxide complex for this purpose.

Yariv and Gordon (1961) and Burgess (1961) suggest the use of $CuSO_4 \cdot 5H_2O$ crystals as an intensity standard [see also Feher (1957)]. Copper sulfate is readily available commercially. Foerster (1960) uses magnesium arsenate.

In Chapter 20 we discuss methods of integrating ESR spectra in order to determine the number of spins, the moments of the line, etc. Wyard (1965) doubly integrates ESR spectra on a desk calculator and obtains a 5% accuracy using intervals equal to a quarter of the linewidth. Burgess (1961) describes an analog method for rapidly determining the integrated area of a spectrum from its first derivative curve. The technique consists of tracing the recorded curve on cardboard and ascertaining its moment on a balance. Burgess recommends copper sulfate pentahydrate ($CuSO_4 \cdot 5H_2O$) as a standard to calibrate the recordings, and thereby determine the absolute number of spins. Aasa and Vanngard (1964) obtained 2% agreement between calculated and measured intensity ratios of copper and cobalt complexes (effective spin $\frac{1}{2}$, axial symmetry, and small hfs energy).

Randolph (1960) made use of the analog computer shown in Fig. 14–37 to determine the total absorption of ESR spectra. Other details on analog integrators are found in Sec. 12-K, and in a paper by Collins (1959). The direct determination of the area by his method is shown in the lower part of Fig. 14–38. The data on Fig. 14–39 demonstrate that a moderate amount of overmodulation does not affect the area, and its effect on the first derivative curve is considerably more pronounced that it is on the straight absorption curve. This is important to know because for barely detectable resonances, it is necessary to overmodulate. Figure 14–38 shows that structure is better resolved with first derivative presentation.

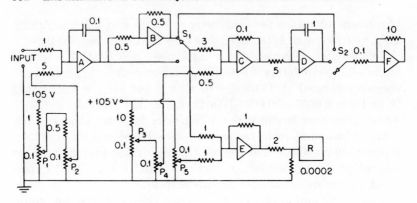

Fig. 14–37. Schematic circuit for the analog computation of ESR spectra. The figure gives typical resistances in MΩ and typical capacitances in microfarads [Randolph (1960)].

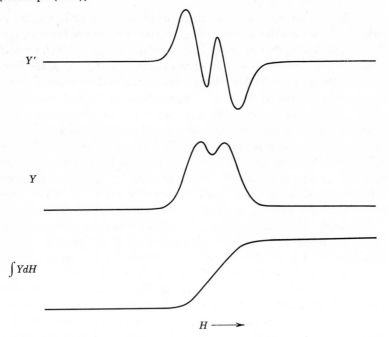

Fig. 14–38. Simultaneous plots of the ESR absorption derivative Y', the ESR absorption Y, and the integral of the ESR absorption $\int Y dH$ of gamma-irradiated glycylglycine vs. the magnetic field H, (H increases from right to left). The peaks are separated by $\sim$17 G on Y, and the modulation amplitude is about 1.2 G [Randolph (1960)].

Johnson and Chang (1965) recorded the third derivative for even greater resolution.

A dual sample cavity for use in comparing an unknown spectrum to a standard is described in Sec. 8-K. One advantage of this arrangement is that it allows one to use a standard sample whose amplitude and line-width is comparable to the unknown. In addition, it obviates the necessity of working with overlapping spectra.

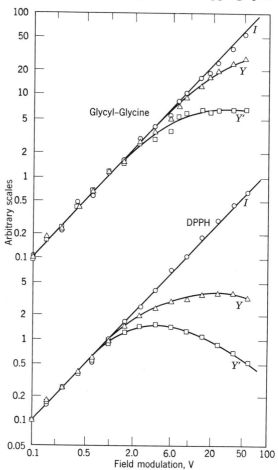

Fig. 14–39. The peak-to-peak derivative amplitude Y', absorption amplitude Y, and integrated area $I = \int Y dH$ vs. the peak-to-peak modulation amplitude. The DPPH sample contained about 2×10^{16} spins. One volt corresponds to a peak-to-peak modulation amplitude of 1.2 G [Randolph (1960)].

Smith and Wilmshurst (1963) provided a rectangular TE_{103} mode dual cavity analogous to the TE_{105} one shown in Fig. 8–32 with separate 465-kc modulation for each sample by means of single-turn hairpin loops. The modulation phase is adjusted to be opposite at each sample, and the spectrometer records the difference between the two signals, as shown on Fig. 14–40. This arrangement is useful for identifying spectra and for separating individual spectra from a mixed material. Incomplete cancellation can reveal small differences in the width, shape, or position of two resonances [Martin (1957)]. Differential techniques have been extensively applied to ultraviolet, visible, and infrared spectroscopy [Powell (1956)].

In this chapter we have discusssed the measurement of intensities and g factors in electron spin resonance. Yariv and Gordon (1961) describe a procedure for determining the number of spins by a measurement of the cavity reflection coefficient Γ. Lacroix, Ryter, and Extermann (1950) worked with a reference cavity whose Q was matched to the sample cavity, but whose frequency was slightly detuned. The reader may be interested in consulting articles which

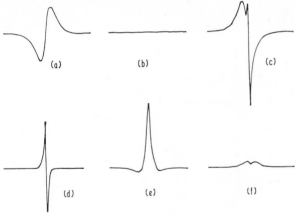

Fig. 14–40.   Electron spin resonance difference spectra obtained using a dual sample cavity from (a) a single sample of powdered coal, (b) two identical samples of coal under exact balance; (c) a single sample of coal to which one crystal of DPPH has been added; (d) the two samples used for (a) and (c) balanced to give the DPPH spectrum; (e) two identical samples of coal which are subjected to a difference in magnetic field; (f) samples as in (e) with equal magnetic fields. (a) to (d) were obtained using the same spectrometer gain, and (e) and (f) were obtained with the gain increased 7 times [Smith and Wilmshurst (1963)].

discuss the measurement of intensities in conventional microwave spectroscopes equipped with a resonant cavity [Verdier (1958); Beers (1959)] or an absorption cell [Hershberger (1948); Baird and Bird (1954)]. Dymanus (1959) and Dymanus, Dijkerman, and Zijderveld (1960) describe the anti-modulation method of determining intensities in a Stark-modulated spectrograph. Scheffler and Stegmann (1963) present a method for determining g factors to a precision of ca. 5×10^{-6}, and Segal, Kaplan, and Fraenkel (1956) report values to within two or three parts per million. See also Blois, Brown, and Maling (1961).

The ESR absorption in an unknown sample may be measured by an NMR spectrometer in a field of about a dozen gauss, and then calibrated against a standard NMR sample under the same instrumental conditions except for an increase in the magnetic field strength by three orders of magnitude.

Belson (1964) describes a method for producing spherical polished samples for ferrimagnetic studies, Howling and Hoskins (1965) present a high speed method for obtaining thin flakes of metal samples, and Schone and Olson (1965) show how to make a hollow metal single crystal.

References

R. Aasa and T. Vänngård, Z. Naturforsch, **19A**, 1425 (1964).

A. Abragam, *The Principles of Nuclear Magnetism*, Clarendon, Oxford, 1961.

L. C. Allen, H. M. Gladney, and S. H. Glarum, *J. Chem. Phys.*, **40**, 3135 (1964).

S. A. Al'tshuler and B. M. Kozyrev, *Electron Paramagnetic Resonance*, trans. from the Russian by Scripta Technica, edited by C. P. Poole, Jr., Academic Press, N. Y., 1964.

R. A. Anderson and H. B. Schulteis, Jr., *Inst. Soc. Am.*, Fourteenth Annual Conf., Sept. 1959.

A. Ye Arbuzov, F. G. Valitova, N. S. Garif'yanov, and B. M. Kozyrev, *Dokl. Akad, Nauk. SSSR*, **126**, 774 (1959).

V. A. Atsarkin, M. E. Zhabotinskii, and A.V. Frantsesson, *Radiotekhn. i Elektron.*, **7**, 866 (820) (1962).

J. N. Aubrun, *Onde Élect.*, (1965).

J. N. Aubrun, P. Veillet, and T. Van Hiep, *Proc. Twelfth Colloque Ampere*, Bordeaux, 1963, p. 534; *C. R. Acad. Sci.*, **256**, 3430 (1963).

D. H. Baird and G. R. Bird, *RSI*, **25**, 319 (1954).

G. W. Barton, Jr., L. E. Gibson, and L. F. Tolman, *Anal. Chem.*, **32**, 1599 (1960).

G. W. Barton, Jr., L. F. Tolman, and R. E. Roulette, *RSI*, **31**, 995 (1960).

Y. Beers, *RSI*, **30**, 9 (1959); **32**, 23 (1961).

H. S. Belson, *RSI*, **35**, 234 (1964).

A. J. Berteaud and H. Le Gall, *Proc. Twelfth Colloque Ampere*, Bordeaux, 1963, p. 507.

G. Berthet, *C. R. Acad. Sci.*, **241**, 1730 (1955); *Ann. Phys. (Paris)*, **3**, 629 (1958).

D. Bijl, H. Kainer, and A. C. Rose-Innes, *J. Chem. Phys.*, **30**, 765 (1959).

A. L. Bil'dyukevich, *PTE*, **6**, 186 (1194) (1963); *ibid.*, **2**, 185 (453) (1964); *Cryogenics* **5**, 205, 277 (1965).

N. Bloembergen and S. Wang, *Phys. Rev.*, **93**, 72 (1954).

M. S. Blois, Jr., H. W. Brown, and J. E. Maling, *Free Radicals in Biological Systems*, Academic, N. Y., 1961, p. 121.

S. Blume, A. Habermehl, and H. Wolter, *Z. Angew. Phys.*, **20**, 149 (1965).

A. Bódi and P. Goara, *Stud. Cercetari Fiz. (Rumania)*, **15**, 385 (1964).

H. C. Bolton, G. J. Troup, and G. V. H. Wilson, *Phil. Mag.*, **9**, 591 (1964).

G. Bonnet, *Arch. Sci. (Spec. No.)*, **14**, 297 (1961).

B. G. Bosch and W. A. Gambling, *J. Brit. Inst. Radio Eng.* **24**, 389 (1962); *ibid.*, **21**, 503 (1961).

S. E. Bresler, E. M. Saminskii, and E. N. Kazbekov, *Zhur. Tekh. Fiz.*, **27**, 2535 (2357) (1958).

M. E. Brodwin and T. J. Burgess, *IEEE Trans. Instr. Meas.*, **IM-12**, 7 (1963).

T. W. P. Brogden and J. Butterworth, *Proc. Phys. Soc.*, **86**, 877 (1965).

H. A. Buckmaster and J. C. Dering, *Can. J. Phys.*, **43**, 1088 (1965).

J. H. Burgess, *J. Phys. Radium*, **19**, 845 (1958).

V. R. Burgess, *JSI*, **38**, 98 (1961).

W. A. Clark, R. M. Brown, M. H. Goldstein, C. E. Molnar, D. F. O'Brien, and H. E. Zieman, *IRE Trans. Bio-Med. Electron.*, **BME-8**, 46 (1961).

M. Clynes and M. Kohn, *Fourth Intern. Conf. Med. Electron.*, N. Y., July 1961.

V. W. Cohen, C. Kikuchi, and J. Turkevich, *Phys. Rev.*, **85**, 379 (1952).

B. A. Coles and D. Bruce, *JSI*, **42**, 532 (1965).

R. L. Collins, *RSI*, **30**, 492 (1959).

P. Cook and J. R. Mallard, *Nature*, **198**, 145 (1963).

D. J. Cram and R. A. Reeves, *J. Am. Chem. Soc.*, **80**, 3094 (1958).

Y. Crosnier and R. Gabillard, *Proc. Twelfth Colloque Ampere*, Bordeaux, 1963, p. 157.

Yu. L. Danilyuk, P. L. Pakhol'chik, and F. A. Koleda, *PTE*, **1**, 213 (222) (1965).

G. D. Dawson, *Electroencephal. Clin. Neurophysiol.*, **6**, 65 (1954).

R. W. DeGrasse, E. O. Schulz-Du Bois, and H. E. D. Scovil, *Bell System Tech. J.*, **38**, 305 (1959).

B. C. Deloach, *Proc. Inst. Elect. Electron. Engr.*, **51**, 1153 (1963).

A. Dymanus, *Physica*, **25**, 859 (1959).

A. Dymanus, H. A. Dijkerman, and G. R. D. Zijderveld, *J. Chem. Phys.*, **32**, 717 (1960).

D. A. Ellerbruch, *J. Res. Nat. Bur. Std.*, **69C**, No. 1, 55 (1965).

J. Engel, *ETP*, **12**, 253 (1964).

R. R. Ernst, *RSI*, **36**, 1689 (1965).

R. R. Ernst and W. A. Anderson, *RSI*, **36**, 1696 (1965); **37**, 93 (1966).

K. M. Evenson and D. S. Burch, *J. Chem. Phys.*, **44**, 1714 (1966).

E. A. Faulkner, *JSI*, **39**, 135 (1962); *Lab. Pract.*, **13**, 1065 (1964).

⌄ G. Feher, *Bell System Tech. J.*, **36**, 449 (1957).

G. Filipovich and T. M. Sanders, Jr., *RSI*, **30**, 293 (1959).

G. v. Foerster, *Z. Naturforsch.*, **15A**, 1079 (1960).

R. H. Frater, *RSI*, **36**, 634 (1965).

R. Gabillard, *Ann. Assoc. Intern. Calcul Analogique*, **6**, 280 (1960).

W. A. Gambling and T. H. Wilmshurst, *Phys. Letters*, **5**, 228 (1963). *Proc. Twelfth Colloque Ampere*, Bordeaux, 1963, p. 171.

S. H. Glarum, *RSI*, **36**, 771 (1965).

J. P. Goldsborough and M. Mandel, *RSI*, **31**, 1044 (1960).

S. Goldschmidt and K. Renn, *Chem. Ber.*, **55**, 628, 694 (1922).

C. J. Gorter and R. deL. Kronig, *Physica*, **3**, 1009 (1936).

A. Gozzini and M. Iannuzzi, *Arch. Sci. (Fasc. Spec.)*, **13**, 178 (1960).

K. H. Hausser, *Ampere Colloquium*, Eindhoven, 1962, p. 420.

K. H. Hausser, *J. Chim. Phys.*, **61**, 1610 (1964).

K. H. Hausser and R. Reinhold, *Z. Naturforsch*, **16A**, 1114 (1961).

P. Hedvig, *Acta Phys. Hung.*, **10**, 115 (1959).

C. L. Hemenway, R. W. Henry, and M. Caulton, *Physical Electronics*, Wiley, N. Y., 1962.

W. D. Hershberger, *J. Appl. Phys.*, **19**, 411 (1948).

⌄ A. N. Holden, C. Kittel, F. R. Merritt, and W. A. Yager, *Phys. Rev.*, **77**, 147 (1950).

T. C. Hollocher, W. H. From, and N. S. Bromberg, *Phys. Med. Biol.*, **9**, 65 (1964).

R. H. Hoskins and R. C. Pastor, *J. Appl. Phys.*, **31**, 1506 (1960).

D. H. Howling and J. M. Hoskins, *RSI*, **36**, 400 (1965).

J. S. Hyde, unpublished notes.

D. J. E. Ingram, *Free Radicals as Studied by Electron Spin Resonance*, Butterworths, London, 1958, Chap. 3.

A. Jelenski, *Ampere Colloquium*, Eindhoven, 1962, p. 734.

C. S. Johnson, Jr. and R. Chang, *J. Chem. Phys.*, **43**, 3183 (1965).

A. E. Karbowiak, *Proc. Inst. Elect. Engr.*, **110**, 2241 (1963).

M. Kent and J. R. Mallard, *JSI*, **42**, 505 (1965).

M. Kent and J. R. Mallard, *Nature*, **207**, 1195 (1965).

J. G. Kenworthy and R. E. Richards, *JSI*, **42**, 675 (1965).

C. Kikuchi and V. W. Cohen, *Phys. Rev.*, **93**, 394 (1954).

M. P. Klein and G. W. Barton, Jr., *RSI*, **34**, 754 (1963); *Paramagnetic Resonance*, **2**, 698 (1963).

P. Kottis and R. Lefebvre, *J. Chem. Phys.*, **39**, 393 (1963); **41**, 379 (1964).

H. A. Kramers, *Atti Congr. Intern. Fis. Como and Rome*, **2**, 545 (1927).

S. Krongelb and M. W. P. Strandberg, *J. Chem. Phys.*, **31**, 1196 (1959).

R. deL. Kronig, *J. Opt. Soc. Am.*, **12**, 547 (1926).

A. F. Krupnov and V. A. Skvortsov, *PTE*, **1**, 212 (230) (1964).

J. B. H. Kuper and M. C. Waltz, *Measurements on Noise from Reflex Oscillators*, Radiation Laboratory Report No. 872, Dec. 21, 1945; see *RLS-24*, p. 113.

R. P. Lacroix, C. E. Ryter, and C. R. Extermann, *Phys. Rev.*, **80**, 763 (1950).

C. Lagercrantz and L. Persson, *RSI*, **35**, 1605 (1964).

H. Lecar and A. Okaya, *Paramagnetic Resonance*, **2**, 675 (1963).

R. Livingston and H. Zeldes, *J. Chem. Phys.*, **24**, 170 (1956).

J. P. Lloyd and G. E. Pake, *Phys. Rev.*, **92**, 1576 (1953); *ibid.*, **94**, 579 (1954).

M. W. Long, *RSI*, **31**, 1286 (1960).

J. J. Lothe and G. Eia, *Acta. Chem. Scand.*, **12**, 1535 (1958).

P. C. Mahendru and R. Parshad, *RSI*, **35**, 1618 (1964).

A. E. Martin, *Nature*, **180**, 231 (1957).

R. D. Mattuck and M. W. P. Strandberg, *RSI*, **29**, 717 (1958).

R. E. Mayo and J. H. Goldstein, *RSI*, **35**, 1231 (1964).

V. J. McBrierty and P. D. Cook, *Nature*, **205**, 1197 (1965).

A. L. McWhorter and F. R. Arams, *Proc. IRE*, **46**, 913 (1958).

P. H. Miller, *Proc. IRE*, **35**, 252 (1947).

M. Misra, *Indian J. Pure Appl. Phys.*, **1**, 37 (1963); **3**, 54 (1965).

R. Mittra, *IEEE Trans. Antennae Propagation* **AP-11**, 585 (1963).

K. E. Mortenson, *J. Appl. Phys.*, **31**, 1207 (1960).

K. A. Müller, *Arch. Sci. (Fasc. Spec.)*, **13**, 342 (1960).

V. Muromtsev, A. K. Piskunov, and N. V. Verein, *Radiotekhn. i Elektron.*, **7**, 1206 (1129) (1962).

A. Okaya, *Paramagnetic Resonance*, **2**, 687 (1963).

G. E. Pake and E. M. Purcell, *Phys. Rev.*, **74**, 1184 (1948).

G. E. Pake, S. I. Weissman, and J. Townsend, *Disc. Faraday Soc.*, **19**, 147 (1955).

J. B. Payne III, *IEEE Trans.*, **MTT-12**, No. 1, 48 (1964).

M. Peter, D. Shaltiel, J. H. Wernick, H. J. Williams, J. B. Mock, and R. C. Sherwood, *Phys. Rev.*, **126**, 1395 (1962).

C. P. Poole, Jr., Thesis, Dept. of Physics, University of Maryland, 1958.

A. M. Portis and D. T. Teaney, *J. Appl. Phys.*, **29**, 1692 (1958).

H. Powell, *J. Appl. Chem.*, **6**, 488 (1956).

R. Rajan, *J. Sci. Ind. Res. (India)*, **21B**, 445 (1962).

M. L. Randolph, *RSI*, **31**, 949 (1960).

RLS-6.

RLS-7.

RLS-11.

RLS-13, Chap. 8.

RLS-16.

RLS-22.

RLS-23.

RLS-24.

G. Roberts and W. Derbyshire, *JSI*, **38**, 511 (1961).

J. D. Robinson and T. Yogi, *RSI*, **36**, 517 (1965).

S. L. Ruby, L. M. Epstein, and K. H. Sun, *RSI*, **31**, 580 (1960).

A. M. Russell and D. A. Torchia, *RSI*, **33**, 442 (1962).

Ch. Ryter, R. Lacroix, and R. Extermann, *Onde Élect.*, **35**, 490 (1955).

K. Scheffler and H. B. Stegmann, *Ber. Bunsengesell. Phys. Chem.*, **67**, 864 (1963).

F. Schneider, *Z. Instrumentenkunde*, **71**, No. 12, 315 (1963).

H. E. Schone and P. W. Olson, *RSI*, **36**, 843 (1965).

E. O. Schulz-Du Bois, *Prog. Cryog.*, **2**, 173 (1961).

R. W. Schumann, *RSI*, **27**, 687 (1956).

R. W. Schumann and J. P. McMahon, *RSI*, **27**, 675 (1956).

A. Scott, *Am. J. Phys.*, **32**, 713 (1964).

B. G. Segal, M. Kaplan, and G. K. Fraenkel, *J. Chem. Phys.*, **43**, 4191 (1965).

M. Sharnoff, *Am. J. Phys.*, **32**, 40 (1964).

K. Shimoda, *J. Phys. Soc. Japan*, **14**, 954, 966 (1959).

K. Shimoda, H. Takahasi, and C. H. Townes, *J. Phys. Soc. Japan*, **12**, 686 (1957).

K. Shimoda and T. C. Wang, *RSI*, **26**, 1148 (1955).

R. S. Sigmond, *JSI*, **42**, 440 (1965).

J. R. Singer, *Masers*, Wiley, N. Y., 1959.

L. S. Singer, *J. Appl. Phys.*, **30**, 1463 (1959).

L. S. Singer and C. Kikuchi, *J. Chem. Phys.*, **23**, 1738 (1955).

L. S. Singer, W. H. Smith, and G. Wagoner, *RSI*, **32**, 213 (1961).

E. L. Sloan, III, A. Ganssen, and E. C. LaVier, *Appl. Phys. Letters*, **4**, 109 (1964).

G. Slomp, *RSI*, **30**, 1024 (1959).

J. Smidt, *Arch. Sci. (Fasc. Spec.)*, **13**, 337 (1960).

R. C. Smith and T. H. Wilmshurst, *JSI*, **40**, 371 (1963).

E. O. Stejskal, *RSI*, **34**, 971 (1963).

K. W. H. Stevens, *JSI*, **37**, 1 (1960).

O. Štirand, *ETP*, **10**, 313 (1962).

L. G. Stoodley, *Nature*, **198**, 1077 (1963).

L. G. Stoodley, *J. Electron. Control*, **14**, 531 (1963).

M. W. P. Strandberg, *Phys. Rev.*, **106**, 617 (1957).

M. W. P. Strandberg, M. Tinkham, I. H. Solt, Jr., and C. F. Davis, Jr., *RSI*, **27**, 596 (1956).

H. Suhl, *J. Appl. Phys.*, **28**, 1225 (1957).

D. T. Teaney, M. P. Klein, and A. M. Portis, *RSI*, **32**, 721 (1961).

P. Thaddeus and L. C. Krisher, *RSI*, **32**, 1083 (1961).

D. S. Thompson and J. S. Waugh, *RSI*, **36**, 552 (1965).

M. Tinkham and M. W. P. Strandberg, *Phys. Rev.*, **97**, 951 (1955).

C. H. Townes, *Phys. Rev. Letters*, **5**, 428 (1960).

C. H. Townes, *Rend. Scuola Intern. Fis. XVII Corso*, **1960**, 39.

C. H. Townes and J. Turkevitch, *Phys. Rev.*, **77**, 148 (1950).

G. J. Troup and J. Walter, *Phil. Mag.*, **11**, 1059 (1965).

Sun Tsung-tang, Chaing Wen-chia, Shun Lien-fong, and Mao Tin-fong, *Acta Phys. Sinica*, **21**, 866 (1965).

J. Uebersfeld, *J. Chim. Phys.*, **56**, 805 (1959).

A. Uhlir, Jr., *Sci. Am.*, **200**, 118 (1959).

A. Valeriu and I. Pascaru, *Rev. Phys. (Rumania)*, **8**, 481 (1963).

P. H. Verdier, *RSI*, **29**, 646 (1958).

S. Visweswaramurthy, *Indian J. Pure Appl. Phys.*, **3**, 316 (1965).

R. H. Webb, *RSI*, **33**, 732 (1962).

J. Weber, *Phys. Rev.*, **108**, 537 (1957).

J. Weber, *Rev. Mod. Phys.*, **31**, 681 (1959).

L. M. Welter, *RSI*, **36**, 487 (1965).

K. Werner, *Hochfrequenztech. ElektAkust. (Germany)*, **73**, 115 (1964).

⤓ J. E. Wertz, D. C. Reitz, and F. Dravnieks, *Free Radicals in Biological Systems*,
M. S. Blois, Jr., et al., Ed., Academic, N. Y., 1961, p. 183.

A. A. Westenberg, *J. Chem. Phys.*, **43**, 1544 (1965); A. A. Westenberg and N.
DeHaas, *ibid.*, **40**, 3087 (1964); **43**, 1550 (1965).

W. E. Willshaw, *Nachrichtentech. Fachber.*, **22**, 6 (1961).

T. H. Wilmshurst, *Nature*, **199**, 477 (1963).

T. H. Wilmshurst, W. A. Gambling, and D. J. E. Ingram, *J. Electron. Control*,
13, 339 (1962).

J. P. Wittke, *Proc. IRE*, **45**, 291 (1957).

S. J. Wyard, *JSI*, **42**, 769 (1965).

A. Yariv and J. P. Gordon, *RSI*, **32**, 462 (1961).

G. M. Zverov, *PTE*, **5**, 109 (930) (1961).

CHAPTER 15

Vacuum Systems

It is frequently desired to provide samples with specialized pre-treatments such as oxidation and reduction, and for this purpose a vacuum system is indispensible. This chapter will briefly introduce the lector to high vacuum techniques; he should consult one of the books listed at the end of the chapter [Barr and Ankorn (1945); Davy (1951); Dushman (1962); Jnanananda (1947); Leck (1957); Yarwood (1955)] for further details.

A. The Necessity of Pretreating Samples

Many systems that produce strong electron spin resonance signals are unaffected by changes in the temperature, pressure, and various environmental conditions. Other systems exhibit remarkable changes in their ESR spectra when one or more of these parameters is changed, as the following examples indicate.

It is well known that α,α'-diphenyl-β-picryl hydrazyl (DPPH) produces a narrow singlet in the solid state, and a quintet with the relative intensity ratios 1–2–3–2–1 in benzene solution. More recently it has been discovered that when one removes all of the oxygen that is disolved in the solvent, then many additional hyperfine lines are resolved, as shown in Fig. 15–1 [see Deguchi (1960); Ueda, Kuri, and Shida (1962)]. Before the removal of the oxygen, only the nitrogen hyperfine coupling constants may be determined, while after the removal of oxygen, the proton hyperfine constants may also be determined.

Various varieties of solid carbons are quite sensitive to the temperature and to the presence of certain gases during the thermal pretreatment that produces and destroys paramagnetic centers. Singer (1963) has given an excellent review of this subject, and a number of pertinent articles may be found in the Proceedings of the Carbon Conferences.

601

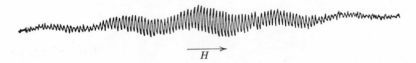

$\overrightarrow{H}$

Fig. 15-1.   Electron spin resonance spectrum of DPPH in tetrahydrofuran after the removal of dissolved oxygen [Deguchi (1960)].

The low-temperature form of chromia-alumina produces ESR spectra from isolated Cr^{+3} ions, clumped Cr^{+3} ions, and Cr^{+5} ions, while Cr^{+6} is detected in this system by its near ultraviolet charge transfer spectrum. These three valence states may be converted reversibly into one another by heating at several hundred degrees centigrade in the presence of oxygen or hydrogen (but not a mixture of both, or an explosion may result!). For further details about this system, see the review article by Poole and MacIver (1965).

The observed ESR spectrum of a free atom such as N, O, and P, or of a simple molecule such as NO and NO_2 in the gaseous state, is dependent upon the pressure, pumping speed, presence of buffer gases, chemical treatment of the gas container walls, etc. The atom or molecule under study is usually generated by dissociation in an electric discharge, and then pumped rapidly through the resonant cavity before it has time to recombine and form a diamagnetic molecule. The spectrometers described in Secs. 13-B and 13-D were employed for the study of paramagnetic gases. The subject is reviewed in the following books: Townes and Schawlow (1955), Chap. 5; Ingram (1955), Sec. 6–18; Ingram (1958); Al'tshuler and Kozyrev (1964), Sec. 7–5.

When an ionic crystal such as an alkali halide is heated in an atmosphere of its cation or anion, the crystal may develop an excess of either constituent, and the result is the formation of a color center such as an F center. Such color centers may also be produced by irradiation with γ-rays, x-rays, neutrons, etc., as discussed in Chap. 17.

The electron spin resonance spectra of the x- or γ-irradiated polymers polyfluoroethylene or Teflon (Rexroad and Gordy (1959)] and polyvinyl chloride [Kuri, Ueda, and Shida (1960)] are dependent both on the gas in contact with the sample during irradiation, and also on various gases introduced after the completion of the irradiation.

Thus we see that some samples require the use of very careful pretreatment and handling procedures. A vacuum system is indispensible for processing such samples. Accordingly, we will devote most of this chapter to the explication of vacuum techniques. The final section will discuss the electrolytic generation of radical ions, because these species require the use of careful pretreatment and handling techniques. For completeness it should also be mentioned that many samples contain paramagnetic species whose ESR spectra are not affected by changes in their physical and chemical environment. For example, the spectra of various minerals such as ruby are insensitive to most of the climatic conditions and geological upheavals to which they have been exposed for countless thousands of years.

B. The Properties of Gases *in Vacuo*

Pressure: Several ranges of pressure may be distinguished:

Soft or low vacuum	760 to 10^{-3} torr
High vacuum	10^{-3} to 10^{-6} torr
Ultra high vacuum	10^{-9} to 10^{-13} torr

One may employ mechanical pumps and rubber hoses in the region of low vacuum, while in the high vacuum region it is necessary to use diffusion pumps and glass or metal systems. Stopcocks and ground glass joints may be used below 10^{-6} torr.

There are several units of pressure in current use: 1 atm = 760 torr = 760 mm Hg = 14.7 lb/in.^{2} = 1.0133 bar. One bar = 10^6 dyn/cm^2 = 7.5×10^{-4} torr.

Ideal Gas Law: The ideal gas law is

$$PV = nRT \tag{1}$$

where P is the pressure, V is the volume, T is the absolute temperature ($273.16 + C°$), n is the number of moles, and the gas constant R is given by

$$R = \begin{cases} 0.082054 & \text{liter atm/mole deg} \\ 8.3144 \times 10^7 & \text{erg/mole deg} \\ 8.3144 & \text{J/mole deg} \\ 1.9865 & \text{cal/mole deg} \end{cases} \tag{2}$$

At high pressures the ideal gas law usually breaks down and it is necessary to employ another relation such as the Van der Waals equation, the Beattie-Bridgeman equation, or the virial coefficients. In the regions of high and ultrahigh vacuum, the ideal gas law usually holds true.

Maxwellian Distribution: The molecules in a gas have a Maxwellian distribution of velocities, and the probability P of finding a molecule with velocity v is given by

$$P = (4/\pi^{1/2}) \, (v/v_p)^2 \exp\left[-(v/v_p)^2\right] \tag{3}$$

where of course

$$\int_0^\infty P d\left(\frac{v}{v_p}\right) = \frac{4}{\pi^{1/2}} \int_0^\infty \left(\frac{v}{v_p}\right)^2 \exp\left[-(v/v_p)^2\right] d\left(\frac{v}{v_p}\right) = 1 \tag{4}$$

and v_p is the most probable velocity since

$$P = \text{maximum} \tag{5}$$

at $v = v_p$. The average velocity v_a and root mean square velocity v_{rms} are given by

$$v_a = \int_0^\infty v P d\left(\frac{v}{v_p}\right) = 1.128 v_p \tag{6}$$

$$v_{\text{rms}} = \left[\int_0^\infty v^2 P d\left(\frac{v}{v_p}\right)\right]^{1/2} = 1.224 v_p \tag{7}$$

The most probable velocity is related to the absolute temperature T and molecular weight M by

$$v_p = 1.29 \times 10^4 \, (T/M)^{1/2} \text{ cm/sec} \tag{8}$$

as shown graphically in Fig. 15–2.

Mean Free Path: The average distance traversed by a molecule between successive collisions is called the mean free path l, and it is given by

$$l = (2^{1/2}\pi \, nd^2)^{-1} \tag{9}$$

where d is the molecular diameter and n is the number of molecules per cubic centimeter. The mean free paths of several common gases are listed in Table 15–1 for 1 and 760 torr. At room temperature and at a pressure of about 3×10^{-3} torr, the mean free path becomes

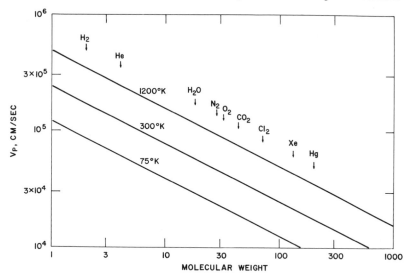

Fig. 15–2. Dependence of the most probable molecular velocity v_p on the molecular weight for three temperatures.

TABLE 15–1

Molecular Diameters and Mean Free Paths (at 25°C) of Several Gases[a]

Gas	Diameter, A	Mean free path, cm	
		1 torr	760 torr
H_2	2.75	0.931×10^{-2}	1.226×10^{-5}
He	2.18	1.472×10^{-2}	1.936×10^{-5}
Ne	2.60	1.045×10^{-2}	1.375×10^{-5}
O_2	3.64	0.540×10^{-2}	0.710×10^{-5}
A	3.67	0.531×10^{-2}	0.667×10^{-5}
Xe	4.91	0.298×10^{-2}	0.393×10^{-5}
air	3.74	0.509×10^{-2}	0.669×10^{-5}

[a] Dushman (1962), p. 32.

comparable to the diameter of a vacuum system manifold so that for $P \ll 10^{-3}$ torr, the average molecule in the system will make many more collisions with the walls than with other molecules. At 10^{-6} torr and 300°K, there are about 3×10^{10} gas molecules per cm^3.

Pumping Speed: If a large volume of V liters which is full of gas at a pressure P is connected to a perfect vacuum through a small aperture of A cm², then the gas will move out of the volume at the rate S [Spangenberg (1948); Dushman (1962), p. 91]

$$S = \frac{V}{P - P_0} \frac{dP}{dt} = -3.64A \, (T/M)^{1/2} \text{ liter/sec} \qquad (10)$$

where T is in °K, M is the molecular weight, and P_0 is the limiting pressure that is attainable. For air at room temperature (300°K)

$$S = -11.7A \text{ liter/sec} \qquad (11)$$

If the gas has the pressure P_i at time $t = 0$, then at a later time t, one has the pressure P_f and

$$t = \frac{V}{S} \int_{P_i}^{P_f} \frac{dP}{P - P_0} \qquad (12)$$

$$= \frac{V}{S} \ln \left(\frac{P_f - P_0}{P_i - P_0} \right) \qquad (13)$$

At low pressures the mean free path exceeds the radius r of glass tubing, and so when gas is pumped through a piece of tubing of length l, the rate of flow (conductance) G is given approximately by

$$G \approx \frac{r^3}{l} \frac{[(T/300) \, (29/M)]^{1/2}}{1 + (8r/3l)} \text{ liter/sec} \qquad (14)$$

where r and l are in millimeters. Several pieces of tubing connected in series have the overall flow rate G

$$\frac{1}{G} = \sum \frac{1}{G_i} \qquad (15)$$

and the composite pumping speed S_c of a pump in series with a piece of tubing is

$$1/S_c = 1/S + 1/G \qquad (16)$$

where S is the speed of the pump alone.   It is important to know the pumping speed associated with a vacuum system in order to evaluate the length of time that one must wait before a desired pressure is reached.   In practice, the pumping speed is often limited by other factors such as the slow desorption of gases from the surface of the sample and the walls of the vacuum system.

C. Pumps

Mechanical Pumps: A forepump or roughing pump is a mechanical pump which is capable of reaching about 10^{-4} torr, as indicated on Fig. 15-3.   It may be employed for low vacua, or for backing-up a diffusion pump.

Diffusion Pumps: A high vacuum is usually produced by a diffusion pump which makes use of the flow of a condensable vapor to draw along molecules from the system being evacuated, and pass them on to the forepump.   To accomplish this task, a diffusion pump makes use of a heater to boil the liquid and a condenser (e.g., of flowing water) to recondense it.   Ordinarily a second cold trap is

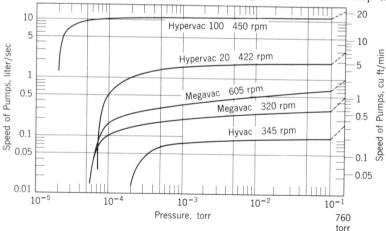

Fig. 15-3.   Pumping speeds of mechanical pumps (data supplied by the Central Scientific Company, Chicago Ill.).

inserted between the diffusion pump and the vacuum system in order to hinder the vapor from diffusing into the system. From its nature, a diffusion pump will not operate unless it is backed-up by a forepump.

A mercury diffusion pump such as the one shown on Fig. 15–4 is frequently employed to obtain pressures down to 10^{-6} torr. The

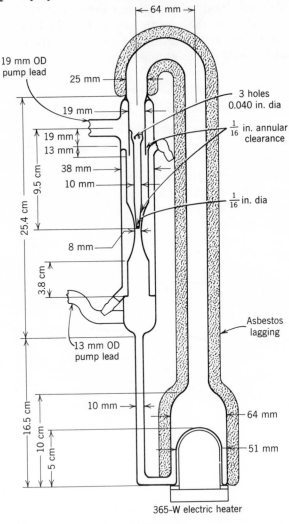

Fig. 15–4.   Mercury diffusion pump [Barr and Ankorn (1959)].

vapor pressure of mercury is about 10^{-3} torr at 18°C as shown on Fig. 15–5, so it is desirable to employ a Dry Ice–acetone or liquid nitrogen cold trap between the pump and the vacuum system to prevent the diffusion of mercury into the system. A typical mercury diffusion pump can pump about 3 liter/sec.

An oil diffusion pump does not need a cold trap if one employs an oil with a vapor pressure less than the overall pressure attained. Oil diffusion pumps are considerably faster than mercury pumps, but they have the disadvantage that the oil may be decomposed by overheating, or by exposure to air when hot.

Cold Trap: Condensable vapors such as water and mercury may be removed from the vacuum system by the use of a cold trap such as the one shown in Fig. 15–6. A Dewar containing liquid nitrogen

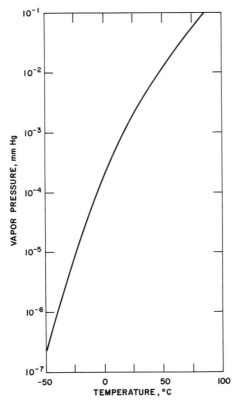

Fig. 15–5. Temperature dependence of the vapor pressure of mercury in millimeters (mm Hg or torr).

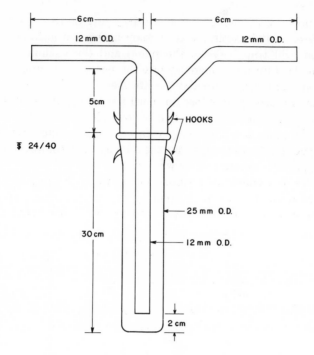

Fig. 15-6.   Cold trap.

(77° K) or a Dry Ice–acetone mixture (195° K) may be employed to condense such vapors in the trap and reduce their pressure in accordance with Fig. 15–5.

D. Pressure Measuring Devices

The pressure ranges covered by several pressure measuring instruments are shown in Table 15–2.   Each of these devices will be discussed briefly.

McLeod Gauge: The McLeod gauge shown in Fig. 15–7 is an absolute pressure measuring device.   It is operated by admitting air to the mercury reservoir.   This raises the mercury level until it fills the volume V_1 and part of the two capillaries C.   The pressure measurement is performed in one of two ways: (1) by lining up the mercury level in the left hand capillary to the top of the right-

TABLE 15-2

Characteristics of Several Pressure Measuring Devices

Name	Pressure in torr		Principle of operation
	Minimum	Maximum	
Monometer	10^{-1}	10^3	Height of Hg column
Spark discharge	10^{-3}	10^2	Color of gas discharge
Pirani gauge	10^{-6}	10^{-2}	Resistance, measured $\left.\begin{array}{l}\text{Heating}\\\text{element}\end{array}\right.$
Thermocouple gauge	10^{-4}	1	Temperature, measured $\left.\begin{array}{l}\text{cooled}\\\text{by gas}\end{array}\right.$
McLeod gauge	10^{-6}	10	Height of Hg column
Ionization gauge	10^{-11}	10^{-3}	Ionization current measured

hand capillary, or (2) by lining up the mercury level in the right-hand closed capillary with the level G_2. The pressure may be calculated from h or from h_1 and h_2. In practice, the pressure is usually read from a scale which is aligned with G or G_2. Since the McLeod gauge is an absolute pressure measuring device, it may be employed to calibrate other gauges. It should not be employed with condensable vapors such as H_2O, or with gases that attack mercury. When not in use, it is best to keep the mercury lowered in the reservoirs. A McLeod gauge may be employed to measure pressures between 10 and 10^{-6} torr.

Spark Discharge: Pressures from 10^{-3} to 100 torr may be estimated by the color of the glow discharge in a vacuum system when a Tesla coil is applied to the glass. If a leak is present the spark will jump to the leak, making the Tesla coil a useful tool in troubleshooting vacuum systems.

Pirani Gauge: The Pirani gauge consists of a heated filament placed in the vacuum system. When gas is present it cools the filament and lowers its resistance, as measured by a Wheatstone bridge. A typical curve of the galvamometer deflection versus the pressure is shown on Fig. 15-8.

Thermocouple Gauge: The thermocouple gauge uses a heated filament and monitors the temperature of the filament by a thermocouple. The pressure dependence of the thermocouple current follows a sigmoid curve such as the one shown on Fig. 15–9. It works in the range 10^{-4} to 1 torr.

Ionization Gauge: The ionization gauge consists of a triode with

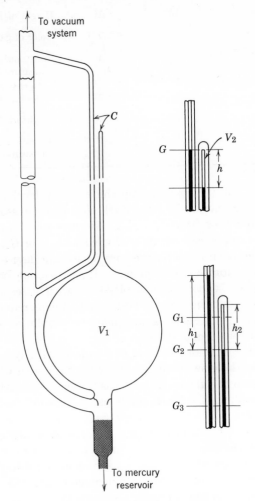

Fig. 15–7.   McLeod gauge [Barr and Ankorn (1959)].

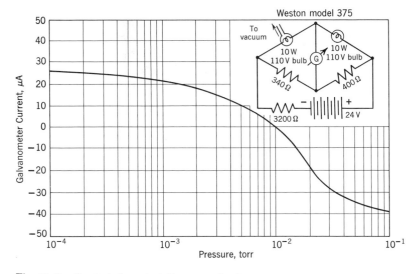

Fig. 15–8.   Typical characteristic curve of galvanometer current versus pressure for a Pirani gauge [Spangenberg (1948)].

a heated filament, a positive grid to collect electrons from the filament, and a negative plate to collect positive ions formed in the gas by collisions of the electrons with gas molecules. The number of positive ions formed is a functon of the pressure. The ionization gauge may be employed to measure pressures between 10^{-11} and 10^{-3} torr, and even lower pressures are reached by some of the more modern gauges.

Manometer: A U tube manometer such as the one shown on Fig. 15–10 is made from two 1-m long glass tubes joined at the bottom to form a U and closed at one end under vacuum. The other end is attached to the vacuum system, and the manometer is filled halfway with mercury so that at high vacuum the two mercury levels are equal. At atmospheric pressure the two levels will differ by 760 torr, and if the length of the tube is made longer than this, the U tube manometer may be employed to measure pressures from about 1 torr to somewhat above 1 atm. It is convenient to provide each manometer with a meter stick for determining the height of the mercury level. A simpler version of the manometer consists of a 1-m long vertical tube inserted into a mercury reservoir at the lower end and attached to the vacuum system at the upper end.

Calibration Curves

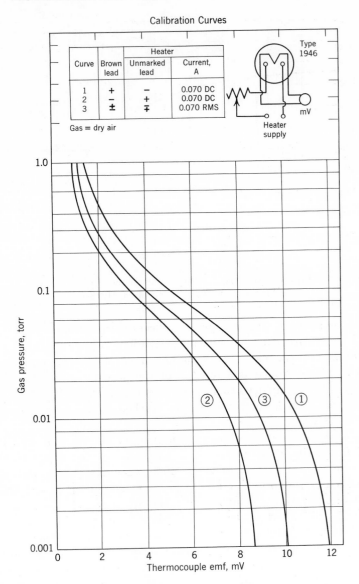

Fig. 15–9.   The gas pressure versus thermocouple voltage characteristic curves of a type 1946 Thermocouple gauge (*RCA Tube Handbook*).

E. Typical Vacuum System

A typical vacuum system for use in pretreating electron spin resonance samples is shown in Fig. 15–10. The diffusion pump at the upper left is backed up by a forepump, and they are separated by a two position stopcock. The cold trap is used with a Dewar of liquid nitrogen (or a Dry Ice–acetone mixture) to remove condensible vapors such as water or mercury from the system. It is not advisable to use this liquid nitrogen cold trap until most of the air has been removed from the vacuum system, since otherwise the air (oxygen) may condense in the trap and take a long time to pump out.

The vacuum system is provided with three pressure measuring devices. In practice, it is convenient to measure the pressure from 10^{-6} to 10^{-3} torr with the McLeod gauge, from 10^{-3} to 1 torr with the thermocouple or Pirani gauge, and from 1 to 10^3 torr with the U tube manometer. One should note that the McLeod gauge is only connected to the vacuum system through a stopcock during a pressure measurement; the thermocouple or Pirani gauge is always physically connected to the system but is only activated electrically during a pressure measurement, while the manometer is operating at all times. The McLeod gauge reservoir is preferably connected to a separate mechanical pump, but it may be operated off the same forepump that backs up the diffusion pump if care is taken to isolate the diffusion pump and the rest of the system during and for several minutes after the evacuation of the reservoir. To minimize leaks, it is advisable to make the vacuum system as simple as is feasible, with all unnecessary stopcocks eliminated. The system shown on Fig. 15–10 is a compromise between simplicity and versatility.

The two sample tube arrangements presented on Figs. 15–11 to 15–13 are shown in position on the main manifold. The gases that are employed to pretreat the samples are supplied from the auxiliary manifold, and they may be dried or purified in the cold trap before use. The two manifolds can be isolated from each other by a stopcock.

The vacuum system may be used to pretreat samples by heating or cooling them *in vacuo* or in the presence of a particular gas such as hydrogen or oxygen (but not both simultaneously or an explosion might occur!). The sample is exposed to the desired gaseous atmosphere by closing the stopcock at the left side of the main manifold

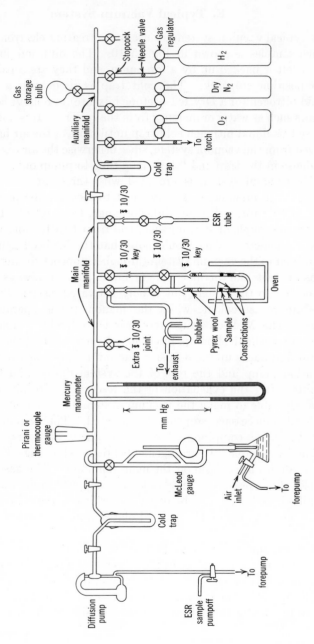

Fig. 15-10. A typical vacuum system.

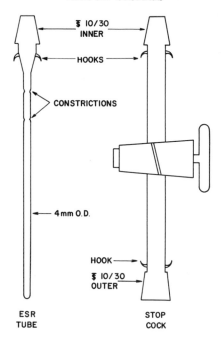

Fig. 15–11. ESR tube and stopcock (KPAH).

in order to isolate the system from the pumps, and then opening the stopcock on the right to introduce the gas. Oxidation and reduction reactions are most efficiently carried out by adjusting the three-way stopcock in the center of the main manifold so that the gas flows into the duplex ESR pretreatment tube from the right and then leaves the system on the left via the bubbler sketched on Fig. 15–14. The rate of flow may be estimated from the number of bubbles per minute. The adapter tube is inserted between the sample and the vacuum system so that the sample may be removed and measured between treatments. For example, one may make use of this arrangement to study the ESR signal as a function of oxygen pressure. The pair of outer tapered joints shown in Fig. 15–13 forms a "key" which mates with the pair of inner joints shown, also. Ball joints may be substituted for the standard taper joints to make the key a little easier to use, but less vacuum tight.

After the completion of the heat or gas treatment, the sample tube may be removed from the vacuum system and the samples shaken

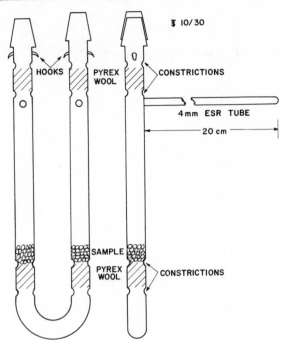

Fig. 15–12.   Duplex ESR pretreatment tube.

into the ESR tubes.   One may then seal them off with a torch* and measure them in the resonant cavity.   It is possible to construct a system similar to the one shown in Fig. 15–12 in which the ESR tubes face the sides rather than the front so that the sample may be placed in the resonant cavity without sealing it off, and then returned to the vacuum system for further treatment.   Systems can also be built which permit the *in situ* pretreatment of samples directly in the resonant cavity.   When powder samples are used, sudden pressure changes should be avoided to prevent the powder from blowing around.   Samples may also be sealed off *in vacuo* sans pretreatment by using the ESR sample pumpoff three-way stopcock if care is exercised to reconnect the diffusion pump to the forepump a minute or two thereafter.

The oven may be conveniently heated to 500°C with Pyrex sample holders, and several hundred degrees higher when quartz or Vycor are

* Dark glasses should be used to protect the eyes when sealing quartz.

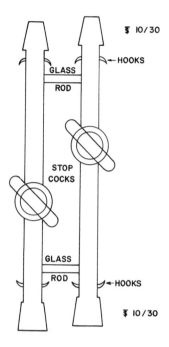

Fig. 15–13. Keyed double stopcock (KPAH) adapter.

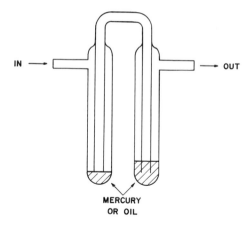

Fig. 15–14. Bubbler for monitoring the rate of flow of a gas.

used. One may construct the entire pretreatment tube out of quartz or Vycor to eliminate the necessity of employing graded seals to the quartz ESR tubes. The oven temperature may be automatically regulated with the aid of a thermocouple and an appropriate controller. Asbestos paper may be placed around the glass at the top of the oven for thermal insulation, and sometimes a small blower or compressed air flow is used to prevent stopcock grease from melting.

The gases that are used for pretreating the sample are obtained from the auxiliary manifold. Each gas tank is supplied with a pressure regulator, and is connected to the auxiliary manifold through a needle valve which provides a fine control adjustment of the gas flow rate. An additional supply of gas may be kept in the gas storage bulb. The cold trap may be used in conjunction with a liquid nitrogen or Dry Ice–acetone bath to dry the gases, or it may be filled with a drying–purifying agent.

Cacciarelli and Stewart (1963) describe a vacuum and pressure system for NMR sample preparation, and Müller-Warmuth (1963) presents a system for free radical solutions. Wamser and Stewart (1965) describe a sample reactor and a sample transfer system for use with liquid samples.

F. The Generation of Radical Ions

The classical method for producing positive radical ions (cations formed by oxidation) is to dissolve the parent compound in sulfuric acid, as shown by Weissman, DeBoer, and Conradi (1957) and Yokozawa and Miyashita (1956). For example, Carrington, Dravnieks, and Symons (1959) used concentrations between 0.01 M and 0.02 M of anthracene, naphthalene, and perylene in 98% sulfuric acid to produce the corresponding positive radical ions. Positive ions have also been produced by air oxidation [Venkataraman and Fraenkel (1955, 1955); Ehrenberg (1957); Adams, Blois, and Sands (1958); Venkataraman, Segal, and Fraenkel (1959)].

The classical method for producing negative radical ions (anions formed by reduction) is to expose the parent compound to an alkali metal. For example, Carrington, Dravnieks, and Symons (1959) prepared negative ions by the vacuum distillation of tetrahydrofuran from phosphoric oxide into a tube containing a piece of kalium and the parent hydrocarbon. The tubes were first sealed off and then heated to melt the potassium. This induced the potassium to transfer electrons to the hydrocarbon and thereby produce the desired radical anions. Negative radical ions have also been produced by reduction with zinc [Ehrenberg (1957); Adams, Blois, and Sands (1958)]. These classical methods of producing both positive and negative radical ions are reviewed by Ingram (1958).

Prior to 1959, most of the ESR studies of radical ions were carried out with ions which had been produced by one of these classical methods. However, these methods are not completely satisfactory. For example, the alkali preparation is laborious, and the presence of the metal in the solution may complicate the spectrum [see Tuttle, Ward, and Weissman (1956); Ward and Weissman (1957); Adams and Weissman (1958)]. Galkin, Shamfarov, and Stefanishina (1957) produced unpaired spins by passing an electric current through NaCl dissolved in liquid ammonia. Austen, Given, Ingram, and Peover (1958) produced free radicals by controlled potential electrolysis, but these radicals were frozen in liquid nitrogen for the ESR measurements. Maki and Geske (1959, 1959) generated free radical ions directly in the resonant cavity (*intra muros* in their terminology) by a polarographic or electrolytic technique, and thereby opened up a new branch of electron spin resonance. Many investigators have followed their example and employed as a selective reducing agent an electrode within a cell located directly in the resonant cavity. Carrington (1963) and Bowers (1964) have recently reviewed the ESR of radical ions, Morosova (1962) reviewed the application of molecular orbital theory to the interpretation of such data, and McClelland (1964) covers the non-ESR aspects of this field.

The electrochemical cell that was employed by Geske and Maki (1960) is shown on Fig. 15–15. They designed a mercury pool electrode A placed in the bottom of a 3-mm OD Pyrex tube B and centered in the microwave reflection cavity. The pool has an exposed area of 2.5 mm^2 and receives its supply voltage by means of a platinum wire C which is sealed into the bottom of B. The tube B is surrounded by a quartz tube D which is cemented to tube E by means of epoxy resin. An aqueous saturated calomel electrode (SCE) placed in the insert tube F makes electrolytic contact with the main solution through its own soft glass-Pyrex Perley seal and a sintered glass disk bottom on the insert tube. The main solution

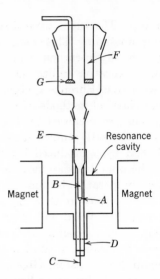

Fig. 15–15. The original electrochemical cell designed for use in an ESR spectrometer [Geske and Maki (1960)].

contains the sample plus a supporting electrolyte of bulky, counterions dissolved in the solvent. It is degassed with the help of a fine capillary which extends through a pinhole in the top down to within 1 mm of the mercury pool. Nitrogen gas is passed through this capillary for preliminary degassing, while a slow flow of nitrogen is maintained through the sintered glass disk G both before and during the electrolysis run. The resistance of the cell was about 20 kΩ for Geske and Maki's solutions.

The radical ions are generated electrolytically by applying the proper voltage V_A between the platinum wire and the calomel anode, and measuring the voltage drop V_C across the cell from the platinum wire to the reference electrode. A typical electrical diagram is shown in Fig. 15–16. The use of a reference electrode placed much closer to the cathode than the calomel electrode helps to correct for polorization effects and the internal voltage drop within the cell. The applied voltage V_A may be varied by means of the potentiometer or voltage divider, and for a typical system the current I through the cell will vary with the cell voltage V_C in the manner shown on the polarogram in Fig. 15–17. The current rises sharply at the half wave potentials denoted by V_1, V_2, and V_3 where there occur transformations from one ionic species to another. For example V_1 might correspond to the formation of a mononegative hydrocarbon radical ion while V_2 indicates the formation of the corresponding dinegative ion. The mononegative ion will be present at the plateau between V_1 and V_2 while the dinegative one is observed on the plateau between V_2 and V_3. It is best to obtain a polarogram such as the one shown in Fig. 15–17 before recording ESR spectra

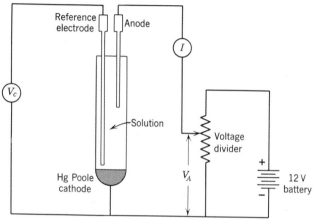

Fig. 15–16. Electrical diagram of an electrolytic cell. The 12-V power supply on the right produces the variable applied voltage drop V_A across the cell while the reference electrode measures the cell voltage V_C which is corrected for polarization effects. The ammeter measures the current I through the cell.

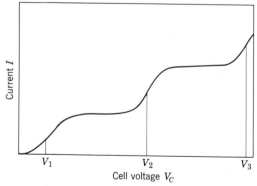

Fig. 15–17. A typical polarogram obtained with a cell of the type shown in Fig. 15–16.

on an unknown system.   A dinegative ion may be in either a singlet or a triplet state, with the former more probable.

The radical ions to be studied are generated electrolytically by applying a voltage V_A corresponding to a cell voltage drop V_C on the plateau between V_1 and V_2.   If the gradual buildup of polarization slowly shifts the actual cell drop V_C for a constant applied voltage V_A, then V_C may be set initially toward one end of the plateau so that the drift will bring it toward the center.   An electron spin resonance run may be made during the electrolysis to record the spectrum of the radical ion.   Pointeau, Favede, and Delhaes (1964) describe the growth and decay of the radical ion concentration during and after the cessation of the electrolysis.

Geske and Maki used the mercury pool electrode to circumvent the high noise level and frequency instabilities that result from allowing small drops of mercury to traverse the resonant cavity periodically.   Most ordinary (i.e., non ESR) polarographic studies make use of a dropping mercury electrode versus an aqueous saturated calomel electrode, with the half wave potential measured relative to a saturated calomel reference electrode.

Various workers have modified the original Geske and Maki cell, and some have employed radically different designs.   Piette, Ludwig, and Adams (1962) generated negative ions by a mercury pool reduction of the type described above.   They also generated positive ions by oxidation at a platinum gauze electrode placed in the resonant cavity.   Their aqueous cells are shown in Fig. 15–18.   Harriman and Maki (1963) also describe a cell which employs a platinum gauze electrode to generate anions.   Jones, LaLancette, and Benson (1964) used a platinum screen in the cavity and a reference electrode of $Ag/AgClO_4$ in acrilonitrile.   Their electrolysis cell was designed by H. G. Hoeve, and is shown in Fig. 15–19.   See also Johnson and Chang (1965).   Levy and Myers (1964) describe an electrolysis cell for use with liquid ammonia.   Lagercrantz and Persson (1964) designed holders for aqueous solution cells.

Bolton and Fraenkel (1964) employed the vacuum electrolytic cell shown on Fig. 15–20.   It is based on the electrolytic technique described by Rieger, Bernal, Reinmuth, and Fraenkel (1963).   The compound (hydrocarbon) under investigation and the tetra-n-butyl ammonium perchlorate (TNBAP) are weighed into tube D to make a 15-ml solution that is 0.1 M in the electrolyte and 0.002 M in the hydrocarbon. The cell is then assembled and attached to the vacuum system at A. After evacuation to a pressure of $\sim 1\ \mu$Hg, the tube D is cooled to 77° K and about 15 ml of the solvent dimethoxyethane (DME) is distilled into D from a storage bulb on the manifold. The apparatus is sealed off from the vacuum system and the warmed up solution is carefully transferred to the rest of the cell by tipping. The apparatus is now attached to the vacuum system at P and evacuated through the stopcock Q. Mercury is admitted from K through the valve H and the electrolysis is initiated at $I = 4$ mA by making the appropriate electrical connections at the cathode J, the anode M, and the Ag/Ag ClO$_4$ reference

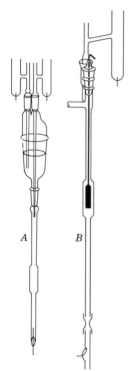

Fig. 15–18. Electrolytic cells: (A) for mercury poole reductions and (B) for platinum electrode oxidations [Piette, Ludwig, and Adams (1962)].

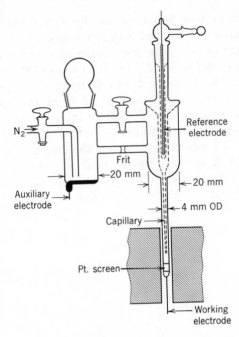

Fig. 15–19.   Electrolytic cell designed for use with short-lived radicals and small quantities (∼1 mg) of the radical precursor [Jones, LaLancette, and Benson (1964)].

electrode E.   Finally the solution is transferred through the valve N to the side arm T for the ESR measurements.   This arrangement does not provide for the *in situ* generation of radical ions.

Bowers, Nolfi, and Greene (1964) designed the electrolytic cell shown on Fig. 15–21 for the rapid routine generation of radical ions. It has been successfully operated with substrates as small as 50 μg. The system on the left with $I = 3$ cm is used for room temperature work, while the tube on the right with $I = 7$ cm is used for variable temperature work.   In the latter case, the electrode connection comes back out of the top of the Dewar.

One of the principal experimental problems encountered in setting up an electrolytic cell results from the high dielectric loss that is an intrinsic property of many of the solvents used in polarography. This loss can have a very deleterious effect on the Q of the resonant cavity, and necessitates a precise alignment of the cell at the point where the microwave electric field is a minimum. This effect on Q may be minimized by employing quartz tubing with a small inner diameter, or a flat quartz cell across a rectangular or cylindrical cavity. For the same size tubing, a cylindrical TE_{011} mode cavity is much less lossy than a rectangular TE_{102} mode cavity. The losses may be considerably reduced by working at S band (3000 Mc) instead of at X band (9500 Mc).

The solutions used in polarography contain three ingredients: (1) the solvent, (2) the supporting electrolyte (bulky counter ions), and

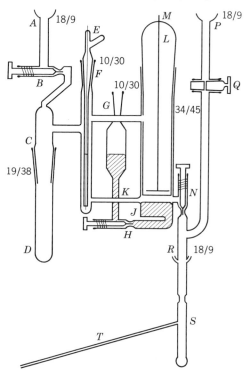

Fig. 15–20. Vacuum electrolytic cell: (A) ball joint connection to vacuum manifold; (B) 1-mm needle valve; (C) mixing chamber; (D) solvent collection tube; (E) connection to (F) reference electrode; (G) mercury storage bulb; (H) mercury admission valve; (J) connection to (K) cathode compartment exit valve; (L) anode compartment; (M) connection to L; (N) cathode compartment; (P) connection to manifold; (Q) stopcock; (R) sample tube connection point (ball joint); (S) sample tube; (T) ESR side arm [Bolton and Fraenkel (1964)].

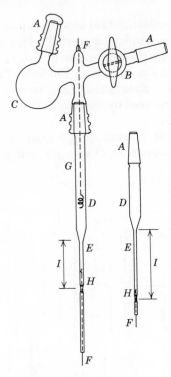

Fig. 15–21.   Electrolytic cell consisting of (A) 12/30 ground glass joint; (B) high vacuum stopcock; (C) 10–50 ml bulb; (D) 11-mm tubing; (E) 3-mm tubing; (F) Pt wire; (G) electrode; (H) electrode [Bowers, Nolfi, and Greene to be published].

(3) the compound to be studied.   The most popular solvents and supporting electrolytes may be deduced from Table 15–3.   Dissolved oxygen produces a strong polarogram as shown on Fig. 15–22, and has a pronounced effect on the ESR relaxation times [Hausser (1960, 1960)].   In addition, a concentration of oxygen that is too small to detect polarographically is still likely to react with the radical ions and produce undesired paramagnetic byproducts.   Therefore, traces of dissolved oxygen must be scrupulously removed from all of the solutions used in polarography.   This may be most easily accomplished by degassing with nitrogen and maintaining a positive pressure of nitrogen in the system during the ESR run.   A more

efficient method of removing oxygen from a solution consists in freezing the solution, evacuating it, closing off the vacuum pump, and allowing the frozen solution to melt. The oxygen is more soluble in the vapor than it is in the liquid, and so several cycles of this freeze-pump-thaw technique are sufficient to remove the dissolved oxygen. As before, a positive pressure of nitrogen gas may be maintained in the system to prevent oxygen from diffusing back in. Lees, Muller, and Noble (1961) describe a gettering technique for the removal of oxygen. Water should also be excluded from electrolytic solutions.

Those who plan to study free radicals by electrolytic generation techniques should familiarize themselves with classical polarographic techniques. The standard two-volume work, *Polarography*, was written by Kolthoff and Lingane (1952), and brought up to date with the more recent pair of volumes entitled *Progress in Polarography* by Zuman and Kolthoff (1962).

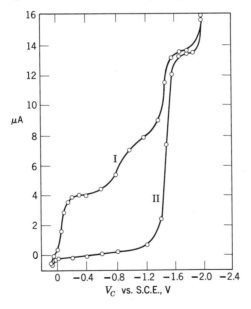

Fig. 15–22. Influence of oxygen on the polarogram of 0.001 N HCl in 0.1 N KCl containing a trace of methyl red: (I) air-free; (II) saturated with air [Kolthoff and Lingane (1952)].

TABLE 15–3

List of Compounds, Solvents, Supporting Electrolytes, and Electrodes Employed in ESR Electrolytic Studies

Samples	Solvents	Supporting electrolytes	Electrodes	Reference
Lithium perchlorate	A	LiClO$_4$	Pt wire	Maki and Geske (1959)
Nitrobenzene	A	TNPAP	Sat. calomel, Hg pool	Geske and Maki (1960)
Substituted nitro benzenes	A	TNPAP	Calomel, Hg pool	Maki and Geske (1961)
o-, m-, and p-Nitroaniline				Piette, Ludwig, and Adams (1961)
p-Nitrophenol	H$_2$O	LiClO$_4$	Hg pool	
p-Nitroanisole		KClO$_4$		
Azulene				Bernal, Rieger, and Fraenkel (1962)
Azulene-1,3 d_2			Ag/AgClO$_4$,	
4,6,8-Trimethylazulene	DMF	TNPAP	Hg pool	
4,6,8-Trimethylazulene 1,3 d_2				
Dinitrodurene	DMF			Freed and Fraenkel (1962)
Dinitrobenzene	DMF			Freed, Rieger, and Fraenkel (1962)
Aromatic and aliphatic		KCl		Piette, Ludwig, and Adams (1962)
nitro compounds	H$_2$O	KOH	Hg pool	
		LiOH		
Benzaldehyde				
Acetophenone				
4-Fluoroacetophenone				

Compound	Solvent	Anion	Reference	Author
Triphenylacetophenone	DMF	TNPAP	Ag/AgClO$_4$, Hg pool	Rieger and Fraenkel (1962)
Benzophenone				
1,4-Diacetylbenzene				
Terephthalamide				
Acetylpyridine, etc.				
Fluorenone				
2,7-Difluorofluorenone				
4,5-Phenanthrylene ketone	DMF	TNBAP	Ag/AgClO$_4$, Hg pool	Dehl and Fraenkel (1963)
o-Phenanthrenequinone				
Acenaphthenequinone				
Benzil				
Bis(p-nitrophenyl) ions	DMSO	TNPAP	Calomel	Harriman and Maki (1963)
Aromatic and aliphatic nitriles	A DMF	TNPAP	Ag/AgClO$_4$, Hg pool	Rieger, Bernal, Reinmuth, and Fraenkel (1963)
Nitrobenzene				
1,4-Dinitrobenzene				
2,6-Dimethylnitrobenzene	DMF	TNPAP	Ag/AgClO$_4$, Hg pool	Rieger and Fraenkel (1963)
4-Nitrophenol				
3-Nitrobenzonitrile				
Nitromesitylene				
Trinitromesitylene				
Dinitromesitylene	DMSO DMF	TNBAP TNPAP	Ag/AgClO$_4$, Hg pool	Bernal and Fraenkel (1964)
Mononitromesitylene				
Dinitrodurene				
Mononitrodurene				
Nitrodurene				

(continued)

TABLE 15–3 (Continued)

Samples	Solvents	Supporting electrolytes	Electrodes	Reference
Anthracene	DME	TNBAP	Ag/AgC10₄, Hg pool	Bolton and Fraenkel (1964)
Paradinitrobenzene o-Dinitrolenzene	DMF	TNPAP	Ag/AgC10₄, Hg pool	Freed and Fraenkel (1964)
Substituted nitrobenzenes and nitroanilines	A DMF DMSO	TNPAP	Calomel, Hg pool	Geske, Ragle, Barnbenek, and Balch (1964)
1,3-Butadiene	Liquid NH₃	TMAI	Pt	Levy and Myers (1964)
Acetophenone Benzaldehyde 4-Fluoroacetophenone	DMSO DMF DME	TNBAP	Ag/AgC10₄, Hg pool	Steinberger and Fraenkel (1964)

(A) acetonitrile; (DME) dimethoxyethane; (DMF) dimethylformamide; (DMSO) dimethylsulfoxide; (TMAI) tetra-methylammoniumiodide; (TNBAP) tetra-n-butylammonium perchlorate; (TNPAP) tetra-n-propylammonium perchlorate. This table was prepared by O. F. Griffith III.

Sometimes it is desired to mix two solutions in predetermined proportions before carrying out an ESR experiment. ESR "mix-flow" cells for use with a continuous flow method for producing short-lived paramagnetic species are described by Piette, Yamazaki, and Mason (1961), Dixon and Norman (1963), Ingram (1963), Bennett and Thomas (1964), and Borg (1964), and reviewed by Norman (1963). Experiments in classical fast reaction chemistry often make use of similar types of apparatus [Roughton and Chance (1963) and Caldin (1964)].

References

F. C. Adams and S. I. Weissman, *J. Am. Chem. Soc.*, **80**, 1518 (1958).

M. Adams, M. S. Blois, and R. H. Sands, *J. Chem. Phys.*, **28**, 774 (1958).

S. A. Al'tshuler and B. M. Kozyrev, *Electron Paramagnetic Resonance*, transl. Scripta Technica, English Edition edited by C. P. Poole, Jr., Academic Press, N. Y., 1964.

D. E. G. Austen, P. H. Given, D. J. E. Ingram, and M. F. Peover, *Nature*, **182**, 1784 (1958).

W. E. Barr and V. J. Ankorn, *Scientific and Industrial Glass Blowing and Laboratory Techniques*, Instruments Publ. Co., Pittsburgh, 1959, pp. 160, 196.

J. E. Bennett and A. Thomas, *Proc. Roy. Soc.*, **A280**, 123 (1964).

I. Bernal and G. K. Fraenkel, *J. Am. Chem. Soc.*, **86**, 1671 (1964).

I. Bernal, P. Rieger, and G. K. Fraenkel, *J. Chem. Phys.*, **37**, 1489 (1962).

J. R. Bolton and G. K. Fraenkel, *J. Chem. Phys.*, **40**, 3307 (1964).

D. C. Borg, *Nature*, **201**, 1087 (1964).

D. C. Borg, *Rapid Mixing and Sampling in Biochemistry*, B. Chance, Ed., Academic Press, N. Y., 1964, p. 135.

K. W. Bowers, G. J. Nolfi, Jr., and F. D. Greene, private communication.

K. W. Bowers, *Advances in Magnetic Resonance*, **1**, 317 (1965).

R. A. Cacciarelli and B. B. Stewart, *RSI*, **34**, 944 (1963).

E. F. Caldin, *Fast Reactions in Solution*, Blackwell, Oxford, 1964, Chap. 3.

A. Carrington, *Quart. Rev.*, **17**, 67 (1963).

A. Carrington, F. Dravnieks, and M. C. R. Symons, *J. Chem. Soc.*, **1959**, 947.

J. R. Davy, *Industrial High Vacuum*, Pitman, London, 1951.

Y. Deguchi, *J. Chem. Phys.*, **32**, 1584 (1960).

R. Dehl and G. K. Fraenkel, *J. Chem. Phys.*, **39**, 1793 (1963).

W. T. Dixon and R. O. C. Norman, *J. Chem. Soc.*, **1963**, 3119.

S. Dushman, *Scientific Foundations of Vacuum Technique*, 2nd ed., Wiley, N. Y., 1962.

A. Ehrenberg, *Acta Chem. Scand.*, **11**, 205 (1957).

J. Freed and G. K. Fraenkel, *J. Chem. Phys.*, **37**, 1156 (1962); **40**, 1815 (1964).

J. Freed, P. Rieger, and G. K. Fraenkel, *J. Chem. Phys.*, **37**, 1881 (1962).

A. A. Galkin, I. L. Shamfarov, and A. V. Stefanishina, *Zh. Eksper. Teor. Fiz.*, **32**, 1581 (1957).

D. H. Geske and A. H. Maki, *J. Am. Chem. Soc.*, **82**, 2671 (1960).

D. H. Geske, J. Ragle, M. Barnbenek, and A. Balch, *J. Am. Chem. Soc.*, **86**, 987 (1964).

J. E. Harriman and A. H. Maki, *J. Chem. Phys.*, **39**, 778 (1963).

K. H. Hausser, *Naturwissenschaften*, **47**, 251 (1960); *Arch. Sci. (Fasc. Spec.)*, **13**, 239 (1960).

D. J. E. Ingram, *Free Radicals as Studied by Electron Spin Resonance*, Butterworths, London, 1958, p. 142ff.

D. J. E. Ingram, *Spectroscopy at Radio and Microwave Frequencies*, Butterworths, London, 1955; *Paramagnetic Resonance*, **2**, 809 (1963).

S. Jnanananda, *High Vacua*, Van Nostrand, N. Y., 1947.

C. S. Johnson, Jr. and R. Chang, *J. Chem. Phys.*, **43**, 3183 (1965).

M. T. Jones, E. A. LaLancette, and R. E. Benson, *J. Chem. Phys.* **41**, 401 (1964).

I. M. Kolthoff and J. I. Lingane, *Polarography*, Interscience, N. Y., 1952, p. 109.

Z. Kuri, H. Ueda, and S. Shida, *J. Chem. Phys.*, **32**, 371 (1960).

C. Lagercrantz and L. Persson, *RSI*, **35**, 1605 (1964).

J. H. Leck, *Pressure Measurement in Vacuum Systems*, The Institute of Physics, London, 1957.

J. Lees, B. H. Muller, and J. D. Noble, *J. Chem. Phys.*, **34**, 341 (1961).

D. H. Levy and R. J. Myers, *J. Chem. Phys.*, **41**, 1062 (1964).

A. H. Maki and D. H. Geske, *Anal. Chem.*, **31**, 1450 (1959); *J. Chem. Phys.*, **30**, 1356 (1959); *J. Am. Chem. Soc.*, **83**, 1852 (1961).

B. J. McClelland, *Chem. Rev.*, **64**, 301 (1964).

I. D. Morosova, *Russ. Chem. Rev.*, **31**, 575 (1962).

W. Müller-Warmuth, *Z. Naturforsch.*, **18A**, 1001 (1963).

R. O. C. Norman, *Lab. Pract.*, **13**, 1084 (1963).

L. H. Piette, P. Ludwig, and R. N. Adams, *J. Am. Chem. Soc.*, **83**, 3909 (1961); **84**, 4212 (1962); *Anal. Chem.*, **34**, 916 (1962).

L. H. Piette, I. Yamazaki, and H. S. Mason, *Free Radicals in Biological Systems*, M. S. Blois, Jr., H. W. Brown, R. M. Lemmon, R. O. Lindblom, and M. Weissbluth, Eds., Academic Press, N. Y., 1961, p. 195.

R. Pointeau, J. Favede, and P. Delhaes, *J. Chim. Phys.*, **61**, 1129 (1964).

C. P. Poole, Jr. and D. S. MacIver, *Advances in Catalysis*, **17**, 1966, to be published.

RCA Tube Handbook, The Radio Corporation of America, Harrison, N. Y.

H. N. Rexroad and W. Gordy, *J. Chem. Phys.*, **30**, 399 (1959).

P. H. Rieger, I. Bernal, W. H. Reinmuth, and G. K. Fraenkel, *J. Am. Chem. Soc.*, **85**, 683 (1963).

P. H. Rieger and G. K. Fraenkel, *J. Chem. Phys.*, **37**, 2811 (1962); **39**, 1793 (1963).

F. J. W. Roughton and B. Chance in *Techniques of Organic Chemistry*, Vol. 8, Part 2, A. Weissberger, Ed., Interscience, N. Y., 1963, p. 704.

L. S. Singer, *Proceedings of the Fifth Carbon Conf.*, Vol. 2, Pergamon, London, 1963, p. 37.

K. R. Spangenberg, *Vacuum Tubes*, McGraw-Hill, N. Y., 1948, p. 754.

N. Steinberger and G. K. Fraenkel, *J. Chem. Phys.*, **40**, 723 (1964).

C. H. Townes and A. L. Schawlow, *Microwave Spectroscopy*, McGraw-Hill, N. Y., 1955.

T. R. Tuttle, Jr., R. L. Ward, and S. I. Weissman, *J. Chem. Phys.*, **25**, 189 (1956).

H. Ueda, Z. Kuri, and S. Shida, *J. Chem. Phys.*, **36**, 1676 (1962).

B. Venkataraman and G. K. Fraenkel, *J. Am. Chem. Soc.*, **77**, 2707 (1955); *J. Chem. Phys.*, **23**, 588 (1955).

B. Venkataraman, B. C. Segal, and G. K. Fraenkel, *J. Chem. Phys.*, **30**, 1006 (1959).

C. A. Wamser and B. B. Stewart, *RSI*, **36**, 397 (1965).

R. L. Ward and S. I. Weissman, *J. Am. Chem. Soc.*, **79**, 2086 (1957).

S. I. Weissman, E. DeBoer, and J. J. Conradi, *J. Chem. Phys.*, **26**, 963 (1957).

J. Yarwood, *High Vacuum Techniques*, Wiley, N. Y., 1955.

Y. Yokozawa and I. Miyashita, *J. Chem. Phys.*, **25**, 796 (1956).

P. Zuman and I. M. Kolthoff, *Progress in Polarography*, Vols. 1 and 2, Interscience, N. Y., 1962.

CHAPTER 16

Variable Temperatures and Pressures

A variable temperature ESR study can provide a great deal of information about a spin system and its interaction with its environment. To first order, the g factor, hyperfine interaction constants, and other terms in the Hamiltonian are independent of the temperature. The line-shape, line-width ΔH, and relaxation times T_1 and T_2 are the principal quantities which are sensitive to the temperature, and these are discussed in detail in Chap. 18. Some spin systems have such short relaxation times that they are only detectable in the liquid helium temperature range. Other spin systems have such long relaxation times that they saturate easily, and microwatt power levels are required for their observation. Particularly dramatic changes in ΔH, T_1, T_2, the line-shape, and the intensity occur at crystallographic phase transitions such as melting, and at magnetic phase transitions such as the passage from the paramagnetic to the antiferromagnetic state.

Several standard temperatures are shown on Table 16–1. They are easy to maintain with constant temperature baths, and may be employed to calibrate thermocouples and other types of thermometers.

A. High Temperatures

High temperature techniques used in pretreating samples were discussed in the previous chapter. The present section deals with electron spin resonance measurements carried out at high temperatures.

There are two general methods of maintaining a high temperature at the ESR sample. The first method consists of inserting the resonant cavity into the oven, as shown on Fig. 16–1. [Poole and O'Reilly (1961); see also Watkins (1959)]. The gold-plated TE_{102} mode X band rectangular resonant cavity changes its frequency by -0.17 Mc/°C over the operating range from 20 to 500°C. A section of thin walled stainless steel waveguide provides thermal isolation from the magic T or circulator. The heating element is made from 300 cm of No. 20 Nichrome wire wound on four Transite plates, and it is activated by the power supply shown in Fig. 16–2. A rectifier is

TABLE 16–1

Several Standard Temperatures for Low Temperature Studies

Substance	Boiling point, °K	Melting point, °K	Triple point, °K	Lambda point, °K
H_2O	373.1	273.1		
NH_3	239.5			
CO_2	194.5[a]			
Xe	165	161		
Ar	87.4	84	83.9	
O_2	90.2		54.4	
N_2	77.4		63.2	
Ne	27.1	24.5	24.6	
H_2	20.3		13.9	
He^4	4.211			2.172
He^3	3.2			

[a] Sublimes.

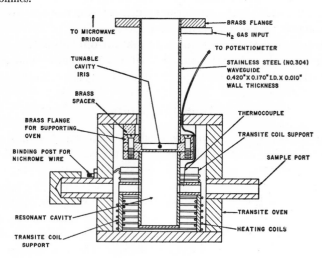

Fig. 16–1.   High-temperature resonant cavity with Transite oven and Nichrome wire heating element [Poole and O'Reilly (1961)].

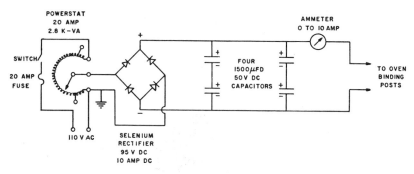

Fig. 16–2. Power supply for oven heating element [Poole and O'Reilly (1961)].

employed in this power supply to minimize the vibrations that may result from an ac source. It requires about 5 A to produce a temperature of 400°C. The resonant cavity is flushed with nitrogen gas to prevent oxidation of its walls. The temperature is measured by a thermocouple which is not ferromagnetic (e.g., copper Constantan). Persyn and Nolle (1965) used an ESR cavity in an oven up to 1000°K, Van Wieringen and Rensen (1963) operated up to 1275°K, and Chaikin (1963) attained spectrometer operation up to 1675°K.

The second method of maintaining a sample at high temperatures is to place it inside a glass or quartz tube which passes through the cavity [Piette and Landgraf (1960); Singer, Smith, and Wagoner (1961); Lebed' and Yakovlev (1962)]. Nitrogen gas passes through a heating element and then through the resonant cavity where it heats the sample, as shown in Fig. 16–3. The temperature may be raised by either increasing the current that flows through the heating elements, or by increasing the gas flow rate. A thermocouple is employed to monitor the sample temperature. It is best to calibrate the thermocouple reading against that of a second thermocouple placed inside an actual sample tube. The Singer (1961) arrangement shown in Fig. 16–3 makes use of water cooling coils to maintain the resonant cavity at room temperature. One may also employ a Dewar made from double walled and evacuated quartz tubing which is silvered everywhere but inside the resonant cavity.

If extra room is required to fit the Dewar in the cavity, then one may increase the small dimension of a TE_{102} rectangular resonant cavity without appreciably effecting the resonant frequency, and use a larger hole. Increasing this dimension will increase Q somewhat,

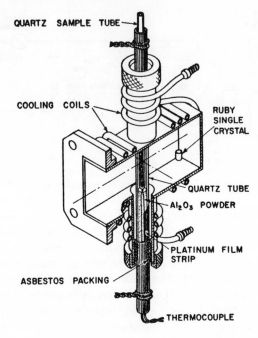

QUARTZ SAMPLE TUBE

COOLING COILS

RUBY
SINGLE
CRYSTAL

QUARTZ TUBE

Al₂O₃ POWDER

PLATINUM FILM
STRIP

ASBESTOS PACKING

THERMOCOUPLE

Fig. 16–3. A microwave resonant cavity for electron spin resonance measurements at high temperature [Singer, Smith, and Wagoner (1961)].

but the losses in the additional glassware will result in a net decrease
in Q. The principal electrical effect of such a dimensional change
will be to lower the energy density in the cavity. A large X band
rectangular resonant cavity may be constructed from oversize
RG 51/U waveguide (2.84 × 1.28 cm i.d.). An easier way to obtain
more room for a Dewar is to employ a TE_{011} mode cylindrical cavity
such as the one discussed in Sec. 8-D.

A temperature control unit may be designed to stabilize the ESR
sample temperature to a predetermined value. This is accomplished
by taking the difference between a standard preset voltage and the
thermocouple voltage, and using this difference as an error signal to
turn on the heating element (or the gas flow). If the temperature
exceeds the desired temperature, then the error voltage will be
opposite in polarity to its low temperature value, and the heater will
not turn on. When the temperature is too low, the heating element
is activated [cf. Fig. 16–7]. The tendency to overshoot the desired

temperature during the initial warmup may be minimized by a periodic application of the power until the operating temperature is reached. A control system of this type is discussed in Sec. 16-C. Veazey and Gordy (1965) describe an oven for observing rotational levels of molecules up to 1100°C. Hafner and Nachtrieb (1964) and Odle and Flynn (1964) describe NMR measurements up to and beyond 1100°C. Schreiber (1964) presents an NMR Dewar for the range 130–820°K.

B. Low Temperatures (77–300°K)

The instrumentation for the low temperature region is similar to that employed above room temperature. Again, there are two general methods of attaining the desired temperature. In the first method the entire resonant cavity is inserted into the Dewar and cooled by the refrigerant, as shown in Fig. 8–6. The resonant cavity shown on this figure may be disassembled at the plane of zero rf current flow for irradiation purposes. A hydrocarbon glass, such as 3-methyl pentane, was employed to seal the cavity by applying it when the lower half of the cavity was immersed in liquid nitrogen. While obtaining ESR data, the entire cavity must be submerged in liquid nitrogen to minimize the noise that results from the bubbling of the refrigerant around the cavity walls. The bubbling can be eliminated by blowing helium gas into the liquid nitrogen [Kohin (1964)]. The cavity is continuously evacuated to prevent oxygen or nitrogen from condensing within. The lead gasket and mica window shown on Fig. 16-4 form a vacuum seal when they are tightly clamped, and such a seal is satisfactory for use above the resonant cavity. An inch or two of thin walled stainless steel waveguide will provide adequate thermal isolation for the resonator. A small air gap in the waveguide may also be used to achieve isolation [Poole (1958)].

The second method of achieving a low temperature is to make use of an arrangement such as that shown in Fig. 16-3. [Piette and Landgraf (1960); Singer, Smith, and Wagoner (1961); Lebed' and Yakovlev (1962)]. The nitrogen gas is precooled by flowing it through a coil of copper tubing immersed in a liquid nitrogen or a Dry Ice–acetone bath. The nitrogen should be passed through a drying tube (e.g., calcium chloride or Drierite) before traversing the

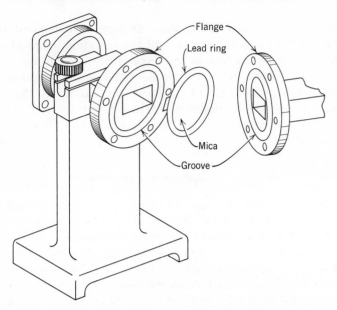

Fig. 16–4.   Lead mica vacuum window.   The mica is sealed by the lead ring clamped in the grooves [Strandberg, Johnson, and Eshbach (1954); see also Strandberg (1954)].

coil in order to prevent moisture condensation from clogging the coil. A typical arrangement will make use of a pressure head of 500 torr ($\sim$10 lb/in^2) stepped down by a needle valve to the desired flow rate. A flow meter may be employed to monitor the gas flow rate.   The needle valve is employed as a coarse control on the temperature, and the current in the heating element constitutes a fine control.

If a double walled evacuated Dewar such as that described in the last section is employed, then the "warming coils" which replace the cooling coils of Fig. 16–3 may be eliminated.   For the most efficient operation, double-walled and evacuated Dewar tubing should be employed to carry the cold gas from the cooling coils to the resonant cavity.   Ball joints or tapered joints may be used for joining several sections of such Dewar tubing.   A temperature stabilization circuit such as the one described in the preceding and following sections may also be employed at low temperatures [see, for example, Gilchrist (1955); Vajda and Hart (1953); Siegel, Baum, Skolnik, and Flournoy (1960); Piette and Landgraf (1960); Piette, Johnson, Booman, and Colburn (1961)].

Another method of maintaining the resonant cavity at temperatures between 77°K and room temperature is to place the bottom surface of the resonant cavity in intimate thermal contact with a copper rod that is several inches long. The lower end of the rod dips into liquid nitrogen, and a heating coil is placed near the top. The temperature of the cavity is determined by the level of the refrigerant and the current through the heating coil [see Ure (1957)]. Bennett and Thomas (1964) describe a liquid flow mixing cell that freezes the mixture at a surface cooled by liquid nitrogen.

A Dewar containing liquid nitrogen can be inserted directly into the resonant cavity, but this is not recommended since the boiling of the nitrogen produces a high noise level.

Homemade containers for liquid nitrogen may be fabricated from Styrofoam (polyfoam or polystyrene foam) [see Froelich and Kenty (1951); Marshall (1955)]. The evaporation rate from polyfoam is greater than that from silvered vacuum vessels. For example, Nelson (1956) quotes an evaporation rate of 3 g/min for polyfoam versus 0.6 g/min for a silvered glass Dewar.

Several constant level-controllers for liquid nitrogen have been described in the literature [e.g., see Lounsbury (1951); Zweig (1951); Sherwood (1952); Maimoni (1956); Bykov and Kostryukov (1959); Roizen and Gannus (1961); Phillips and Owens (1963); Nelson (1963)]. It is usually best to shield the tops of Dewars so that moisture will not condense within (see Skvarla and Evans (1951); Svec (1956); Kunzler (1956)].

Recent low temperature NMR apparatus is described by Sauzade and Kan (1963), Müller and Schnabel (1964), and Blears Warren and Allen (1965).

C. Very Low Temperatures (Below 77°K)

Most very low temperature studies are carried out at the temperature of liquid hydrogen (20°K) or liquid helium (4.2°K). Temperatures somewhat below 4.2°K such as the λ-point of helium (2.172°K) are obtained by reducing the pressure above the helium, while extremely low temperatures are achieved only by specialized techniques such as adiabatic demagnetization [de Klerk (1956); Steenland and Tolhoek (1957); Ambler (1960); Hudson (1961); Huiskams and Tolhoek (1961); Hess, Greenebaum, Pipkin, and Weyhmann (1965)]. These very low temperature experiments are much more difficult to carry out than those at 77°K and above. The books listed at the end of the chapter may be referred to for general background material on cryogenics [Mendelssohn (1960); Vance and Duke (1962); Sittig and Kidd (1963); Vance (1964); Rose-Innes (1964); Johnson (1961)].

Refrigerants: Liquid hydrogen and liquid helium are available commercially, but some institutions which consume large quantities build their own liquifiers [Scott (1959); Croft (1961)]. Many large scale consumers find it economical to install a helium recovery system. Liquid neon may be used between 20 and 30°K [Dillon and Jaccarino (1959)].

Storage Vessels: Both liquid hydrogen and liquid helium are ordinarily stored in the inner chamber of a double walled Dewar [Wexler and Jacket (1951)]. Liquid nitrogen fills the outer chamber, and it is necessary to maintain a minimum level of liquid nitrogen to prevent excessive evaporation of the helium. Whitehouse, Callcott, Naber, and Raby (1965) describe an economical homemade cryostat. Fradkov (1960, 1961) has described a liquid helium cryostat design in which the escaping helium vapor cools a shield to between 72 and 80°K, and thereby obviates the necessity of using liquid nitrogen. The inner sections of Dewars are ordinarily evacuated to minimize heat loss, although powder insulation [Fulk (1959)] has also been used. Liquid helium cryostats are available commercially. A special transfer tube is employed to transfer the liquid helium to the cryostat where the low temperature experiment will be carried out [Stout (1954)]. The efficiency of a cryostat depends on the evaporation rate of the liquid helium, which is discussed by Wexler (1951). Bewilogua and Lippold (1962) describe a simple apparatus for checking the evaporation rate from Dewars.

Sometimes it is desirable to perform irradiation experiments at liquid helium temperatures. Rieckhoff and Weissbach (1962) describe an X band cavity for such optical studies. A large number of literature articles have been written which describe Dewars provided with transparent windows for ultraviolet, visible, and infrared irradiation [e.g., see Schoen, Kuntzel, and Broida (1958); Schoen and Broida (1962); Lotkova and Fradkov (1961)]. Such Dewars are commercially available.

Temperatures below 4.2°K may be reached by several methods such as by pumping on liquid helium and by adiabatic demagnetization. Several recent articles on this subject are by Kogan, Reinov,

Sokolov, and Stel'makh (1959), Peshkov, Zinov'eva, and Filiminov (1959), Arp and Kropschot (1961), Ambler and Dove (1961), Esel'son, Shvets, and Bereznyak (1961), Esel'son, Lazarev, and Shvets (1960); Brewer (1960) has reported on a Physical Society Symposium held in 1959 on the subject of generating temperatures below 1°K.

Thermometers: A number of different thermometric principles have been employed for measuring temperatures in the liquid helium region. The *1958 He⁴ Scale of Temperatures* has been established so that all laboratories can employ a uniform temperature scale [Brickwedde, van Dijk, Durieux, Clement, and Logan (1960); Van Dijk (1961)]. It is based on the vapor pressure of He^4 between 0.5 and 5.22°K, but was compiled only after considering the available data obtained from paramagnetic susceptibility and carbon resistor thermometers. Slack (1956) describes a vacuum gauge for measuring helium pressures at low temperatures.

Thermocouples such as copper–Constantan or Chromel-P are useful at very low temperatures, but close to liquid helium temperature, their thermoelectric power becomes very small. A copper–gold thermocouple [Scott (1959) p. 124] is more sensitive at low temperatures but not so reproducible [Mauer (1960)]. The thermoelectric power of all thermocouples vanishes at absolute zero, and the low sensitivity at extremely low temperatures requires the use of expensive apparatus (e.g., a potentiometer) to detect the thermal EMF. It is best to calibrate a thermocouple at two or more of the fixed points shown on Table 16–1.

Pure metals at high temperatures normally exhibit an electrical resistivity which is approximately proportional to the temperature. As a result, the change in resistivity per degree is constant. At low temperatures the rate of change of resistivity with temperature becomes much less, and the metal approaches a constant resistivity at the lowest temperatures. Therefore the resistivity of a metal is a poorer thermometer at liquid helium temperature than it is above liquid nitrogen temperature. Alloys have also been used as resistance thermometers. Metallic resistance thermometers are discussed by Scott (1959, p. 128 ff.), Mikhailov and Govor (1962), and Golovashkin and Motulevich (1962).

In contrast to the behavior of metals, carbon resistors increase their resistance as the temperature T is lowered. Clement and Quinnell

(1952) studied the resistance R of a series of 1 W Allen Bradley resistors with room temperature values between 10 and 270 Ω. As shown on Fig. 16–5 their data in the range 2 to 20°K fit the equation

$$\log R + K/\log R = A + B/T \tag{1}$$

where K, A, and B are experimentally determined constants. Clement (1955) later proposed the equation

$$[(\log R)/T]^{1/2} = a + b \log R \tag{2}$$

where a and b are constants for a closer fit to the data. Carbon resistance thermometers are very useful for measuring the temperature inside Dewars, and usually only require the use of an inexpensive ohmmeter instead of the expensive precision potentiometer that is ordinarily used with thermocouples and metallic thermometers. Pearce, Markham, and Dillinger (1956) used carbon resistors down to 0.3°K. Blake, Chase, and Maxwell (1958) describe a resistance thermometer bridge for measuring temperatures in the liquid helium range. Ambler and Plumb (1960) have discussed the effect of stray

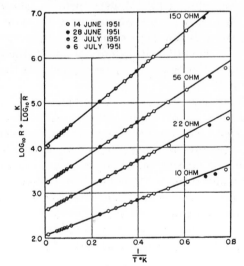

Fig. 16–5. Graph of eq. (16–C–1) for four carbon resistors [Clement and Quinnell (1952)].

rf fields on carbon resistor thermometers. Strips of carbon have also been employed as thermometers [Van Dijk, Keesom, and Steller (1938); Giauque, Stout, and Clark (1938); Fairbank and Lane (1947)].

Other semiconducting resistance thermometers suitable for low temperature work are germanium [Friedberg (1956); Kunzler (1957)] and metallic oxide thermistors [Becker, Green, and Pearson (1946)].

A resistance thermometer may be conveniently employed for indicating the level of liquid helium in a Dewar [Blanpain (1961); Rovinskii (1961, 1961)]. Nechaev (1961) and Meiboom and O'Brien (1963) employ a capacitor for this purpose.

ESR Apparatus: Now that some background has been presented on cryogenic techniques, several specific experimental arrangements will be discussed in detail. Flournoy, Baum, and Siegel (1960) employed an adaptation of the commercial Varian liquid helium V-4545A EPR Dewar assembly, as shown in Fig. 16–6. The unmodified Varian system consists of an X band TE_{101} mode rectangular reflection cavity and a centered circular iris. The cavity is screwed together at the iris. It is electrically coupled to the input waveguide above the Dewar by means of a thin-walled stainless steel waveguide which has the standard X band inner dimensions. The stainless steel cover at the top of the Dewar is provided with inputs for electrical leads to thermometers and heaters, and is designed to permit pumping on the liquid helium for the attainment of temperatures below 4.2°K. The resonant cavity is filled with liquid helium during the experiment. The Varian system employs a double walled glass Dewar with an unsilvered strip down the side to permit observation of the refrigerant levels. The O ring seal at the top allows for pumping on the liquid helium in the center Dewar. The outer Dewar is filled with liquid nitrogen. The helium transfer tube at the upper lefthand side of Fig. 16–6 terminates at the "helium inlet."

The arrangement of Flournoy, Baum, and Siegel employs cold helium from the transfer tube to cool the lower brass section of the waveguide assembly. Thermal isolation is achieved through the upper stainless steel waveguide. The helium source is slightly pressurized by the gas flow through the valve V_1, as shown on Fig. 16–7. The gas flow through valve V_2 is adjusted to maintain a temperature near the desired value. The heater below the resonant cavity counteracts the cooling produced by the helium, and the two effects may be balanced to provide any temperature between 4.2 and 77°K. The switches S_1 and S_2 are both open for manual operation. Automatic temperature control is activated by the thermocouple (T.C.) voltage, and it may be achieved in two ways: (1) by closing switch S_1 to provide intermittent gas flow through the solenoid valve, and (2) by closing switch S_2 to provide intermittent heat that supplements the current obtained directly from the Variac. In the first method, the valves V_1 and V_2 are set to provide the proper balance between constant and intermittent flow of cold helium gas, and in the

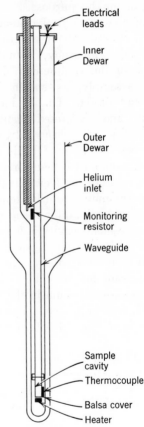

Fig. 16–6.　ESR–Dewar assembly showing the locations of the heating, cooling, and temperature-sensing elements [Flournoy, Baum, and Siegel (1960)].

second method, the 100-Ω variable potentiometer adjusts the balance between constant and intermittent heat.   The resistance reading on the carbon resistor may be employed to monitor the liquid helium transfer rate.   Thompson, Persyn, and Nolle (1963) [see also Persyn and Nolle (1965)] and Wartewig, Welter, and Windsch (1964) also provided for temperature control in their studies.

When the Flournoy system is to be operated at 4.2°K with the resonant cavity immersed in liquid helium, it is only necessary to evacuate the inner Dewar to 1 or 2 torr before admitting the liquid helium, because the low temperature automatically condenses the remaining gas.   For use at intermediate temperatures, however, such residual gas can cause a serious heat leak, and to prevent this, the inner Dewar must be pumped to at least 10^{-5} torr while at liquid nitrogen temperature.   In either case, the inner part of the Dewar may be precooled by filling the evacuated space between the inner and outer Dewars with nitrogen gas, and then filling the outer Dewar with liquid nitrogen.   Thermal conduction between the two Dewar sections will precool the center part to almost 77°K.

The Flournoy arrangement places the entire resonant cavity into the Dewar.   Jen, Foner, Cochran, and Bowers (1958, 1960), and

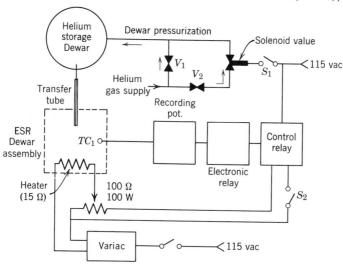

Fig. 16–7.   Block diagram of low temperature control system [Flournoy, Baum, and Siegel (1960)].

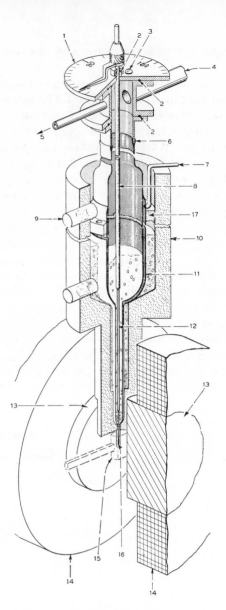

Fig. 16–8.   Tip Dewar with the following components: (*1*) indicator showing sample orientation; (*2*) O ring seal; (*3*) plugged hole for transfer of liquid helium; (*4*) pump lead to helium vessel; (*5*) tube to manometer; (*6*) glass to Kovar seal; (*7*) pump line to vacuum interspace; (*8*) fused quartz rod; (*9*) evacuated glass window; (*10*) Styrofoam outer vessel containing liquid nitrogen; (*11*) Dewar containing liquid helium; (*12*) brass connecting rod; (*13*) pole piece; (*14*) magnet winding; (*15*) TE_{013} cavity; (*16*) specimen; (*17*) spacer [Dillon, Geschwind, Jaccarino, and Machalett (1959)].

Dillon, Geschwind, Jaccarino, and Machalett (1959) employed the opposite approach by placing the sample on a refrigerated sapphire rod which is inserted into the room temperature resonant cavity. The Dillon et al. experimental arrangement shown on Fig. 16–8 included a glass inner Dewar (*11*) to hold liquid helium and a Styrofoam (polyfoam or polystyrene foam) outer Dewar (*10*) to contain the liquid nitrogen. The sample (*16*) is bonded to a rod of sapphire (*16*) which is connected to a mechanism for rotating the sample (*1*) through a brass rod (*12*) and a quartz rod (*8*). Sapphire is employed because of its exceedingly high thermal conductivity and low dielectric loss. The inner Dewar has an unsilvered tip which is inserted into the cavity, and an unsilvered strip down the side to allow observation of the refrigerant levels through several windows (*9*). An expanded view of the Dewar tip in the K band TE_{013} mode transmission resonant cavity is shown on Fig. 16–9. The cavity is continuously flushed with dry nitrogen from (9) in order to prevent moisture condensation. One liability of the Dillon setup is that vibrations of the quartz tip in the cavity produce considerable noise

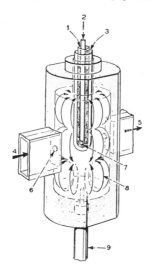

Fig. 16–9. Positioning of the Dewar tip in the K band cylindrical resonant cavity: (*1*) liquid helium; (*2*) single crystal sapphire rod; (*3*) vacuum interspace; (*4*) microwave input; (*5*) microwave output; (*6*) coupling iris; (*7*) specimen; (*8*) arrows which represent the rf magnetic field; (*9*) tube for dry flushing gas [Dillon, Geschwind, Jaccarino, and Machalett (1959)].

which is troublesome when working with weak samples under high sensitivity operating conditions. Zhitnikov and Kolesnikov (1964, 1965) describe an analogous arrangement for trapping atoms in inert matrices at 77°K.

Abkowitz and Honig (1962) describe a K band ESR apparatus which operates at a steady-state temperature of 0.48°K using continuously recycled He^3. The upper part of the waveguide contains two aperiodic bends to prevent infrared radiation from passing down the waveguide. The system has been operated at 0.3°K by pumping on the liquid He^3. Svare and Seidel (1964) and Cowen, Spence, Van Till, and Weinstock (1964) also describe a He^3 system.

Henry and Dolecek (1950) describe a stainless steel Dewar which is suitable for use with an ESR resonant cavity immersed under liquid helium.

Seven of the spectrometers described in Chap. 13 have been operated at liquid helium temperature: (1) Feher and Kip (1955) (Sec. 13-G); (2) Buckmaster and Scovil (1956) (Sec. 13-H); (3) Feher (1957) (Sec. 13-M); (4) Rose-Innes (1957) (Sec. 13-N); (5) Mock (1961) (Sec. 13-P); (6) Teaney, Klein, and Portis (1961) (Sec. 13-Q); (7) Llewellyn, Whittlestone, and Williams (1962) (Sec. 13-R), and many others are listed in Table 13-1. Zverev (1961) describes an X band spectrometer for measuring spin lattice relaxation times between 2 and 60°K, and Federov (1963, 1965) discusses a radio frequency (42 Mc) ESR spectrometer which operates between 0.15 and 4.2°K using adiabatic demagnetization. A stub tuner for impedance matching coaxial cables to a resonant cavity in liquid helium is described by de Klerk (1963). Maxwell and Schmidt (1958) described a superconducting cavity resonator made by electroplating lead on brass. This cavity operates at several hundred megacycles, and has a Q of 400,000. It incorporates a demountable cryostat for operation at liquid helium temperatures. Fuschillo (1956), Mulay (1957), Babenko and Baisa (1964), Hecht (1965), and Franconi and Fraenkel (1960) describe NMR instrumentation for use at these low temperatures.

A number of articles have appeared in the literature which describe methods of maintaining temperatures at any value between the boiling points of liquid helium and liquid nitrogen. For example, see Larson and Mayer (1952), Flournoy, Baum, and Siegel (1960), Cataland, Edlow, and Plumb (1961), Adkins (1961), Shimashek

(1961), and Blake and Chase (1963). Vetchinkin (1961) and Lutes (1962) discuss the attainment of controlled temperatures below 4.2°K.

The mechanical properties of metals at low temperatures are discussed by Klyavin and Stepanov (1959) and Parker and Sullivan (1963). Plastics are treated by Giauque, Stout, and Clark (1952) and epoxy resin cements by Netzel and Dillinger (1961). Wheatley, Griffing, and Estle (1956) cover thermal contact and insulation below 1°K. Salinger and Wheatley (1961) measured the magnetic susceptibilities of materials which are commonly incorporated into cryogenic apparatus. Horwitz and Bohm (1961) recommend an indium O ring seal that remains leak-tight when immersed in liquid helium. Wexler, Corak, and Cunningham (1950) had previously employed gold gaskets for this purpose. Schulte (1965) recommends a Teflon ribbon as a self-adhesive tape from liquid helium temperature to 350°K. Mathes (1963) discusses the low temperature properties of dielectrics.

D. Electron Spin Resonance at High Pressures

The lattice parameters of solids and fluids depend upon both the temperature and the pressure. Since it is easier to vary the temperature in an experiment, most investigators follow this procedure. The present section will describe some experimental techniques that may be used to carry out electron spin resonance studies at high pressures. This field has been reviewed by Benedek (1963) and Smith (1963). It should be mentioned in passing that the lattice parameters may be varied over an even wider range by the use of isomorphous solid solutions [Poole, Kehl, and MacIver (1962); Poole and Itzel (1964)]. Recent reviews on general high pressure techniques are Bradley (1963) and Dadson, Greig, and Horner (1965).

Birnbaum (1950), Birnbaum and Maryott (1951), David, Hammer, and Pearce (1952), and Philips (1955) describe microwave devices for studying the complex dielectric constant of compressed gases up to 100 bars. Cacciarelli and Stewart (1963) and Veigele and Bevan (1963) discuss NMR measurements at high pressures. Lawson and Smith (1959) employed two conically tapered single crystals of alumina as a high pressure microwave window which is capable of supporting a pressure of 10 or more kilobars in a circular waveguide

and its terminating high Q resonator.   At the same time, the window
provides an impedance match from a standard 1-cm circular waveguide at atmospheric pressure to the cavity which sustains an
internal hydrostatic pressure of up to 10 kilobars.   Vallauri and
Forsbergh (1957) describe a wide band dielectric cell for use at S band
at pressures up to 1500 atm.

Walsh   and   Bloembergen   (1957)   studied   nickel   fluorosilicate
($NiSiF_6 \cdot 6H_2O$)   under   high   pressure   and   observed   the   pressure

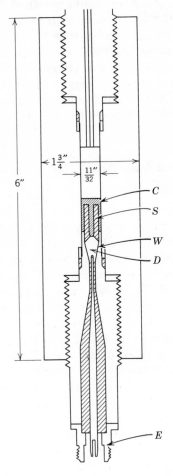

Fig. 16–10.   Experimental arrangement for studying electron spin resonance
at high pressures [Walsh and Bloembergen (1957)].

dependence of the zero field splitting parameter D. They employed
the high-pressure cell shown in Fig. 16–10 which is good up to 10
kilobars. The assembly is enclosed in a nonmagnetic Be–Cu cylinder
with a pressure feed plug [Bridgman (1952)] at one end. The brass
TEM coaxial microwave cavity C with a pressure seal consisting of
a cone D and washer W is supplied with power at the type-N connector E. The cavity center conductor is $\sim 3\lambda/4$ long. The sample
S is pressed against the Teflon that fills the cavity. The cavity has a
loaded Q of about 500 and is immersed in the pressure transmitting
fluid petroleum ether. The high pressure generating and measuring
equipment are described by Bridgman (1952) and Kushida, Benedek,
and Bloembergen (1956). The uniaxial stress equipment and spectrometer shown on Figs. 16–11 and 16–12, respectively, were used by
Walsh (1959, 1961) in conjunction with this high-pressure cell.

Gardner, Hill, Johansen, Larson, Murri, and Nelson (1963)
describe the high pressure ESR spectrometer shown in Fig. 16–13.
It consists of four subsystems: (1) the microwave apparatus (lower
right), (2) the magnetic field and modulation components, (3) the
low temperature apparatus (upper left), and (4) the high-pressure
system (top center). The X band superheterodyne microwave bridge
couples microwave energy via a coaxial cable into the alumina-filled
cavity both by means of a loop and by a straight probe. The modulating field at the sample is supplied by a single strip of silver wire

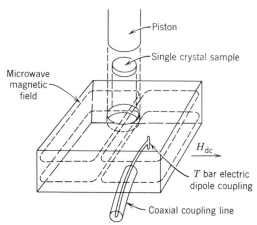

Fig. 16–11. Apparatus for applying uniaxial stress to a sample in a resonant
cavity [Walsh (1959)].

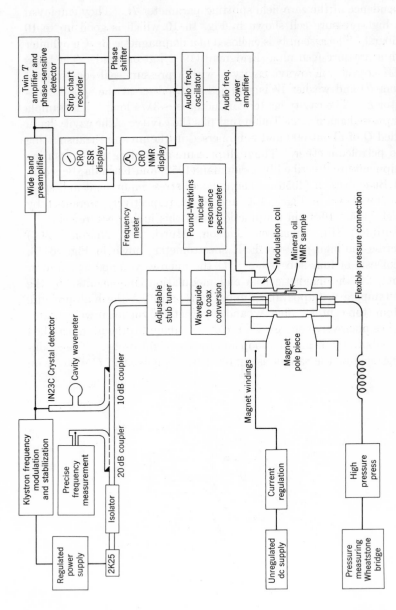

Fig. 16-12.   Block diagram of ESR spectrometer used for high-pressure research [Walsh (1959)].

placed perpendicular to the large applied magnetic field, as shown in Fig. 16–14. Comparable sensitivities were obtained with both 100-kc modulation and superheterodyne detection. The sample may be cooled by flowing liquid nitrogen at a controlled rate onto the lower anvil of the high pressure head shown on Fig. 16–15.

The sample cell is a copper disk placed between a pair of Bridgman anvils. The lower anvil is silver-coated and serves as a resonant

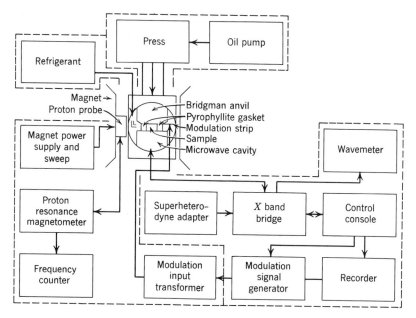

Fig. 16–13. Block diagram of complete high-pressure ESR spectrometer [Gardner, Hill, Johansen, Larson, Murri, and Nelson (1963)].

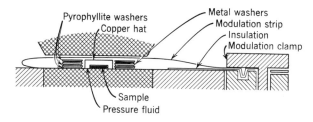

Fig. 16–14. Modulation system in high-pressure sample cell [Gardner, Hill, Johansen, Larson, Murri, and Nelson (1963)].

cavity.   The sample cell is filled with either Viscasil 100,000 silicon fluid or with mineral oil for the pressure transmitting medium. The anvils are placed in a pressure head as shown on Fig. 16–15.   The original article should be consulted for further details of the high pressure apparatus.   Clark and Wait (1964) describe an ESR spectrometer for studying pressure effects up to 10 kilobars, and Goodrich,

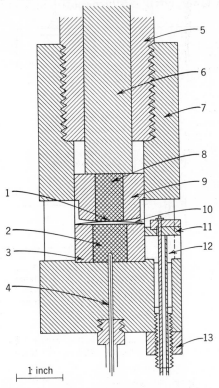

Fig. 16–15.   Schematic diagram of high-pressure head: (1) sample cell; (2) combined pressure anvil and microwave cavity; (3) beryllium–copper binding ring for pressure anvil; (4) coaxial line for coupling microwaves; (5) beryllium–copper sleeve for coupling to hydraulic press; (6) beryllium–copper pressure ram; (7) beryllium–copper pressure head; (8) Bridgman type tapered pressure anvil; (9) beryllium–copper binding ring for pressure anvil; (10) silver modulation strip; (11) modulation clamp; (12) plastic insulating support for modulation clamp; (13) locking nut for modulation clamp [Gardner, Hill, Johansen, Larson, Murri, and Nelson (1963)].

Everett, and Lawson (1964) present a K band high pressure cavity. Watkins and Corbett (1961, 1964) measured the effect of uniaxial stress down to 20°K. One confusing aspect of high-pressure research is the fact that various investigators use different units of pressure. Benedek (1963) gives the conversion factors 1 kg/cm² = 0.9678 atm = 0.9807 bar = 14.22 lb/in.² = 0.9807 × 10⁶ dyn/cm².

References

M. Abkowitz and A. Honig, *RSI*, **33**, 568 (1962).

C. J. Adkins, *JSI*, **38**, 305 (1961).

E. Ambler, *Progr. Cryogenics*, **2**, 235 (1960).

E. Ambler and H. Plumb, *RSI*, **31**, 656 (1960).

E. Ambler and R. B. Dove, *RSI*, **32**, 737 (1961).

V. D. Arp and R. H. Kropschot, *RSI*, **32**, 217 (1961).

V. P. Babenko and D. F. Baisa, *Cryogenics*, **4**, 40 (1964).

J. A. Becker, C. B. Green, and G. L. Pearson, *Elect. Eng.*, **65**, 711 (1946).

G. B. Benedek, *Magnetic Resonance at High Pressure*, Interscience, N. Y., 1963.

J. E. Bennett and A. Thomas, *Proc. Roy. Soc.*, **A280**, 123 (1964).

L. Bewilogua and H. Lippold, *ETP*, **10**, 373 (1962).

G. Birnbaum, *RSI*, **21**, 169 (1950).

G. Birnbaum and A. A. Maryott, *J. Appl. Phys.*, **22**, 95 (1951).

C. Blake and C. E. Chase, *RSI*, **34**, 984 (1963).

C. B. Blake, C. E. Chase, and E. Maxwell, *RSI*, **29**, 715 (1958).

R. Blanpain, *Bull. Soc. Roy. Sci. Liege*, **30**, 310 (1961).

D. J. Blears, R. F. Warren, and G. Allen, *JSI*, **42**, 292 (1965).

R. S. Bradley, *High Pressure Physics and Chemistry*, Vols. 1, 2, Academic Press, N. Y., 1963.

D. F. Brewer, *Nature*, **185**, 349 (1960).

F. G. Brickwedde, H. van Dijk, M. Durieux, J. R. Clement, and J. K. Logan, *Nat. Bur. Stand. (USA) Monograph*, **10**, 1 (1960); see also *J. Res. Nat. Bur. Std.*, **64A**, 1 (1960).

P. W. Bridgman, *The Physics of High Pressure*, Bell, London, 1952.

H. A. Buckmaster and H. E. D. Scovil, *Can. J. Phys.*, **34**, 711 (1956).

V. P. Bykov and V. N. Kostryukov, *PTE*, 154 (1959).

R. A. Cacciarelli and B. B. Stewart, *RSI*, **34**, 944 (1963).

G. Cataland, M. H. Edlow, and H. H. Plumb, *RSI*, **32**, 980 (1961).

A. M. Chaikin, *PTE*, **6**, 178 (1185) (1963).

A. F. Clark and D. F. Wait, *RSI*, **35**, 863 (1964).

J. R. Clement and E. H. Quinnell, *RSI*, **23**, 213 (1952); J. R. Clement, *Temperature, Its Measurement and Control*, **2**, 380 (1955).

J. A. Cowen, R. D. Spence, H. Van Till, and H. Weinstock, *RSI*, **35**, 914 (1964).

A. J. Croft, *Progr. Cryogenics*, **3**, 1 (1961).

R. S. Dadson, R. G. P. Greig, and A. Horner, *Metrologia*, **1**, 55 (1965).

J. de Klerk, *RSI*, **34**, 183 (1963).

J. de Klerk, *Handbuch der Physik*, Vol. XV, Part II, S. Flügge, Ed., Springer-Verlag, Berlin, 1956, p. 38.

J. F. Dillon, Jr., S. Geschwind, V. Jaccarino, and A. Machalett, *RSI*, **30**, 559 (1959).

J. F. Dillon, Jr., and V. Jaccarino, *RSI*, **30**, 132 (1959).

B. N. Esel'son, A. D. Shvets, and N. G. Bereznyak, *PTE*, **6**, 123 (1160) (1961).

B. N. Esel'son, B. G. Lazarev, and A. D. Shvets, *PTE*, **5**, 160 (980) (1961).

H. A. Fairbank and C. T. Lane, *RSI*, **18**, 525 (1947).

B. V. Federov, *PTE*, **4**, 98 (686) (1963); *Cyorgenics*, **5**, 12 (1965).

G. Feher, *Bell System Tech. J.*, **36**, 449 (1957).

G. Feher and A. F. Kip, *Phys. Rev.*, **98**, 337 (1955).

J. M. Flournoy, L. H. Baum, and S. Siegel, *RSI*, **31**, 1133 (1960).

A. B. Fradkov, *Dokl. Akad. Nauk. SSSR*, **133**, 829 (1960); Engl. Trans. *Soviet Phys.-Dokl.* **5**, 888 (1961).

A. B. Fradkov, *PTE*, **4**, 170 (796) (1961).

C. Franconi and G. Fraenkel, *RSI*, **31**, 657 (1960).

S. A. Friedberg, *Temperature, Its Measurement and Control in Science and Industry*, Vol. 2, Reinhold, N. Y., 1956, p. 359.

H. C. Froelich and C. Kenty, *RSI*, **22**, 214 (1951).

M. M. Fulk, *Progr. Cryogenics*, **1**, 63 (1959).

N. Fuschillo, *RSI*, **27**, 394 (1956).

J. H. Gardner, M. W. Hill, C. Johansen, D. Larson, W. Murri, and N. Nelson, *RSI*, **34**, 1043 (1963).

W. F. Giauque, J. W. Stout, and C. W. Clark, *J. Am. Chem. Soc.*, **60**, 1053 (1938).

W. F. Giauque, T. H. Geballe, D. N. Lyon, and J. J. Fritz, *RSI*, **23**, 169 (1952).

A. Gilchrist, *RSI*, **26**, 773 (1955).

A. I. Golovashkin and G. P. Motulevich, *PTE*, **2**, 182 (404) (1962).

R. G. Goodrich, G. E. Everett, and A. W. Lawson, *RSI*, **35**, 1596 (1964).

S. Hafner and N. H. Nachtrieb, *RSI*, **35**, 680 (1964).

A. M. Hecht, *J. Phys.*, *(France)*, **26**, Suppl. No. 4, 167A (1965).

W. E. Henry and R. L. Dolecek, *RSI*, **21**, 496 (1950).

J. Hess, B. Greenebaum, F. M. Pipkin, and W. Weyhmann, *RSI*, **36**, 21 (1965).

N. H. Horwitz and H. V. Bohm, *RSI*, **32**, 857 (1961).

R. P. Hudson, *Progr. Cryogenics*, **3**, 99 (1961).

W. J. Huiskams and H. A. Tolhoek, *Progr. Low Temp. Phys.*, **3**, 333 (1961).

C. K. Jen, S. N. Foner, E. L. Cochran, and V. A. Bowers, *Phys. Rev.*, **112**, 1169 (1958); *J. Chem. Phys.*, **32**, 963 (1960).

V. J. Johnson, Ed., *Properties of Materials at Low Temperatures*, Pergamon, N.Y., 1961.

S. D. Kaitmazov and A. M. Prokhorov, *PTE*, **5**, 107 (1959).

O. V. Klyavin and A. V. Stepanov, *Fiz. Tverd. Tela, Suppl., Sbornik*, **1**, 241 (1959).

A. V. Kogan, N. M. Reinov, I. A. Sokolov, and M. F. Stel'makh, *Zh. Tekh. Fiz.*, **29**, 1039 (1959).

R. P. Kohin, 1964, private communication.

J. E. Kunzler, *RSI*, **27**, 879 (1956).

J. E. Kunzler, T. H. Geballe, and G. W. Hull, *RSI*, **28**, 96 (1957).

T. Kushida, G. B. Benedek, and N. Bloembergen, *Phys. Rev.*, **104**, 1364 (1956).

E. V. Larson and R. Mayer, *RSI*, **23**, 692 (1952).

A. W. Lawson and G. E. Smith, *RSI*, **30**, 989 (1959).

B. M. Lebed' and Yu. M. Yakovlev, *PTE*, **6**, 107 (1171) (1962).

P. M. Llewellyn, P. R. Whittlestone, and J. M. Williams, *JSI*, **39**, 586 (1962).

E. N. Lotkova and A. B. Fradkov, *PTE*, **1**, 188 (1961).

N. Lounsbury, *RSI*, **22**, 533 (1951).

O. S. Lutes, *RSI*, **33**, 1008 (1962).

A. Maimoni, *RSI*, **27**, 1024 (1956).

L. Marshall, *RSI*, **26**, 614 (1955).

K. N. Mathes, *Dielectrics in Space Symposium*, Westinghouse Electric Corp., Pittsburgh, 1963, p. 14.

F. A. Mauer, "Low Temperature Equipment and Techniques," Chapter in *Formation and Trapping of Free Radicals*, A. M. Bass and H. P. Broida, Eds., Academic Press, N. Y., 1960.

E. Maxwell and A. F. Schmidt, *Bull. Inst. Froid*, Annexe 95, (1958–61).

S. Meiboom and J. P. O'Brien, *RSI*, **34**, 811 (1963).

K. Mendelssohn, *Cryophysics*, Interscience, N. Y., 1960.

N. N. Mikhailov and A. Ya. Gover, *PTE*, **2**, 180 (402) (1962).

J. B. Mock, *RSI*, **31**, 551 (1960).

L. N. Mulay, *RSI*, **28**, 279 (1957).

R. Müller and B. Schnabel, *ETP*, **12**, 106 (1964).

Yu. I. Nechaev, *PTE*, **4**, 174 (801) (1961).

L. S. Nelson, *RSI*, **27**, 655 (1956).

L. C. Nelson, *JSI*, **40**, 428 (1963).

R. G. Netzel and J. R. Dillinger, *RSI*, **32**, 855 (1961).

R. L. Odle and C. P. Flynn, *RSI*, **35**, 1611 (1964).

C. M. Parker and J. W. W. Sullivan, *Ind. Eng. Chem.*, **55**, 18 (1963).

D. C. Pearce, A. H. Markham, and J. R. Dillinger, *RSI*, **27**, 240 (1956).

G. A. Persyn and A. W. Nolle, *Phys. Rev.*, **140**, A1610 (1965).

V. P. Peshkov, K. N. Zinov'eva, and A. I. Filimonov, *Zh. Eksper. Teor. Fiz.*, **36**, 1034 (734) (1959).

C. S. E. Philips, *J. Chem. Phys.*, **23**, 2388 (1955).

T. R. Phillips and D. R. Owens, *JSI*, **40**, 426 (1963).

L. H. Piette and W. C. Landgraf, *J. Chem. Phys.*, **32**, 1107 (1960).

L. H. Piette, F. A. Johnson, K. A. Booman, and C. B. Colburn, *J. Chem. Phys.*, **35**, 1481 (1961).

C. P. Poole, Jr., Thesis, University of Maryland, 1958.

C. P. Poole, Jr., and J. F. Itzel, Jr., *J. Chem. Phys.*, **41**, 287 (1964).

C. P. Poole, Jr., W. L. Kehl, and D. S. MacIver, *J. Catalysis*, **1**, 407 (1962).

C. P. Poole, Jr. and D. E. O'Reilly, *RSI*, **32**, 460 (1961).

A. M. Portis and D. Teaney, *J. Appl. Phys.*, **29**, 1692 (1958).

K. E. Rieckhoff and R. Weissbach, *RSI*, **33**, 1393 (1962).

L. I. Roizen and V. K. Gannus, *PTE*, **2**, 191 (399) (1961).

A. C. Rose-Innes, *JSI*, **34**, 276 (1957).

A. C. Rose-Innes, *Low Temperature Techniques*, The English University Press, London, 1964.

A. E. Rovinskii, *PTE*, **2**, 190 (398) (1961).

A. E. Rovinskii, *Cryogenics*, **2**, 115 (1961).

G. L. Salinger and J. C. Wheatley, *RSI*, **32**, 872 (1961).

M. Sauzade and S. K. Kan, *C. R. Acad. Sci.*, **257**, 3344 (1963).

L. J. Schoen, L. E. Kuntzel, and H. P. Broida, *RSI*, **29**, 633 (1958).

L. J. Schoen and H. P. Broida, *RSI*, **33**, 470 (1962).

D. S. Schreiber, *RSI*, **35**, 1582 (1964).

E. Schulte, *RSI*, **36**, (706) (1965).

R. B. Scott, *Cryogenic Engineering*, Van Nostrand, N. Y., 1959.

J. E. Sherwood, *RSI*, **23**, 446 (1952).

E. Shimashek, *PTE*, **4**, 173 (800) (1961).

S. Siegel, L. Baum, S. Skolnik, and J. M. Flournoy, *J. Chem. Phys.*, **32**, 1249 (1960).

L. S. Singer, W. H. Smith, and G. Wagoner, *RSI*, **32**, 213 (1961); see also L. S. Singer, *J. Appl. Phys.*, **30**, 1463 (1959).

M. Sittig and S. Kidd, *Cryogenic Research and Applications*, Van Nostrand, N. Y., (1963).

J. E. Skvarla and E. C. Evans, *RSI*, **22**, 341 (1951).

G. A. Slack, *RSI*, **27**, 241 (1956).

J. A. S. Smith, *High Pressure Physics and Chemistry*, Vol. 2, Academic Press, N. Y., 1963, p. 293.

M. J. Steenland and H. A. Tolhoek, *Progr. Low Temp. Phys.*, **2**, 292 (1957).

J. W. Stout, *RSI*, **25**, 929 (1954).

M. W. P. Strandberg, *Microwave Spectroscopy*, Wiley, N.Y., 1954

M. W. P. Strandberg, H. R. Johnson, and J. R. Eshbach, *RSI*, **25**, 776 (1954).

I. Svare and G. Seidel, *Phys. Rev.*, **134**, A172 (1964).

H. J. Svec, *RSI*, **27**, 969 (1956).

D. T. Teaney, M. P. Klein, and A. M. Portis, *RSI*, **32**, 721 (1961); see Portis and Teaney (1958).

B. C. Thompson, G. A. Persyn, and A. W. Nolle, *RSI*, **34**, 943 (1963).

R. W. Ure, Jr., *RSI*, **28**, 836 (1957).

J. Vajda and D. P. Hart, *RSI*, **24**, 354 (1953).

M. G. Vallauri and P. W. Forsbergh, Jr., *RSI*, **28**, 198 (1957).

R. W. Vance, Ed., *Cryogenic Technology*, Wiley, N. Y., 1964.

R. W. Vance and W. M. Duke, Eds., *Applied Cryogenic Engineering*, Wiley, N. Y., 1962.

H. van Dijk, W. H. Keesom, and J. P. Steller, *Physica*, **5**, 625 (1938).

H. van Dijk, *Progr. Cyrogenics*, **2**, 121 (1961).

J. S. van Wieringen and J. G. Rensen, *Proceedings of the Twelfth Colloque Ampere*, Bordeaux, 1963, p. 229.

S. E. Veazey and W. Gordy, *Phys. Rev.*, **138**, A1303 (1965).

W. J. Veigele and A. W. Bevan, Jr., *J. Chem. Phys.*, **34**, 21, 1158 (1963).

A. N. Vetchinkin, *PTE*, **1**, 192 (1961).

W. M. Walsh, *Phys. Rev.*, **114**, 1473, 1485 (1959); **122**, 762 (1961).

W. M. Walsh and N. Bloembergen, *Phys. Rev.*, **107**, 904 (1957).

S. Wartewig, M. Welter, and W. Windsch, *ETP*, **12**, 354 (1964).

G. D. Watkins, *Phys. Rev.*, **113**, 79 (1959).

G. D. Watkins and J. W. Corbett, *Phys. Rev.*, **121**, 1001 (1961); **134**, A1359 (1964).

A. Wexler, *J. Appl. Phys.*, **22**, 1463 (1951).

A. Wexler, W. S. Corak, and G. T. Cunningham, *RSI*, **21**, 259 (1950).

A. Wexler and H. S. Jacket, *RSI*, **22**, 282 (1951).

W. C. Wheatley, D. F. Griffing, and T. L. Estle, *RSI*, **27**, 1070 (1956).

J. E. Whitehouse, T. A. Callcott, J. A. Naber, and J. S. Raby, *RSI*, **36**, 768 (1965).

P. A. Zhitnikov and N. V. Kolesnikov, *Cryogenics*, **5**, 129 (1965); *PTE*, **3**, 189 (682) (1964).

G. M. Zverev, *PTE* **5**, 109 (930) (1961).

B. Zweig, *RSI*, **22**, 431 (1951).

CHAPTER 17

Irradiation

A. Types of Irradiation

When a fluid or solid is irradiated, the type of radiation damage that can occur is dependent on the energy of the incoming photons or other particles. Table 17–1 gives the energy associated with various bombarding photons and particles, and Table 17–2 lists the energies associated with several crystallographic and molecular quantities. The energy units used in these two tables are electron volts (eV) and kilocalories per mole (kcal/mole) since these are the two units generally employed by physicists and chemists, respectively, for most of the quantities listed in Table 17–2. Appendix A and Sec. 17–K discuss the relations between the various energy units. The energy of thermal neutrons (0.025 eV) corresponds to kT at room temperature.

The first thing to notice about Table 17–1 is that the energies associated with γ-rays, x-rays, and the bombarding particles (except thermal neutrons) are many orders of magnitude greater than a typical bond energy (50–100 kcal/mole). When these high energy particles pass through matter, they gradually lose their energy by producing radiation damage such as displacing atoms from their lattice positions, ionizing atoms, and electronically exciting atoms. The last two effects are dominant in dielectrics such as ionic crystals, polymers, and glasses, while bombarding charged particles usually produce atomic displacements in metals. In liquids and non-crystalline solids, it is usually the whole molecule which is ionized or electronically excited.

Most radiation damage studies employ an external source for the irradiation of the substance under study. It is also possible to synthesize compounds that contain short-lived radioactive isotopes which spontaneously decay into different nuclei by emitting neutrons, electrons, protons, α-particles, or γ-rays. Such *in situ* radiation products produce radiation damage, while the new nuclei that are

665

TABLE 17-1

Typical Energies per Photon or per Particle of Several Types of Irradiation Sources

Radiation	Energy		Typical source
	kcal/mole	eV	
γ-rays	10^6–10^8	10^5–10^7	Co^{60}
X-rays	10^3–10^6	40–40,000	X-ray tube
Ultraviolet	70–350	3.2–15	Arc lamp
Visible	35–70	1.6–3.2	Incandescent lamp
Infrared	1–35	0.04–1.6	Incandescent lamp
Electrons	$\sim 2 \times 10^7$	$\sim 1 \times 10^6$	Van de Graaff
Protons	$\sim 4 \times 10^8$	$\sim 2 \times 10^7$	Cyclotron
Thermal neutrons	~ 0.6	~ 0.025	Nuclear reactor
Fast neutrons	$\sim 10^8$	$\sim 5 \times 10^6$	Nuclear reactor
α-particles	4×10^8	$\sim 2 \times 10^7$	Cyclotron

TABLE 17-2

Typical Energies Associated with Several Molecular and Lattice Characteristics

System	Energy		Comments
	kcal/mole	eV	
Bonding energy per nucleon in nucleus	2×10^8	8×10^6	Nuclear excited states are in this energy range
Activation energy of diffusion in ionic lattice	20	1	
Lattice energy of ionic solid	~ 200	~ 9	Approximate energy to completely remove atom from ionic lattice
F center energy in alkali halide lattice	50–100	2–4	From optical spectra
Covalent bond energy	50–100	2–4	Organic compounds
Activation energy of thermal conductivity	$\begin{cases} 20\text{–}70 \\ 7\text{–}20 \end{cases}$	$\begin{cases} 1\text{–}3 \\ 0.3\text{–}0.9 \end{cases}$	Intrinsic $\big\}$ Alkali halide Extrinsic $\big\}$ lattice defects
Electronic transitions of organic molecules	50–150	2–6	
Characteristic group vibrational frequencies	1–10	0.04–0.4	Vibrational frequencies of organic chemical groups
Lattice vibrations of ionic solid	0.2	10^{-2}	
Rotations of diatomic molecules	10^{-3}–10^{-2}	10^{-4}–10^{-3}	Region of microwave spectroscopy

formed constitute impurities in the lattice. For example, Kroh, Green, and Spinks (1962) studied the tritium-produced radiation damage in THO.

B. Neutrons

Neutrons are produced in a nuclear reactor, and most neutron irradiation experiments are carried out at such a reactor. Neutrons may also be obtained in other ways such as by bombarding certain materials with charged particles from high energy accelerators, and from natural radioactive sources such as the α-emitter, beryllium. Fast neutrons have energies of several million electron volts (MeV), while thermal neutrons are in thermal equilibrium with their environment and have energies of the order of 1/40 of an electron volt (eV).

Since neutrons are not charged particles, they do not experience a coulombic attraction or repulsion when they approach atoms or ions, but rather their collisions are of the hard sphere type at energies where the nucleus itself is not excited. Fast neutrons may collide with and knock ionized atoms out of their lattice sites. When a fast neutron passes through a solid, it leaves a trail of radiation damage behind it. The displaced atoms have a considerable amount of kinetic energy which they may dissipate by ionization and by production of localized high frequency lattice vibrations. The latter corresponds to a thermal spike or a localized heating of the neighborhood of the displaced atom which lasts for a very small fraction of a microsecond.

A neutron may penetrate a nucleus in its path and produce a nuclear disintegration with the emission of one or more γ-rays, protons, additional neutrons, etc. The fission fragments will go on to produce additional damage, and the transformed nucleus will become a foreign atom in the host lattice. Thermal neutrons are particularly effective in producing nuclear reactions. Fast neutrons are easily thermalized by collisions with protons in hydrogen rich materials such as hydrocarbons, since the maximum energy transfer from a bombarding particle takes place when it strikes a particle of equal mass, as will be explained in the next section.

C. Charged Particles

The following charged particles listed in the order of increasing mass are often used for irradiation projectiles: electrons (e), positrons (e^+), protons (p or $^1H^+$), deuterons (d, D^+, or $^2H^+$), tritons (T or $^3H^+$), and α-particles (α or He^{++}). The masses of both an electron and a positron are several thousand times less than that of the other particles listed. Heavier nuclei may also be accelerated and used for irradiation sources.

The energy E_c required to displace an atom from its lattice site permanently (perhaps to an intersticial site) is about 25 eV, and for such a displacement to take place, it is necessary to transfer at least this threshold energy E_c to the atom. If the incident particle of mass M_1 possesses the energy E, then the maximum energy E_m transferred by a collision to an atom of mass M_2 is given by

$$E_m = \frac{4M_1M_2}{(M_1 + M_2)} E \qquad (1)$$

An atomic displacement can take place when $E_m > E_c$. Relativistic effects must be taken into account in the case of electron bombardment, which leads to the following expression [Harwood, Hausner, Morse, and Rauch (1958), p. 7]

$$E_m = \frac{2(E + 2mc^2)}{M_2c^2} E \qquad (2)$$

where $M_1 = m$ is the electronic mass and c is the velocity of light. The most important rest energies are

$$mc^2 = 0.511 \text{ MeV} \qquad \text{electrons} \qquad (3)$$

$$M_pc^2 = 938 \text{ MeV} \qquad \text{protons} \qquad (4)$$

and for an atom of atomic weight N, one has to a high approximation

$$M_2c^2 = 931N \qquad \text{MeV} \qquad (5)$$

Both the rate at which a charged particle loses energy in a solid, and the range of the particle are strongly dependent upon the particle's mass, as shown in Figs. 17–1 and 17–2. It is of interest to know the ranges of various particles in ESR sample tubes and samples. Ranges are usually expressed in the units mg/cm^2 or g/cm^2, and the latter may be converted to centimeters by dividing by the density ρ g/cm^3. Protons in aluminum have a range of 0.5 g/cm^2

at 17.5 MeV and 10 g/cm² at 100 MeV. Electrons in aluminum have a range of 1 g/cm² at 2 MeV and 10 g/cm² at 20 MeV. Since aluminum has a density of 2.7 g/cm², both 48-MeV protons and 5-MeV electrons have a range of 1 cm. These data may be found in Sec. 8 of the *American Institute of Physics Handbook*. Ranges expressed in the units g/cm² are approximately independent of the particular absorber, so the above data may be employed to estimate the extent to which charged particles will penetrate shields and samples. For example, if a sample is irradiated within an ESR tube, the irradiation

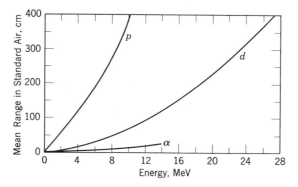

Fig. 17–1. Mean ranges of (p) protons, (d) deuterons, and (α) α-particles in air [adapted from Halliday (1950)].

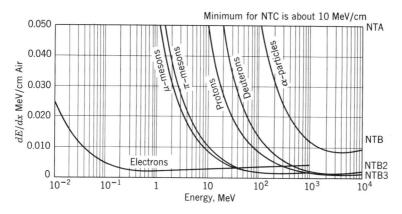

Fig. 17–2. The stopping power of standard air for several particles as a function of their energy. The numbers on the right refer to Eastman Kodak nuclear track emulsions (courtesy of the Eastman Kodak Co.).

must be energetic enough to penetrate the sample tube and reach the specimen within.

The wavelength λ associated with a particle of mass M and energy E is

$$\lambda = h/(2ME)^{1/2} \tag{6}$$

where h is Planck's constant. In terms of the Compton wavelength λ_0

$$\lambda_0 = h/mc = 0.0242621 \quad \text{Å} \tag{7}$$

this becomes

$$\lambda = \lambda_0 \, (mc^2/2E)^{1/2} \, (m/M)^{1/2} \tag{8}$$

where mc^2 is given by eq. (3). The ratio of the proton mass M_p to the electron mass m is given by

$$M_p/m = 1837 \tag{9}$$

Putting numerical values into eq. (8) one obtains for $M = M_p$

$$\lambda = 2.86 \times 10^{-4}/E^{1/2} \quad \text{for protons} \tag{10}$$

and for $M = m$

$$\lambda = 1.23 \times 10^{-2}/E^{1/2} \quad \text{for electrons} \tag{11}$$

where the particle energy E is in MeV, and λ is in Å (10^{-8} cm). It is interesting to note that the circumference $2\pi a_0$ of the first Bohr orbit in a hydrogen atom is

$$2\pi a_0 = h^2/2\pi m e^2 = 3.32 \text{ Å} \tag{12}$$

which is identical with the wavelength λ calculated from eq. (11) using the energy of the first Bohr orbit or hydrogen ground state

$$E = 1 \text{ Rydberg} = e^2/2a_0 = 13.54 \text{ eV} \tag{13}$$

Electron diffraction studies are made with wavelengths of the order of typical crystallographic spacings or several angstrom units, and the energies employed are about 100 eV. Such low energy electrons only penetrate the first few atomic surface layers of the solid under investigation, and so electron diffraction studies are useful for the investigation of the crystallographic structure of surfaces. The structure of the entire lattice is provided by x-ray diffraction since x-rays of the same wavelength are so much more penetrating.

D. Gamma Rays and X-Rays

It may be seen from Table 1–1 that γ-rays are photons whose wavelength λ

$$\lambda = hc/E = c/f \tag{1}$$

is usually much less than atomic spacings (0.1 to 0.4 mμ), while x-rays are photons whose wavelengths are often comparable to atomic spacings. The wavelengths of γ-rays are much greater than nuclear radii which lie between 2×10^{-13} and 9×10^{-13} cm. The dielectric constant ϵ and permeability μ of most materials for γ-rays and x-rays are close to the free space values ϵ_0 and μ_0, respectively, so these photons will traverse matter at close to the speed of light *in vacuo* $[1/(\mu_0\epsilon_0)^{1/2}]$. Lower frequency photons such as those in the visible region travel through matter slower than light in free space since in this case $\epsilon > \epsilon_0$.

When high energy photons traverse matter, they become scattered (i.e., change their direction of propagation), lose intensity (i.e., the number of photons decreases), and loose energy (i.e., the photon frequency decreases) by the photoelectric effect, Compton effect, and pair production.

Gamma rays possess nuclear energies, and are produced in some types of nuclear transformations when one nucleus is converted to another. A convenient source of γ-rays is Co^{60} which emits an electron and two γ-rays of 1.332 and 1.172 MeV, and thereby decays to Ni^{60} with the suitable halflife of 5.27 yr. The nuclear transformation follows the scheme

$$Co^{60} \rightarrow Ni^{60*} + e \tag{2}$$

$$Ni^{60*} \rightarrow Ni^{60} + \gamma \tag{3}$$

where the asterisk (*) indicates a Ni^{60} nucleus in an excited nuclear energy state.

When fast moving electrons strike matter, they interact with the matter to produce x-rays with energies up to their own energy. Such bombarding electrons produce a broad, continuous x-ray spectrum known as Bremstrahlen. This spectrum will have superimposed upon it fairly sharp regions of greater intensity corresponding to the characteristic x-ray wavelengths of the target. X-rays of a particular wavelength, called monochromatic x-rays, may be produced by preferentially suppressing the continuous background relative to the sharp lines.

In practice, monochromatic x-rays are produced in a Coolidge tube by thermionically emitting electrons from a heated cathode, accelerating them to a high velocity, and focusing them on to a heavy metal target. The x-rays emitted by the target have energies (wavelengths) which are dependent upon the particular target element which is employed. X-ray tubes are available commercially. Naryadchikov, Grishina, and Bakh (1962) present an experimental arrangement for *in situ* ESR measurements during x-irradiation.

E. Ultraviolet and Visible Radiation

The photons in the visible and ultraviolet spectral regions, called optical photons, are treated separately from the γ-rays and x-rays for several reasons. In the first place, they traverse matter at velocities below the velocity of light *in vacuo* c because the relative dielectric constant ϵ/ϵ_0 exceeds unity. They may be produced without the use of specialized equipment, they may be diffracted by prisms and gratings, and they are easily separated into monochromatic beams. In addition, they may be plane polarized or elliptically polarized. Ultraviolet transmission filters are discussed by Kasha (1948).

The most important characteristic of optical photons that causes them to merit a separate classification is the fact that their energies are comparable to the electronic and bond energies of molecules, as shown in Tables 17–3 to 17–7. The arrangement of the data in these tables is convenient for comparison purposes. Additional bond energy data given by Farmer and Lossing (1955), Cottrell (1958), Harrison and Lossing (1955), Mortimer (1962), and Neale (1964) have been used to bring Tables 17–4 and 17–5 up to date [see also Field and Franklin (1957); Walling (1957)]. Benson (1965) has published a recent tabulation of bond energies.

An optical photon may be absorbed by a transition from a bonding level G to an antibonding level E_A of a diatomic molecule as shown on Fig. 17-3a, and in this case, spontaneous bond rupture will result since the antibonding energy state has its lowest energy when the atoms are separated at infinity. Another predissociation mechanism

TABLE 17-3

Optical Absorption Maxima λ_m and Extinction Coefficients ϵ_m for Organic Compounds[a]

Compounds	$\lambda_m, m\mu$	ϵ_m
Ethylene[b]	162.5	15,000
Octene-2-*cis*[b,c]	183	13,000
Cyclohexene	182	6,600
1,3 butadiene[d]	217	21,000
2,4,6-Octatriene-1-ol[d]	265	53,000
Octyne-1 and octyne-2[b]	222.5	4,800
Benzene[e]	{ 254 {~195	204 } 6,900 }
Naphthalene	{ ~297.5 { ~275	230 } 9,300 }
Anthracene	~365	9,000
Mesitylene	270	300
1,3-pentadiene[d]	224	24,000
Acetaldehyde[f]	285	15
Acetone[g]	279.5	15
Benzaldehyde[f]	330	20
p-Benzoquinone[f]	{ 445 { 276	20 300
Nitromethane[i]	270	15
Nitrobenzene[j]	350	200
Phenol[e]	270	1,450
Aniline[e]	280	1,430

[a] The data are for the longest wavelength band.
[b] Platt, Klevens, and Price (1949).
[c] Octene-1 and octene-2-trans have slightly lower λ_{max} values.
[d] Broude (1945, 1950).
[e] Doub and Vanderbelt (1947, 1949).
[f] Henri (1929).
[g] Scheibe and Frömel (1937).
[h] McMurray (1941), Smakula (1934).
[i] Körtum (1939).
[j] Dede and Rosenberg (1934).

TABLE 17–4

R'—R'' Bond Dissociation Energies (kcal/mole) of Hydrocarbons [Steacie (1954), p. 98]

R'	R''											
	H	CH_3	C_2H_5	$CH_2{=}CH$	$CH{\equiv}C$	$n\text{-}C_3H_7$	$iso\text{-}C_3H_7$	CH_2CHCH_2	$n\text{-}C_4H_9$	$tert\text{-}C_4H_9$	C_6H_5	$C_6H_5CH_2$
CH_3	101	83	82	93[c]	110?	79	74.5?	60	78	74?	89[a]	63
C_2H_5	98	85[b]	78[b]	104[c]	109?	79	75?	61[a]	78	73?	91?	62
$CH_2{=}CH$	104[a]	93[c]	104[c]	101?		87?	85?	68.5?	86?	81?	101?	
$CH{\equiv}C$	114[a]	110?	109?			106?	103?				119?	
$n\text{-}C_3H_7$	95	79	79	87?	106?	76	72?	57.5	75	70?	88?	59
$iso\text{-}C_3H_7$	94[a]	74.5?	75?	85?	103?	72?	66.5?	54.5?	71?	65?	83?	54.5?
$CH_2{=}CHCH_2$	77	60	61[a]	68.5?		57.5	54.5?	38	56.5			
$n\text{-}C_4H_9$	94	78	78	86?		75	71?	56.5	74	69?	87?	57.5
$(CH_3)_3C$	90[a]	74?	73?	81?		70?	65?		69?	60?	78?	
$CH{=}C(CH_3)CH_2$	76?	60?	60?									
C_6H_5	102[a]	89[a]	91?	101?	119?	88?	83?		87?	78?	103?	76.5?
$C_6H_5CH_2$	77.5	63	62			59	54.5?		57.5		76.5?	47
$o\text{-}CH_3C_6H_4CH_2$	74	58	58									
$m\text{-}CH_3C_6H_4CH_2$	77.5	62	62.5									
$p\text{-}CH_3C_6H_4CH_2$	75	60	60									

[a] Values from Neale (1964).
[b] Values from Mortimer (1962).
[c] Values from Harrison and Lossing (1960).

TABLE 17-5

R'—R'' Bond Dissociation Energies (kcal/mole) of Miscellaneous Compounds [Steacie (1954), p. 97]

R'	R''									
	H	Cl	Br	I	OH	NH_2	CN	CHO	$COCH_3$	NO_2
CH_3	101	80	67[a]	53[a]	89[b]	91[b]	104	71–75	77?	57
C_2H_5	98	80	65	53[b]	90[b]	78	107[b]	71?	77?	52
$n\text{-}C_3H_7$	95	77?	59[d]	50	93[b]	77?	104[b]	71?	77?	
$(CH_3)_2CH$	94[a]	73[d]	61?	~42[d]	~92[b]				73?	
$(CH_3)_3C$	90[a]	75?	73[c]	~45?	91[b]	76?				
$CH_2{=}CH$	104[a]	86[c]	73[c]	41[c]	71	64?	121?	84?		
$CH_2{=}CHCH_2$	77	58	48	35–37	107?	94?	92?	50?		
C_6H_5	102[a]	88?	71[b]	57[e]	73?	59	109[b]	83?		
$C_6H_5CH_2$	77.5	68[e]	50.5	39?	~90[e]	89?	95?		63	
CHO	79?								59?	
CH_3CO	85?	82?	67?	51?	102? (90)	98?		59	60	

[a] Values from Neale (1964).
[b] Values from Mortimer (1962).
[c] Values from Harrison and Lossing (1960).
[d] Values from Farmer and Lossing (1955).
[e] Values from Cottrell (1958).

TABLE 17-6

Values of Bond Dissociation Energies for Single Bonds [Pauling (1960), p. 85]

Bond	Bond energy, kcal/mole	Bond	Bond energy, kcal/mole	Bond	Bond energy, kcal/mole
H—H	104.2	P—H	76.4	Si—Cl	85.7
C—C	83.1	As—H	58.6	Si—Br	69.1
Si—Si	42.2	O—H	110.6	Si—I	50.9
Ge—Ge	37.6	S—H	81.1	Ge—Cl	97.5
Sn—Sn	34.2	Se—H	66.1	N—F	64.5
N—N	38.4	Te—H	57.5	N—Cl	47.7
P—P	51.3	H—F	134.6	P—Cl	79.1
As—As	32.1	H—Cl	103.2	P—Br	65.4
Sb—Sb	30.2	H—Br	87.5	P—I	51.4
Bi—Bi	25	H—I	71.4	As—F	111.3
O—O	33.2	C—Si	69.3	As—Cl	68.9
S—S	50.9	C—N	69.7	As—Br	56.5
Se—Se	44.0	C—O	84.0	As—I	41.6
Te—Te	33	C—S	62.0	O—F	44.2
F—F	36.6	C—F	105.4	O—Cl	48.5
Cl—Cl	58.0	C—Cl	78.5	S—Cl	59.7
Br—Br	46.1	C—Br	65.9	S—Br	50.7
I—I	36.1	C—I	57.4	Cl—F	60.6
C—H	98.8	Si—O	88.2	Br—Cl	52.3
Si—H	70.4	Si—S	54.2	I—Cl	50.3
N—H	93.4	Si—F	129.3	I—Br	42.5

entails the absorption or a photon in a transition from the ground state bonding level G to an excited bonding level E_B which intersects an antibonding level E_A. As the diatomic molecule in the level E_B vibrates back and forth between the internuclear separations r_0 and r_3, as shown on Fig. 17–3b, it passes through the intersection with the antibonding level E_A. At this point the molecule may cross over from the state E_B to the state E_A, and spontaneously dissociate. The process of breaking up a molecule into its component free radicals or ions by optical irradiation is called photolysis.

Figure 17–3 is drawn in accordance with the Franck-Condon principle which states that electronic transitions occur so much more rapidly than the motions of the nuclei during molecular vibrations that the nuclei may be considered as fixed during the electronic transition. In the ground vibrational level g of the ground electronic level G, the molecule vibrates between the internuclear separations r_1 and r_2 shown on Fig. 17–3a. The electronic transitions shown on Fig. 17–3 are assumed to occur when the molecule is at the midpoint r_0.

A comparison of Tables 17–3 to 17–7 shows that in many cases the longest wavelength optical absorption maximum listed on Table 17–3

TABLE 17–7

Values of Bond Dissociation Energies for Multiple Bonds [Pauling (1960), p. 185]

Bond	Bond energy, kcal/mole	Compounds
$C{=}C$	147	
$N{=}N$	100	Azoisopropane[a]
$O{=}O$	96	$^1\Delta$ state of O_2
$C{=}N$	147	n-Butylisobutylideneamine[a]
$C{=}O$	164	Formaldehyde
	171	Other aldehydes
	174	Ketones
$C{=}S$	114	
$C{\equiv}C$	194	
$N{\equiv}N$	226	N_2
$C{\equiv}N$	207	Hydrogen cyanide
	213	Other cyanides

[a] From heats of combustion reported by Coates and Sutton (1948).

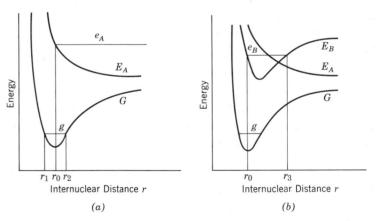

(a)   (b)

Fig. 17–3. Predissociation of a diatomic molecule when excitation is from the ground level to (a) an antibonding level and (b) a bonding level which intersects an antibonding level [Poole (1958)].

exceeds typical C—H and C—C bond energies, and when it does not do so, there are shorter wavelength absorptions which do have this property. In aromatics such as benzene and naphthalene, the shorter wavelength absorption is much more intense, i.e., a much greater percentage of the incident photons is absorbed. The amount of absorption is expressed in terms of the extinction coefficient ϵ (liter/mole cm) which relates the intensity of the incident light I_0 to the transmitted I light in terms of the concentration C (mole/liter) and sample thickness d (cm) by the relation

$$I = I_0 10^{-\epsilon C d} \tag{1}$$

Some authors define an absorption coefficient α in terms of the equation

$$I = I_0 e^{-\alpha d} \tag{2}$$

and, of course,

$$\alpha = 2.303 \, \epsilon C \tag{3}$$

Table 17–3 does not include the shorter wavelength absorption maxima, and it is important to emphasize that in many cases they have much greater extinction coefficients than the longest wavelength transition which is tabulated.

Ultraviolet light sometimes produces free radicals through a photosensitization mechanism whereby one molecular species absorbs the photons and passes the energy on to another species which dissociates into two free radicals. For example, Gibson, Ingram, Symons, and Townsend (1957) and Smith and Wyard (1961) added hydrogen peroxide H_2O_2 to organic "glasses" and interpreted their results in terms of the two-step process (1) the absorption of a photon by H_2O_2 with the production of OH radicals, and (2) the extraction of a hydrogen atom from the surrounding rigid solvent with the formation of H_2O and the free radical that they detected by ESR. They produced free radicals with irradiation at both the 253.7 and the 365 mμ ultraviolet bands of mercury vapor.

After dissociation occurs, the "cage effect" of Franck-Rabinowitch (1934) causes the photolysis products to become trapped by the surrounding medium at the site of the photodecomposition, and thereby to recombine rapidly. This is the main quantum yield limiting mechanism since as a result only a very small fraction of the incident photons actually produces stabilized free radicals. This cage effect is less important with higher energy radiation which is more capable of transferring to the free radical fragment sufficient kinetic energy to permit its escape from the "cage".

Several authors have described resonant cavities [e.g., see Rieckhoff and Weissbach (1962)] and Dewars [e.g., see Schoen, Broida, and Kuentzel (1958, 1962); Lotkova and Fradkov (1961)] suitable for low temperature irradiation studies (cf. Chap. 16).

F. Infrared, Microwave, and Radiofrequency Irradiation; Gas Discharges

High power infrared (ir) and microwave radiation is capable of heating solids and fluids to high temperatures, and as a result many free radicals and lattice defects will anneal out by migration, recombination, and neutralization processes. Ultraviolet (uv) and visible light sources frequently emit a considerable amount of infrared radiation, and it is best to interpose a filter between the lamp and the sample to remove the ir. For high powers, it may be necessary to water cool the filter. A convenient method of filtering out infrared radiation is to employ two quartz plates cemented to a Pyrex cylinder by means of black wax or some other cement. Such a cylinder filled with distilled water forms an effective filter, and it may be prevented from overheating by the use of flowing water.

A commonly used method of producing free radicals in the gaseous state is by means of a gas discharge. Such a discharge may be produced by a high voltage (e.g., 2500 V) between two electrodes in a Wood discharge tube [Wood (1922); Beringer and Heald (1954)]. Dehmelt (1955) employed a Universal dissociator which utilized an ac voltage (~ 800 V) to start the arc by heating the cathode to about 3000°K, where it emitted a current of several amperes. After starting, the arc was sustained by about 50 V dc. An electrodeless discharge may be produced by winding a coil around the glass tubing which carries the gas and connecting it to a high power transmitter with a frequency of several megacycles. Jen, Foner, Cochran, and Bowers (1956) employed 4 Mc at 100 W. A higher frequency electrodeless discharge may be produced by placing the evacuated quartz tube in an S band resonant cavity and supplying several hundred watts of microwave power to the cavity from a diathermy unit [e.g., see McCarthy (1954); Bass and Broida (1956); Cole, Harding, and Pellam (1957); Radford (1959)]. McCarthy (1954) obtained up to 1500 W at 2460 Mc. Experimental details pertaining to these methods of producing gas discharges are shown in Table 17–8. Papazian (1957) produced free radicals in a gas discharge generated by a Tesla coil. See also Kleppner, Berg, Crampton, Ramsey, Vessot, Peters, and Vanier (1965).

Krongelb and Strandberg (1959) [see also Hacker, Marshall, and Steinberg (1961)] discuss a method of measuring atomic recombination times, and they present data on the recombination kinetics of atomic oxygen. They produced the discharge by means of a QK-62 magnetron that supplied 20 W to the discharge cavity which was placed either in a side arm to the main flow stream, or in series with the main flow stream, as shown in Fig. 17–4. Another flow-type arrangement is shown in Fig. 13–4. Most discharge tube experimental setups pump the gas through both the discharge tube and the resonant cavity, as shown in Figs. 13–4 and 17–4b. It is important to allow sufficient space between the discharge and the resonant cavity so that the discharge is not actually in the cavity. Sometimes a very broad cyclotron resonance such as the one reported by Ingram and Tapley (1955) may be observed in the discharge itself. See also Fukuda, Matumoto, Uchida, and Yoshimura (1959), Lazukin (1960), Collins (1961), Bayes, Kivelson, and Wong (1962) and Kivelson, Bayes, and Wong (1962). On the other hand, it is also important not to place the resonant cavity too far from the discharge since this would allow most of the atoms to recombine before reaching the cavity. An inert carrier gas such as argon may be employed to prevent recombination of the radicals in the gas, and the wall of the tube between the discharge and the resonant cavity may be coated with a substance to prevent the destruction of free radicals during surface collisions [Dehmelt (1955); Wittke and Dicke (1956); Kleppner, Berg, Crampton, Ramsey, Vessot, Peters, and Vanier (1965)]. Examples of such substances are listed in the last column of Table 17–8.

A number of authors [e.g., see Jen, Foner, Cochran, and Bowers (1958, 1960, 1962); Goldsborough and Koehler (1964)] have condensed the products of electric discharges on cold surfaces down to liquid helium temperature and studied the ESR spectra of the atoms

TABLE 17-8

Data on Several Types of Gas Discharges

Discharge type	Voltage, V	Current, A	Power supplied, W	Gas flow rate[a]	Gas pressure, torr	Systems studied	Investigators	Comments
dc	2200	0.050	—	10^{-4} g/sec	0.05[b]	H atoms gas	Beringer and Heald (1954)	Glass coated with fused metaphosphoric acid
dc[c]	45	4	—	—	10–100 (A and He)[d] 0.02–1 (P)	P atoms gas	Dehmelt (1955)	—
4 Mc r.f. electrodeless	—	—	100	15 m/sec	—	H atoms trapped	Jen, Foner, Cochran, and Bowers (1956)	—
dc	3000	0.1–3	—	—	0.1[b]	H atoms gas	Wittke and Dicke (1956)	Glass coated with Dri Film[e]
Microwave 2460 Mc	—	—	1500	—	50	—	McCarthy (1954)	—

[a] In units of g/sec or m/sec.
[b] At resonant cavity.
[c] Arc started with 800 V ac.
[d] Buffer gas.
[e] General Electric Co. trade name for mixture of dimethyldichlorosilane and methyldichlorosilane.

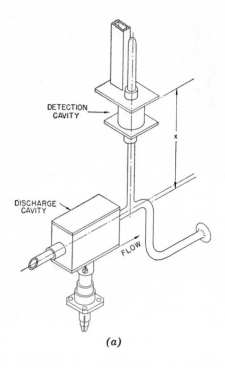

(a)

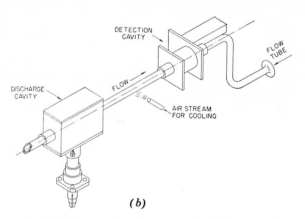

(b)

Fig. 17–4.   The dissociation of molecules in a discharge cavity: (a) side arm method; (b) flow method [Krongelb and Strandberg (1959)].

and free radicals that are thereby trapped. The refrigeration techniques employed in these investigations are discussed in Sec. 16-C. Zhitnikov and Kolesnikov (1962) trapped free atoms in matrices at 77°K.

Molecules may be dissociated thermally by heating them in an oven to a high temperature (e.g., 2500°K). This dissociation method has been used extensively in atomic and molecular beam experiments, and is described for example by Rabi, Zacharias, Millman, and Kusch (1938), Lamb and Retherford (1950, 1951), and Heberle, Reich, and Kusch (1956). Noon, Holt, and Reynolds (1965) describe a waveguide cell for studying magnetoplasmas.

G. Time and Temperature Effects

When a material is irradiated, the rate of production of radiation damage is greatest at the start of the irradiation, and gradually decreases with time. The accumulated or integrated radiation damage, on the other hand, monotonically or continuously increases with irradiation time, and eventually approaches an asymptotic value for prolonged irradiations. An example of this behavior is shown in Fig. 17-5 [Alger, Anderson, and Webb (1959)]. When a particular system is under investigation, it is best to obtain a graph of the spin concentration as a function of time in order to decide upon the best exposure time. The approach to an asymptotic number of spins at

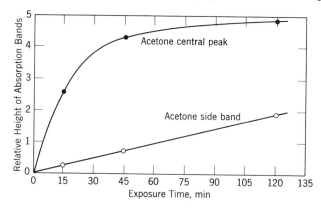

Fig. 17-5. Growth of ESR signals in irradiated acetone [Alger, Anderson, and Webb (1959)].

long irradiation times is sometimes referred to as a saturation phenomenon, and this should not be confused with the ESR saturation that occurs at high microwave powers, as discussed in Sec. 18-C. Sometimes one observes a more complex dependence of the spin concentration on irradiation time as illustrated by Fig. 17-6. There are other possibilities, such as the predominance of one ESR species at short irradiation times, and another, after long exposures.

The rate of production of paramagnetic centers may be expressed in terms of the quantum yield or number of centers produced per

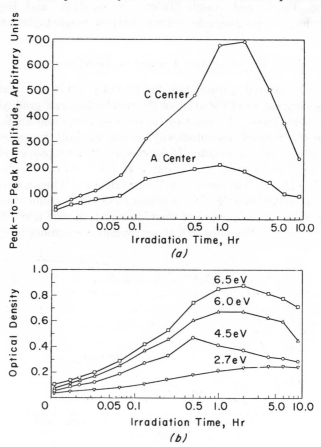

Fig. 17-6. Growth of (a) ESR signal and (b) optical absorption in Ge-doped quartz with x-irradiation time [Anderson and Weil (1959)].

incident photon (or particle). Optical irradiation rates are ordinarily expressed in terms of quantum yield, and this is usually very much less than one since a given optical photon usually does not have enough energy to produce more than one bond rupture, and the cage effect makes immediate recombination much more likely than radical stabilization. One should recall that the 253.7 mμ mercury resonance line corresponds to 113 kcal/mole or 4.9 eV if one wishes to compare the quantum yield unit to the G value defined in the next paragraph.

High energy photons (x-rays and γ-rays) and high energy particles (electrons, protons, etc.) are capable of undergoing many ionizing and replacement collisions as they traverse matter, and the primary radiation products usually are energetic enough to produce secondary radiation damage, with the result that quantum yields may greatly exceed unity. For such high energy radiations it is customary to express the rate of radiation damage in terms of the G value or number of free radicals formed per 100 eV of energy absorbed in a material. It was mentioned earlier that the threshold energy per atomic displacement is about 25 eV, so one expects the G value to be of the order of unity. Such G values are often observed.

After termination of the irradiation, the ESR signal will often decay with time. In most cases it merely decays, while in other cases it is converted to an ESR signal from a new paramagnetic species. The decay is referred to as annealing, and usually one may accelerate the annealing process by heating the specimen [Livingston, Zeldes, and Taylor (1955)], as illustrated in Fig. 17-7. This figure demonstrates that a small temperature change is often capable of changing the rate of decay by more than an order of magnitude. Sometimes, one can produce annealing by exposure to ultraviolet or visible light, a process referred to as bleaching, since it is often employed to decolorize alkali halide crystals by the removal of color centers. The apparatus required for variable temperature studies is discussed in Chap. 16.

H. Experimental Techniques

If one is not worried about the effect of air, a sample may be irradiated first, and then afterwards placed in an ESR tube. One often prefers to carry out the irradiation *in vacuo* or in a particular atmosphere, and in this case the sample may be sealed in an ESR

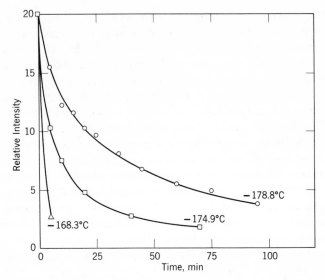

Fig. 17–7.   The disappearance of atomic hydrogen in concentrated sulfuric acid irradiated with γ-rays at low temperature [Livingston, Zeldes, and Taylor (1955)].

tube before beginning the irradiation.   Quartz ESR tubes are transparent in the near uv from the visible to about 220 mμ.   When high energy radiation is employed, it will produce paramagnetic centers in the ESR tube, as is evidenced by the pronounced coloration of the tube.   One may anneal away these centers by shaking the sample to the upper end of the ESR tube and heating the lower end with a Bunsen burner or torch, taking care not to warm the sample.   The annealing process will decolorize the tube and render it completely transparent.   The efficacy of the annealing technique may be tested by recording and comparing ESR spectra of unirradiated, irradiated, and annealed ESR tubes.   At the end of this chapter are listed several references [Anderson and Weil (1959); Castle, Feldman, Klemens, and Weeks (1963); Dienes (1960); Fröman, Pettersson, and Vänngard (1959); Hines and Arndt (1960); Jacobsen, Shiren, and Tucker (1959); Mackey (1963); Molin and Voevodsky (1958); Shamfarov and Smirnova (1963); Silsbee (1961); Weeks (1956, 1963); van Wierningen and Kats (1957, 1963)] to the spectra of irradiated quartz since quartz is the material customarily employed for constructing ESR tubes. Several articles on irradiated silica are found in *J. Phys. Chem. Solids*, **13**, No. 3–4 (1960).

Low temperature irradiation may be carried out by placing ESR tubes in a Dewar under an ice–water mixture, a Dry Ice–acetone bath, or liquid nitrogen. Care should be exercised not to have too thick a layer of refrigerant above the sample when employing irradiation with low penetrating power. The transmittance of distilled water is 85% down to 200 mμ [Hodgman (1933)]. Near ultraviolet radiation can also penetrate several centimeters of liquid nitrogen.

When silica ESR sample tubes are irradiated with 2 MeV electrons from a van de Graaff generator at 77°K and then removed from the liquid nitrogen bath, they gradually warm up, and during this warmup process they go through a certain temperature range where they glow. This glowing is an example of thermoluminescence. The ESR tubes are still darkly colored when they reach room temperature and must be heated in a Bunsen burner to completely anneal away the coloration.

Some workers have recorded ESR spectra while simultaneously irradiating the sample with electrons [Fessenden and Schuler (1963); Molin, Koritskii, Semenov, Buben, and Shamshev (1960)], x-rays [Naryadchikov, Grishina, and Bakh (1962)], ultraviolet light [Piette and Landgraf (1960)], and other irradiations. A light pipe may be employed to conduct visible and ultraviolet radiation to the sample position for such studies. Slots in the cavity endplate may also be used for this purpose as discussed in Sec. 8-C.

I. The Effect of Irradiation on Materials

High energy irradiation produces lattice damage which alters a number of physical and chemical properties of the irradiated material. This section will briefly mention some of the principal effects of irradiation. The comments made are very general, and are subject to numerous exceptions. Different results are often obtained with neutrons, charged particles, γ-rays, and x-rays.

Electrical Properties: The electrical resistivity of most materials is strongly depended upon the irradiation time.

Optical Properties: Many of the centers produced by irradiation have ultraviolet, visible, and infrared absorption bands, and a study of these bands helps to differentiate and identify the various centers. It is often possible to selectively anneal a specific center by irradiation at a particular band of optical wavelengths.   The various optical bands often anneal at different temperatures.   One sometimes observes luminescence (optical irradiation at one wavelength with emission at another), phosphorescence (delayed luminescence), electroluminescence (luminescence induced by the application of an electric field), and other forms of luminescence.   Many investigators study the optical absorption spectra and ESR spectra simultaneously.

Dimensional Changes: The bulk density tends to decrease with irradiation.   Part of this may be due to lattice expansion in the neighborhood of interstitial atoms.   Anisotropy effects often occur; for example, during the irradiation period, graphite expands considerably along the crystallographic (interplanar) c direction and contracts slightly perpendicular to it.   [Harwood, Hausner, Morse, and Rauch (1958)].

Stored Energy: Energy is stored in the lattice during irradiation and released during annealing.

Mechanical Properties: Mechanical properties such as strength, ductibility, hardness, brittleness, etc. are strongly influenced by irradiation.   The effect of irradiation on the mechanical properties is of considerable practical importance in reactor design, and other applications.

Magnetic Properties: Many radiation-produced centers are paramagnetic and contribute to the overall magnetic susceptibility. Structure sensitive properties such as the permeability are more

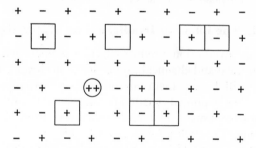

Fig. 17–8.   Vacancies and vacancy clusters which play a prominent role in the theory of the alkali halides.   As displayed from upper left to lower right and reading across, the centers are: Positive ion vacancy; negative ion vacancy; coupled pair of vacancies of opposite sign; divalent ion present substitutionally with associated positive ion vacancy; cluster of two positive ion vacancies and one negative ion vacancy [Seitz (1954)].

affected by irradiation than nonstructive-sensitive properties such as saturation magnetization.

Crystal Structure: Radiation tends to render a crystal lattice more disordered, and sometimes gross changes in structure are produced.

Surface Properties: The catalytic and adsorption properties, as well as the corrosion resistance, are sensitive to irradiation.

Chemical Properties: Polymeric and catalytic properties are sensitive to irradiation.

J. Color Centers

Several of the common types of centers will be defined. Some of them are illustrated on Figs. 17–8 and 17–9.

A Center: This is believed to be an *F* center associated with an impurity anion [see Mieher (1962) and Ohkura, Murase, and Sugimoto (1962)].

F Center: This is an electron associated with a negative ion vacancy. The letter *F* stands for the German word for color, Farbe [see Seitz (1954)].

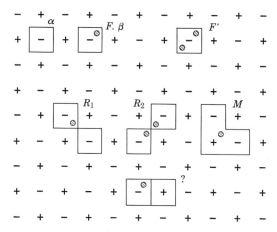

Fig. 17–9. Centers believed to give prominent absorption bands in the pure alkali halides. Reading across and from the upper lefthand corner to the lower right, they are: the negative ion vacancy presumed to be responsible for the α band; the F center consisting of the negative ion vacancy and an associated electron, responsible for the F band and β band; the F' center obtained by adding a second electron to the F center; the R_1 and R_2 centers; the M center; a hypothetical center consisting of a pair of vacancies and an associated electron [Seitz (1954)].

F' Center: This consists of a doubly charged *F* center, or two electrons associated with a negative ion vacancy [see Seitz (1954)].

Frenkel Defect: This is produced by removing an atom from its regular lattice position to an interstitial location [see Seitz (1954)].

H Center: This is considered to be two *V* centers adjacent to each other along the (110) axis and interacting magnetically with each other [see Känzig and Woodruff (1958)].

M Center: This consists of an association of an electron with a positive ion vacancy and two adjacent negative ion vacancies [see Seitz (1954)].

N Center: [see Ohlsen and Holcomb (1962)].

R_1 *Center:* This consists of two adjacent negative ion vacancies which share a single electron [see Seitz (1954)].

R_2 *Center:* This is a doubly charged R_1 center [see Seitz (1954)].

Shottky Defect: This is a vacant lattice site. Electrical neutrality may be maintained by producing both positive and negative ion vacancies [see Seitz (1954)].

V Center (sometimes called V_k center): This consists of an $(X_2)^-$ molecule ion oriented along the (110) direction of a fcc alkali halide lattice where *X* is a halide ion. It may be considered as a trapped hole shared by two adjacent halide ions (see Castner and Känzig (1957), Woodruff and Känzig (1958), and Castner (1959)].

V_F *Center:* This is a hole trapped on a positive ion vacancy (see Känzig (1960)].

Z_1 *Center:* [see Kawamura and Ishiwatari (1958)].

Z_2 *Center:* [see Takeuchi, Mizuno, Sasakura, and Ishiguro (1963)].

These color centers have been extensively studied in alkali halide crystals, and seven are discussed in the excellent review of Seitz (1954). Similar centers are observed in other types of lattices, and new ones are continuously being discovered.

K. Units and Definitions of Terms

There are several systems of units currently employed in the irradiation literature. This section will define the more common units and relate them to each other.

Quantum Yield: The number of free radicals or other irradiation products produced per incident photon.

G Value: The number of free radicals or other irradiation products produced per 100 eV of energy absorbed from the incident beam of radiation.

Extinction Coefficient ϵ: This is defined by eq. (17-E-1). It has the units liter/mole cm where C is in moles per liter and d is in centimeters. This unit is often employed in optical irradiation studies.

Absorption Coefficient α: This is defined by eq. (17-E-2) and has the units cm^{-1}. It is often referred to as the linear absorption coefficient. One should note that $\alpha = 2.303\epsilon C$.

Optical Density ϵCd: This is defined by eq. (17-E-1).

Mass Absorption Coefficient α_m: This is also employed for high energy radiation, and is defined in terms of the density ρ g/cm^3 by the relation

$$\alpha_m = \alpha/\rho \tag{1}$$

It has the units cm^2/g, and tends to be roughly independent of the nature of the absorbing material. The areal density ρd has the units g/cm^2, and for thin films it is easily measured by weighing. Sometimes, α_m is referred to simply as an absorption coefficient.

Rad: This corresponds to the absorption of 100 erg/g in a material. A megarad equals 10 J/g.

There are two principal units which express the activity or the rate of production of disintegration products such as electrons, protons, neutrons, or γ-rays. They are:

Rutherford (rd): This is defined as a disintegration rate of 10^6 disintegrations/sec.

Curie (c): The curie was originally defined as the amount of radon in equilibrium with 1 g of radium, but its current definition is 3.7 $\times$ 10^{10} disintegrations/sec. It has its submultiples the millicurie (mc) and microcurie (μc).

Relative Biological Effectiveness (RBE): A dimensionless number is assigned to each type of radiation; namely 1 for electrons, x-rays, and γ-rays, 10 for neutrons, and 20 for α-particles.

Linear Energy Transfer (LET): or linear density of ionization is the fractional part of the stopping power (energy lost per unit distance, dE/dx) that does not go into the production of δ-rays [Burch (1957)].

References

R. S. Alger, T. H. Anderson, and L. A. Webb, *J. Chem. Phys.*, **30**, 695 (1959).

American Institute of Physics Handbook, 2nd Ed., N. Y., Sec. 8.

J. H. Anderson and J. A. Weil, *J. Chem. Phys.*, **31**, 427 (1959).

A. M. Bass and H. P. Broida, *Phys. Rev.*, **101**, 1740 (1956).

K. D. Bayes, D. Kivelson, and S. C. Wong, *J. Chem. Phys.*, **37**, 1217 (1962).

S. W. Benson, *J. Chem. Ed.*, **42**, 502 (1965).

R. Beringer and M. A. Heald, *Phys. Rev.*, **95**, 1474 (1954).

P. R. J. Burch, *Rad. Res.*, **6**, 289 (1957).

E. A. Broude, *Ann. Rept. Progr. Chem.*, **42**, 105 (1945); *J. Chem. Soc.*, **1950**, 379.

J. G. Castle, Jr., D. W. Feldman, P. G. Klemens, and R. A. Weeks, *Phys. Rev.*, **130**, 577 (1963).

T. G. Castner, *Phys. Rev.*, **115**, 1506 (1959).

T. G. Castner and W. Känzig, *J. Phys. Chem. Solids*, **3**, 178 (1957).

G. E. Coates and L. E. Sutton, *J. Chem. Soc.*, **1948**, 1187.

T. Cole, J. T. Harding, J. R. Pellam, and D. M. Yost, *J. Chem. Phys.*, **27**, 593 (1957).

R. L. Collins, *J. Chem. Phys.*, **34**, 1425 (1961).

T. L. Cottrell, *The Strengths of Chemical Bonds*, 2nd Ed., Butterworths, London, 1958.

L. Dede and A. Rosenberg, *Ber.*, **67**, 147 (1934).

H. G. Dehmelt, *Phys. Rev.*, **99**, 527 (1955).

G. J. Dienes, *J. Phys. Chem. Solids*, **13**, 272 (1960).

L. Doub and J. M. Vanderbelt, *J. Am. Chem. Soc.*, **69**, 2714 (1947); **71**, 2414 (1949).

J. D. Farmer and F. P. Lossing, *Can. J. Chem.*, **33**, 861 (1955).

R. W. Fessenden and R. H. Schuler, *J. Chem. Phys.*, **39**, 2147 (1963).

F. H. Field and J. L. Franklin, *Electron Impact Phenomena*, Academic Press, N. Y., 1957, p. 140.

J. Franck and E. Rabinowitch, *Trans. Faraday Soc.*, **30**, 120 (1934).

P. O. Fröman, R. Pettersson, and T. Vänngard, *Ark. Fys.*, **15**, 559 (1959).

K. Fukuda, H. Matumoto, Y. Uchida, and H. Yoshimura, *J. Phys. Soc. Japan*, **14**, 543 (1959).

J. F. Gibson, D. J. E. Ingram, M. C. R. Symons, and M. G. Townsend, *Trans. Faraday Soc.*, **53**, 914 (1957).

J. P. Goldsborough and T. R. Koehler, *Phys. Rev.*, **133**, A135 (1964).

D. S. Hacker, S. A. Marshall, and M. Steinberg, *J. Chem. Phys.* **35**, 1788 (1961).

D. Halliday, *Introductory Nuclear Physics*, Wiley, N. Y., 1950, Sec. 6–5.

A. G. Harrison and F. P. Lossing, *J. Am. Chem. Soc.*, **82**, 519 (1960).

J. J. Harwood, H. H. Hausner, J. G. Morse, and W. G. Rauch, *The Effects of Radiation On Materials*, Reinhold, N. Y., 1958, pp. 7, 26.

J. W. Heberle, H. A. Reich, and P. Kusch, *Phys. Rev.*, **101**, 612 (1956).

V. Henri, *International Critical Tables*, Vol. 5, McGraw-Hill, N. Y., 1929, pp. 359ff.

R. L. Hines and R. Arndt, *Phys. Rev.*, **119**, 623 (1960).

C. D. Hodgman, *J. Opt. Soc. Am.*, **23**, 426 (1933).

D. J. E. Ingram and J. G. Tapley, *Phys. Rev.*, **97**, 238 1955).

E. H. Jacobsen, N. S. Shiren, and E. B. Tucker, *Phys. Rev. Letters*, **3**, 81 (1959).

C. K. Jen, S. N. Foner, E. L. Cochran, and V. A. Bowers, *Phys. Rev.*, **104**, 846 (1956); **112**, 1169 (1958); **126**, 1749 (1962); *J. Chem. Phys.*, **32**, 963 (1960).

W. Känzig and T. O. Woodruff, *Phys. Rev.*, **109**, 220 (1958); W. Känzig, *J. Phys. Chem. Solids*, **17**, 80, 88 (1960).

M. Kasha, *J. Opt. Soc. Am.*, **38**, 929 (1948).

H. Kawamura and K. Ishiwatari, *J. Phys. Soc. Japan*, **13**, 574 (1958).

D. Kivelson, K. D. Bayes, and S. C. Wong, *11th Ampere Colloquium*, Eindhoven, 1962, p. 531.

D. Kleppner, H. C. Berg, S. B. Crampton, N. F. Ramsey, R. F. C. Vessot, H. E. Peters, and J. Vanier, *Phys. Rev.*, **138**, 972 (1965).

G. Körtum, *Z. Phys. Chem.*, **B43**, 271 (1939).

J. Kroh, B. C. Green, and J. W. T. Spinks, *Can. J. Chem.*, **40**, 413 (1962).

S. Krongelb and M. W. P. Strandberg, *J. Chem. Phys.*, **31**, 1196 (1959).

W. E. Lamb, Jr., and R. C. Retherford, *Phys. Rev.*, **79**, 549 (1950); **81**, 222 (1951).

V. N. Lazukin, *Dokl. Akad. Nauk. SSSR*, **131**, 1064 (1960).

R. Livingston, H. Zeldes, and E. H. Taylor, *Disc. Faraday Soc.*, **19**, 166 (1955).

E. N. Lotkova and A. B. Fradkov, *PTE*, **1**, 188 (1961).

R. L. McCarthy, *J. Chem. Phys.*, **22**, 1360 (1954).

J. H. Mackey, Jr., *J. Chem. Phys.*, **39**, 74 (1963).

H. L. McMurray, *J. Chem. Phys.*, **9**, 231, 241 (1941).

R. L. Mieher, *Phys. Rev. Letters*, **8**, 362 (1962).

Yu. N. Molin, A. T. Koritskii, A. G. Semenov, N. Ya Buben, and V. N. Shamshev, *PTE*, **6**, 73 (931) (1960).

Yu. N. Molin and V. V. Voevodsky, *Zhur. Tek. Fiz.*, **28**, 143 (1958).

C. T. Mortimer, *Reaction Heats and Bond Strengths*, Pergamon, N. Y., 1962.

D. I. Naryadchikov, A. D. Grishina, and N. A. Bakh, *PTE*, **3**, 192 (1962).

R. S. Neale, *J. Phys. Chem.*, **68**, 143 (1964).

J. H. Noon, E. H. Holt, and J. F. Reynolds, *RSI*, **36**, 622 (1965).

H. Ohkura, K. Murase, and H. Sugimoto, *J. Phys. Soc. Japan*, **17**, 708 (1962).

W. D. Ohlsen and D. F. Holcomb, *Phys. Rev.*, **126**, 1953 (1962).

H. A. Papazian, *J. Chem. Phys.*, **27**, 813 (1957).

L. Pauling, *The Nature of the Chemical Bond*, 3rd Ed., Cornell University Press, Ithaca, N. Y., 1960, p. 131.

L. H. Piette and W. C. Landgraf, *J. Chem. Phys.*, **32**, 1107 (1960).

J. R. Platt, H. B. Klevens, and W. C. Price, *J. Chem. Phys.*, **17**, 466 (1949).

C. P. Poole, Jr., Thesis, University of Maryland, 1958, p. 9.

I. I. Rabi, J. R. Zacharias, S. Millman, and P. Kusch, *Phys. Rev.*, **53**, 318 (1938).

H. E. Radford, *Nuovo Cimento*, **14**, 245 (1959).

K. E. Rieckhoff and R. Weissbach, *RSI*, **33**, 1393 (1962).

G. Scheibe and W. Fromel, in *Hand-und Jahrbuch der chemischen Physik*, A. Eucken and K. L. Wolf, eds, Vol. 9, Part IV, Akademische Verlagsgesell-schaft, Leipzig, 1937, pp. 167, 169.

L. J. Schoen and H. P. Broida, *RSI*, **33**, 470, (1962).

L. J. Schoen, L. E. Kuentzel, and H. P. Broida, *RSI*, **29**, 633 (1958).

F. Seitz, *Rev. Mod. Phys.*, **26**, 7 (1954).

Ya. L. Shamfarov and T. A. Smirnova, *Fiz. Tverd. Tela*, **5**, 1046 (1963).

R. H. Silsbee, *J. Appl. Phys.*, **32**, 1459 (1961).

A. Smakula, *Angew. Chem.*, **47**, 657 (1934).

R. C. Smith and S. J. Wyard, *Nature*, **191**, 897 (1961).

E. W. R. Steacie, *Atomic and Free Radical Reactions*, Vol. 1, 2nd Ed., Reinhold, N. Y., 1954, pp. 97, 98.

N. Takeuchi, T. Mizuno, H. Sasakura, and M. Ishiguro, *J. Phys. Soc. Japan*, **18**, 743 (1963).

J. S. van Wieringen and A. Kats, *Philips Res. Rept.*, **12**, 432 (1957); J. S. van Wieringen, Y. Haven, and A. Kats, *11th Ampere Colloquium*, Eindhoven, 1963, p. 403.

C. Walling, *Free Radicals in Solution*, Wiley, N. Y., 1957, pp. 48–50.

R. A. Weeks, *J. Appl. Phys.*, **27**, 1376 (1956); *Phys. Rev.*, **130**, 570 (1963).

J. P. Wittke and R. H. Dicke, *Phys. Rev.*, **103**, 620 (1956).

R. W. Wood, *Phil. Mag.*, **44**, 538 (1922).

T. O. Woodruff and W. Känzig, *J. Phys. Chem. Solids*, **5**, 268 (1958)

R. A. Zhitnikov and N. V. Kolesnikov, *PTE*, **3**, 189 (682) (1964).

CHAPTER 18

Relaxation Times

A. General Description of Relaxation Times

Consider a paramagnetic sample located in a magnetic field. The sample contains two types of electronic spins S_1 and S_2 and two types of nuclear spins I_3 and I_4. The electronic and nuclear spins constitute four spin systems each of which is in thermodynamic equilibrium within itself and possesses a distribution of spin energy corresponding to the characteristic temperatures θ_1, θ_2, θ_3, and θ_4, respectively.* Let these four spin systems be completely isolated from each other, and from the lattice. The spins in each system are distributed among their Zeeman energy levels in accordance with the Boltzmann distribution (see Sec. 14-E). Let us assume that the four spin systems are initially at the same temperature θ_0.

$$\theta_1 = \theta_2 = \theta_3 = \theta_4 = \theta_0 \tag{1}$$

Now if the sample is irradiated at a microwave frequency which corresponds to the resonance condition for the S_1 spins, then these spins will gradually undergo transitions from the lower to the upper energy levels until eventually the populations of all of the S_1 Zeeman levels will be equal.† The S_1 spin system now is said to be saturated, and can absorb no more microwave energy. Quantum mechanically, we say that the Einstein coefficient for induced emission is equal for the transitions up and down between each pair of levels, and thermodynamically we say that the spin system S_1 is at an infinite temperature ($\theta_1 = \infty$). The Einstein coefficient for spontaneous emission may be neglected at microwave frequencies.

* In this section only, the symbol θ is used for temperature to avoid confusion with the use of T_1 and T_2 for relaxation times. In the remainder of the book, the symbol T is used for temperature.

† Technically speaking, an infinite time is needed to equalize the populations completely.

If the inhomogeneities in the magnetic field exceed the line-width, then only some of the S_1 spins will be at resonance, and as a result the remainder cannot absorb energy. The individual spins within each spin system may transfer energy among themselves at the rate $1/T_2$ by means of the dipolar and exchange interactions. This process of energy transfer causes all of the S_1 spins to maintain a constant temperature θ_1 as long as the microwave power is sufficiently low so that the rate at which the spins absorb microwave photons does not exceed $1/T_2$. Physically, we say that the resonant S_1 spins slowly absorb microwave energy, and rapidly pass it on to the nonresonant S_1 spins. If the spins do absorb energy at a greater rate than $1/T_2$, then the S_1 spin system will not be in internal thermal equilibrium during the irradiation process until saturation sets in. As saturation is approached, the rate of energy absorption will slow down and eventually cease, thereby restoring internal thermal equilibrium at an infinite temperature. Since the other three spin systems do not interact with S_1 spins, and they are not in resonance at the same microwave frequency, it follows that the spin systems are now described by the following temperatures

$$\theta_1 = \infty \qquad (2)$$

$$\theta_2 = \theta_3 = \theta_4 = \theta_0 \qquad (3)$$

If we now allow the spin system S_1 to interact with S_2 at the rate $1/T_\chi{}^{12}$, then "spin energy" will pass from S_1 to S_2 until both spin systems reach equilibrium with each other. The sample is now characterized by the temperatures

$$\theta_1 = \theta_2 \qquad (4)$$

$$\theta_3 = \theta_4 = \theta_0 \qquad (5)$$

The characteristic time $T_\chi{}^{12}$ is called the cross relaxation time between the spin systems S_1 and S_2 [see Bloembergen, Shapiro, Pershan, and Artman (1959); Kaplan (1960)] and may arise from dipolar or exchange interactions. In general, the cross relaxation time between the ith and jth spin systems is denoted by $T_\chi{}^{ij}$. Five additional cross relaxation times, $T_\chi{}^{13}$, $T_\chi{}^{14}$, $T_\chi{}^{23}$, and $T_\chi{}^{34}$ may also be defined for this system, where we assume $T_\chi{}^{ij} = T_\chi{}^{ji}$.

In a given sample which contains both nuclear and electronic spins, the electronic spin-spin relaxation time T_2^e is usually much less than the nuclear spin-spin relaxation time T_2^n. If these two spin systems interact with the cross relaxation time T_χ^{en}, which is also much less than T_2^n, then the measurement of T_2 in a nuclear magnetic resonance experiment will produce a value much shorter than the actual T_2^n. This is because the NMR experiment measures the rate of interchange of energy between the nuclear spins, and the slow process of energy transfer

$$\text{nucleus} \xrightarrow{T_2^n} \text{nucleus} \tag{6}$$

is now short-circuited by much more rapid processes of the type

$$\text{nucleus} \xrightarrow{T_\chi^{en}} \text{electron} \xrightarrow{T_2^e} \text{electron} \xrightarrow{T_\chi^{en}} \text{nucleus} \tag{7}$$

since

$$T_2^e, \; T_\chi^{en} \ll T_2^n \tag{8}$$

If, on the other hand, the electronic spins are saturated so that

$$\theta^e \sim \infty \tag{9}$$

then in some cases the mechanism for energy exchange between the electrons and nuclei permits the nuclei to be polarized by a double resonance experiment. Such experiments are discussed in Chap. 19. Tumanov (1962) and Grant (1964) discuss the calculation of moments in the presence of cross relaxation.

If the only mechanisms for the transferal of spin energy were of the spin-spin and cross relaxation type, then resonance experiments would serve to heat up spin systems, and they would stay "hot" forever. Actually each spin system is imbedded in a fluid or solid "lattice" characterized by a temperature θ_L which ordinarily arises from vibrations in a solid and rotations and translations in a fluid. The spin system transfers energy to the lattice at the rate $1/T_1$, where T_1 is the spin lattice relaxation time. If more than one spin system is present, then one may use the notation T_1^i to distinguish each one. In solids one usually has

$$T_1^i \gg T_2^i \tag{10}$$

for each spin system. Mechanisms for producing spin lattice relaxation at low temperatures are discussed in Sec. 18-E. Jeener, du Bois, and Broekaert (1965) discuss the existence of noninteracting Zeeman and dipolar temperatures.

In a liquid, the rate at which molecules migrate is characterized by the correlation time τ_c which is a function of the viscosity η through the Debye-like relation [Abragam (1961)]

$$\tau_c = 4\pi\eta a^3/3k\theta_L \tag{11}$$

where a is the molecular radius. In liquids, the spin lattice relaxation time T_1 is given in terms of the magnetic resonance angular frequency ω_0 by [Bloembergen, Purcell, and Pound (1948)]

$$\frac{1}{T_1} = C\left[\frac{\tau_c}{1 + (\omega_0\tau_c)^2} + \frac{2\tau_c}{1 + (2\omega_0\tau_c)^2}\right] \tag{12}$$

where C is a constant. In the proton NMR of water, one has explicitly

$$C = \frac{2}{5}\frac{g^4\beta_N^4}{\hbar^2}\frac{I(I+1)}{b^6} \tag{13}$$

where b is the proton-proton distance in the water molecule and $I = \frac{1}{2}$. [Bloembergen, Purcell, and Pound (1948)]. The minimum value of T_1 occurs where

$$\tau_c\omega_0 = (\frac{1}{2})^{1/2} \tag{14}$$

as Fig. 18-1 indicates.

When $\tau_c\omega_0 \ll (\frac{1}{2})^{1/2}$, then T_1 equals T_2 and is inversely proportional to τ_c. When, on the other hand, $\tau_c\omega_0 \gg (\frac{1}{2})^{1/2}$, then T_1 becomes directly proportional to τ_c and in addition $T_1 \ll T_2$.

A resonance absorption line has a finite shape $Y(H)$ where H_0 is the center of the spectral line and the absorption is a maximum at $Y(H_0)$ (cf. Sec. 20-A). A line-shape may be normalized as follows

$$\int_{-\infty}^{\infty} Y(\omega)\, d\omega = \int_{-\infty}^{\infty} Y(H)\, dH = 1 \tag{15}$$

and Bloch (1946) defined the spin-spin relaxation time T_2 by the relation

$$\gamma T_2 = \frac{1}{2}Y(H_0) = \frac{1}{2}\gamma Y(\omega_0) \tag{16}$$

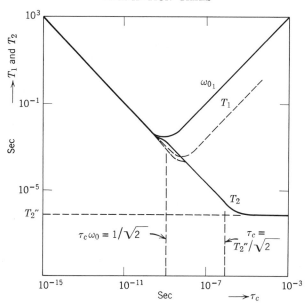

Fig. 18–1. Dependence of the relaxation times T_1 and T_2 on the correlation time τ_c [Bloembergen, Purcell, and Pound (1948)].

Thus the quantity $1/Y(\omega_0)$ is approximately equal to the line-width in frequency units, and $1/Y(H_0)$ approximates the line-width in gauss. This definition of T_2 differs from the more precise one given in Sec. 18-C.

The preceding discussion of relaxation times presented some general aspects of the theory to allow the reader to put into perspective the experimental techniques that will be presented later in the chapter. The actual theory of relaxation times is very complicated, and a discussion of the ranges of validity of the above formulae is beyond the scope of this book.

B. Homogeneous and Inhomogeneous Broadening

The distinction between homogeneous and inhomogeneous broadening in ESR was clarified by Portis (1953, 1955) and applied to the experimental results on F centers by Kip, Kittel, Levy, and Portis (1953). Homogeneous broadening occurs when the ESR signal results from a transition between two spin levels which are not sharply defined, but instead are somewhat broadened. Several sources of homogeneous broadening are [Portis (1953)]: (1) dipolar interaction between like spins; (2) spin-lattice interaction; (3) interaction with the radiation field; (4) motion of carriers in the microwave field; (5) diffusion of excitation throughout the sample; (6) motionally narrowed fluctuations in the local field.

An inhomogeneously broadened resonant line is one which consists of a spectral distribution of individual resonant lines merged into one overall line or envelope, as shown in Fig. 18-2. For example, if the applied magnetic field inhomogeneities over the volume of the sample exceed the natural line-width $1/\gamma T_2$, then the spins in various parts of the sample find themselves in different field strengths, and the resonance is artifically broadened in an inhomogeneous manner. Other sources of inhomogeneous broadening include unresolved fine structure, hyperfine structure, and the dipolar interaction between spins with different Larmor frequencies.

Portis (1955) has presented a mathematical treatment of inhomogeneously broadened lines under the following assumptions

$$H_1 < \Delta H_{env} \tag{1}$$

$$H_m < \Delta H_{env} \tag{2}$$

$$\gamma H_1 T_2 > 1 \quad \text{for saturation} \tag{3}$$

$$\omega_m H_m / H_1 < \gamma H_1 \quad \text{adiabatic condition} \tag{4}$$

$$1/H_1 (dH_0/dt) < \gamma H_1 \quad \text{adiabatic condition} \tag{5}$$

$$dH_0/dt < \omega_m \Delta H_{env} \tag{6}$$

where H_1 is the applied rf field, H_m and ω_m, respectively, are the modulation amplitude and angular frequency, ΔH_{env} is the overall line-width of the envelope, γ is the gyromagnetic ratio, T_2 is the spin-spin relaxation time, H_0 is the applied "constant" magnetic field, and t is the time. The amplitude of the dispersion signal χ' for various conditions (cases) is given in Table 18-1, and the actual line-shapes are sketched by Portis (1955).

Kip, Kittel, Levy, and Portis (1953) showed that the ESR resonances of F centers in KCl, NaCl, and KBr are inhomogeneously broadened by unresolved hyperfine structure. Portis (1953, 1956) analyzed these results and showed that when the individual spin packets are narrow compared to the inhomogeneous broadening, then saturation reduces the intensity of the absorption χ'' in agreement with the experimental results shown on Fig. 18-3. He showed that

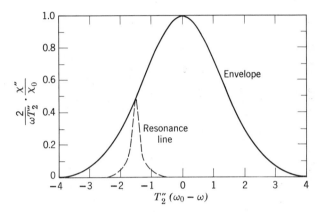

Fig. 18-2. Absorption envelope and one of its individual resonant lines [Portis (1953)].

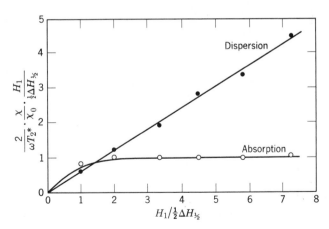

Fig. 18-3. Saturation behavior of the absorption and dispersion modes of F centers in KCl [Portis (1953)].

TABLE 18-1

The Amplitude of the rf Susceptibility χ' when Recorded under Various Conditions [Portis (1955)]

General conditions [a]

$$H_1 \& H_m < \Delta H \qquad \gamma H_1 \tau > 1$$
$$dH_0/dt \& \omega_m H_m < \gamma H_1^2 \qquad dH_0/dt < \omega_m \Delta H$$

Case	Conditions		Amplitude of χ'	Description	Phase
I	$\omega_m T_2 < H_1/\Delta H < 1$	$H_m < H_1/\omega_m T_2$ $\quad T_2 \, dH_0/dt < H_1$	$\chi_0(\omega/\Delta\omega)(H_m/\Delta H)\cos\omega_m t$	Dispersion derivative	0
IIA	$H_1/\Delta H < \omega_m T_2 < 1$	$H_m < H_1/\omega_m T_2$ $\quad T_2 \, dH_0/dt < H_1$	$\chi_0(\omega/\Delta\omega)\omega_m T_2(H_m/H_1)\sin\omega_m t$	Absorption	$\pi/2$
IIB	$H_1/H_m < \omega_m T_2 < 1$	$H_m > H_1/\omega_m T_2$ $\quad T_2 \, dH_0/dt < \omega_m H_m$	$\chi_0(\omega/\Delta\omega)\ln(2H_m\omega_m T_2/H_1)\sin\omega_m t_2$	Absorption	$\pi/2$
IIIA	$\omega_m T_2 > 1$	$T_2 \, dH_0/dt < H_1$	$-\chi_0(\omega/\Delta\omega)(H_m/H_1)\cos\omega_m t$	Absorption	π
IIIB	$\omega_m T_2 > 1$	$T_2 \, dH_0/dt < H_m$	$-\chi_0(\omega/\Delta\omega)\ln(2H_m/H_1)\cos\omega_m t$	Absorption	π
IV	$\omega_m T_2 > 1$	$T_2 \, dH_0/dt > H_1 \& H_m$	$\mp\chi_0(\omega/\Delta\omega)(H_m/\Delta H)\ln(2\Delta H/H_1)\cos\omega_m t$	Absorption derivative (sign reverses with direction of travel)	π

[a] ΔH denotes ΔH_{env}.

under the conditions of power modulation, the microwave power P_c incident on the crystal has the form

$$P_c = F\chi_0\omega_0 T_2 P_w \frac{\chi''(\omega, H_1)}{\chi''(\omega, 0)} (1 + \sin \omega_m t) \qquad (7)$$

where P_w is the microwave power incident on the cavity, ω is the microwave resonant frequency, and F is a function of the Q of the cavity, the filling factor, and other quantities. The saturation factor $\chi''(\omega, H_1)/\chi''(\omega, 0)$ is the ratio of the imaginary part of the susceptibility at the rf field amplitude H_1 to its value at $H_1 = 0$. The detected signal P_c may be expanded in a Fourier series

$$P_c = F\chi_0\omega_0 T_2 P_w \sum (a_n \cos n\omega_m t + b_n \sin n\omega_m t) \qquad (8)$$

and the lock-in detector is tuned to detect only the $b_1 \sin \omega_m t$ term. Portis (1953) showed that the results for the following four cases are:

Case 1: Homogeneous broadening and $\omega_m T_1 < 1$. The system follows the variations in microwave power, and

$$b_1 = (2/s'^2)[(1 + s')/(1 + 2s')^{1/2}] \qquad (9)$$

Case 2: Homogeneous broadening and $\omega_m T_1 > 1$. The system does not follow the variations in the average microwave power, but saturates at the average power level, and

$$b_1 = 1/(1 + s') \qquad (10)$$

Case 3: Inhomogeneous broadening and $\omega_m T_1 < 1$. The spin packets will individually follow the periodic variations in power level, and will saturate individually rather than transferring power at once to the entire spin system. The quantity b_1 will have the form

$$b_1 \cong (1 + 0.60s')/(1 + s')^{3/2} \qquad (11)$$

Case 4: Inhomogeneous broadening and $\omega_m T_1 > 1$. This gives

$$b_1 = 1/(1 + s')^{1/2} \qquad (12)$$

where

$$s' = \tfrac{1}{4}\gamma^2 H_1^2 T_1 T_2 = -1 + 1/s \qquad (13)$$

and s is the saturation factor used in the next section. These functions are plotted in Fig. 18–4.

Numerous authors have discussed inhomogeneously broadened magnetic resonance lines. For example, Hyde (1960), Kiel (1962), and van Gerven (1963) have treated the subject theoretically; Drain (1962) considered the effect of sample inhomogeneities and Bugai (1962) discussed passage effects when high frequency modulation is employed. Motchane (1962), Motchane and Uebersfeld (1960, 1960), and Kessenikh and Manenkov (1963) discuss the double resonance of inhomogeneously broadened lines, while Richter and Schwind (1963) mention that the square of the observed line-width is approximately equal to the square of the natural line-width in a homogeneous field plus a term that is proportional to the square of the range of resonance frequencies that result from the magnetic

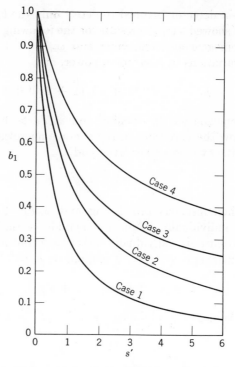

Fig. 18–4. The dependence of the observed signal amplitude b_1 on the parameter s' [Portis (1953)].

field inhomogeneities. Kaplan (1965) discusses cross relaxation of inhomogeneous lines. In a review article, Weger (1960) classified the ESR signals from inhomogeneously broadened lines occurring under various experimental conditions. See also Timerov (1961) and Gill and Meredith (1965).

Castner (1959) generalized Portis' theory by omitting the assumption that the individual spin packet width is very much less than the envelope width. He assumed that each spin packet had a Lorentzian shape, and showed that only those spins within $1/T_2$ or γH_1, whichever is larger, of the Larmor frequency will be saturated at sufficient microwave power levels. Spin diffusion [Anderson (1959)] is too slow to modify this. Moran, Christensen, and Silsbee (1961) obtained experimental evidence in support of Castner's more general theory.

C. Saturation Methods of Determining Relaxation Times

If one assumes that the Bloch equations are valid, then the magnetic resonance absorption Y and its first derivative Y' have a Lorentzian line-shape [Bloch (1946); Bloembergen, Purcell, and Pound (1948)], and in the notation of Chap. 20 we may write

$$Y = \frac{y_m^0}{1 + \left(\dfrac{H - H_0}{\frac{1}{2}\Delta H_{1/2}}\right)^2} \tag{1}$$

$$Y' = \frac{\left(\frac{4}{3}\right)^2 (H - H_0)\, y_m^{0\prime}}{\frac{1}{2}\Delta H_{pp}\left[1 + \frac{1}{3}\left(\dfrac{H - H_0}{\frac{1}{2}\Delta H_{pp}}\right)^2\right]^2} \tag{2}$$

for normalized line-shapes. If one writes these relations as functions of the spin lattice and spin-spin relaxation times T_1 and T_2, and includes the effect of the microwave amplitude, H_1, they assume the form

$$Y = \frac{H_1 y_m^0}{1 + (H - H_0)^2 \gamma^2 T_2^2 + \frac{1}{4}H_1^2 \gamma^2 T_1 T_2} \tag{3}$$

and

$$Y' = \frac{16}{3^{3/2}} \frac{(H - H_0)\gamma T_2 H_1 y_m^{0'}}{[1 + (H - H_0)^2 \gamma^2 T_2^2 + \frac{1}{4}H_1^2\gamma^2 T_1 T_2]^2} \tag{4}$$

where y_m^0 and $y_m^{0'}$ are the maximum amplitudes below saturation ($\frac{1}{4}H_1^2\gamma^2 T_1 T_2 \ll 1$), and γ is the gyromagnetic ratio given by

$$\gamma = g\beta/\hbar = 0.87934 \times 10^7 \, g \text{ cps/G} \tag{5}$$

If the saturation factor s is defined by

$$s = \frac{1}{1 + \frac{1}{4}H_1^2\gamma^2 T_1 T_2} \tag{6}$$

then Y and Y' have the forms

$$Y = \frac{sH_1 y_m^0}{1 + s(H - H_0)^2 \gamma^2 T_2^2} \tag{7}$$

and

$$Y' = \frac{16(H - H_0) \gamma T_2 s^2 H_1 y_m^{0'}}{3^{3/2}[1 + s(H - H_0)^2 \gamma^2 T_2^2]^2} \tag{8}$$

Note that below saturation $s \sim 1$. The half power line-width $\Delta H_{1/2}$ of Y and the peak-to-peak line-width ΔH_{pp} of Y' are given in terms of their unsaturated ($s = 1$) values $\Delta H_{1/2}^0$ and ΔH_{pp}^0, respectively, by

$$\Delta H_{1/2} = [\Delta H_{1/2}^0]s^{-1/2} = [2/(\gamma T_2)]s^{-1/2} \tag{9}$$

$$\Delta H_{pp} = [\Delta H_{pp}^0]s^{-1/2} = [2/(3^{1/2}\gamma T_2)]s^{-1/2} \tag{10}$$

The amplitude y_m of the center of the absorption line is obtained by letting $H = H_0$ in eq. (7), and has the form

$$(y_m/H_1) = [y_m^0]s \tag{11}$$

while the peak-to-peak amplitude of the first derivative curve $Y' = y_m'$ at $H - H_0 = \pm\frac{1}{2}\Delta H_{pp}$ [i.e., at $H - H_0 = \pm(3\gamma^2 T_2^2 s)^{-1/2}$] has the form

$$(y_m'/H_1) = [y_m^{0'}]s^{3/2} \tag{12}$$

Since below saturation $s = 1$, it follows that under this condition both y_m/H_1 and y_m'/H_1 are independent of the power level. Equations (9)–(12) are all of the general form $A = Bs^n$ and so

$$1/s = [B/A]^{1/n} \tag{13}$$

where B is a constant. Below saturation $s = 1$, so that

$$1/s = \left[\frac{\lim_{H_1 \to 0} (A)}{A} \right]^{1/n} = 1 + \tfrac{1}{4}\gamma^2 H_1^2 T_1 T_2 \tag{14}$$

and one has explicitly

$$1/s = \begin{cases} \left[\dfrac{\Delta H_{1/2}}{\lim\limits_{H_1 \to 0} \Delta H_{1/2}} \right]^2 & \text{using eq. (9)} \\[2em] \left[\dfrac{\Delta H_{pp}}{\lim\limits_{H_1 \to 0} \Delta H_{pp}} \right]^2 & \text{using eq. (10)} \\[2em] \left[\dfrac{\lim\limits_{H_1 \to 0} (y_m/H_1)}{y_m/H_1} \right] & \text{using eq. (11)} \\[2em] \left[\dfrac{\lim\limits_{H_1 \to 0} (y_m'/H_1)}{y_m'/H_1} \right]^{2/3} & \text{using eq. (12)} \end{cases} \tag{15}$$

The shorthand notation $y_m{}^0$ corresponds to $\lim\limits_{H_1 \to 0} y_m$ and similarly for $y_m{}^{0\prime}$, $\Delta H_{1/2}{}^0$ and $\Delta H_{pp}{}^0$. Note that the terms in parentheses have different exponents (2, 2, 1, and 2/3, respectively). It is best to use the amplitudes y_m/H_1 or y_m'/H_1 for computing $1/s$ in eq. (14) since they can be more accurately measured than the line-widths.

The peak-to-peak amplitude y_m' is proportional to the microwave magnetic field H_1 below saturation. Experimentally, one observes a linear dependence on the square root of the power, and a power independent line-width in this region, as shown on Figs. 18–5a and 18–5b. When the resonant line is strongly saturated, the amplitude y_m' becomes proportional to H_1^{-2} or P^{-1}, and therefore it decreases with increasing power in the manner shown in Fig. 18–5a. At these high

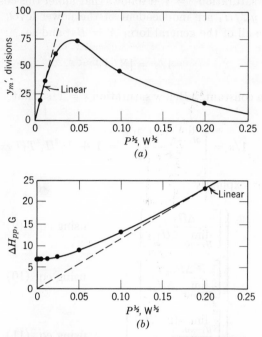

Fig. 18–5. (a) Peak-to-peak amplitude y_m' plotted as a function of the square root of the microwave power P. The dotted line is an extrapolation of the linear dependence at low powers. (b) Peak-to-peak line-width ΔH_{pp} plotted as a function of the square root of the microwave power P. The dotted line gives the linear asymptotic behavior at very high powers.

power levels the line-width becomes proportional to H_1, as shown in Fig. 18–5b. The width ΔH_{pp} will follow the dotted straight line for powers greater than those shown.

From eq. (14) we see that a plot of $1/s$ against $H_1{}^2$ will give a straight line with the slope $\gamma^2 T_1 T_2/4$ and the intercept 1. Figures 18–5c and 18–5d show plots of $1/s$ versus $H_1{}^2$ using the derivative amplitude and the line-width expressions, respectively. [The denominators of the ordinate functions $(1/3)^{2/3}$ and 7 are $(H_1/y_m{}^{0\prime})^{2/3}$ and $\Delta H_{pp}{}^0$, respectively]. This is of course equivalent to plotting $1/s$ against the microwave power P because P is proportional to $H_1{}^2$. The slope of the line in either Fig. 18–5c or 18–5d may be used to calculate the product $T_1 T_2$.

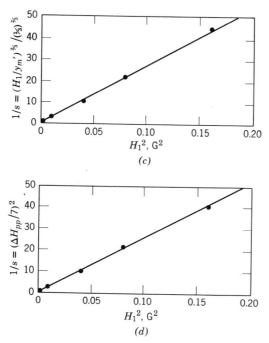

Fig. 18–5. (c) The normalized quantity $(y_m'/H_1)^{-2/3}$ depends linearly on the square of the microwave field strength H_1^2, as shown. The slope of the line is $\gamma^2 T_1 T_2/4$, and $1/s = 1$ when $H_1 = 0$. (d) The linear dependence of $(\Delta H_{pp})^2$ normalized relative to the value 7^2 below saturation depends linearly on H_1^2 as shown. The slope of the line is $\gamma^2 T_1 T_2/4$ and $1/s = 1$ when $H_1 = 0$. The data points shown in Figs. 18–5 are obtained from Table 18–2.

In order to determine the relaxation times T_1 and T_2, a series of ESR spectra is recorded with the power varying from a condition of negligible saturation ($\frac{1}{4}H_1^2\gamma T_1 T_2 \ll 1$) to one of pronounced saturation ($\frac{1}{4}H_1^2\gamma^2 T_1 T_2 \gg 1$). If necessary, one may set the leakage at $4\mu A$ or less for these measurements. The spin-spin relaxation time T_2 is calculated from the line-width below saturation (i.e., $\Delta H_{1/2}^0$ or ΔH_{pp}^0) by means of the expression

$$T_2 = \frac{2}{\gamma\Delta H_{1/2}^0} = \frac{2}{3^{1/2}\gamma\Delta H_{pp}^0} = \frac{2.2742 \times 10^{-7}}{g\Delta H_{1/2}^0}$$

$$= \frac{1.3131 \times 10^{-7}}{g\Delta H_{pp}^0} \tag{16}$$

and eq. (6) allows us to write for T_1

$$T_1 = \left(\frac{(3)^{1/2}\Delta H_{pp}^{0}}{2\gamma}\right)\left(\frac{1/s - 1}{\frac{1}{4}H_1^2}\right) \tag{17}$$

$$= \frac{3.9392 \times 10^{-7}\Delta H_{pp}^{0}}{g}\left(\frac{1/s - 1}{H_1^2}\right) \tag{18}$$

where both ΔH_{pp}^{0} and H_1 are in gauss. A similar expression may be written by substituting $\Delta H_{1/2}^{0}$ for $3^{1/2}\Delta H_{pp}^{0}$. Equation (18) may be used to calculate T_1 from the data. Note that below saturation the term $(1/s - 1)/H_1^2$ becomes very difficult to measure because $(1/s - 1)$ becomes much less than one, while far above saturation, the amplitude y_m' (or y_m) is very weak and the width ΔH_{pp} (or $\Delta H_{1/2}$) is very large so that the ratio $(1/s - 1)\,\Delta H_{pp}/H_1^2$ cannot be accurately evaluated. The best results are obtained when eq. (18) is used for power levels that are only moderately above saturation. One of the principal experimental advantages of this saturation method of determining relaxation times is that it may be carried out with routine spectrometers using very low leakages (e.g., $\sim 4\mu A$), while the pulse methods to be discussed in the next section require the use of specialized microwave and electronic components.

A sample calculation of T_1 and T_2 by the saturation method is presented in Table 18-2. The raw data consist of the microwave power P_w measured on a power meter, the line-widths ΔH_{pp}, and the peak-to-peak amplitudes of the derivative spectrum y_m' in arbitrary units. These data are plotted on Figs. 18-5a and 18-5b. The microwave magnetic field H_1 at the sample may be computed from the microwave power P_w incident on the resonant cavity by the methods described in Sec. 8-H, and will have the functional dependence

$$H_1^2 = KP_w \tag{19}$$

where H is in gauss, P_w is in watts, and in a typical case, K is of the order of unity. Equation (19) with $K = 1^1\ \text{G}^2/\text{W}$ is used to compute the second column from the first column. Then the fifth column is calculated by dividing the values of the fourth column by those in the second column. The two top entries in the third column and also the two top entries in the fifth column are close to each other, which indicates that they correspond to the condition of negligible saturation. Therefore, they are used to determine $\Delta H_{pp}{}^0$ and $\lim\limits_{H_1 \to 0} (y_m'/H_1)$. The sixth column is calculated by dividing $\lim\limits_{H_1 \to 0} (y_m'/H_1)$ by the entries in the fifth column since

$$(1/s)^{3/2} = \frac{\lim\limits_{H_1 \to 0} (y_m'/H_1)}{y_m'/H_1} = \frac{3.0}{y_m'/H_1} \tag{20}$$

Only three entries are given for $(1/s - 1)/H_1{}^2$ in the seventh column since at low powers $1/s$ is too close to unity, and at the highest powers the amplitude y_m' is too small for accuracy. The saturation factor s computed from the calculated T_1 and T_2 values is listed in the eighth column for completeness. Figure 18-5c shows values of $1/s$ computed from the sixth column, and data from the third column are plotted in Fig. 18-5d.

A simpler way to calculate T_1 is to determine either y_m or y_m' as a function of power, and ascertain where a maximum is reached. For example, we might deduce from Fig. 18-5a or from the data on Table 18-2 that the maximum value of y_m' is obtained for H_1 between 0.025 and 0.05 G, and somewhat closer to the higher value. A reasonable estimate is 0.04 G. The maxima in eqs. (11) and (12), respectively, come where

$$\frac{dy_m}{dH_1} = 0 \quad \text{and} \quad \frac{dy_m'}{dH_1} = 0 \tag{21}$$

One may easily show that these maxima occur when

$$s = 1/2 \qquad \text{max in } y_m \tag{22}$$

$$s = 2/3 \qquad \text{max in } y_m' \tag{23}$$

Using eqs. (18), (22), and (23), one may show that at the maxima

$$T_1 = 2.28 \times 10^{-7} \Delta H_{1/2}{}^0/(gH_1{}^2) \qquad \text{max in } y_m \tag{24}$$

$$T_1 = 1.97 \times 10^{-7} \Delta H_{pp}{}^0/(gH_1{}^2) \qquad \text{max in } y_m' \tag{25}$$

TABLE 18-2

Typical Saturation Curve Data and Illustrative Calculation of T_1 and T_2

P, W	H_1, G	ΔH_{pp}, G	y'_m divisions	y'_m/H_1 [b]	$(1/s)^{3/2}$	$(1/s - 1)/H_1^2$	s
3.9×10^{-5}	0.0063	7.0	19	3.0	0.98	—	0.99
1.56×10^{-4}	0.0125	7.1	36	2.9	1.02	—	0.96
6.25×10^{-4}	0.025	7.4	61	2.4	1.23	—	0.86
2.5×10^{-3}	0.05	8.9	73	1.5	1.97	—	0.59
1.0×10^{-2}	0.1	13.1	46	0.46	6.4	244	0.23
4.0×10^{-2}	0.2	23.	17	0.085	35	242	0.083
8.0×10^{-2}	0.28	33.	8	0.029	103	263	0.044
1.6×10^{-1}	0.4	45.	4	0.01	300	—	0.023
6.4×10^{-1}	0.8	90.	1	1.3×10^{-3}	2000	—	0.006

$$y_m^{0'} = \lim_{H_1 \to 0} \left(\frac{y'_m}{H_1} \right) = \frac{1}{2} \left(\frac{19}{0.063} + \frac{36}{0.0125} \right) \sim 3 \times 10^3 \text{ divisions/G}$$

$$(1/s)^{3/2} = \left(\frac{\lim_{H_1 \to 0} (y'_m/H_1)}{y'_m/H_1} \right) \text{ using amplitude data in the fourth column}^a$$

$$\frac{1/s - 1}{H_1^2} = \frac{1}{3} (244 + 242 + 274) \approx 250$$

$$\Delta H_{pp}^0 = \lim_{H_1 \to 0} \Delta H_{pp} = 7 \text{ G}$$

$$g = 2.00$$

$$T_2 = \frac{1.3 \times 10^{-7}}{g \Delta H_{pp}^0} = \frac{1.3 \times 10^{-7}}{2 \times 7} \sim 10^{-8} \text{ sec}$$

$$T_1 = 3.9 \times 10^{-7} \, \Delta H_{pp}^0 / g \left(\frac{1/s - 1}{H_1^2} \right) = 3.9 \times 10^{-7} \times \tfrac{1}{2} \times 7 \times 250 \sim 3.5 \times 10^{-4} \text{ sec}$$

$$\gamma = \beta/\hbar = 0.88 \times 10^7 \, g \text{ cps/G}$$

$$s = \frac{1}{1 + \tfrac{1}{4}\gamma^2 H_1^2 T_1 T_2} = \frac{1}{1 + 0.78 \times 10^{14} \times 10^{-8} \times 3.5 \times 10^{-4} H_1^2} = \frac{1}{1 + 275 H_1^2}$$

a A less accurate calculation may be made using $(1/s)^{1/2} = (\Delta H_{pp}/\Delta H_{pp}^0)$ in the sixth column.
b Divisions per milligauss.

In the example under consideration, $\Delta H_{pp}{}^0 = 7$ G and we estimated $H_1 = 0.04$ G, so from eq. (25)

$$T_1 \sim (1.96 \times 10^{-7} \times \tfrac{1}{2} \times 7)/(0.04)^2 \sim 4 \times 10^{-4} \text{ sec} \qquad (26)$$

in reasonable agreement with the estimate obtained from Table 18–2. One may of course determine the maximum in $y_m{}'$ more precisely by a graphical method with data obtained at intermediate power settings.

Some authors such as Singer and Kommandeur (1961) display saturation data by plotting the amplitude $y_m{}'$ relative to a (ruby) standard $y_{ms}{}'$ against the logarithm of the power, as shown in Fig. 18–6 for iodine complexes. This has the advantage of fitting on one graph power data which span several orders of magnitude. Singer and Kommandeur determined the product T_1T_2 of an unknown sample relative to that of solid DPPH from the relation

$$T_1T_2 = (P_{\text{DPPH}}/P)\ T_1{}^2{}_{\text{DPPH}}$$

where for DPPH Lloyd and Pake (1953) and Bloembergen and Wang (1954) found [see also Berthet (1955)]

$$T_1 = T_2 = 6 \times 10^{-9} \text{ sec}$$

The powers P_{DPPH} and P of DPPH and the unknown are determined at the same amount of saturation, e.g., where $y_m{}'/y_{ms}{}'$ on Fig. 18–6 reaches 0.5. The value of T_2 for the unknown is deduced from eq. (16). The paper of Singer and Kommandeur may be consulted for other practical methods of interpreting ESR data.

Two difficulties involved in the saturation method of determining relaxation times are the conversion of power P_w incident on the cavity to $H_1{}^2$ values, and the measurement of P_w. The former is difficult to do accurately, and Sec. 8-H may be consulted for the theory behind it [see also Marr and Swarup (1960)]. A calibration of $H_1{}^2$ may be carried out experimentally from saturation data on a sample such as DPPH whose relaxation times are known.

The value of P may be measured by means of a power meter and bolometer which monitors the microwave power through a directional coupler. One may also use a nonsaturating standard sample in the same resonant cavity, and the Singer method [Singer (1959); Singer,

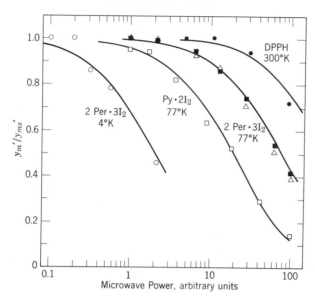

Fig. 18–6. Saturation curves for pyrene and perylene complexes at low temperatures. The ordinate is the radical ion amplitude y_m' divided by the amplitude of the ruby standard y_{ms}' normalized to one at low power [Singer and Kammandeur (1961)].

Smith, and Wagoner (1961)], described in Sec. 14-K is useful. This has the advantage of monitoring the actual H_1 field and automatically correcting for the impedance mismatch that is inevitable at low power levels. In other words, when the slide screw tuner is inserted very far to achieve the desired leakage level at low powers, the cavity pip on the mode is raised close to the top, and a much smaller percentage of the incident microwave power actually enters the cavity. This causes the power meter to give a false indication of the energy density $(\mu H_1^2/2)$ in the cavity. A standard sample must be used to check H_1^2 accurately. The use of a very low leakage (e.g., $4\mu A$) at these low powers will minimize the mismatch difficulty. A dual sample cavity such as the one shown on Fig. 8–32 is convenient for use with the standard sample [Kramer and Müller-Warmuth (1963)].

Mandel (1962) describes a continuous wave saturation method which is useful for systems with long relaxation times when the lattice-bath bottleneck rather than the spin-lattice bottleneck controls the equilibrium temperature of the spin system.

McConnell (1958) generalized the Bloch equations to include a system in which the observed spins are reversibly exchanging between two sites such as might occur in a simple chemical exchange system. Swift and Connick (1962) and O'Reilly and Poole (1963) applied these equations to NMR systems. Sohma (1962) discusses the effect of free radical lifetimes on ESR relaxation, and shows how to estimate either T_1 or the radical lifetime when the other is known.

The saturation method of determining relaxation times assumes the validity of the Bloch equations and a Lorentzian line-shape. It should be emphasized that not all systems obey the Bloch equations, and in particular, the dispersion mode χ' often saturates at much higher power levels than the absorption mode χ'' as shown in Fig. 18–3 [see, e.g., Portis (1953); Redfield (1955, 1957)]. When a resonant line is inhomogeneously broadened, then equations such as (9), (10), and (16) are only valid for the individual component spin-packet line-width, not for the overall (envelope) width.

When a saturation study is carried out with a large sample such as one along the axis of a cavity, then the microwave field will vary throughout the sample. Some spins will be saturated, while others are not. Many samples such as the one shown on Fig. 8–5 have a sinusoidal variation of the microwave field strength H_1 of the type $\sin \pi x/a$, so the saturation factor s has a $\sin^2 \pi x/a$ term. The filling factor is smallest where the saturation is least at the top and bottom of the tube. One should use only the center $\frac{1}{3}$ or $\frac{1}{4}$ of the tube for best results.

The modulation frequency will influence the detected ESR signal, as discussed in Sec. 10-F [see also Andrew (1956), p. 109]. When audio modulation frequencies are used which satisfy the conditions $f_{mod} \ll 1/T_1$, and a fortiori, $f_{mod} \ll 1/T_2$, then the saturation factor (spin system) will follow the modulation cycle. The data tabulated in Table 18–2 and displayed in Fig. 18–5 were recorded under these conditions. When the modulation frequency becomes comparable to or exceeds the reciprocal of the relaxation time, then the magnetic field changes too rapidly for the spin system to follow it, and the spins "see" an average applied magnetic field. This produces a change in the amplitude of the detected signal. The relaxation time T_1 may be determined by modulating the microwave field H_1 and observing the detected amplitude as a function of f_{mod} in the neighborhood of $f_{mod} \sim 1/T_1$ [Pescia and Hervé (1961); Bassompierre and

Pescia (1962); Hervé and Pescia (1962, 1963); Hervé (1963); Pescia (1965); Zueco and Pescia (1965)]. Hervé (1963) used modulation frequencies up to 30 Mc. Halbach (1954) also described a modulation method for determining relaxation times. Carruthers and Rumin (1965) evaluated the spin lattice relaxation time from a measurement of the phase and amplitude of the detected ESR signal. This method does not require a knowledge of the power level or linewidth.

D. Pulse Methods for Determining Relaxation Times

Relaxation times are routinely determined by pulse methods in the field of nuclear magnetic resonance, and one may consult a standard text on NMR [e.g. Andrew (1956); Lösche (1957); Pople, Schneider, and Bernstein (1959); Abragam (1961); Slichter (1963)] for some of the general theory behind this technique. Woonton (1961) has reviewed ESR pulse techniques. In essence, the pulse method consists in (1) exposing the sample to a very high-power, short-duration pulse of microwave energy, and (2) measuring the strength and decay rate of the induced magnetization. Pulsed microwave spectroscopy is discussed by Dicke and Romer (1955). An early study of ESR relaxation times by means of pulse techniques with H_1 up to 50 G was carried out by Bloembergen and Wang (1954) using the apparatus of Fig. 18–7. Magnetrons are well suited as sources for such pulse work.

Davis, Strandberg, and Kyhl (1958) emphasized that the saturation method of determining ESR relaxation times employs "cw techniques in the frequency domain," and that the interpretation of such data depends upon the assumption of a physical model such as the Bloch theory (1946). They measured electron spin-lattice relaxation times in the time domain by a pulse technique using the apparatus shown in Fig. 18–8. A 3-cm magnetron supplies ~ 1 μsec pulses at ~ 1 sec intervals through a high-power attenuator and circulator to the resonant cavity. A low-power (millimicrowatt) cw (i.e., nonpulsed) klystron is coupled into the magnetron transmission line, and the reflected signal from this klystron traverses a TR switch and is detected by a superheterodyne receiver with micromicrowatt sensitivity. The entire measurement is carried out at liquid helium temperature with the resonance condition $\hbar\omega_0 = g\beta H_0$ satisfied.

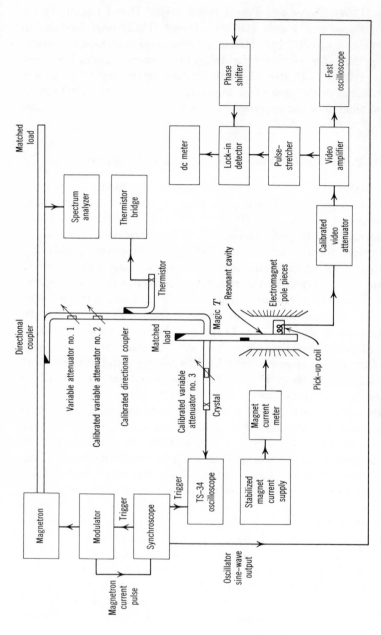

Fig. 18–7.   Block diagram of one of the first ESR spectrometers designed for measuring relaxation times by the pulse method [Bloembergen and Wang (1954)].

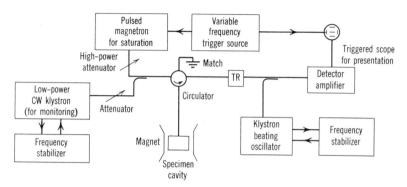

Fig. 18–8.   Block diagram of ESR equipment for determining T_1 by the pulsed saturation method [Davis, Strandberg, and Kyhl (1958)].

Paxman (1961) also employed the method of Davis, Strandberg, and Kyhl (1958).

Before applying the pulse, the Davis, Strandberg, and Kyhl system is tuned up to resonance, and the detected power is a measure of the unsaturated absorption (rf susceptibility χ''_∞). When the pulse is applied, the absorption χ'' increases to an initial high value $\chi''(0)$ and then decays with time $[\chi''(t)]$ to χ''_∞ at a rate that is determined by the spin-lattice relaxation time, as shown on Fig. 18–9. The relaxation time is determined from the slope of the straight line that is obtained by plotting log $(1 - \chi''(t)/\chi''_\infty)$ against time.

A number of additional ESR spectrometers have been designed specifically for use in measuring relaxation times. The block diagram of Zverev's (1961) X band system is shown in Fig. 18–10. The power from the klystron K_1 is fed through two attenuators A_1 and A_2 to arm 1 of the circulator. The sample under study is placed in the resonator R which is located in the bottom of the liquid helium Dewar D, and situated between the pole pieces of the magnet M.

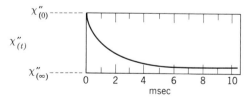

Fig. 18–9.   Typical oscilloscope trace obtained with La(Gd) $(C_2H_5SO_4)_3 \cdot 9H_2O$ at 4.2°K [Davis, Strandberg, and Kyhl (1958)].

The signal reflected from the cavity beats against the local oscillator klystron K_2 and then undergoes superheterodyne detection. This spectrometer is provided with a klystron power supply (B_1) and systems for stabilizing the klystron frequency (B_2), the sample temperature (B_3), and the magnetic field strength (B_4). This spectrometer is employed for measuring T_1 by the continuous saturation method, and should more properly have been described in the last section. Dionne (1965) and Kipling, Smith, Vanier, and Woonton (1961) describe instrumentation for cw relaxation experiments.

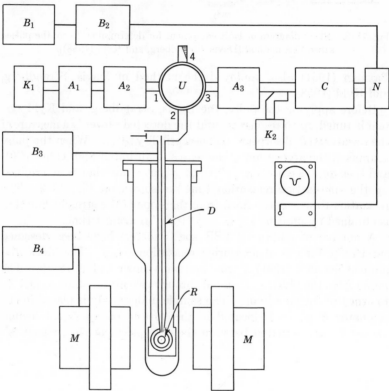

Fig. 18–10. Block diagram of a radio frequency spectrometer: (A_1, A_2, A_3) attenuators; (B_1) klystron power supply; (B_2) klystron stabilizer; (B_3) temperature measurement and regulation; (B_4) system for stabilizing the magnetic field; (C) mixer of the superheterodyne receiver; (D) vacuum housing; (M) magnet; (R) resonator; (K_1, K_2) klystrons; (U) circulator; (N) intermediate frequency amplifier [Zverev (1961)].

ESR spectrometers for relaxation time studies were designed by Leifson and Jeffries (1961), Ruby, Benoit, and Jeffries (1962), and Scott and Jeffries (1962). The block diagram of one of them is shown in Fig. 18–11. The sample was placed in the bottom of a cylindrical TE_{111} reflection cavity. The diode switch is used to provide the high power pulse and the monitor power which is used to observe the recovery of the magnetization after the pulse. The monitor power level was ordinarily set at about 10^{-10} W. The transient recovery of the signal was photographed on an oscilloscope and replotted on semilog paper to determine if the decay was exponential. Relaxation times were determined from the slopes of such plots.

Leifson and Jeffries' (1961) spectrometer used the cylindrical TE_{011} transmission cavity shown in Fig. 19–11. They estimated that the microwave field strength in gauss at the sample H_1 was related to the

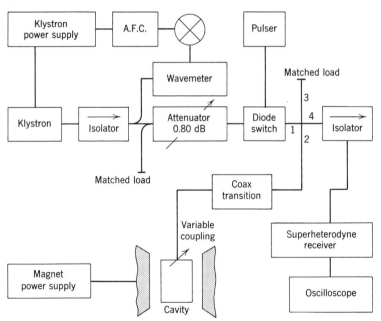

Fig. 18–11. Block diagram of ESR spectrometer designed for measuring relaxation times [Ruby, Benoit, and Jeffries (1962); see also Scott and Jeffries (1962)].

incident microwave power P_w in watts the expression [cf. Sec. 8–H]

$$H_1{}^2 \approx 0.1\ P_w \tag{1}$$

Pashinin and Prokhorov (1961) employed the X band spectrometer shown on Fig. 18–12 for determining spin-lattice relaxation times by both pulsed and continuous saturation methods. For pulse measurements, the klystron K_1 provides 25 μsec duration pulses, with a rise time of <1 μsec at a repetition rate of between 0.1 and 100 pulses/sec. For continuous saturation measurements, the klystron K_1 supplies cw power which is measured by the low power meter (LPM) that is fed by the directional coupler. The rest of the apparatus consists of a superheterodyne spectroscope similar to the one that was designed by Manenkov and Prokhorov (1956), discussed in Sec. 13-J and shown on Fig. 13–12. The signal klystron K_2 works at a low power level and beats against the reference klystron K_3 in the hybrid ring (HR) to produce the intermediate frequency that is detected by the balanced mixer in the other two arms of HR.

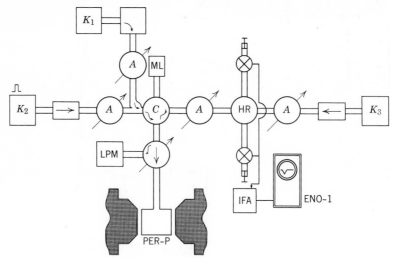

Fig. 18–12. Block diagram of spectrometer for determining T_1 by the continuous saturation and pulse techniques. It employs three klystrons K_1, K_2, and K_3, four variable attenuators A, a circulator C, a hybrid ring HR, a resonant cavity PER-P, a low-power meter LPM, an intermediate frequency amplifier IFA, a matched load ML, and an ENO-1 oscilloscope [Pashinin and Prokhorov (1961)].

Kaplan (1962) [Kaplan, Browne, and Cowen (1961)] designed the dual source spectrometer shown on Fig. 18–13. The magnetrons produce 200 W of peak power at 9300 Mc in pulses whose duration may be made as short as 10^{-8} sec. The two magnetrons produce pulses at 90°- and 180°-intervals. The modulators employ an

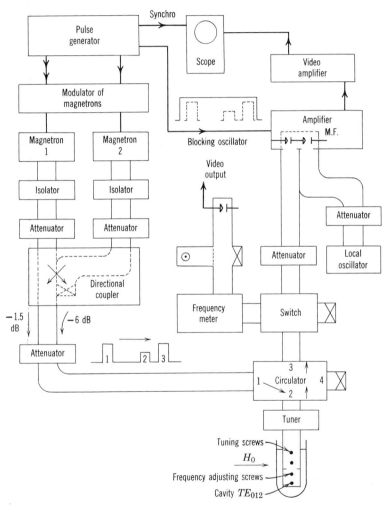

Fig. 18–13. Dual source spectrometer for pulse measurements of spin lattice and spin-spin relaxation times between 10^{-7} and 1 sec [Kaplan (1962)].

amplifier which consists of two stages of blocking oscillators. The microwave power traverses an isolator, a directional coupler, two attenuators, and a ferrite circulator before reaching the TE_{102} rectangular cavity. The cavity is considerably overcoupled to the waveguide through a large diameter iris which limits the Q to 600. Two screws for adjusting the resonant frequency are located within the cavity at points of maximum electric field strength, and two impedance matching screws separated by $\lambda_g/4$ are located outside the iris. The free precession signal that is emitted by the resonant cavity traverses the circulator to the superheterodyne receiver.

Llewellyn, Whittlestone, and Williams (1962) designed the pulse spectrometer shown on Fig. 13–34 for use in measuring relaxation times between 1 μsec and 100 msec at temperatures in the interval 1 to 20°K in samples containing as few as 10^{16} spins/cm^3. It uses only one klystron. The pulses have rise times of 0.1 μsec or less [Kaplan, Browne, and Cowen (1961)]. The authors give a good discussion of pulse circuitry and techniques.

Mims, Nassau, and McGee (1961) studied systems in which diffusion was sufficiently slow to permit the use of the spin echo technique which is extensively used in NMR [Gordon and Bowers (1958); Hahn (1950); Herzog and Hahn (1956)]. They employed both normal two-pulse echos and a "stimulated echo" method. In the latter arrangement, three pulses of microwave energy are applied at the times $t = 0$, $t = \tau$, and $t = \tau + T$, and an echo is observed at $t = 2\tau + T$. The echo may be studied as a function of both τ and T. This procedure consists in "burning holes" of simple form and controllable width in an inhomogeneously broadened line, and observing the rate at which these holes are filled in. Mims, Nassau, and McGee discuss the theoretical background required for understanding the spin echo technique.

A spectrometer similar to Kaplan's [Kaplan (1962); Kaplan, Browne, and Cowen (1961)] was employed by Rowan, Hahn, and Mims (1965) to study a transient electron-nuclear coupling effect [Mims, Nassau, and McGee (1961)]. The transient method was employed to produce an electron-spin echo whose envelope exhibited amplitude beat modulation. The modulation contained periods corresponding to the NMR frequencies of nuclei which are coupled to the electrons. This technique provides information similar to the ENDOR method. The present experiment provides an echo which contains contributions from all close neighboring nuclei regardless of their resonant frequencies, and so it is more difficult to analyze than the ENDOR signal which arises from a single nuclear transition. Under some circumstances, the present method may be more sensitive than ENDOR. The original article should be consulted for further details. See also Mims (1965, 1965).

Faughnan and Strandberg (1961) unsuccessfully attempted to detect the presence of nonequilibrium phonons by placing one end of the sample in a cavity coupled to the klystron generator, the center of the sample in a waveguide beyond cutoff with 40-dB isolation, and the other end in a cavity coupled to the detector, as shown in Fig. 18–14.

The apparatus shown in Fig. 18–15 was used by Fletcher, LeCraw, and Spencer (1960) for determining the electron spin relaxation in ferromagnetic insulators [single crystal spheres of yttrium iron garnet (YIG)]. Since the subject of ferromagnetic resonance is beyond the scope of this book, the reader is referred to the original article for a description of the spectrometer [see also Masters and Roberts (1959)]. Van Vleck (1964, 1964) discusses ferromagnetic relaxation.

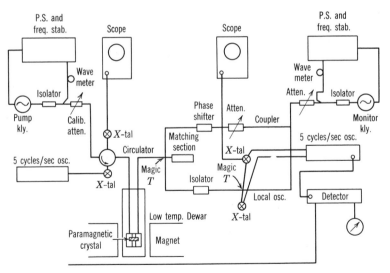

Fig. 18–14. Experimental apparatus in which a sample has one end in a cavity coupled to the klystron and the other in a cavity coupled to the detector [Faughnan and Strandberg (1961)].

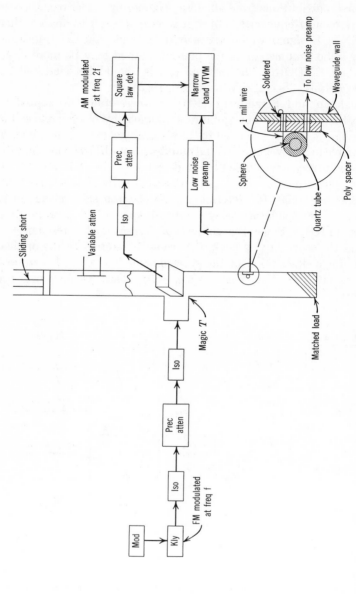

Fig. 18–15.   Experimental arrangement for studying electron spin relaxation in ferromagnetic insulators.   The dc magnetic field goes into the page [Fletcher, LeCraw, and Spencer (1960)].

Shamfarov (1963) describes an experimental arrangement for studying spin lattice relaxation at low temperatures by the pulse inversion method. Bölger (1959) gives a detailed discussion of pulse saturation techniques. Favret and Meister (1965) designed a pulse pattern generator for transient NMR experiments. Candela and Mundy (1965) combined ESR and magnetic susceptibility techniques to measure T_1 (see Sec. 13-S). Bolef, deKlerk, and Gosser (1962) describe an ultrasonic spectrometer for studying spin phonon interactions in solids (see Sec. 19-F). NMR transitions may also be studied by acoustic modulation or saturation methods [Denison, James, Currin, Tanttila, and Mahler (1964); Tewari and Verma (1965)].

E. Miscellaneous Comments on Relaxation Times

A considerable amount of experimental work has been carried out ascertaining the temperature dependence of relaxation times, and this field has been reviewed by Al'tshuler and Kozyrev (1964). In solids at low temperature, relaxation can occur by the direct process which entails the resonance exchange of a quantum between the spin system and the lattice, or by the Raman process which consists of the inelastic scattering of a phonon with the change in phonon energy being supplied by the spins. Kronig (1939) [see Van Vleck (1940)] estimated the spin lattice relaxation times via these two mechanisms for $S = \frac{1}{2}$ and obtained the expressions

$$T_1 \approx \frac{10^4 (E_2 - E_1)^4}{\lambda^2 H^4 T} \text{ sec} \quad \text{direct process} \quad (1)$$

$$T_1 \approx \frac{10^4 (E_2 - E_1)^6}{\lambda^2 H^2 T^7} \text{ sec} \quad \text{Raman process} \quad (2)$$

where E_1 and E_2 are the ground and first excited crystal field orbital levels respectively in cm^{-1}, λ is the spin-orbit coupling coefficient in cm^{-1}, H is the applied magnetic field, and T is the absolute temperature. Ordinarily the direct process predominates at very low temperatures and the Raman process is dominant at relatively higher temperatures, although both processes are usually studied in the liquid helium temperature range.

Van Vleck (1940, 1941) [see Temperley (1939)] has developed a more detailed theory of spin-lattice relaxation, and he emphasizes that the electron spins relax by transferring energy selectively to those lattice modes with which they are resonant. Van Vleck says that the resonant lattice modes are on "speaking terms" with the spins. Only a narrow portion of the phonon spectrum may take part in the spin lattice relaxation. Strandberg (1958) shows that for some systems the cw saturation method which is designed to measure the spin lattice relaxation time may measure the lattice-phonon relaxation rate instead. This will explain why sometimes pulse and saturation measurements of T_1 agree, and sometimes they do not. Anderson (1959) discusses the "phonon bottleneck" whereby the rate-determining step in the spin-lattice relaxation is the rate at which the energetically excited phonons dispose of the energy that is transferred to them by the spins. Mattuck and Strandberg (1960) discuss the theory for the iron group and Orbach (1961) for the rare earths. Sometimes a distribution of relaxation times is observed (e.g., see Benzie and Cooke (1951)].

Giordmaine, Alsop, Nash, and Townes (1958), Collins (1959), Bowers and Mims (1959), Mims, Nassau, and McGee (1961), and Klauder and Anderson (1962) discuss details of how the excited spin system rids itself of its energy. For example, Bowers and Mims show in Fig. 18–16 the possible relaxation processes that ultimately

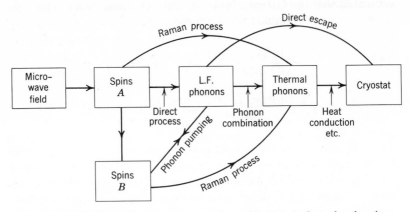

Fig. 18–16.   Relaxation processes for resonant spins A that absorb microwave energy and pass it on via spins B, low-frequency (LF) phonons, and thermal phonons to the heat bath cryostat [Bowers and Mims (1959)].

transfer the energy from the microwave field via the resonant spins A to the cryostat heat bath. These phonon relaxation processes will probably be intensively studied for years to come. Burns (1964) found ESR intensities proportional to $(1 - c)^n$ where c is the impurity concentration and n is the wipe-out number.

A number of workers have discussed the possible dependence of the spin lattice relaxation time on the size and shape of the sample. Giordmaine, Alsop, Nash, and Townes (1958) mention that if the dominant method of energy conduction from the spins to the cryostat bath is diffusion, then T_1 should be proportional to the square of the sample's linear dimensions, while it should be proportional to the linear dimension itself if the phonon paths to the bath are uninterrupted by collisions. Scott and Jeffries (1962) observed a sample size dependence in their relaxation time studies.

The relaxation times that were determined by the pulse method for Gadolinium by Davis, Strandberg, and Kyhl (1958) were about fifty times as long as those reported by Feher and Scovil (1957) from cw saturation measurements. Davis, Strandberg, and Kyhl (1958) found that T_1 in Gadolinium decreases with increasing power and with increasing temperature and varies with the individual energy transition. Giordmaine, Alsop, Nash, and Townes (1958), on the other hand, studied $Gd_2Mg_3(NO_3)_{12} \cdot 24H_2O$, $K_3Cr(CN)_6$, and $Cu(NH_4)_2(SO_4)_2 \cdot 6H_2O$ and measured their spin-lattice relaxation times in three ways: (1) by the saturation method, (2) by a pulse method, and (3) by saturating the spin system with cw power and then using a weak microwave source to measure the rate at which equilibrium is restored after the saturating signal has been removed. The relaxation times determined by these three methods agreed within a factor of three. Pashinin and Prokhorov (1961) measured T_1 of Fe^{+3} and Cr^{+3} in $K_3M(CN)_6$ by both the saturation and pulse methods and found very little difference between the two results.

The presence of paramagnetic gases such as oxygen can have a very pronounced effect on the relaxation times of spin systems. The usual result of the presence of O_2 is a shortening of T_1 since the paramagnetic O_2 molecule affords an efficient relaxation path. Several systems in which this oxygen effect has been observed include (1) free radicals and radical ions in solution [Hausser (1960, 1960); Deguchi (1960); Müller-Warmuth (1963)]; (2) carbons [Spackman (1962); Singer (1963); Poole, DiCarlo, Noble, Itzel, and Tobin (1965)];

(*3*) irradiated solids [Rexroad and Gordy (1956); Kuri, Ueda, and Shida (1960)]; (*4*) petroleum oils [Saraceno and Coggeshall (1961)]; (*5*) NMR of protons [Chiarotti, Christiani, and Giulotto (1955); standard texts on NMR]. Techniques for removing oxygen from solution are discussed in Sec. 15-F.

Most theories of ESR relaxation in solution assume that the relaxing species is a sphere. McConnell (1956) assumed that his "microcrystalline model" had an axis of symmetry. Several authors such as Perrin (1934), Favro (1960), Woessner (1962, 1962), Shimizu (1962, 1964), Valiev and Zaripov (1962), Valiev, Timerov, and Yulmet'ev (1963), and Moniz, Steele and Dixon (1963) have considered relaxation from spheroidal, asymmetric top, and other molecules in solution, but space does not permit a discussion of their results.

Theoretical treatments of relaxation may be found in the Scottish Summer School Proceedings [ter Haar (1961)], and in a book by Caspers (1964). Additional discussions of apparatus have been given by Combrisson and Uebersfeld (1953) and van Gerven, van Itterbeek, and Stals (1960).

References

A. Abragam, *The Principles of Nuclear Magnetism*, Clarendon, Oxford, 1961.
S. A. Al'tshuler and B. M. Kozyrev, *Electron Paramagnetic Resonance*, translated by Scripta Technica, C. P. Poole, Jr., Ed., Academic Press, N.Y., 1964.
P. W. Anderson; *Phys. Rev.*, **109**, 1492 (1958); **114**, 1002 (1959).
E. R. Andrew, *Nuclear Magnetic Resonance*, Cambridge University Press, Cambridge, 1956.
A. Bassompierre and J. Pescia, *C. R. Acad. Sci.*, **254**, 4439 (1962).
R. J. Benzie and A. H. Cooke, *Proc. Phys. Soc.*, **A64**, 507 (1951).
G. Berthet, *C. R. Acad. Sci.*, **241**, 1730 (1955).
F. Bloch, *Phys. Rev.*, **70**, 460 (1946).
N. Bloembergen, E. M. Purcell, and R. V. Pound, *Phys. Rev.*, **73**, 679 (1948).
N. Bloembergen, S. Shapiro, P. S. Pershan, and J. O. Artman, *Phys. Rev.*, **114**, 445 (1959).
N. Bloembergen and S. Wang, *Phys. Rev.*, **93**, 72 (1954).
D. I. Bolef, J. de Klerk, and R. B. Gosser, *RSI*, **33**, 631 (1962).
B. Bölger, *Proc. K. Ned. Akad. Wetensch.*, **B62**, 315, 329, 348 (1959).
K. D. Bowers and W. B. Mims, *Phys. Rev.*, **115**, 285 (1959).
A. A. Bugai, *Fiz. Tverd. Tela*, **4**, 3027 (2218) (1962).
G. Burns, *Phys. Rev.*, **135**, 481A (1964).
G. A. Candela and R. E. Mundy, *RSI*, **36**, 338 (1965).

J. A. Carruthers and N. C. Rumin, *Can. J. Phys.*, **43**, 576 (1965).

W. J. Caspers, *Theory of Spin Relaxation*, Interscience, N. Y., 1964.

T. G. Castner, Jr., *Phys. Rev.*, **115**, 1506 (1959).

G. Chiarotti, G. Cristiani, and L. Giulotto, *Nuovo Cimento*, **1**, 863 (1955).

S. A. Collins Jr., R. L. Kyhl, and M. W. P. Strandberg, *Phys. Rev. Letters*, **2**, 88 (1959).

J. Combrisson and J. Uebersfeld, *J. Phys. Radium*, **14**, 724 (1953).

C. F. Davis Jr., M. W. P. Strandberg, and R. L. Kyhl, *Phys. Rev.*, **111**, 1268 (1958).

V. Deguchi, *J. Chem. Phys.*, **32**, 1584 (1960).

A. B. Denison, L. W. James, J. D. Currin, W. H. Tanttila, and R. J. Mahler, *Phys. Rev. Letters*, **12**, 244 (1964).

R. H. Dicke and R. H. Romer, *RSI*, **26**, 915 (1955).

G. F. Dionne, *Phys. Rev.*, **139**, A1648 (1965).

L. E. Drain, *Proc. Phys. Soc.*, **80**, 1380 (1962).

B. W. Faughnan and M. W. P. Strandberg, *J. Phys. Chem. Solids*, **19**, 155 (1961).

A. G. Favret and R. Meister, *RSI*, **36**, 154 (1965).

L. D. Favro, *Phys. Rev.*, **119**, 53 (1960).

G. Feher and H. E. D. Scovil, *Phys. Rev.*, **105**, 760 (1957).

R. C. Fletcher, R. C. LeCraw, and E. G. Spencer, *Phys. Rev.*, **117**, 955 (1960).

J. C. Gill and D. J. Meredith, *Phys. Letters*, **15**, 201 (1965).

J. A. Giordmaine, L. E. Alsop, F. R. Nash, and C. H. Townes, *Phys. Rev.*, **109**, 302 (1958).

J. P. Gordon and K. D. Bowers, *Phys. Rev. Letters*, **1**, 368 (1958).

W. J. C. Grant, *Phys. Rev.*, **134**, A1554, A1565, A1574 (1964); **135**, A1265 (1964).

E. L. Hahn, *Phys. Rev.*, **80**, 580 (1950).

K. Halbach, *Helv. Phys. Acta*, **27**, 259 (1954).

K. H. Hausser, *Naturwissenschaften*, **47**, 251 (1960); *Arch. Sci. Genève (Fasc. Spec.)*, **13**, 239 (1960).

J. Hervé, *Paramagnetic Resonance*, **2**, 689 (1963).

J. Hervé and J. Pescia, *Proc. Twelfth Colloque Ampere*, Bordeaux, 1963, p. 335.

J. Hervé and J. Pescia, *C. R. Acad. Sci.*, **255**, 2926 (1962).

B. Herzog and E. L. Hahn, *Phys. Rev.*, **103**, 148 (1956).

J. S. Hyde, *Phys. Rev.*, **119**, 1483, 1492 (1960).

J. Jeener, R. duBois, and P. Broekaert, *Phys. Rev.*, **139**, A1959 (1965).

D. E. Kaplan, *J. Phys. Radium Suppl. No. 3*, **23**, 21A (1962).

D. E. Kaplan, M. E. Browne, and J. A. Cowen, *RSI*, **32**, 1182 (1961).

J. I. Kaplan, *Am. J. Phys.*, **28**, 491 (1960).

J. I. Kaplan, *J. Chem. Phys.*, **42**, 3789 (1965).

A. V. Kessenikh and A. A. Manenkov, *Fiz. Tverd. Tela*, **5**, 1143 (1963).

A. Kiel, *Phys. Rev.*, **125**, 1451 (1962).

A. F. Kip, C. Kittel, R. A. Levy, and A. M. Portis, *Phys. Rev.*, **91**, 1066 (1953).

A. L. Kipling, P. W. Smith, J. Vanier, and G. A. Woonton, *Can. J. Phys.*, **39**, 1859 (1961).

J. R. Klauder and P. W. Anderson, *Phys. Rev.*, **125**, 912 (1962).

K. D. Kramer and W. Müller-Warmuth, *Z. Angew. Phys.*, **16**, 281 (1963).

R. de L. Krönig, *Physica*, **6**, 33 (1939).

Z. Kuri, H. Ueda, and S. Shida, *J. Chem. Phys.*, **32**, 371 (1960).

O. S. Leifson and C. D. Jeffries, *Phys. Rev.*, **122**, 1781 (1961).

P. M. Llewellyn, P. R. Whittlestone, and J. M. Williams, *JSI*, **39**, 586 (1962).

J. P. Lloyd and G. E. Pake, *Phys. Rev.*, **92**, 1576 (1953).

A. Lösche, *Kerninduktion*, Veb. Deutscher Verlag der Wissenschaften Berlin, East Germany, 1957.

H. M. McConnell, *J. Chem. Phys.*, **25**, 709 (1956); **28**, 430 (1958).

M. Mandel, *RSI*, **33**, 247 (1962).

A. A. Manenkov and A. M. Prokhorov, *Radiotechn. i Elektron. CCCP*, **1**, 469 (1956).

G. V. Marr and P. Swarp, *Can. J. Phys.*, **38**, 495 (1960).

J. I. Masters and R. M. Roberts, Jr., *J. Appl. Phys. (Suppl.)*, **30**, 179S (1959).

R. D. Mattuck and M. W. P. Strandberg, *Phys. Rev.*, **119**, 1204 (1960).

W. B. Mims, *Proc. Royal Soc.*, **283**, 452 (1965); *RSI*, **36**, 1472 (1965).

W. B. Mims, K. Nassau, and J. D. McGee, *Phys. Rev.*, **123**, 2059 (1961).

W. B. Moniz, W. A. Steele, and J. A. Dixon, *J. Chem. Phys.*, **38**, 2418 (1963).

P. R. Moran, S. H. Christensen, and R. H. Silsbee, *Phys. Rev.*, **124**, 442 (1961).

J. L. Motchane, *C. R. Acad. Sci.*, **254**, 1614 (1962).

J. L. Motchane and J. Uebersfeld, *C. R. Acad. Sci.*, **251**, 709 (1960); *Arch. Sci. (Fasc. Spec.)*, **13**, 682 (1960).

W. Müller-Warmuth, *Z. Naturforsch.*, **18A**, 1001 (1963).

R. Orbach, *Proc. Roy. Soc.*, **A264**, 456 (1961).

D. E. O'Reilly and C. P. Poole, Jr., *J. Phys. Chem.*, **67**, 1762 (1963).

P. P. Pashinin and A. M. Prokhorov, *Zh. Eksper. Teor. Fiz.*, **40**, 49 (33) (1961).

D. H. Paxman, *Proc. Phys. Soc.*, **78**, 180 (1961).

F. Perrin, *J. Phys. Radium*, **5**, 497 (1934).

J. Pescia, *Ann. Phys.*, (*Paris*), **10**, 389 (1965).

J. Pescia and J. Hervé, *Arch. Sci. (Spec. No.)*, **14**, 123 (1961).

C. P. Poole, Jr., E. N. DiCarlo, C. S. Noble, J. F. Itzel, Jr., and H. H. Tobin, *J. Catalysis*, **4**, 518 (1965).

J. A. Pople, W. G. Schneider, and H. J. Bernstein, *High Resolution Nuclear Magnetic Resonance*, McGraw-Hill, N. Y., 1959.

A. M. Portis, *Phys. Rev.*, **91**, 1071 (1953).

A. M. Portis, *Magnetic Resonance in Systems with Spectral Distributions*, Technical Note No. 1, Sarah Mellon Scaife Radiation Laboratory, University of Pittsburgh, 1955.

A. G. Redfield, *Phys. Rev.*, **98**, 1787 (1955); *IBM J. Res. Dev.*, **1**, 19 (1957).

H. N. Rexroad and W. Gordy, *J. Chem. Phys.*, **30**, 399 (1959).

G. Richter and A. E. Schwind, *Ann. Phys. (Germany)*, **11**, 405 (1961).

L. G. Rowan, E. L. Hahn, and W. B. Mims, *Phys. Rev.*, **137**, A61 (1965).

R. H. Ruby, H. Benoit, and C. D. Jeffries, *Phys. Rev.*, **127**, 52 (1962).

A. J. Saraceno and N. D. Coggeshall, *J. Chem. Phys.*, **34**, 260 (1961).

P. L. Scott and C. D. Jeffries, *Phys. Rev.*, **127**, 32 (1962).

Ya. L. Shamfarov, *PTE*, **5**, 134 (914) (1963).

H. Shimizu, *J. Chem. Phys.*, **37**, 765 (1962); **40**, 754 (1964).

L. S. Singer, *J. Appl. Phys.*, **30**, 1463 (1959).

L. S. Singer, *Proc. Fifth Carbon Conf.*, Vol. 2, Pergamon, London, 1963, p. 37.

L. S. Singer and J. Kommandeur, *J. Chem. Phys.*, **34**, 133 (1961).

L. S. Singer, W. H. Smith, and G. Wagoner, *RSI*, **32**, 213 (1961).

C. P. Slichter, *Principles of Magnetic Resonance*, Harper and Row, N. Y., 1963.

J. Sohma, *J. Chem. Phys.*, **37**, 2151 (1962).

J. W. C. Spackman, *Nature*, **195**, 764 (1962).

M. W. P. Strandberg, *Phys. Rev.* **110**, 65 (1958).

T. J. Swift and R. E. Connick, *J. Chem. Phys.*, **37**, 307 (1962).

H. N. V. Temperley, *Proc. Cambridge Phil. Soc.*, **35**, 256 (1939).

D. ter Haar, Ed., *Fluctuation Relaxation and Resonance in Magnetic Systems*, Scottish Summer School in Physics, Oliver and Boyd, London, 1961.

D. P. Tewari and G. S. Verma, *Nuovo Cimento*, **38**, 197 (1965).

R. Kh. Timerov, *Zh. Eksper. Teor. Fiz.*, **40**, 1101 (777) (1961).

V. S. Tumanov, *Fiz. Tverd. Tela.*, **4**, 2419 (1773) (1962).

K. A. Valiev, R. Kh. Timerov, and R. M. Yulmet'ev, *Zh. Eksper. Teor. Fiz.*, **44**, 522 (356) (1963).

K. A. Valiev and M. M. Zaripov, *Zh. Eksper. Teor. Fiz.*, **42**, 503 (353) (1962).

L. van Gerven, *Ampère Colloquium*, Eindhoven, 1963, p. 566.

L. van Gerven, A. van Itterbeek, and L. Stals, *Med. K. Vlaamse Acad. Wetensch.*, **22**, 44 (1960).

J. H. Van Vleck, *Phys. Rev.*, **57**, 426, 1052 (1940); **59**, 724, 730 (1941).

J. H. Van Vleck, *J. Appl. Phys.*, **35**, 882 (1964); *Proc. Intern. Conf. Magnetism, Nottingham*, The Physical Society, London, 1965, p. 401.

M. Weger, *Bell System Tech. J.*, **39**, 1013 (1960).

D. E. Woessner, *J. Chem. Phys.*, **36**, 1 (1962); **37**, 647 (1962).

G. A. Woonton, *Advan. Electron. Electron Phys.*, **15**, 163 (1961).

E. Zueco and J. Pescia, *C. R. Acad. Sci.*, **260**, 3605 (1965).

G. M. Zverev, *PTE*, **5**, 105 (930) (1961).

CHAPTER 19

Double Resonance

Since this book is primarily concerned with electron spin resonance we will discuss in detail those types of apparatus that are employed in double resonance experiments which include an ESR transition. The chapter begins with a description of the nature of ESR–NMR double resonance, touches upon other polarization studies, and then presents a detailed exposition of the required apparatus. For convenience, most of the experiments of this type are carried out at X band, but Borghini and Abragam (1959) and Richards and White (1964) worked at 12,000 G (35,000 Mc) to pick up almost a factor of four in the amount of polarization.

A. The ESR–NMR Polarization Schemes

Several types of ESR–NMR double resonance have been studied, and a brief description of each will be presented. The emphasis in this discussion will be on the distinguishing features of each polarization scheme. Further details may be found in Chaps. 8 and 9 of Abragam's book (1961), in Chap. 8 of the book by Al'tshuler and Kozyrev (1964), and in the review articles by Series (1959), Khutsishvili (1960a), Jeffries (1961, 1964), Webb (1961b), and Uebersfeld (1963).

The Overhauser Effect: Overhauser (1953) showed that in metals the dominant nuclear spin lattice relaxation mechanism is via the conduction electrons through the isotropic Fermi contact interaction $A\mathbf{I}\cdot\mathbf{S}$. The populations of the electronic spin system may be equalized by saturating the ESR transition. As a result, the nuclear spins distribute themselves among their Zeeman levels in accordance with the electronic level Boltzmann distribution, and the NMR signal is enhanced by the factor $g\beta/g_N\beta_N$ where the numerator contains the electronic g factor and magneton, and the denominator contains their nuclear counterparts.

More precisely, the ratio n_+/n_- of the number of nuclei in the upper to those in the lower nuclear Zeeman level is given by

$$n_+/n_- = \exp\left[(E_F{}^+ - E_F{}^- - \hbar\omega_n)/kT\right] \tag{1}$$

where the Fermi energies $E_F{}^+$ and $E_F{}^-$ of spin up and spin down electrons, respectively, are measures of the kinetic energies of the conduction electrons. In the absence of a resonant microwave field $E_F{}^+ = E_F{}^-$ and

$$n_+/n_- = \exp\left[-\hbar\omega_n/kT\right] \tag{2}$$

as in a standard NMR experiment, where ω_n is the NMR frequency. This is the standard nuclear Boltzmann factor. When the electronic or ESR transition is saturated at the resonant frequency, ω_e then the Fermi levels shift slightly to satisfy the relation

$$E_F{}^+ - E_F{}^- = \hbar\omega_e \tag{3}$$

and the nuclear population ratio is governed by the electronic Boltzmann factor

$$n_+/n_- = \exp\left[(\hbar\omega_e - \hbar\omega_n)/kT\right] \tag{4}$$

Since

$$\omega_e/\omega_n \sim 10^3$$

an enhancement results.

The relaxation transitions are more probable from the upper Zeeman level to the lower one under saturation conditions. The continuity of the conduction electrons' kinetic energy ensures the possibility of conserving energy during these nuclear–electronic relaxation transitions [see, e.g., Kaplan (1954, 1955); Little (1957); Carver and Slichter (1953, 1956)].

Azbel', Gerasimenko, and Lifshitz (1957, 1957) showed that the Overhauser effect permits polarization of particles whose average diameter is either large or small relative to the skin depth, and they calculated the polarization in samples of arbitrary thickness. The Overhauser effect may also be observed in semiconductors and other nonmetals [Overhauser (1954); Bloch (1954); Korringa (1954, 1954); Abragam (1955); Valiev (1958); Bashkirov and Valiev (1958);

Khutsishvili (1958, 1958)]. The Underhauser effect [Underhauser and Abragam (1955); Underhauser, Bennett, and Torrey (1957); Underhauser and Seiden (1957)] produces half the polarization of the Overhauser effect, but in the opposite sense. It can occur in dipole coupled liquids.

The Electron Nuclear Double Resonance (ENDOR) or Fast Passage Effect: Feher (1956) proposed an enhancement scheme for spin systems with resolved hyperfine structure which places no requirements on the detailed relaxation processes. The energy level scheme in Fig. 19–1 shows the population of the four energy levels for $I = \frac{1}{2}$, $S = \frac{1}{2}$ in terms of the electronic Boltzmann factor $\epsilon = g\beta H/2kT$. The nuclear Boltzmann factor is neglected since it is three orders of magnitude smaller. As a result, the initial state of the system shown on the right or high field side of Fig. 19–1 consists of two lower levels with the population $\frac{1}{4}N(1 + \epsilon)$ and two upper levels with the population $\frac{1}{4}N(1 - \epsilon)$, where N is the total number of electronic spins in the sample. In region II an adiabatic fast passage sweep [Bloch (1946)] is used to induce the indicated ESR transition with $\Delta m_I = 0$,

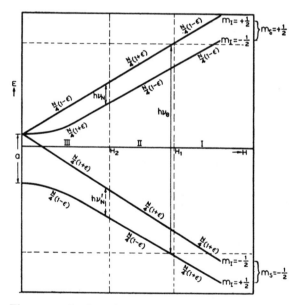

Fig. 19–1. The energy levels and corresponding populations $\frac{1}{4}N(1 \pm \epsilon)$ for a spin system with $I = \frac{1}{2}$ and $S = \frac{1}{2}$ [Feher (1956)] where $\epsilon = g\beta H/2kT$.

and thereby to invert the populations of the top and bottom energy levels. A net nuclear polarization in the sample is established by performing an adiabatic fast passage through either the upper ν_N or lower ν_N' NMR transition. The Breit-Rabi formula [Breit and Rabi (1931)] predicts that $\nu_N' > \nu_N$ so it is necessary for the difference $\nu_N' - \nu_N$ to exceed the NMR line-width to be able to induce only one of these transitions at a time. The polarization that is obtained will decay with a time constant comparable to the nuclear relaxation time.

In liquids the condition for an adiabatic fast passage is

$$1/T_2 \ll (1/H_1)\,|\,(dH_0/dt)\,| \ll \gamma H_1 \qquad (5)$$

This means that the normalized sweep rate or the rate of change of the applied field H_0 normalized relative to the microwave field H_1 must be much less than the "frequency" γH_1. In other words, the normalized sweep rate must change slowly or adiabatically relative to the strength of the microwave field H_1 expressed in frequency units. This is the adiabatic condition. In addition, the normalized sweep rate is fast enough so that the rate of relaxation is negligible during the passage through resonance. More specifically, the rate of passage through resonance is slow or adiabatic enough so that it does not disturb the alignment of the spins along H_1, and at the same time it is fast enough so that the spins do not have time to relax. In solids, the adiabatic fast passage has been observed under conditions compatible with the weaker requirement

$$1/T_1 \ll (1/H_1)\,|\,(dH_0/dt)\,| \ll \gamma H_1 \approx 1/T_2 \qquad (6)$$

For further details see Abragam (1961), p. 66.

The ENDOR enhancement was observed experimentally by Feher and Gere (1956). Since the details of the energy level diagram differ for positive and negative nuclear moments this scheme will distinguish the two polarities [Feher, Fuller, and Gere (1957)]. Bleaney (1958) discussed the use of ENDOR to measure hyperfine structure. The experimental results of Eisinger and Feher (1958) on antimony isotopes are shown on Table 19–1, and the corresponding energy levels are sketched on Fig. 19–2. Rowan, Hahn, and Mims (1965) describe a spin-echo experiment which provided information similar to that of the ENDOR method [see Sec. 18-D].

TABLE 19–1

Determination of the Hyperfine Interaction Constant A for Sb^{121} and Sb^{123} by the ENDOR Technique [Eisinger and Feher (1958)]

Saturated electronic transition $m_J,m_I \leftrightarrow m_J,m_I$	ν_e Mc/sec	H, Oe	Hyperfine transitions $m_J,m_I \leftrightarrow m_J,m_I$	ν_N, Mc/sec	A, Mc/sec
			Sb^{121}		
$\frac{1}{2},\ \frac{5}{2} \leftrightarrow -\frac{1}{2},\ \frac{5}{2}$	906 6.3	3072.1	$\frac{1}{2},\ \frac{5}{2} \leftrightarrow \frac{1}{2},\ \frac{3}{2}$	93.457	186.809
			$-\frac{1}{2},\ \frac{5}{2} \leftrightarrow -\frac{1}{2},\ \frac{3}{2}$	85.402	186.784
$\frac{1}{2},\ \frac{3}{2} \leftrightarrow -\frac{1}{2},\ \frac{3}{2}$	906 6.3	3136.2	$\frac{1}{2},\ \frac{5}{2} \leftrightarrow \frac{1}{2},\ \frac{3}{2}$	85.441	186.805
			$-\frac{1}{2},\ \frac{5}{2} \leftrightarrow -\frac{1}{2},\ \frac{3}{2}$	93.583	186.803
			$\frac{1}{2},\ \frac{3}{2} \leftrightarrow \frac{1}{2},\ \frac{1}{2}$	87.190	186.803
			$-\frac{1}{2},\ \frac{3}{2} \leftrightarrow -\frac{1}{2},\ \frac{1}{2}$	95.434	186.789
$\frac{1}{2},\ \frac{1}{2} \leftrightarrow -\frac{1}{2},\ \frac{1}{2}$	905 6.5	3197.9	$\frac{1}{2},\ \frac{3}{2} \leftrightarrow \frac{1}{2},\ \frac{1}{2}$	87.190	186.812
			$-\frac{1}{2},\ \frac{3}{2} \leftrightarrow -\frac{1}{2},\ \frac{1}{2}$	95.523	186.791
			$\frac{1}{2},\ \frac{1}{2} \leftrightarrow \frac{1}{2},\ -\frac{1}{2}$	89.004	186.791
			$-\frac{1}{2},\ \frac{1}{2} \leftrightarrow -\frac{1}{2},\ -\frac{1}{2}$	97.464	186.795
$\frac{1}{2},\ -\frac{1}{2} \leftrightarrow -\frac{1}{2},\ -\frac{1}{2}$	904 5.7	3261.2	$\frac{1}{2},\ \frac{1}{2} \leftrightarrow \frac{1}{2},\ -\frac{1}{2}$	88.973	186.808
			$-\frac{1}{2},\ \frac{1}{2} \leftrightarrow -\frac{1}{2},\ -\frac{1}{2}$	97.522	186.808
			$\frac{1}{2},\ -\frac{1}{2} \leftrightarrow \frac{1}{2},\ -\frac{3}{2}$	90.868	186.794
			$-\frac{1}{2},\ -\frac{1}{2} \leftrightarrow -\frac{1}{2},\ -\frac{3}{2}$	99.547	186.807

(continued)

TABLE 19–1 (*continued*)

Saturated electronic transition $m_J, m_I \leftrightarrow m_J, m_I$	ν_e Mc/sec	H, Oe	Hyperfine transitions $m_J, m_I \leftrightarrow m_J, m_I$	ν_N, Mc/sec	A, Mc/sec
$\frac{1}{2}, -\frac{3}{2} \leftrightarrow -\frac{1}{2}, -\frac{3}{2}$	904 4.5	3328.8	$\frac{1}{2}, -\frac{1}{2} \leftrightarrow \frac{1}{2}, -\frac{3}{2}$	90.791	186.804
			$-\frac{1}{2}, -\frac{1}{2} \leftrightarrow -\frac{1}{2}, -\frac{3}{2}$	99.561	186.809
			$\frac{1}{2}, -\frac{3}{2} \leftrightarrow \frac{1}{2}, -\frac{5}{2}$	92.779	186.816
			$-\frac{1}{2}, -\frac{3}{2} \leftrightarrow -\frac{1}{2}, -\frac{5}{2}$	101.668	186.799
$\frac{1}{2}, -\frac{5}{2} \leftrightarrow -\frac{1}{2}, -\frac{5}{2}$	904 2.3	3397.5	$\frac{1}{2}, -\frac{3}{2} \leftrightarrow \frac{1}{2}, -\frac{5}{2}$	92.646	186.800
			$-\frac{1}{2}, -\frac{3}{2} \leftrightarrow -\frac{1}{2}, -\frac{5}{2}$	101.639	186.806
			Avg.		186.802±0.005
			Sb^{123}		
$\frac{1}{2}, \frac{7}{2} \leftrightarrow -\frac{1}{2}, \frac{7}{2}$	906 6.3	3113.2	$\frac{1}{2}, \frac{7}{2} \leftrightarrow \frac{1}{2}, \frac{5}{2}$	47.034	101.506
			$-\frac{1}{2}, \frac{7}{2} \leftrightarrow -\frac{1}{2}, \frac{7}{2}$	51.010	101.515
$\frac{1}{2}, \frac{5}{2} \leftrightarrow -\frac{1}{2}, \frac{5}{2}$	905 6.5	3136.6	$\frac{1}{2}, \frac{7}{2} \leftrightarrow \frac{1}{2}, \frac{5}{2}$	47.042	101.520
			$-\frac{1}{2}, \frac{7}{2} \leftrightarrow -\frac{1}{2}, \frac{5}{2}$	51.040	101.529
			$\frac{1}{2}, \frac{5}{2} \leftrightarrow -\frac{1}{2}, \frac{3}{2}$	47.566	101.509
			$-\frac{1}{2}, \frac{5}{2} \leftrightarrow -\frac{1}{2}, \frac{3}{2}$	51.584	101.522
$\frac{1}{2}, \frac{3}{2} \leftrightarrow -\frac{1}{2}, \frac{3}{2}$	905 6.5	3180.0	$\frac{1}{2}, \frac{5}{2} \leftrightarrow \frac{1}{2}, \frac{3}{2}$	47.565	101.516
			$-\frac{1}{2}, \frac{5}{2} \leftrightarrow -\frac{1}{2}, \frac{3}{2}$	51.614	101.508
			$\frac{1}{2}, \frac{3}{2} \leftrightarrow \frac{1}{2}, \frac{1}{2}$	48.106	101.517
			$-\frac{1}{2}, \frac{3}{2} \leftrightarrow -\frac{1}{2}, \frac{1}{2}$	52.170	101.504

½, ½↔ −½, ½	904 7.0	3213.7	½, ³⁄₂↔ ½, ½	48.096	101.515
			−½, ³⁄₂↔ −½, ½	52.196	101.512
			½, ½↔ ½, −½	48.644	101.505
			−½, ½↔ −½, −½	52.774	101.525
½, −½↔ −½, −½	904 7.0	3249.1	½, ½↔ ½, −½	48.633	101.515
			−½, ½↔ −½, −½	52.789	101.519
			½, ½↔ ½, −³⁄₂	49.202	101.523
			−½, −½↔ −½, −³⁄₂	53.336	101.504
½, −³⁄₂↔ −½, −³⁄₂	904 5.7	3285.5	½, −½↔ ½, −³⁄₂	49.178	101.519
			−½, −½↔ −½, −³⁄₂	53.384	101.517
			½, −³⁄₂↔ ½, −⁵⁄₂	49.756	101.519
			−½, −³⁄₂↔ −½, −⁵⁄₂	53.982	101.516
½, −⁵⁄₂↔ −½, −⁵⁄₂	904 4.5	3322.1	½, −³⁄₂↔ ½, −⁵⁄₂	49.730	101.524
			−½, −³⁄₂↔ −½, −⁵⁄₂	53.990	101.523
			½, −⁵⁄₂↔ ½, −⁷⁄₂	50.319	101.520
			−½, −⁵⁄₂↔ −½, −⁷⁄₂	54.598	101.515
½, −⁷⁄₂↔ −½, −⁷⁄₂	904 3.1	3358.9	½, −⁵⁄₂↔ ½, −⁷⁄₂	50.284	101.521
			−½, −⁵⁄₂↔ −½, −⁷⁄₂	54.598	101.520
			Avg.		101.516±0.004

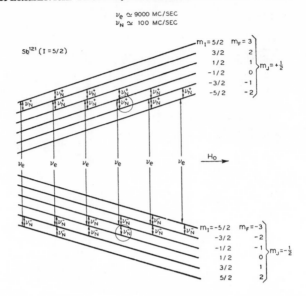

Fig. 19-2.   The hyperfine energy levels for Sb^{121} in antimony-doped silicon [Eisinger and Feher (1958)].

Dynamic Polarization of Forbidden Transitions or Method of Parallel Fields: The hyperfine interaction $A\mathbf{I}\cdot\mathbf{S}$ mixes states with different values of M_I and M_s so forbidden transitions for which $\Delta M_I = \pm 1$ and $\Delta M_s = \pm 1$ may be observed when the microwave magnetic field vector is parallel to the applied constant magnetic field. When these two fields are perpendicular, as is the case in ordinary ESR experiments, the allowed transitions for which $\Delta M_I = 0$ and $\Delta M_s = \pm 1$ are observed. Fig. 19-3 shows an ESR spectrum which exhibits a strong allowed and weaker forbidden transitions. The nuclear polarization arises only from the forbidden transitions. Jeffries (1957, 1963) proposed the use of the forbidden nuclear transitions for aligning nuclei. The alignment of Co^{60} nuclei obtained by this method was detected by the resulting γ-ray anisotropy [Abragam, Jeffries, and Kedzie (1960)].

The detailed analysis of a system of $S = \frac{1}{2}$ electronic spins and $I = 1$ nuclear spins is given in Fig. 19-4 [Jeffries (1961, 1963)]. The resulting ESR spectrum, nuclear polarization p_1 and nuclear align-

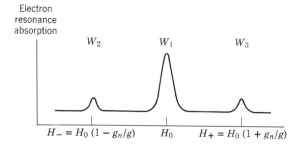

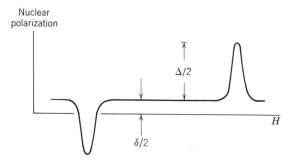

Fig. 19–3. An idealized double resonance spectrum showing the allowed center line W_1 and the two weaker forbidden transitions W_2 and W_3. The latter two transitions produce nuclear polarization in the positive and negative senses [Leifson and Jeffries (1961)].

ment p_2 defined by the sums over the i levels [Blin-Stoyle, Grace, and Halban (1957); Steenland and Tolhoek (1957)] as follows:

$$p_1 = \frac{\sum_i \langle \Psi_i | I_z | \Psi_i \rangle N_i}{I \sum_i N_i} \qquad (7)$$

and

$$p_2 = \frac{1}{I(2I-1)} \left[\frac{\sum_i 3 \langle \Psi_i | I_z^2 | \Psi_i \rangle}{\sum_i N_i} - I(I+1) \right] \qquad (8)$$

are tabulated in Fig. 19–4 and illustrated in Fig. 19–5. We shall illustrate the use of these expressions by calculating p_1 and p_2 for case (a) of Fig. 19–4 using the conditions*

$$\epsilon = g\beta H/kT \ll 1 \tag{9}$$

$$\delta \cong A/2kT \ll 1 \tag{10}$$

For this system the nuclear spin $I = 1$, and the diagonal matrix elements are

$$\langle \Psi_i | I_z | \Psi_i \rangle = \begin{cases} 1 & I_z = 1 \\ 0 & I_z = 0 \\ -1 & I_z = -1 \end{cases} \tag{11}$$

$$\langle \Psi_i | I_z{}^2 | \Psi_i \rangle = \begin{cases} 1 & I_z = \pm 1 \\ 0 & I_z = 0 \end{cases} \tag{12}$$

The populations N_{Mm} are given in Fig. 19–4 where the letters M and m denote, respectively, the projections of the electronic spin $S = \frac{1}{2}$ and the nuclear spin $I = 1$ along the magnetic field direction. From eq. (7) we have for the nuclear polarization

$$p_1 = \frac{+ e^{-\delta} - e^{+\delta} - e^{\epsilon-\delta} + e^{\epsilon+\delta}}{e^{-\delta} + 1 + e^{\delta} + e^{\epsilon-\delta} + e^{\epsilon} + e^{\epsilon+\delta}} = \epsilon\delta/3 \tag{13}$$

using power series expansions and only retaining the leading terms. The nuclear alignment p_2 from eq. (8) for this case is

$$p_2 = \frac{3[e^{-\delta} + e^{\delta} + e^{\epsilon-\delta} + e^{\epsilon+\delta}]}{e^{-\delta} + 1 + e^{\delta} + e^{\epsilon-\delta} + e^{\epsilon} + e^{\epsilon+\delta}} - 2 = \delta^2/3 \tag{14}$$

The theoretical and experimental details of dynamic nuclear orientation by forbidden transitions are elaborated upon by Jeffries (1960, 1961) and Leifson and Jeffries (1961).

The Solid Effect, Double Effect, or Abragam and Proctor Method: The double effect [Abragam and Proctor (1958); Erb, Motchane, and Uebersfeld (1958); Abragam (1961), p. 392; Burget, Odelhnal,

---

* The electronic Boltzmann factor ϵ is defined differentially in Figs. 19–1 and 19–4.

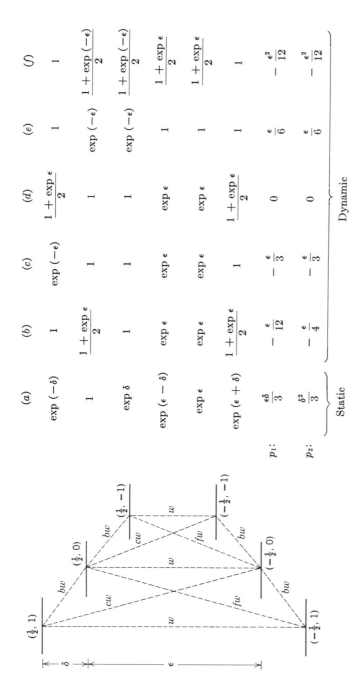

	(a)	(b)	(c)	(d)	(e)	(f)
	$\exp(-\delta)$	1	$\exp(-\epsilon)$	$\dfrac{1+\exp\epsilon}{2}$	1	1
	1	$\dfrac{1+\exp\epsilon}{2}$	1	1	$\exp(-\epsilon)$	$\dfrac{1+\exp(-\epsilon)}{2}$
	$\exp\delta$	1	1	1	$\exp(-\epsilon)$	$\dfrac{1+\exp(-\epsilon)}{2}$
	$\exp(\epsilon-\delta)$	$\exp\epsilon$	$\exp\epsilon$	$\exp\epsilon$	1	$\dfrac{1+\exp\epsilon}{2}$
	$\exp\epsilon$	$\exp\epsilon$	$\exp\epsilon$	$\exp\epsilon$	1	$\dfrac{1+\exp\epsilon}{2}$
	$\exp(\epsilon+\delta)$	$\dfrac{1+\exp\epsilon}{2}$	1	$\dfrac{1+\exp\epsilon}{2}$	1	1
$p_1:$	$\dfrac{\epsilon\delta}{3}$	$-\dfrac{\epsilon}{12}$	$-\dfrac{\epsilon}{3}$	0	$\dfrac{\epsilon}{6}$	$-\dfrac{\epsilon^2}{12}$
$p_2:$	$\dfrac{\delta^2}{3}$	$-\dfrac{\epsilon}{4}$	$-\dfrac{\epsilon}{3}$	0	$\dfrac{\epsilon}{6}$	$-\dfrac{\epsilon^2}{12}$
	Static	Dynamic				

Fig. 19–4. Energy levels of a nuclear spin ($I = 1$) and an electron spin ($S = \frac{1}{2}$) with $A\mathbf{I}\cdot\mathbf{S}$ hfs coupling in a magnetic field. The levels are characterized by (M, m) in zero order, and $\epsilon = g\beta H/kT$, $\delta \simeq A/2kT$. The relaxation rates are w, bw, cw, and fw. The populations, nuclear polarization p_1, and alignment p_2, are shown for (a) thermal equilibrium; (b) and (c) rf saturation of allowed transitions; (d), (e), and (f) rf saturation of forbidden transitions [Jeffries (1961)].

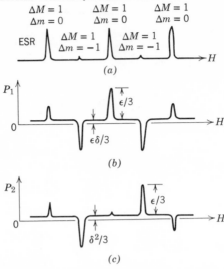

Fig. 19–5. (a) The ESR absorption, (b) the nuclear polarization p_1, and (c) the nuclear alignment p_2 vs. the applied magnetic field H for a microwave frequency ν applied to the spectrum of Fig. 19–4 assuming $b = c = 0$. It is assumed that both allowed and forbidden transitions are saturated [Jeffries (1961)].

Petřicek, and Sacha (1961); Motchane (1962); Kramer and Müller-Warmuth (1963)] requires two spin systems which interact with each other by some mechanism such as the dipolar interaction. If a system of electronic spins S and nuclear spins I have the resonant frequencies ω_e and ω_n, respectively, then the frequency $\omega = \omega_e + \omega_n$ is used to simultaneously flip an electronic and a nuclear spin. When dynamic equilibrium is established during this irradiation, the nuclear spin levels will be populated in the same ratio as the electronic spin levels. This polarization may also be set up by the frequency difference $\omega = \omega_e - \omega_n$. It is required that the microwave power level be adjusted so that microwave transitions $\omega_e \pm \omega_n$ are induced at a rate faster than $1/T_{1n}$ and slower than $1/T_{1e}$ where T_{1n} and T_{1e} are the respective nuclear and electronic spin lattice relaxation rates. This condition causes the nuclear spins to acquire an electronic Boltzmann distribution. Figure 19–6 shows the proton polarization that results from the solid effect at $\omega = \omega_e \pm \omega_n$ with an additional polarization at $\omega = \omega_e$ due to thermal mixing [Goldman and Landesman (1963)].

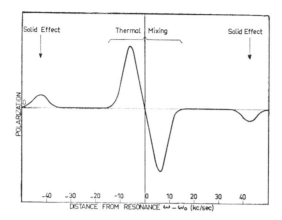

Fig. 19–6. Proton polarization in p-dichlorobenzene as a result of the solid effect and thermal mixing [Goldman and Landesman (1963)].

The energy level diagrams of Figs. 19–1 and 19–2 correspond to a strong scalar coupling $A\mathbf{I} \cdot \mathbf{S}$ between the electronic and nuclear spins. In each diagram, the upper set of energy levels corresponds to the upward orientation of the electronic spin ($M_s = \frac{1}{2}$, where the notation $M_s = M_J$ is used on the figures). The nuclear spin levels M_I are labeled with opposite polarities, since the positive values of M_I lie highest for the $M_s = \frac{1}{2}$ state, and the negative values of M_I lie highest for $M_s = -\frac{1}{2}$. In the case of weak dipolar coupling, the two sets of M_I levels are labeled in the same order for each electronic spin state (i.e., $M_I = \frac{1}{2}$ lies above $M_I = -\frac{1}{2}$ for $M_s = \pm\frac{1}{2}$.) This is discussed by Abraham, McCausland, and Robinson (1959), Schmugge and Jeffries (1962), and Poindexter (1963).

Thermal Mixing between Spin Systems: Thermal mixing between two spin systems occurs when mutual spin flips induced by spin-spin interactions between these systems can take place without a change in the total energy [Abragam and Proctor (1958b); Schumacher (1958); Goldman and Landesman (1963); Goldman (1962, 1965)]. This condition may prevail at low fields where the spin-spin energy and the Zeeman energy are comparable. Experiments by Goldman and Landesman on p-dichlorobenzene produced a maximum proton polarization eight times larger than that arising from a full solid effect, as exemplified in the $\omega = \omega_e$ center line on Fig. 19–6.

Comparison of Polarization Schemes: The Overhauser and Solid Effects are compared by Borghini (1960), Uebersfeld (1961), and Solomon (1962). The use of forbidden versus allowed transitions is treated by Buishvili (1959), Khutsishvili (1960), and Narchal and Barker (1963). Webb (1961b) found that Wurster's blue perchlorate exhibited an Overhauser enhancement above 77°K, but a solid effect below this temperature. Hausser and Reinhold (1962) describe the triple dynamical polarization of a three-spin system. General theories of double resonance have been advanced by a number of authors such as Combrisson (1958), Tomita (1958), Solomon (1958, 1962), Khutsishvili (1958, 1958, 1959) and Korringa, Seevers, and Torrey (1962).

B. Several Additional Polarization Schemes

Many NMR experiments are carried out by observing the NMR signal from one nuclear species, while simultaneously irradiating another species at or near its own particular NMR frequency [Baldeschwieler and Randall (1963)]. Anderson and Baldeschwieler (1962) have shown that, in principle, a nuclear magnetic double resonance experiment is capable of determining the relative signs of all the coupling constants between non-equivalent nuclei in a spin system.' Some of the theory that has been developed for nuclear double resonance experiments can be adapted to the interpretation of ESR–NMR double resonance studies.

Feher (1959) produced nuclear polarization via "hot" conduction electrons by employing an electric field to increase the average kinetic energy of the electrons and thereby raise them to a higher effective temperature than the nuclei. In this polarization scheme, the electric field effectively takes the place of the usual saturating microwave power. Feher (1959) obtained the predicted nuclear polarization using phosphorus-doped silicon at a lattice temperature of 1.3°K.

Pipkin (1958) used double resonance techniques to study radioactive Sb^{122} donors in silicon. The ESR transition was saturated and then the γ-rays emitted parallel and perpendicular to the magnetic field were studied as a function of the saturation of the nuclear transitions [see also Pipkin and Culvahouse (1958)]. Eisinger and Feher (1958) determined the hyperfine structure anomaly Δ of Sb^{121} and Sb^{123} doped silicon, where Δ is defined in terms of the ratios of the respective hyperfine coupling constants A and the g factors by the relation [see Kopferman (1940); Bitter (1949); and Bohr and Weisskopf (1950)]

$$\Delta = (A_{121}/A_{123})\,(g_{123}/g_{121}) - 1 \tag{1}$$

Honig (1954) studied arsenic-doped silicon and found that when a single hyperfine line is swept through twice in succession, the amplitude y_2 recorded during the second sweep is decreased relative to the amplitude y_1 recorded in the first sweep in accordance with the relation

$$y_2/y_1 = 1 - e^{-t/\tau} \tag{2}$$

where t is the time between sweeps and τ is about 16 sec. In addition, he found that when two successive hyperfine components are swept through sufficiently rapidly, the second line is enhanced by about a factor of two relative to the first line. This is discussed further by Honig and Combrisson (1956).

Abragam (1956) showed that when a solid containing paramagnetic centers is demagnetized in a time much less than the spin lattice relaxation time T_1, then a nuclear polarization is induced which decays with a time constant approximately equal to T_1.

A number of authors [such as Kittel (1954), Brovetto and Cini (1954), Brovetto and Ferroni (1954), Klein (1955), Barker and Mencher (1956), Motchane and Uebersfeld (1960), and Goldman and Landesman (1963)] have published discussions of nuclear polarization and double resonance from the viewpoint of thermodynamics.

A considerable number of double resonance experiments have been carried out by using a combination of an optical and an rf or microwave source. This optical–magnetic resonance technique is used to study atoms with paramagnetic ground states, and also to study atoms with nonmagnetic ground states by employing the optical irradiation to excite them to a paramagnetic state which exhibits magnetic resonance absorption. This field of research has been reviewed by Al'tshuler and Kozyrev (1964), and Skrotsky and Izyumova (1961). Space does not permit an elaboration on the theory or experimental techniques that are employed in these studies.

A number of investigators [such as, Kaplan (1955); Burgess and Norberg (1955); Provotorov (1962); Heeger, Portis, and Witt (1962)] have discussed the line-shapes obtained in ESR–NMR double resonance. Bloch (1958) extended Van Vleck's theory of moments (1948) to double resonance, and Sarles and Cotts (1958) obtained experimental data in agreement with the Bloch theory. In carrying out double resonance experiments the modulation amplitude should be kept below the ESR line-width to prevent distortion [Rädler (1961)]. Doyle (1962) discusses how to eliminate undesirable modulation effects from double resonance experiments.

C. Double Resonance at Microwave Frequencies

Motchane, Erb, and Uebersfeld (1958) ennumerate the three arrangements of the ESR cavity and NMR coil that are *a priori* possible:

(*a*) The resonant cavity and NMR coil may be physically separated. With this arrangement the electronic spin system is first saturated in the resonant cavity, and then it is transferred to the NMR coil to detect the nuclear polarization. Years ago, Pound (1951) found that the nuclear polarization of Li^7 in a lithium fluoride crystal exhibited only a small decay when removed from the magnet for a few seconds [see also Pershan (1960); Blumberg (1960)]. However, this is an exceptional case, and ordinarily the nuclear spin-lattice relaxation time is too short for the nuclear spins to retain their polarization during a transfer to the NMR coil [Abragam, Combrisson, and Solomon (1957)], so this experimental arrangement is not used in practice.

(*b*) The NMR coil may be placed around or outside the cavity.

(*c*) The NMR coil may be placed within the cavity.

(*d*) The NMR coil forms the resonator walls [cf. Fig. 19–10; Sec. 14–G].

The second and third methods are frequently used, and examples of each will be given in turn.

An ordinary microwave cavity cannot be placed in an NMR coil because the cavity wall thickness prevents the NMR signal that is generated in the coil from entering the cavity from reaching the coil. This difficulty may be obviated by constructing the lower half of a cylindrical TE_{111} mode cavity from Pyrex glass that is silvered either by painting or by chemical depositon, as shown in Fig. 19–7 [Jeffries (1961)]. The thickness of the silver is small relative to the skin depth δ at the modulation frequency of 10^5 cps. A thin stripe in the silvering permits the NMR frequency to penetrate the cavity walls,

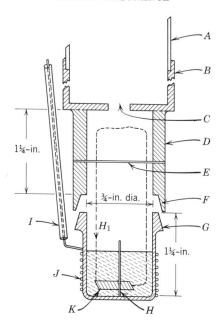

Fig. 19–7. TE_{111} mode cylindrical microwave cavity used for double resonance studies at X band (9500 Mc). Microphonics from bubbling helium may be reduced by filling the cavity with Styrofoam when operating at temperatures above the lambda point (between 2.17 and 4.2°K). (A) 0.015-in. stainless steel (types 321) waveguide; (B) rectangular brass waveguide 1 × ½ in., (C) 5/16-in. diameter iris; (D) brass cylinder; (E) copper wire mode suppressor; (F) silicone-greased ground joint; (G) Pyrex glass cavity 24/40 taper joint; (H) stripe in cavity silvering; (I) miniature coaxial cable (Microdot type 503947); (J) rf coil; (K) sample crystal in Styrofoam plug (1 in. = 2.54 cm) [Jeffries 1961)].

but the Q of the coil is too low to pick up an NMR polarization. A similar glass cavity described by Feher (1959) is shown on Fig. 19–8. This cavity has the coupling hole to the waveguide on top, and also employs a slit for the NMR frequency penetration of the cavity walls [see also Feher and Gere (1956, 1959) and Eisinger and Feher (1958)]. All three of these cavities may be used in the liquid helium temperature range.

Pipkin and Culvahouse (1957, 1958) and Culvahouse and Pipkin (1958) made use of a rectangular resonant cavity with the sides constructed from Lucite silvered to a thickness which permits a fluorescent light to be barely seen through the silvering. A 0.25-mm

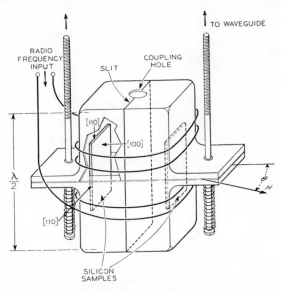

Fig. 19–8.   Microwave resonant cavity fabricated from Pyrex coated with silver on the inside.   The slit in the coating reduces rf eddy currents.   Silicon samples are shown mounted in the cavity (Feher (1959)].

scratch is made lengthwise along the center of the Lucite, and the rf coil surrounds the cavity.

Hardeman (1960) performed his double resonance experiment by placing the sample over a relatively large hole in the center of the bottom of a rectangular X band cavity.   The coil for measuring the NMR signal at about 13 Mc was wound around the cavity at the level of the coil.   A cylindrical cap covered the lower part of the cavity and was adjusted to maintain a high Q in the cavity, and at the same time to concentrate the rf field for the NMR on the sample.

Grützediek, Kramer, and Müller-Warmuth (1965) employed a 493-Mc quarter wavelength coaxial cavity surrounded by an NMR coil.

Jeffries (1961) used the microwave helix J and nuclear resonance coil H to observe double resonance with the sample I shown in Fig. 19–9.   Hausser and Reinhold (1962) [see Van Steenwinkel and Hausser (1965)] made use of an alternate form of a helix which serves both as a short section of helical waveguide and as an NMR receiver coil, as shown in Fig. 19–10. The microwave part of their experimental arrangement also included an attenuator, a power meter, a directional coupler, and a tuning element as shown in Fig. 19–10a. One may consult Fig. 19–10b for the arrangement of the quarter wavelength choke, helix, shield, and tuning plunger. Kenworthy and Richards (1965) [see Richards and White (1962, 1964); Werner (1963)] describe a helix ENDOR spectrometer and compare it to their spectrometer with cavity operation. Helices are discussed in Sec. 14-G.

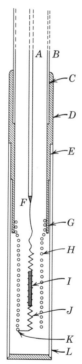

Fig. 19–9. X band microwave helix and rf coil arrangement for double resonance studies. (A) Inner conductor, 1 mm German silver, copper-plated; (B) outer conductor, 10 mm German silver, copper-plated on the inside; (C) Wood's metal joint between B and sleeve D; (D) brass sleeve; (E) Wood's metal joint between sleeve D and L; (F) soft-soldered joint connecting J to A; (G) soft-soldered joint connecting H to D; (H) nuclear resonance coil; (I) specimen; (J) microwave helix; (K) soft-soldered joint connecting J to H; (L) cap, 12 mm German silver with brass base [Jeffries (1961)].

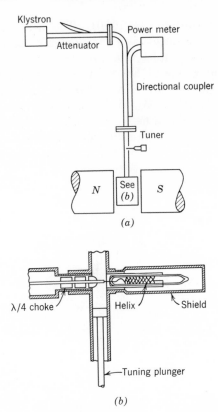

Fig. 19–10.   An experimental arrangement for the simultaneous use of a helix as both an rf coil for the NMR spectrometer and as a substitute for the resonant cavity of the ESR spectrometer: (a) microwave components, and (b) details of the helix [Hausser and Reinhold (1961)].

When the NMR coil is placed in the resonant cavity it should be mounted so that it surrounds the sample at a position of maximum microwave magnetic field intensity and minimum microwave electric field intensity.   In addition, it ought to be mounted perpendicular to the electric lines of force, and often this necessitates a rectangular form for the coil [Motchane (1962)].   When a source of 5 W excites an X band cavity with a Q of 5000, then Motchane (1962) deduced that the microwave magnetic field strength in the cavity reaches a value of 1.7 G.

A method of inserting the NMR coil within the resonant cavity is illustrated by the arrangement of Leifson and Jeffries (1961) shown on Fig. 19–11. The 15-mm quartz Dewar tip placed in the TE_{011} mode cylindrical resonant cavity encloses a sample that is maintained at liquid helium temperature. Most of the microwave power is dissipated in the cavity walls, and so very little liquid helium is boiled away by it. The sample may be changed without the necessity of refilling the liquid helium reservoir in the center of the Dewar.

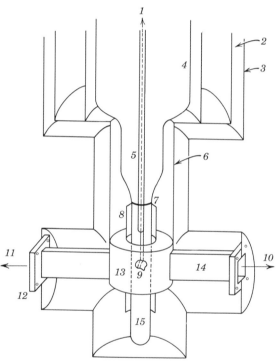

Fig. 19–11. Double resonance cryostat with thermal shields and vacuum jackets shown cut away. (1) Connection to nuclear resonance detector; (2) brass liquid nitrogen reservoir; (3) outer vacuum jacket; (4) silvered Pyrex liquid helium container; (5) coaxial cable; (6) copper thermal shield; (7) Pyrex-to-quartz seal; (8) sleeve to reduce coupling of cavity through port holes; (9) rf coil and sample; (10) connection to klystron oscillator; (11) connection to microwave resonance detector; (12) mica vacuum window; (13) TE_{011} mode cavity; (14) thin-wall stainless steel waveguide 2.54 cm × 1.27 cm; (15) quartz tube [Leifson and Jeffries (1961)].

The double resonance arrangement of Lambe, Laurance, McIrvine, and Terhune (1961) and Terhune, Lambe, Kikuchi, and Baker (1961) is shown on Fig. 19–12.   The upper NMR coil that is actuated by the marginal oscillator was used to induce Cr^{53} NMR transitions in the upper part of the ruby sample, and the rectangular microwave cavity [Lambe and Ager (1959)] was employed to induce Cr^{+3} ESR transitions in the lower part of the sample while simultaneously observing the Al ^{27} NMR resonance with the rf oscillator coupled to the coil inside the cavity.   This arrangement was also used without the marginal oscillator and upper coil to carry out conventional double resonance experiments.   Lambe et al. (1961) detected "distant

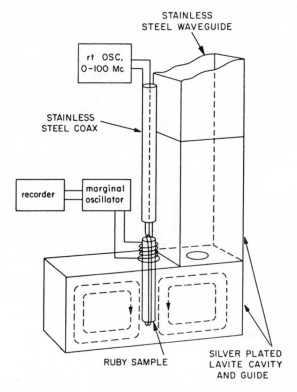

Fig. 19–12.   Apparatus for carrying out a simultaneous ESR microwave absorption and a 0 to 100-Mc NMR absorption experiment while a marginal oscillator auxiliary source induces nuclear transitions [Lambe, Laurance, McIrvine, and Terhune (1961); see also Terhune, Lambe, Kikuchi, and Baker (1961)].

ENDOR" effects whereby Zeeman transitions are induced in nuclei far removed from the saturated paramagnetic spins.

Watkins and Corbett (1964) performed ENDOR studies at 4.2°K by placing a single-turn coil in a cylindrical TE_{011} cavity, as shown on Fig. 19–13. The coil was driven by a General Radio oscillator. Schacher (1964) employed a similar arrangement.

Baker and Williams (1962) placed two vertical rods in their TE_{011} mode cylindrical X band resonant cavity shown on Fig. 19–14, and supplied them with both the 115 kc magnetic field modulation and the 50 to 900-Mc NMR frequency. The latter was derived from a General Radio oscillator which provided up to 200 MW of power. The NMR signal was modulated between 30 and 200 cps. Hall and Schumacher (1962) made use of a similar arrangement and supplied the vertical wire with several amperes of 12-Mc current.

Holton and Blum (1962) describe an X band ENDOR spectrometer for use at 1.3°K. Their resonator is shown on Fig. 8–41. Kramer, Müller-Warmuth, and Schindler (1965) designed the double resonance cavity shown on Fig. 8–40.

Several other authors have described experiments wherein the NMR coil was placed within the cavity [e.g., Kessenikh (1961, 1961); Jacubowicz, Motchane, and Uebersfeld (1961)]. Parker, McLaren,

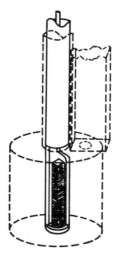

Fig. 19–13. TE_{011} mode microwave cavity with a single-turn coil introduced for ENDOR studies [Watkins and Corbett (1964)].

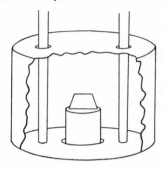

Fig. 19–14.   View of the parallel rods that simultaneously introduce the 50 to 900-Mc NMR and 115-Kc modulation frequencies into the resonant cavity. The sample is shown mounted in the center of the cavity [Baker and Williams (1962)].

and Conradi (1960) assembled a double resonance spectrometer by coupling a Varian V-4500 EPR unit to a Varian V-4200 wide line NMR spectrometer.   A bridge circuit was substituted for the Varian probe, and the rf coil was placed in the cavity.   The microwave power incident on the cavity was increased by a factor of four by eliminating the hybrid bridge and by operating the klystron with excessive beam and filament voltages (cf. Sec. 6–G).

This section was devoted to describing the modifications that must be made in the resonant cavity of an electron spin resonance spectrometer in order to be able to perform an NMR experiment while simultaneously carrying out an ESR absorption.   In addition to the cavity modification, it is, of course, necessary to incorporate an NMR spectrometer into the apparatus to generate or detect the nuclear polarization.   This NMR spectrometer should be the single-coil type rather than the double coil (transmitter and receiver) Bloch or induction type.   Either a commercial NMR spectrometer or a commercial NMR magnetometer (gaussmeter) may be adapted to this purpose by making only minor modifications in the circuitry [e.g., see Parker, McLaren, and Conradi (1960)].

Several of the NMR spectrometer types that have been employed by workers in this field include (a) the Autodyne method [Bruin and Schimmel (1955); Berthet, Imbaud, Ackermann, and Rondet (1960); Bruin and Van Soest (1960); Tchao (1960, 1961); De Martini (1963)]; (b) the modified or unmodified Pound-Knight circuit [Pound and Knight (1950); Watkins and Pound (1951; Pound (1952);

Motchane, Erb, and Uebersfeld (1958); Mays, Moore, and Schulman (1958); Leifson and Jeffries (1961); Motchane (1962); Schacher (1964); Howling (1965)]; (c) The bridge circuit [Bloembergen, Purcell, and Pound (1948); Parker, McLaren, and Conradi (1960); Imbaud and Berthet (1962)]; (d) a marginal oscillator was used by Lambe, Laurance, McIrvine, and Terhune (1961) [i.e., Terhune, Lambe, Kikuchi, and Baker (1961)]; (e) a Thomas oscillator [Thomas (1952)] was employed by Beljers, Van Der Kint, and Van Wieringen (1954); (f) Pipkin and Culvahouse (1958) made use of Commercial Hewlett-Packett and General Radio oscillators; (g) Müller-Warmuth and Parikh (1960) used a modified Q meter.

Many of the earlier references included in the last paragraph were to the papers which described prototype circuits, and a standard text on nuclear magnetic resonance [e.g., Andrew (1956); Lösche (1957); Pople, Schneider, and Bernstein (1959)] should be consulted for details on more up-to-date NMR instrumentation.

Moran (1964) studied inhomogeneously broadened resonant lines in KCl F centers [Portis (1953); Castner (1959); Wolf and Gross (1961);

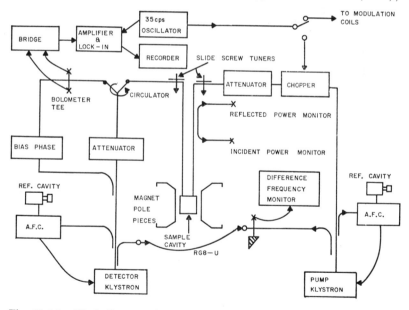

Fig. 19–15. Block diagram of a double resonance spectrometer employing two microwave frequencies [Moran (1964)].

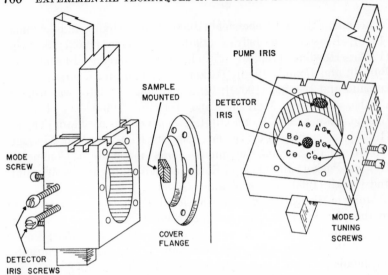

Fig. 19–16.   Bimodal sample cavity with resistive $(A–A')$ and reactive $(C–C')$ tuning screws.   The frequency difference between the two modes is adjusted by the B and B' tuning screws [Moran (1964)].

Moran, Christensen, and Silsbee (1961)] by saturating one point of the resonance and probing its intensity with a weak power level at other parts of the resonance.   The cylindrical sample cavity was operated in two orthogonal TM_{110} modes for the pump and detector frequencies. A block diagram of the apparatus is shown in Fig. 19–15, and details of the sample cavity are shown in Fig. 19–16.   Bowers and Mims (1959) carried out a similar double resonance experiment with a pump frequency of 3.9 Gc and a monitor frequency of 4.1 Gc.   They describe their apparatus and the bimodal cavity (cf. Sec. 8–J).

Cox, Flynn, and Wilson (1965) describe a double resonance microwave spectrometer with an X band pump frequency and a K band observing frequency.   Mims (1964) designed a pulsed ENDOR spectrometer [cf. Sec. 18-D].

D. Double Resonance at Radio Frequencies

Many investigators have employed one radio frequency to saturate the electronic spin system and a lower radio frequency to detect the nuclear polarization.   It is often easier to saturate the electronic spin system at radio frequencies than at microwave frequencies [Müller-Warmuth and Haupt (1962)]. The experimental techniques that are required for such studies are typical of those encountered in the field of NMR, and so they lie beyond the scope of this tome. The standard NMR texts mentioned toward the end of the last section may be consulted for further details.

The following articles discuss recent double resonance apparatus in the radio frequency region; the ESR frequency and applied magnetic field are given for each case. (a) Carver and Slichter (1956), 33 to 124 Mc, 10 to 50 G; (b) Landesman (1958), 25 to 200 Mc, 6 to 50 G; a resonant cavity for use at the upper part of the frequency range is illustrated; (c) Battut, Berthet, and Imbaud (1961, 1961), 200 Mc, 78 G; (d) Poindexter (1959, 1962, 1962), 52.6 Mc, 18.6 G; (e) Kubarev and Mezenev (1959), 1 to 125 Mc; 1 to several hundred G; (f) Müller-Warmuth (1960, 1964) and Müller-Warmuth and Haupt (1962), 10 to 100 Mc, 3 to 30 G; (g) Hashi (1961), 150 Mc, 54 G. Several of these systems are discussed in the next section.

E. Block Diagrams of Double Resonance Spectrometers

Block diagrams of four rf double resonance spectrometers are presented in Figs. 19–17 to 19–20. Baker and Williams (1962) employed the spectrometer shown in Fig. 19–17 for microwave range double frequency experiments. It is patterned after the Llewellyn (1957) spectrometer described in Sec. 13-L, and incorporates the resonant cavity shown in Fig. 19–14.

In the Carver and Slichter (1956) spectrometer shown in Fig. 19–18a, a push-pull oscillator supplies up to 59 W of rf power in the range from 84 to 124 Mc to saturate the electrons. Only a small fraction of this power is actually absorbed by the sample which is placed in the tank coil. Narrow band detection of the 50-kc nuclear resonance signal was accomplished in the twin T, preamplifier, and converter which converts the 50-kc signal to 600 kc for use in a standard communications receiver, as shown on Fig. 19–18b. The entire 50-kc NMR spectrometer was shielded from the output of the high frequency oscillator. The magnetic field of 10–50 G was produced by a solenoid provided with end windings to improve the homogeneity [Garrett (1951)]. Both scope and recorder presentation of the data may be used.

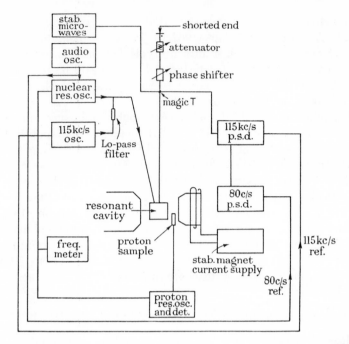

Fig. 19–17. Block diagram of an ESR–NMR double resonance spectrometer which operates at X band. It employs an audio frequency (80 cps) and a high frequency (115 kc) phase-sensitive detector (p.s.d.). The resonant cavity shown in Fig. 19–14 was incorporated into this spectrometer [Baker and Williams (1962)].

The Müller-Warmuth (1960) spectrometer shown in Fig. 19–19 employs a 15 to 100-Mc power oscillator provided with a frequency meter to saturate the electrons. The 25 to 90-kc nuclear resonance spectrometer employs a Q meter [Müller-Warmuth and Servoz-Gavin (1958); Grützediek, Kramer, and Müller-Warmuth (1965)], demodulator, phase-sensitive detector, and three amplifiers, one of which is a dc amplifier. The magnetic field is provided by Helmholtz coils which are current-stabilized [Müller-Warmuth (1958)]. The magnetic field modulation is derived from either a sawtooth current generator or a sine wave generator. Either oscillograph or recorder presentation may be employed.

The Hashi (1961) rf double resonance spectrometer is illustrated on Fig. 19–20. The static magnetic field is supplied by a current-stabilized generator. The 150-Mc generator produces an rf magnetic field of up to 4 G in the Helmholtz coil. The Pound-Knight (1950) marginal oscillator operates at 4.5 to 30 Mc. The magnetic field is modulated at 20 cps. Both narrow band and visual presentation may be employed.

Reichert and Townsend (1965) argue that at 1 Gc it takes 10^4 W to produce an 8-G saturating microwave field in a rectangular TE_{012} cavity, which is prohibitively expensive. They reduced the volume over which the microwave energy is stored by the use of a line resonator which has a high filling factor. The original article describes their ESR and NMR double resonance system.

F. Acoustic Electron Spin Resonance

In an ordinary electron spin resonance experiment, the spins absorb microwave energy and then relax by passing on this energy to the lattice vibrations which are "on speaking terms" with the spins. The inverse process is also possible if one irradiates the sample with ultrasonic energy at the resonant frequency ω_0 where

$$h\omega_0 = g\beta H \qquad (1)$$

Al'tshuler and Kozyrev (1964) have reviewed the theory of this effect [see Al'tshuler (1952, 1955); Al'tshuler, Zaripov, and Shekun (1952); Al'tshuler and Bashkirov (1960); Averbuch and Proctor (1963)].

The effect of ultrasonic energy on magnetic resonance absorption was first observed indirectly by its disturbing influence on the resonance absorption in NMR [Proctor and Tanttila (1955, 1956); Proctor and Robinson (1956); Kraus and Tanttila (1958); Jennings and Tanttila (1958); Taylor and Bloembergen (1959)]. The first direct acoustic excitation of nuclear spins was made by means of an ultrasonic continuous wave (cw) resonance technique in which a marginal rf oscillator was locked in to a high Q mechanical resonator [Menes and Bolef (1958, 1961); Bolef and Menes (1959); see also Barnes (1963) and Tewari and Verma (1964, 1965)].

One of the principal experimental difficulties in studying acoustic ESR in the microwave region is the problem of generating such high frequencies. Marginal oscillators are useful only up to about 200 Mc [Bolef, De Klerk, and Gosser (1962)]. Baranskii (1957), Bömmel and

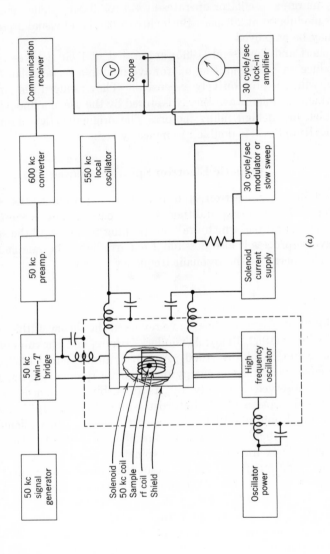

(a)

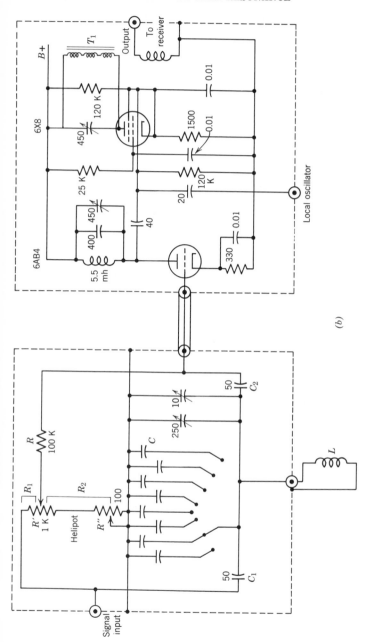

Fig. 19–18. A double resonance spectrometer which saturates the electrons spins between 84 and 124 Mc, and covers a magnetic field range from 10 to 50 G. (a) Block diagram; (b) details of the NMR 50-kc twin T bridge preamplifier and converter. The ferrite-tuned i.f. transformer T_1 has its secondary replaced by matched link coupling to the receiver antenna. Carver and Slichter (1956)].

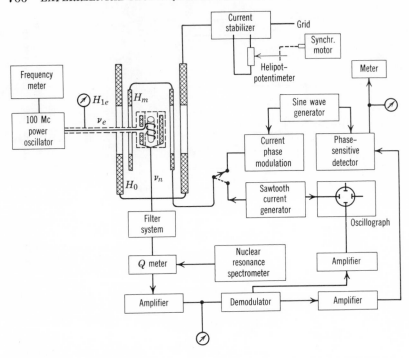

Fig. 19–19.   Block diagram of a double resonance spectrometer which saturates the ESR transitions between 15 and 100 Mc [Müller-Warmuth (1960)].

Dransfeld (1960), Jacobsen, Shiren, and Tucker (1959) and Dorland (1963) discuss the generation of microwave ultrasonics in a piezo-electric quartz rod which has a free surface at a point of maximum electric field strength in a microwave resonant cavity.   In a second resonant cavity at the other end of the rod, the ultrasonic energy is reconverted into electromagnetic energy.   The ESR absorption aris-ing from electron spins in the rod was found to decrease when the microwave phonons interacted with the electron spins [Jacobsen, Shiren, and Tucker (1959)].   At the ESR resonant condition, the ultrasonic waves transmitted along the rod were found to be attenu-ated [Tucker (1961)].   Using acoustic pulse-echo techniques, Tucker was able to operate at both X band and K band frequencies.   De Klerk (1964) designed a resonant cavity for use between 1 and 8 Gc in ultrasonic studies.

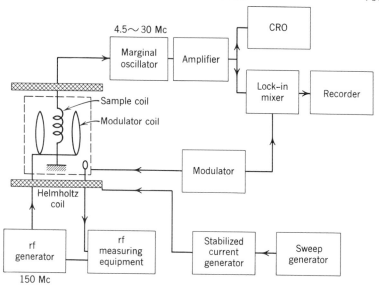

Fig. 19–20. Block diagram of a double resonance spectrometer which operates at an ESR frequency of 150 Mc [Hashi (1961)].

Bolef, De Klerk, and Gosser (1962) designed the acoustic analog of an ESR microwave transmission spectrometer, and their block diagram is shown in Fig. 19–21. It operates from 10 to 1000 Mc at temperatures between 1.5 and 300°K. The spectrometer is built around an acoustic transmission probe which attaches the sample to piezoelectric quartz transducers. The end faces of the specimen are rendered optically flat to produce an acoustic composite resonator. This resonator may be represented by an equivalent electrical circuit [Hueter and Bolt (1955); Williams and Lamb (1958)]. The cw ultrasound is generated by a commerical swept-frequency rf signal source which actuates one of several available types of transducers (i.e., overtone, surface excitation, externally tuned probe, or cavity excitation types).

Conventional ultrasonic pulse-echo techniques measure relative changes $\Delta\alpha/\alpha$ in the ultrasonic attenuation constant α of the order of 10^{-3}, while magnetic resonance techniques detect relative changes in electromagnetic attenuation of the order of 10^{-6}. To achieve this figure in the acoustic ESR spectrometer, one utilizes the Q of the

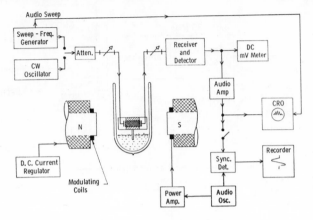

Fig. 19–21. Block diagram of an acoustic cw spectrometer. The swept-frequency oscillator is used for oscilloscope presentation while for high sensitivity, the cw oscillator, magnetic field modulation, and recorder display are used [Bolef, De Klerk, and Gosser (1962)].

mechanical resonator which ranges from low values to 10^6. High sensitivity is obtained with magnetic field modulation. The cw oscillator should be stable in frequency to one part in a million. The Bolef, De Klerk, and Gosser (1962) spectrometer has been operated with video, narrow band, and superheterodyne detection.

A number of recent articles have discussed ultrasonic ESR. Jacobsen and Stevens (1963) and Kopvillem and Mineeva (1963) present theoretical background material. Ultrasonic line-widths and shapes are treated by Shiren (1963) and Meyer, Bennett, Donoho, and Daniel (1966) and compared with ordinary ESR results. Guermeur, Joffrin, Levelut, and Penne (1965) describe saturation phenomena. Experimental apparatus is discussed by Dobrov and Browne (1962, 1963) and Ganapol'skii and Chernets (1964). See also Shiren and Tucker (1961), Denison, James, Currin, Tanttila, and Mahler (1964), Lewis (1965), Pomerantz (1965), and Wetsel and Donoho (1965).

References

A. Abragam, *Phys. Rev.*, **98**, 1729 (1955); *C. R. Acad. Sci.*, **242**, 1720 (1956).

A. Abragam, *The Principles of Nuclear Magnetism*, Clarendon, Oxford, 1961.

A. Abragam, J. Combrisson, and I. Solomon, *C. R. Acad. Sci.*, **245**, 157 (1957).

A. Abragam and W. G. Proctor, (a) *C. R. Acad. Sci.*, **246**, 2253 (1958); (b) *Phys. Rev.*, **109**, 1441 (1958).

M. Abraham, C. D. Jeffries, and R. W. Kedzie, *Phys. Rev.*, **117**, 1070 (1960).

M. Abraham, M. A. H. McCausland, and F. N. H. Robinson, *Phys. Rev. Letters*, **2**, 449 (1959).

S. A. Al'tshuler, *Dokl. Akad. Nauk SSSR*, **85**, 1235 (1952); *Zh. Eksper. Teor. Fiz.*, **28**, 49 (1955).

S. A. Al'tshuler and Sh. Sh. Bashkirov, *Conference on Paramagnetic Resonance*, Kazan, 1960, p. 78.

S. A. Al'tshuler and B. M. Kozyrev, *Electron Paramagnetic Resonance*, trans. by Scripta Technica, C. P. Poole, Jr., Ed., Academic Press, N. Y., 1964.

S. A. Al'tshuler, M. M. Zaripov, and L. Ya Shekun, *Izv. Akad. Nauk., Ser. Fiz.*, **21**, 844 (1957).

J. M. Anderson and J. D. Baldeschwieler, *J. Chem. Phys.*, **37**, 39 (1962).

E. R. Andrew, *Nuclear Magnetic Resonance*, Cambridge University Press, Cambridge, 1956.

P. Averbuch and W. G. Proctor, *Phys. Letters*, **4**, 221 (1963).

M. Ya. Azbel', V. I. Gerasimenko, and E. M. Lifshitz, *Zh Eksper. Teor. Fiz.*, **32**, 1212 (986) (1957); *ibid.*, **33**, 792 (609) (1957).

J. M. Baker and F. I. B. Williams, *Proc. Roy. Soc.*, **A267**, 283 (1962).

J. D. Baldeschwieler and E. W. Randall, *Chem. Rev.*, **63**, 81 (1963).

K. A. Baranskii, *Dokl. Akad. Nauk. SSSR*, **114**, 517 (1957); translation in *Soviet Phys. Dokl.* **2**, 237 (1958).

W. A. Barker and A. Mencher, *Phys. Rev.*, **102**, 1023 (1956).

D. J. Barnes, *Nature*, **200**, 253, 253 (1963).

Sh. Sh. Bashkirov and K. A. Valiev., *Zh. Eksper. Teor. Fiz.*, **35**, 678 (471) (1958).

R. Battut, G. Berthet, and J. P. Imbaud, *C. R. Acad. Sci.*, **253**, 638 (1961); *Arch. Sci. Spec. No.*, **14**, 490 (1961).

H. G. Beljers, L. Van Der Kint, and J. S. Van Wieringen, *Phys. Rev.*, **95**, 1683 (1954).

G. Berthet, J. P. Imbaud, P. Ackermann, and R. Rondet, *Arch. Sci., Fasc. Spec.*, **13**, 674 (1960).

F. Bitter, *Phys. Rev.*, **76**, 150 (1949).

B. Bleaney, *J. Phys. Radium*, **19**, 826 (1958).

R. J. Blin-Stoyle, M. A. Grace, and H. Halban, *Progr. Nucl. Phys.*, **3**, 63 (1957).

F. Bloch, *Phys. Rev.*, **70**, 460 (1946); **96**, 496 (1954); **111**, 841 (1958).

N. Bloembergen, E. M. Purcell, and R. V. Pound, *Phys. Rev.*, **73**, 679 (1948).

W. E. Blumberg, *Phys. Rev.*, **119**, 1842 (1960).

A. Bohr and V. F. Weisskopf, *Phys. Rev.*, **77**, 94 (1950)

D. I. Bolef and J. De Klerk, *IRE Trans.*, **UE-10**, 19 (1963).

D. I. Bolef, J. De Klerk, and R. B. Gosser, *RSI*, **33**, 631 (1962).

D. I. Bolef and M. Menes, *Phys. Rev.*, **114**, 1441 (1959).

H. E. Bömmel and K. Dransfeld, *Phys. Rev.*, **117**, 1245 (1960).

M. Borghini, *Arch. Sci., Fasc. Spec.*, **13**, 664 (1960).

M. Borghini and A. Abragam, *C. R. Acad. Sci.*, **248**, 1803 (1959).

K. D. Bowers and W. B. Mims, *Phys. Rev.*, **115**, 285 (1959).

G. Breit and I. I. Rabi, *Phys. Rev.*, **38**, 2072 (1931).

P. Brovetto and G. Cini, *Nuovo Cimento*, **11**, 618 (1954).

P. Brovetto and S. Ferroni, *Nuovo Cimento*, **12**, 90 (1954).

F. Bruin and F. M. Schimmel, *Physica*, **21**, 867 (1955).

F. Bruin and P. C. Van Soest, *RSI*, **31**, 909 (1960).

L. L. Buishvili, *Zh. Eksper. Teor. Fiz.*, **36**, 1926 (1369) (1959).

J. H. Burgess and R. E. Norberg, *Phys. Rev.*, **100**, 752 (1955).

J. Burget, M. Odelhnal, V. Petřicek, and J. Sacha, *Arch. Sci., Spec. No.*, **14**, 487 (1961).

T. R. Carver and C. P. Slichter, *Phys. Rev.*, **92**, 212 (1953); **102**, 975 (1956).

T. G. Castner, *Phys. Rev.*, **115**, 1506 (1959).

J. Combrisson, *J. Phys. Radium*, **19**, 840 (1958).

J. W. Culvahouse and F. M. Pipkin, *Phys. Rev.*, **109**, 319 (1958).

A. P. Cox, G. W. Flynn, and E. B. Wilson, Jr., *J. Chem. Phys.*, **42**, 3094 (1965).

J. de Klerk, *Ultrasonics*, **2**, 137 (1964).

F. De Martini, *Energia Nucl.*, **10**, 626 (1963).

A. B. Denison, L. W. James, J. D. Currin, W. H. Tanttila, and R. J. Mahler, *Phys. Rev. Letters*, **12**, 244 (1964).

W. I. Dobrov and M. E. Browne, *Proc. 11th Colloque Ampère*, Eindhoven, 1962, p. 129.

W. I. Dobrov and M. E. Browne, *Paramagnetic Resonance*, **2**, 447 (1963).

M. Dorland, *J. Phys. (France), Suppl. No. 10*, **24**, 191A (1963).

W. T. Doyle, *RSI*, **33**, 118 (1962).

J. Eisinger and G. Feher, *Phys. Rev.*, **109**, 1172 (1958).

E. Erb, J. L. Motchane, and J. Uebersfeld, *C. R. Acad. Sci.*, **246**, 2121, 3050 (1958).

G. Feher, *Phys. Rev.*, **103**, 500, 834 (1956); **114**, 1219 (1959); *Phys. Rev. Letters*, **3**, 135 (1959).

G. Feher, C. S. Fuller, and E. A. Gere, *Phys. Rev.*, **107**, 1462 (1957).

G. Feher and E. A. Gere, *Phys. Rev.*, **103**, 501 (1956); **114**, 1245 (1959).

E. M. Ganapol'skii and A. N. Chernets, *Zh. Eksper. Teor. Fiz.*, **47**, 1677 (1964).

M. W. Garrett, *J. Appl. Phys.*, **22**, 1091 (1951).

M. Goldman, *Proc. 11th Ampère Colloquium*, Eindhoven, 1962, p. 688; *Phys. Rev.*, **138**, A1668 (1965).

M. Goldman and A. Landesman, *Phys. Rev.*, **132**, 610 (1963).

H. Gross and H. C. Wolf, *Naturwiss.*, **8**, 299 (1961).

H. Grützediek, K. D. Kramer, and W. Müller-Warmuth, *RSI*, **36**, 1418 (1965).

R. Guermeur, J. Joffrin, A. Levelut, and J. Penne, *Phys. Letters*, **13**, 107 (1964); **15**, 203 (1965).

J. L. Hall and R. T. Schumacher, *Phys. Rev.*, **127**, 1892 (1962); *erratum*, **131**, 2839 (1963).

G. E. G. Hardeman, *Philips. Res. Rept.*, **15**, 587 (1960).

T. Hashi, *J. Phys. Soc., Japan*, **16**, 1243 (1961).

K. H. Hausser and F. Reinhold, *Z. Naturforsch.*, **16A**, 1114 (1961); *Phys. Letters*, **2**, 53 (1962).

A. J. Heeger, A. M. Portis, and G. Witt, *Proc. 11th Ampère Colloquium*, Eindhoven, 1962, p. 694.

W. C. Holton and H. Blum, *Phys. Rev.*, **125**, 89 (1962).

A. Honig, *Phys. Rev.*, **96**, 234 (1954).

A. Honig and J. Combrisson, *Phys. Rev.*, **102**, 917 (1956).

D. H. Howling, *RSI*, **36**, 660 (1965).

T. F. Hueter and R. H. Bolt, *Sonics*, Wiley, N. Y., 1955.

J. P. Imbaud and G. Berthet, *Proc. 11th Ampère Colloquium*, Eindhoven, 1962, p. 705.

E. H. Jacobsen, N. S. Shiren, and E. B. Tucker, *Phys. Rev. Letters*, **3**, 81 (1959).

E. H. Jacobsen and K. W. H. Stevens, *Phys. Rev.*, **128**, 2036 (1963).

J. Jacubowicz, J. L. Motchane, and J. Uebersfeld, *Arch. Sci. Spec. No.*, **14**, 476 (1961).

C. D. Jeffries, *Ann. Rev. Nucl. Sci.*, **14**, 101 (1964).

C. D. Jeffries, *Dynamic Nuclear Orientation*, Interscience, N. Y., 1962.

C. D. Jeffries, *Phys. Rev.*, **106**, 164 (1957); **117**, 1056 (1960); *Progr. Cryogenics*, **3**, 129 (1961).

D. A. Jennings and W. H. Tanttila, *Phys. Rev.*, **109**, 1059 (1958).

J. I. Kaplan, *Phys. Rev.*, **96**, 238 (1954); **99**, 1322 (1955).

J. G. Kenworthy and R. E. Richards, *JSI*, **42**, 675 (1965).

A. V. Kessenikh, *Zh. Eksper. Teor. Fiz.*, *PTE*, **40**, 32 (21) (1961); **3**, 107 (521) (1961).

G. R. Khutsishvili, *Zh. Eksper. Teor. Fiz.*, **34**, 1653 (1136) (1958); **35**, 1031 (720) (1958); **38**, 942 (679) (1960); *Nuovo Cimento*, **11**, 186 (1959); *Uspekhi Fiz. Nauk.*, **71**, 9 (285) (1960).

C. Kittel, *Phys. Rev.*, **95**, 589 (1954).

M. J. Klein, *Phys. Rev.*, **98**, 1736 (1955).

H. Kopfermann, *Kernmomente*, Akademische Verlagsgesellschaft, Leipzig, 1940.

U. Kh. Kopvillem and R. M. Mineeva, *Izv. Akad. Nauk. SSSR Ser. Fiz.*, **27**, 93 (98), 95 (101) (1963).

J. Korringa, *Phys. Rev.*, **94**, 1388 (1954).

J. Korringa, D. O. Seevers, and H. C. Torrey, *Phys. Rev.*, **127**, 1143 (1962).

K. D. Kramer and W. Müller-Warmuth, *Z. Naturforsch.*, **18A**, 1129 (1963).

K. D. Kramer, W. Müller-Warmuth, and J. Schindler, *J. Chem. Phys.*, **43**, 31 (1965); *Z. Naturforsch.* **19A**, 375 (1964).

O. Kraus and W. H. Tanttila, *Phys. Rev.*, **109**, 1052 (1958).

A. V. Kubarev and Yu. A. Mezenev, *PTE*, **2**, 86 (268) (1960).

J. Lambe and R. Ager, *RSI*, **30**, 599 (1959).

J. Lambe, N. Laurance, E. C. McIrvine, and R. W. Terhune, *Phys. Rev.*, **122**, 1161 (1961).

A. Landesman, *C. R. Acad. Sci.*, **246**, 1538 (1958); *J. Phys. Radium*, **20**, 937 (1959).

O. S. Leifson and C. D. Jeffries, *Phys. Rev.*, **122**, 1781 (1961).

M. F. Lewis, *Phys. Letters*, **17**, 183 (1965).

W. A. Little, *Proc. Phys. Soc.*, **B70**, 785 (1957).

P. M. Llewellyn, *JSI*, **34**, 236 (1957).

A. Lösche, *Kerninduktion*, Veb. Deutscher Verlag des Wissenschaften, Berlin, East Germany, 1957.

J. M. Mays, H. R. Moore, and R. G. Schulman, *RSI*, **29**, 300 (1958).

M. Menes and D. I. Bolef, *Phys. Rev.*, **109**, 218 (1958); *J. Phys. Chem. Solids*, **19**, 79 (1961).

H. C. Meyer, J. S. Bennett, P. L. Donoho, and A. C. Daniel, *Bull. Am. Phys. Soc.*, **11**, 202 (1966).

W. B. Mims, *Proc. Roy. Soc.*, **A283**, 452 (1964); *Phys. Rev.*, **141**, 499 (1964).

P. R. Moran, *Phys. Rev.*, **135**, A247 (1964).

P. R. Moran, S. H. Christensen, and R. H. Silsbee, *Phys Rev.*, **124**, 442 (1961).

J. L. Motchane, *Ann. Phys. (France)*, **7**, 139 (1962).

J. L. Motchane, E. Erb, and J. Uebersfeld, *C. R. Acad. Sci.*, **246**, 1833 (1958).

J. L. Motchane and J. Uebersfeld, *J. Phys. Radium*, **21**, 194 (1960).

W. Müller-Warmuth, *Z. Agnew. Phys.*, **10**, 497 (1958); *Z. Naturforsch.*, **15A**, 927 (1960); **19A**, 1309 (1964).

W. Müller-Warmuth and J. Haupt, *Proc. 11th Ampère Colloquium*, Eindhoven, 1962, p. 714; *Z. Naturforsch.* **17A**, 1011 (1962).

W. Müller-Warmuth and P. Parikh, *Arch. Sci. Fasc. Spec.*, **13**, 680 (1960).

W. Müller-Warmuth and P. Servoz-Gavin, *Z. Naturforsch.*, **13A**, 194 (1958).

M. Lal Narchal and W. A. Barker, *Appl. Optics*, **2**, 787 (1963).

A. W. Overhauser, *Phys. Rev.*, **89**, 689 (1953); **92**, 411 (1953); **94**, 1388 (1954).

D. J. Parker, G. A. McLaren, and J. J. Conradi, *J. Chem. Phys.*, **33**, 629 (1960).

P. S. Pershan, *Phys. Rev.*, **117**, 109 (1960).

F. M. Pipkin, *Phys. Rev.*, **112**, 935 (1958).

F. M. Pipkin and J. W. Culvahouse, *Phys. Rev.*, **106**, 1102 (1957); **109**, 1423 (1958).

E. H. Poindexter, *J. Chem. Phys.*, **31**, 1477 (1959); **36**, 507 (1962); **37**, 463 (1962).

M. Pomerantz, *Phys. Rev.*, **139**, A501 (1965).

J. A. Pople, W. G. Schneider, and H. J. Bernstein, *High Resolution Nuclear Magnetic Resonance*, McGraw-Hill, N. Y., 1959.

A. M. Portis, *Phys. Rev.*, **91**, 1071 (1953).

R. V. Pound, *Phys. Rev.*, **81**, 156 (1951); *Progr. Nucl. Phys.*, **2**, 21 (1952).

R. V. Pound and W. D. Knight, *RSI*, **21**, 219 (1950).

W. G. Proctor and W. A. Robinson, *Phys. Rev.*, **104**, 1344 (1956).

W. G. Proctor and W. H. Tanttila, *Phys. Rev.*, **98**, 1854 (1955); **101**, 1757 (1956).

B. N. Provotorov, *Phys. Rev.*, **128**, 75 (1962).

K. H. Rädler, *Ann. Phys. (Germany)*, **7**, 45 (1961).

J. F. Reichert and J. Townsend, *Phys. Rev.*, **137**, A476 (1965).

R. E. Richards and J. W. White, *Proc. Roy. Soc.*, **A269**, 287 (1962); **A279**, 474, 481 (1964).

L. G. Rowan, E. L. Hahn, and W. B. Mims, *Phys. Rev.* **137**, A61 (1965).

R. H. Ruby, H. Benoit, and C. D. Jeffries, *Phys. Rev.*, **127**, 51 (1962).

L. R. Sarles and R. M. Cotts, *Phys. Rev.*, **111**, 853 (1958).

T. J. Schmugge and C. D. Jeffries, *Phys. Rev. Letters*, **9**, 268 (1962).

R. T. Schumacher, *Phys. Rev.*, **112**, 837 (1958).

P. L. Scott and C. D. Jeffries, *Phys. Rev.*, **127**, 32 (1962).

G. W. Series, *Repts. Prog. Phys.*, **22**, 280 (1959).

N. S. Shiren, *Paramagnetic Resonance*, **2**, 482 (1963).

N. S. Shiren and E. B. Tucker, *Phys. Rev. Letters*, **6**, 105 (1961).

G. E. Schacher, *Phys. Rev.*, **135**, A185 (1964).

G. V. Skrotsky and T. G. Izyumova, *Usp. Fiz. Nauk.*, **73**, 423 (177) (1961).

I. Solomon, *J. Phys. Radium*, **19,** 837 (1958); *Proc. 11th Ampère Colloquium*, Eindhoven, 1962, p. 25.

M. J. Steenland and H. A. Tolhoek, *Progr. Low Temperature Phys.*, **2,** 292 (1957).

E. K. Taylor and N. Bloembergen, *Phys. Rev.*, **113,** 431 (1959).

Y. H. Tchao, *Arch. Soc., Fasc. Spec.*, **13,** 686 (1960); *Arch. Sci. Spec. No.*, **14,** 479 (1961).

A. L. Terhune, J. Lambe, C. Kikuchi, and J. Baker, *Phys. Rev.*, **123,** 1265 (1961).

D. P. Tewari and G. S. Verma., *Phys. Letters*, **12,** 97 (1964).

D. P. Tewari and G. S. Verma, *Nuovo Cimento*, **38,** 197 (1965).

H. A. Thomas, *Electronics*, **25,** 114 (1962).

K. Tomita, *Progr. Theor. Phys.*, **20,** 743 (1958).

E. B. Tucker, *Phys. Rev. Letters*, **6,** 183 (1961).

J. Uebersfeld, *Arch. Sci. Spec. No.*, **14,** 456 (1961).

J. Uebersfeld, *12th Colloque Ampère*, Bordeaux, 1963, p. 109.

V. M. Underhauser and A. Abragam, *Phys. Rev.*, **98,** 1729 (1955).

V. M. Underhauser, L. H. Bennett, and H. C. Torrey, *Phys. Rev.*, **108,** 449 (1957).

V. M. Underhauser and J. Seiden, *C. R. Acad. Sci.*, **245,** 1528 (1957).

K. A. Valiev, *Fiz. Metal. i. Metalloved.*, **6,** 193 (1958).

R. Van Steenwinkel and K. H. Hausser, *Phys. Letters*, **14,** 24 (1965).

J. H. Van Vleck, *Phys. Rev.*, **74,** 1168 (1948).

G. D. Watkins and J. W. Corbett, *Phys. Rev.*, **134,** A1359 (1964).

G. D. Watkins and R. V. Pound, *Phys. Rev.*, **82,** 343 (1951).

R. H. Webb, (a) *Phys. Rev. Letters*, **6,** 611 (1961); (b) *Am. J. Phys.*, **29,** 428 (1961).

K. Werner, *Hochfrengztech. Elekt. Akust.*, **73,** 115 (1964).

G. C. Wetsel, Jr. and P. L. Donoho, *Phys. Rev.*, **139,** A334 (1965).

J. Williams and J. Lamb, *J. Acoust. Soc. Am.*, **30,** 308 (1958).

H. C. Wolf and H. Gross, *Naturwiss.*, **8,** 299 (1961).

CHAPTER 20

The Characteristics of Spectral Line-Shapes

A great deal of information can be obtained from a careful analysis of the width and shape of a resonant absorption line. The first few sections of this chapter analyze in detail the two most common line-shapes, the Lorentzian and the Gaussian, when they are detected and recorded under various types of instrumental conditions which faithfully reproduce their true shape. The remainder of the chapter discusses various mechanisms which broaden spectral lines. The broadening (and narrowing) that arises under the influence of the measuring arrangement is discussed in Chaps. 10, 14, and 18 [see also Flynn and Seymour (1960); Štirand (1962)]. Homogeneous and inhomogeneous broadening is discussed in Sec. 18-B. A general review of the various theories of line-breadths is given by Van Vleck (1957).

In this chapter, unless otherwise stated, we shall assume that the microwave power level is sufficiently low so that saturation is avoided. As a result the integrated area A of a resonance absorption line is proportional to the number of spins, and the measured moments of the lines are physically significant in terms of the theories of Van Vleck (1948) and others. We shall also assume that the modulation amplitude is much less than the line-width. If the recorded spectrum is distorted by either saturation or overmodulation, then the methods described in Secs. 18-C, and 10-E, respectively, may be used to convert the observed area and moments to the physically meaningful ones discussed in this chapter.

Line broadening in gases is similar to that ordinarily observed in microwave spectroscopy studies, and so it will not be discussed here [see Van Vleck and Weisskopf (1945); Townes and Schawlow (1955); Breen (1961); Tobler, Bauder, and Günthard (1965); Ben-Reuven (1965)]. A microwave spectrograph for line-width measurements is described by Rinehart, Legan, and Lin (1965). Kiel (1962, 1963) discusses line-shapes in the ESR spectra of optically excited crystal field levels, but almost all published spectra are for the optical ground states of the type discussed in this chapter.

A. Area and Moments of a Resonance Absorption Curve

The area A under the resonance absorption curve Y shown in Fig. 20-1a and 20-1c is given by

$$A = \sum_{j=1}^{m} y_j (H_j - H_{j-1}) \tag{1}$$

where y_j is the amplitude of the resonance absorption line at the magnetic field H_j, as shown on Fig. 20–1c. In practice it is convenient to select equal intervals $(H_j - H_{j-1})$ along the field direction so that

$$A = (H_j - H_{j-1}) \sum_{j=1}^{m} y_j \tag{2}$$

where there are m intervals in all. This area is usually proportional to the number of unpaired spins in the sample. The precision of the area determination is increased by increasing m and decreasing the interval $(H_j - H_{j-1})$.

The nth moment $\langle H^n \rangle$ of a resonance absorption is defined by

$$\langle H^n \rangle = \frac{H_j - H_{j-1}}{A} \sum_{j=1}^{m} (H_j - H_0)^n y_j \tag{3}$$

where the summation limits are the same as in eq. (2), and in general, these moments are functions of the field H_0. If a resonance absorption line is symmetrical, then H_0 is the magnetic field which divides the line into two halves, each of which contains half the area A

$$\int_{-\infty}^{H_0} Y(H) dH = \tfrac{1}{2} A = \int_{H_0}^{\infty} Y(H) dH \tag{4}$$

where Y is the line shape function. This criterion may be used to determine H_0, and we shall use this definition even for unsymmetrical lines. Another method for determining H_0 of a symmetric line entails the computation of the first moment

$$\langle H^1 \rangle = \frac{H_j - H_{j-1}}{A} \sum_{j=1}^{m} (H_j - H_0) y_j \tag{5}$$

which vanishes for the proper choice of H_0.   If this expression is not zero, then let

$$\langle H^1 \rangle = B = \frac{\sum\limits_{j=1}^{m} (H_j - H_0)\, y_j}{\sum\limits_{j=1}^{m} y_j} \qquad (6)$$

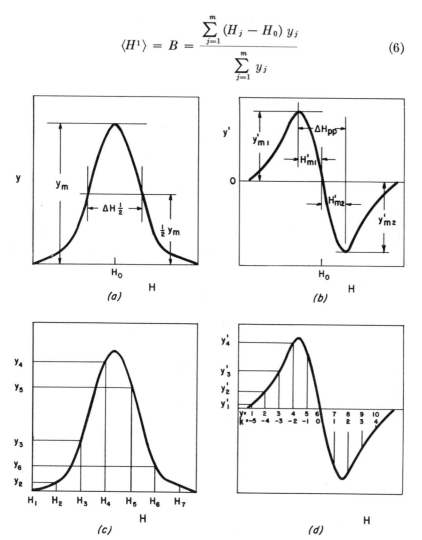

Fig. 20–1. (a,c) Absorption and (b,d) absorption derivative line-shapes. The line-shape parameters are defined in (a) and (b) and the method of integration is illustrated in (c) and (d).

and when B is inserted into eq. (5), the corrected value of $\langle H^1 \rangle$ will vanish since

$$\langle H^1 \rangle_{\text{corr}} = \frac{H_j - H_{j-1}}{A} \sum_{j=1}^{m} (H_j - H_0 - B) y_j = 0 \qquad (7)$$

The correction factor B is the displacement shown on Fig. 20-2. As a result, eq. (3) may be rewritten as

$$\langle H^n \rangle_{\text{corr}} = \frac{H_j - H_{j-1}}{A} \sum_{j=1}^{m} (H_j - H_0 - B)^n y_j \qquad (8)$$

In practice one can usually select H_0 so that $B = 0$, and use eq. (3), but eq. (6) plus (8) may be employed if a more refined computation of A or $\langle H^n \rangle$ is desired. It should be emphasized that the vanishing of the first moment and all other odd moments is a property of symmetric absorption lines, so B cannot be defined in a physically meaningful way for an asymmetric absorption line.

The use of eqs. (2), (7), and (8) is illustrated by the calculation with a Gaussian line-shape $^G Y$ that is shown on Table 20-1.

$$^G Y(H_j) = {}^G y_j = y_m \exp\left[-0.693\left(\frac{H_j - H_0}{\frac{1}{2}\Delta H_{1/2}}\right)^2 \right] \qquad (9)$$

where more generally

$$^G Y(H) = y_m \exp\left[-0.693\left(\frac{H - H_0}{\frac{1}{2}\Delta H_{1/2}}\right)^2 \right] \qquad (9a)$$

where $\ln 2 = 0.693$. We let $y_m = 1$, and compute the correction B, obtaining from Table 20-1

$$\frac{B}{\frac{1}{2}\Delta H_{1/2}} = \frac{\sum_{j=1}^{m} (H_j - H_0) y_j}{\sum_{j=1}^{m} y_j} = \frac{4.253}{4.259} \sim 1 \qquad (10)$$

For this calculation we selected the convenient increments

$$H_j - H_{j-1} = \frac{1}{4}\Delta H_{1/2} \qquad (11)$$

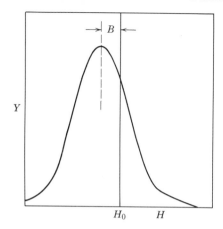

Fig. 20-2. Correction factor B that results from an improper choice of the resonant field H_0. When the resonant line is unsymmetrical, the proper choice of H_0 is not as obvious as it is in this case.

where $\Delta H_{1/2}$ is the full line-width between half amplitude points (i.e., the half amplitude line-width) defined in Fig. 20-1a. The use of smaller increments will considerably improve the accuracy of the results. Since the line-shape is symmetrical, the calculation of A, $\langle H^2 \rangle$, and $\langle H^4 \rangle$ can be limited to a calculation with half the line if one doubles the result. (It is important to use only half the amplitude of y at the center point in this abbreviated calculation).

From Table 20-1 and eq. (2), we obtain

$$A = 1.065 \Delta H_{1/2} \tag{12}$$

and from eq. (8)

$$\langle H^2 \rangle = \frac{H_j - H_{j-1}}{A} \left(\tfrac{1}{2}\Delta H_{1/2}\right)^2 \sum_{j=1}^{m} \left(\frac{H_j - H_0 - B}{\tfrac{1}{2}\Delta H_{1/2}}\right)^2 y_j \tag{13}$$

$$= 0.721 \left(\tfrac{1}{2}\Delta H_{1/2}\right)^2 \tag{14}$$

$$\langle H^4 \rangle = \frac{H_j - H_{j-1}}{A} \left(\tfrac{1}{2}\Delta H_{1/2}\right)^4 \sum_{j=1}^{m} \left(\frac{H_j - H_0 - B}{\tfrac{1}{2}\Delta H_{1/2}}\right)^4 y_j \tag{15}$$

$$= 1.56 \left(\tfrac{1}{2}\Delta H_{1/2}\right)^4 \tag{16}$$

TABLE 20-1

Computation of Correction Factor B, Area A and Second and Fourth Moments of a Gaussian Line-Shape Using Eqs. (6), (2), and (8) of Sec. 20-A

j	y_i	$\left(\dfrac{H_i - H_0}{\frac{1}{2}\Delta H_{1/2}}\right)$	$y_i\left(\dfrac{H_i - H_0}{\frac{1}{2}\Delta H_{1/2}}\right)$	$\left(\dfrac{H_i - H_0 - B}{\frac{1}{2}\Delta H_{1/2}}\right)$	$y_i\left(\dfrac{H_i - H_0 - B}{\frac{1}{2}\Delta H_{1/2}}\right)^2$	$y_i\left(\dfrac{H_i - H_0 - B}{\frac{1}{2}\Delta H_{1/2}}\right)^4$
1	0.000015	-3.0	-0.0000	-4.0	0.0002	0.0038
2	0.00020	-2.5	-0.0005	-3.5	0.0015	0.0300
3	0.00195	-2.0	-0.0039	-3.0	0.0178	0.1600
4	0.0131	-1.5	-0.0197	-2.5	0.0819	0.5117
5	0.0626	-1.0	-0.0626	-2.0	0.2508	1.0032
6	0.2101	-0.5	-0.1051	-1.5	0.4727	1.0630
7	0.5000	0.0	0.0000	-1.0	0.5000	0.5000
8	0.8380	0.5	0.4190	-0.5	0.2095	0.0524
9	1.0000	1.0	1.0000	0	1.5353	3.3241
10	0.8380	1.5	1.2570	0.5	$\times\,2$	$\times\,2$
11	0.5000	2.0	2.0000	1.0	3.0706	6.6482
12	0.2101	2.5	0.5253	1.5		
13	0.0626	3.0	0.1881	2.0		
14	0.0131	3.5	0.0459	2.5		
15	0.00195	4.0	0.0078	3.0		
16	0.00020	4.5	0.0018	3.5		
17	0.000015	5.0	0.0001	4.0		
	4.259		5.4450			
			-0.1919			
			4.2531			

$$B = \frac{\frac{1}{2}\Delta H_{1/2} \sum_{j=1}^{m} y_j \left(\dfrac{H_i - H_0}{\frac{1}{2}\Delta H_{1/2}} \right)}{\sum_{j=1}^{m} y_j} = \frac{4.2531}{4.259} \left(\tfrac{1}{2}\Delta H_{1/2} \right) = 0.5\Delta H_{1/2}$$

$$H_j - H_{j-1} = \tfrac{1}{2}(\tfrac{1}{2}\Delta H_{1/2}) = \tfrac{1}{4}\Delta H_{1/2}$$

$$A = |\, H_j - H_{j-1} \,| \sum_{j=1}^{m} y_j = (\tfrac{1}{4}\Delta H_{1/2})\,(4.259) = 1.065\Delta H_{1/2}$$

$$\langle H^2 \rangle = \frac{H_j - H_{j-1}}{A} (\tfrac{1}{2}\Delta H_{1/2})^2 \sum_{j=1}^{m} \left(\frac{H_i - H_0 - B}{\frac{1}{2}\Delta H_{1/2}} \right)^2 y_j = \frac{(\frac{1}{2}\Delta H_{1/2})^2}{4.259}\,(3.0706) = 0.18(\Delta H_{1/2})^2$$

$$\langle H^4 \rangle = \frac{H_j - H_{j-1}}{A} (\tfrac{1}{2}\Delta H_{1/2})^4 \sum_{j=1}^{m} \left(\frac{H_i - H_0 - B}{\frac{1}{2}\Delta H_{1/2}} \right)^4 y_j = \frac{(\frac{1}{2}\Delta H_{1/2})^4}{4.259}\,(6.6482) = 0.097(\Delta H_{1/2})^4$$

The preceding summations may be represented more elegantly by means of the following two integrals:

$$A = \int_{-\infty}^{\infty} Y dH = 2 \int_{0}^{\infty} Y dH \qquad (17)$$

and

$$\langle H^n \rangle = \begin{cases} 0 & n \text{ odd} \\ \dfrac{2}{A} \displaystyle\int_{0}^{\infty} (H - H_0)^n Y dH & n \text{ even} \end{cases} \qquad (18)$$

The change in the lower limit ($-\infty \to 0$) is only valid for symmetrical lines. For a Gaussian line-shape (9a), the change of variable $x = [(H - H_0)/(\frac{1}{2}\Delta H_{1/2})](\ln 2)^{1/2}$ yields

$$A = \frac{2 y_m (\frac{1}{2}\Delta H_{1/2})}{(\ln 2)^{1/2}} \int_{0}^{\infty} \exp(-x^2)\, dx \qquad (19)$$

$$= [\tfrac{1}{2}\sqrt{\pi}/(\ln 2)^{1/2}]\, y_m \Delta H_{1/2} \qquad (12)$$

$$= 1.0643\, y_m \Delta H_{1/2} \qquad (12a)$$

To evaluate the moments, one may employ the expression

$$\int_{-\infty}^{\infty} x^n \exp[-(x/a)^{1/2}]dx = a^{n+1}\Gamma[(n+1)/2] \qquad (20)$$

where the gamma function $\Gamma[(n+1)/2]$ is defined by

$$\Gamma[(n+1)/2] = \frac{1 \cdot 3 \cdot 5 \ldots (n-1)}{(2)^{n/2}} \pi^{1/2} = \frac{(n-1)!!}{2^{n/2}} \pi^{1/2} \qquad (21)$$

for the even moments (even n), while from symmetry the odd moments (odd n) vanish. Since $dH = d(H - H_0)$, we have

$$\langle H^n \rangle = \frac{(\frac{1}{2}\Delta H_{1/2})^n}{\pi^{1/2}(\ln 2)^{n/2}} \Gamma[(n+1)/2] = \frac{(\frac{1}{2}\Delta H_{1/2})^n (n-1)!!}{(2 \ln 2)^{n/2}} \qquad (22)$$

with the result that

$$\langle H^2 \rangle = 0.721 (\tfrac{1}{2}\Delta H_{1/2})^2 \qquad (14)$$

and

$$\langle H^4 \rangle = 1.56(\tfrac{1}{2}\Delta H_{1/2})^4 \qquad (16)$$

as found above.

For a Lorentzian line-shape

$$^{L}Y(H) = \frac{y_m}{1 + [(H - H_0)/\tfrac{1}{2}\Delta H_{1/2}]^2} \qquad (23)$$

one may let $x = 2(H - H_0)/\Delta H_{1/2}$, and obtain from eq. (17)

$$A = y_m \Delta H_{1/2} \int_0^\infty \frac{dx}{1 + x^2} \qquad (24)$$

and letting $x = \tan \theta$, and $dx = \sec^2 \theta d\theta$ the integral becomes

$$A = y_m \Delta H_{1/2} \int_0^{\pi/2} d\theta \qquad (25)$$

$$= (\pi/2)\ y_m \Delta H_{1/2} \qquad (26)$$

$$= 1.57 y_m \Delta H_{1/2} \qquad (26a)$$

Since the Lorentzian line-shape is symmetrical, all odd moments vanish, e.g., for the second moment we have

$$\langle H^2 \rangle = \frac{y_m}{A} \int_{-\infty}^\infty \frac{(H - H_0)^2 dH}{1 + [(H - H_0)/\tfrac{1}{2}\Delta H_{1/2}]^2} \qquad (27)$$

$$= \frac{2}{\pi}(\tfrac{1}{2}\Delta H_{1/2})^2 \int_0^\infty \frac{x^2 dx}{1 + x^2} \qquad (28)$$

which diverges to an infinite result. This is evident if one considers that for large x, the integral behaves like $\int_0^\infty dx$, Thus, for a Lorentzian line-shape all odd moments vanish, and all even moments are infinitely large.

It is important to note that the area of an absorption line is proportional to the amplitude times the line-width $\Delta H_{1/2}$, and the constant of proportionality depends on the line-shape. The units of the area are amplitude units $\times$ gauss, or number of unpaired spins. Of particular interest is the fact that for the same amplitude y_m and the same line-width $\Delta H_{1/2}$, a Lorentzian line corresponds to $(1.56/1.06)$ or 1.48 times as many spins as a Gaussian line. One should bear in mind that this factor of 1.48 applies only to absorption lines themselves, since the derivative line-shape requires a different normalization factor, $4(2\pi/3e)^{1/2} = 3.51$, from Table 20–5.

We have emphasized the vanishing of all the odd moments of symmetrical absorption lines such as those with Gaussian and Lorentzian shapes. It is the even moments which vanish for the corresponding dispersion mode line-shapes. The moments of the first derivative of an absorption line are defined to agree with the corresponding moments of the absorption line itself, as discussed in the next section.

To record the actual absorption line one may either perform a dc experiment (sans modulation) as discussed in Sec. 10-B, or an electronic integrator may be employed to integrate the ESR signal before it is recorded (*vide* Sec. 12-K). Divers methods of integrating spectra are discussed in Sec. 14-K. A quick integration method is given by Charlier, Danan, and Taglang (1964).

The extent to which an unsymmetrical resonant line is asymmetric may be expressed quantitatively by giving the dimensionless ratio

$$\text{Anisotropy} = \frac{\langle H^3 \rangle}{\langle H^2 \rangle^{3/2} + \langle H^3 \rangle} \tag{29}$$

Svare (1965) calculated third moments for $g\beta H \geqslant kT$ and showed that paramagnetic lines are asymmetric at low temperatures. Equation (7) states that experimental line-shapes are defined with vanishing first moments. If instead the line center is selected as an unperturbed resonant field, then first moments may exist (e.g., see Svare and Seidel (1964)].

B. Area and Moments of a First Derivative Absorption Curve

If the narrow band amplifier and phase-sensitive detector are tuned to the modulation frequency, and the modulation amplitude H_m is much less than the line-width, then the recorded line-shape becomes the first derivative Y' of the absorption line Y (see Sec. 10-D)

$$Y' = (d/dH)\, Y \tag{1}$$

shown in Fig. 20–1b. Again we use equal intervals $(H_j - H_{j-1})$ as shown in Fig. 20–1d, so we may write

$$y_j = (H_j - H_{j-1}) \sum_{i=j}^{m} y'_i \tag{2}$$

From eq. (20-A-2), the area A becomes

$$A = (H_j - H_{j-1})^2 \sum_{j=1}^{m} \sum_{i=j}^{m} y'_i \tag{3}$$

$$= (H_j - H_{j-1})^2 \sum_{j=1}^{m} j y'_j \tag{4}$$

The 2nd and 4th moments are given by:

$$\langle H^2 \rangle = \frac{(H_j - H_{j-1})^2}{A} \sum_{j=1}^{m} \sum_{i=j}^{m} (H_j - H_0)^2 y'_i \tag{5}$$

$$\langle H^4 \rangle = \frac{(H_j - H_{j-1})^2}{A} \sum_{j=1}^{m} \sum_{i=j}^{m} (H_j - H_0)^4 y'_i \tag{6}$$

Equations (2)–(4) presuppose that the baseline is chosen properly, so that

$$\sum_{j=1}^{m} y'_j = 0 \tag{7}$$

If this is not the case, then we redefine Y'_j by subtracting a correction term B_1 defined by the displacement shown on Fig. 20–3a

$$\sum_{j=1}^{m} (y'_j - B_1) = 0 \tag{8}$$

whence

$$B_1 = \frac{1}{m} \sum_{j=1}^{m} y'_j \tag{9}$$

Using this, the area is given by

$$A = (H_j - H_{j-1})^2 \sum_{j=1}^{m} \sum_{i=j}^{m} (y'_i - B_1) \tag{10}$$

$$= (H_j - H_{j-1})^2 \sum_{j=1}^{m} j(y'_j - B_1) \tag{11}$$

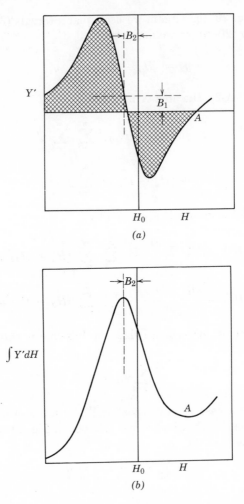

Fig. 20-3. (a) The derivative line for an improper choice of baseline and resonant field H_0, and (b) the shape of the resonant line (a) after integration. A is the point where Y' crosses the incorrect baseline for the second time, and thereby causes the integrated curve to begin to rise again. The shaded areas above and below the baseline of (a) will be equal for the proper choice of baseline (i.e., when $B_1 = 0$).

Equations (5) and (6) presuppose the proper choice of crossover point, and if it is not properly chosen, then a second correction factor B_2 defined by Fig. 20–3a and the relation

$$\sum_{j=1}^{m} (H_j - H_0 - B_2)^2 (y_j' - B_1) = 0 \qquad (12)$$

or more explicitly

$$B_2 = \frac{1}{2} \frac{\displaystyle\sum_{j=1}^{m} (H_j - H_0)^2 (y_j' - B_1)}{\displaystyle\sum_{j=1}^{m} (H_j - H_0)(y_j' - B_1)} \qquad (13)$$

may be included, to give

$$\langle H^2 \rangle = \frac{(H_j - H_{j-1})^2}{A} \sum_{j=1}^{m} \sum_{i=j}^{m} (H_j - H_0 - B_2)^2 (y_i' - B_1) \qquad (14)$$

The fourth moment has the form

$$\langle H^4 \rangle = \frac{(H_j - H_{j-1})^2}{A} \sum_{j=1}^{m} \sum_{i=j}^{m} (H_j - H_0 - B_2)^4 (y_i' - B_1) \qquad (15)$$

An improper choice of the baseline (i.e., $B_1 \neq 0$) will produce an integrated shape of the type shown on Fig. 20–3b. The baseline of the integrated shape will be the same at both ends of the line only if the derivative area (shaded on Fig. 20–3a) is equal above and below the baseline. An improper choice of H_0 (i.e., $B_2 \neq 0$) will not effect the area or integrated shape, but will produce erroneous values of the moments.

The use of eqs. (10)–(14) is illustrated by the calculations shown on Table 20–2. They are performed with a Gaussian line-shape $^G Y'(H)$

$$^G Y'(H_j) = {}^G y_j' = 1.649\, y_m' \left(\frac{H_j - H_0}{\frac{1}{2}\Delta H_{pp}} \right)$$

$$\exp\left[-\frac{1}{2} \left(\frac{H_j - H_0}{\frac{1}{2}\Delta H_{pp}} \right)^2 \right] \qquad (16)$$

TABLE 20-2

Computation of the Correction Factors B_1 and B_2 Illustrated for a Gaussian Derivative Line-Shape, Using Eqs. (9) and (13) of Sec. 20-B

j	y_i'	$(y_i' - B_1)$	$\left(\dfrac{H_i - H_0}{\frac{1}{2}\Delta H_{pp}}\right)$	$\left(\dfrac{H_i - H_0}{\frac{1}{2}\Delta H_{pp}}\right)(y_i' - B_1)$	$\left(\dfrac{H_i - H_0}{\frac{1}{2}\Delta H_{pp}}\right)^2 (y_i' - B_1)$	$\left(\dfrac{H_i - H_0 - B_1}{\frac{1}{2}\Delta H_{pp}}\right)$
1	0.1022	0.0022	-3.0	-0.0066	0.020	-4.0
2	0.1126	0.0126	-2.5	-0.032	0.079	-3.5
3	0.155	0.055	-2.0	-0.110	0.220	-3.0
4	0.280	0.180	-1.5	-0.270	0.405	-2.5
5	0.546	0.446	-1.0	-0.446	0.446	-2.0
6	0.903	0.803	-0.5	-0.401	0.200	-1.5
7	1.100	1.000	0.0	0	0	-1.0
8	0.828	0.728	0.5	0.303	0.152	-0.5
9	0.100	0.000	1.0	0	0	0
10	-0.628	-0.728	1.5	-1.058	-1.587	0.5
11	-0.900	-1.000	2.0	-2.000	-4.000	1.0
12	-0.703	-0.803	2.5	-2.008	-5.020	1.5
13	-0.346	-0.446	3.0	-1.338	-4.014	2.0
14	-0.080	-0.180	3.5	-0.630	-2.205	2.5
15	0.045	-0.055	4.0	-0.220	-0.880	3.0
16	0.0874	-0.0126	4.5	-0.057	-0.255	3.5
17	0.0978	-0.0022	5.0	-0.011	-0.055	4.0
	1.700			-8.285	-16.494	

$$B_1 = \sum_{j=1}^{m} \frac{y_j'}{m} = \frac{1.700}{17} = 0.1$$

$$B_2 = \frac{1}{2} \frac{\sum_{j=1}^{m} (H_j - H_0)^2 (y_j' - B_1)}{\sum_{j=1}^{m} (H_j - H_0) (y_j' - B_1)} = \frac{1}{4} (\Delta H_{pp}) \left(\frac{16.494}{8.285} \right) = 0.996 \ (\tfrac{1}{2} \Delta H_{pp}) \approx 1.00 \ (\tfrac{1}{2} \Delta H_{pp})$$

where $1.649 = e^{1/2}$, and the quantities y_m' and ΔH_{pp} are the derivative half amplitude and the peak-to-peak full line-width (cf. Fig. 20–1 with $y_{m1}' = y_{m2}' = y_m'$. For the sample calculation given in Table 20–2, we let $y_m' = 1$ and $|H_j - H_0| = \frac{1}{4}\Delta H_{pp}$ so that $y'_j = \pm 1$ at the peaks of the line. We deliberately displace the baseline and crossover point from their true values as shown in Fig. 20–3 to illustrate the calculation of the correction factors B_1 and B_2.

From the sum of the second column in Table 20–2 and eq. (9), we find that the first correction factor B_1 equals 0.1, and we subtract 0.1 from each number in the second column to obtain the third column. The fourth column lists the values of $2(H_j - H_0)/\Delta H_{pp}$ obtained with the incorrect choice of crossover point, and the sums of the fifth and sixth columns are put into eq. (13) to obtain $B_2 = 1.00$. This is subtracted from the fourth column to give the seventh column. A proper choice of baseline and crossover point would have given the third and seventh columns directly. The calculations themselves are given in the lower part of the table.

The next step is to compute the area, second moment, and fourth moment, and this is done in Table 20–3 after adjusting the values of y_j' and $(H_j - H_0)$ so that the correction factors B_1 and B_2 vanish. The computations carried out in the table are self-explanatory. The use of eqs. (3), (5), and (6) to calculate A, $\langle H^2 \rangle$, and $\langle H^4 \rangle$ is illustrated at the lower part of the table. Note that the subtotals in the seventh and eighth columns differ considerably for the first half ($1 \leq j \leq 8$) and the second half ($9 \leq j \leq 17$) of the line. If one chooses much smaller magnetic field increments so that $|H_j - H_{j-1}| \ll \Delta H_{pp}$, then the subtotals for each half of the line will become equal, instead of differing by a factor of two or three. It is interesting that the calculated moments are so close to the theoretical ones shown in Table 20–5, despite the large size of the increments $|H_j - H_{j-1}|$. This occurs because the errors on the two halves of the resonance line are in opposite directions, and tend to cancel. If the increments are made sufficiently small, then it is only necessary to carry out the calculation shown on Table 20–3 with half of the lineshape, as was done in the previous section (cf. Table 20–1). When $(H_j - H_{j-1})$ is not much less than ΔH_{pp}, then it is important to select one point at each peak in the resonant line [i.e., the ratio $\frac{1}{2}\Delta H_{pp}/(H_j - H_{j-1})$ should be an integer]. More care is required in calculations with the first derivative Y' because errors can accumulate in the double summation more easily than in the single summation of the straight absorption line Y.

The calculation presented on Table 20–3 may be called the even moment first derivative method, since it entails summations of the type

$$\sum_{j=1}^{m} \sum_{i=1}^{j} (H_j - H_0)^n y'_i$$

with even n. The odd moment method of calculating the area and moments makes use of the following equations, and is illustrated on Table 20–4.

$$A = |H_j - H_{j-1}| \sum_{j=1}^{m} (H_j - H_0) y'_j \tag{17}$$

$$\langle H^2 \rangle = \frac{|H_j - H_{j-1}|}{3A} \sum_{j=1}^{m} (H_j - H_0)^3 y'_j \tag{18}$$

$$\langle H^4 \rangle = \frac{|H_j - H_{j-1}|}{5A} \sum_{j=1}^{m} (H_j - H_0)^5 y'_j \tag{19}$$

$$\langle H^n \rangle = \frac{|H_j - H_{j-1}|}{(n+1)A} \sum_{j=1}^{m} (H_j - H_0)^{n+1} y'_j \tag{20}$$

These relations are the summation analogs to their integral counterparts which will be discussed next. Since eqs. (17)–(20) are completely symmetrical, it is only necessary to calculate for half of the resonance line, as is done on Table 20–4.

If the line-shape is unsymmetrical, then one may treat each half separately with the numbering convention shown in Fig. 20–4. It is best to use smaller intervals ($|H_j - H_{j-1}| \ll \Delta H_{pp}$) for asymmetric lines.

The first derivative line-shape formulae may also be put in integral form. Recall that the absorption amplitude Y is related to the derivative amplitude Y' by the expression

$$Y(H) = \int_{-\infty}^{H} Y'(H) dH \tag{21}$$

TABLE 20-3

Sample Calculation of the Area and Second and Fourth Moments of a Gaussian First Derivative Line-Shape by the Method of Even Moments, Using Eqs. (3), (5), and (6) of Sec. 20-B[a]

j	y_i'	$\sum_{i=1}^{i} y_i'$	$\left(\dfrac{H_i - H_0}{\frac{1}{2}\Delta H_{pp}}\right)$	$\left(\dfrac{H_i - H_0}{\frac{1}{2}\Delta H_{pp}}\right)^2$	$\left(\dfrac{H_i - H_0}{\frac{1}{2}\Delta H_{pp}}\right)^4$	$\left(\dfrac{H_i - H_0}{\frac{1}{2}\Delta H_{pp}}\right)^2 \sum_{i=1}^{i} y_i'$	$\left(\dfrac{H_i - H_0}{\frac{1}{2}\Delta H_{pp}}\right)^4 \sum_{i=1}^{i} y_i'$
1	0.002	0.002	4.0	16.0	256.0	0.03	0.51
2	0.013	0.015	3.5	12.25	150.0	0.18	2.25
3	0.055	0.070	3.0	9.0	81.0	0.63	5.67
4	0.180	0.250	2.5	6.25	39.1	1.56	9.78
5	0.446	0.716	2.0	4.0	16.0	2.86	11.46
6	0.803	1.519	1.5	2.25	5.06	3.42	7.69
7	1.000	2.519	1.0	1.00	1.00	2.52	2.52
8	0.728	3.247	0.5	0.25	0.063	0.81	0.20
		(8.338*)				(12.01*)	(39.88*)
9	0	3.247	0	0	0	0	0
10	−0.728	2.519	0.5	0.25	0.063	0.63	0.16
11	−1.000	1.519	1.0	1.00	1.00	1.52	1.52
12	−0.803	0.716	1.5	2.25	5.06	1.63	3.62
13	−0.446	0.250	2.0	4.0	16.0	1.00	4.00
14	−0.180	0.070	2.5	6.25	39.1	0.44	2.74
15	−0.055	0.015	3.0	9.0	81.0	0.14	1.22
16	−0.013	0.002	3.5	12.25	150.0	0.02	0.30
17	−0.002	0	4.0	16.0	256.0	0	0
		(8.338*)				(5.38*)	(13.56*)
		16.676**				17.39**	53.44**

$$H_j - H_{j-1} = \tfrac{1}{4}\Delta H_{pp}$$

$$A = |H_j - H_{j-1}|^2 \sum_{j=1}^{m} \sum_{i=1}^{j} {y_i}' = (\tfrac{1}{4}\Delta H_{pp})^2 (16.68) = 1.04(\Delta H_{pp})^2$$

$$\langle H^2 \rangle = \frac{|H_j - H_{j-1}|^2}{A} \sum_{j=1}^{m} \sum_{i=1}^{j} (H_i - H_0)^2 {y_i}' = \frac{17.39}{16.68} (\tfrac{1}{2}\Delta H_{pp})^2 = 0.266(\Delta H_{pp})^2$$

$$\langle H^4 \rangle = \frac{|H_j - H_{j-1}|^2}{A} \sum_{j=1}^{m} \sum_{i=1}^{j} (H_i - H_0)^4 {y_i}' = \frac{53.44}{16.68} (\tfrac{1}{2}\Delta H_{pp})^4 = 0.203(\Delta H_{pp})^4$$

[a] Subtotals are indicated by asterisks (*), and grand totals by (**).

TABLE 20–4

Sample Calculation of the Area and Second and Fourth Moments of a Gaussian First Derivative Line-Shape by the Method of Odd Moments, Using Eqs. (17)–(19) of Sec. 20-B

j	y_i'	$\left(\dfrac{H_i - H_0}{\frac{1}{2}\Delta H_{pp}}\right)$	$\left(\dfrac{H_i - H_0}{\frac{1}{2}\Delta H_{pp}}\right)^3$	$\left(\dfrac{H_i - H_0}{\frac{1}{2}\Delta H_{pp}}\right)^5$	$y_i'\left(\dfrac{H_i - H_0}{\frac{1}{2}\Delta H_{pp}}\right)$	$y_i'\left(\dfrac{H_i - H_0}{\frac{1}{2}\Delta H_{pp}}\right)^3$	$y_i'\left(\dfrac{H_i - H_0}{\frac{1}{2}\Delta H_{pp}}\right)^5$
1	0.002	4.0	64.0	1024	~0	0.13	2.05
2	0.013	3.5	42.9	525	0.05	0.56	6.83
3	0.055	3.0	27.0	243	0.17	1.49	13.37
4	0.180	2.5	15.6	98	0.45	2.81	17.64
5	0.446	2.0	8.0	32	0.93	3.73	14.91
6	0.803	1.5	3.4	7.6	1.20	2.73	6.10
7	1.000	1.0	1.0	1	1.00	1.00	1.00
8	0.728	0.5	0.1	~0	0.36	0.07	~0
9	0	0	0	0	0	0	0
					$\overline{4.16}$	$\overline{12.52}$	$\overline{61.90}$
					$\times\,2$	$\times\,2$	$\times\,2$
					$\overline{8.32}$	$\overline{25.04}$	$\overline{123.8}$

$$H_i - H_{i-1} = \tfrac{1}{4}\Delta H_{pp}$$

$$A = |H_i - H_{i-1}| \sum_{j=1}^{m} (H_i - H_0)y_i' = (\tfrac{1}{4}\Delta H_{pp})(8.32)(\tfrac{1}{2}\Delta H_{pp}) = 1.04(\Delta H_{pp})^2$$

$$\langle H^2 \rangle = \left(\frac{H_i - H_{i-1}}{3A}\right)\sum_{j=1}^{m} (H_i - H_0)^3 y_i' = \frac{\tfrac{1}{4}\Delta H_{pp}(25.04)}{3 \times 1.04(\Delta H_{pp})^2}\,(\tfrac{1}{2}\Delta H_{pp})^3 = 0.253(\Delta H_{pp})^2$$

$$\langle H^4 \rangle = \left(\frac{H_i - H_{i-1}}{5A}\right)\sum_{j=1}^{m} (H_i - H_0)^5 y_i' = \frac{\tfrac{1}{4}\Delta H_{pp}(123.8)}{5 \times 1.04(\Delta H_{pp})^2}\,(\tfrac{1}{2}\Delta H_{pp})^5 = 0.187(\Delta H_{pp})^4$$

and the area A and nth moment $\langle H^b \rangle$ are obtained through integrating by parts

$$A = \int_{-\infty}^{\infty} Y dH \tag{22}$$

$$= -\int_{-\infty}^{\infty} (H - H_0)\, Y' dH + (H - H_0)\, Y \Big|_{-\infty}^{\infty} \tag{23}$$

$$= -\int_{-\infty}^{\infty} (H - H_0)\, Y' dH \tag{24}$$

since for all line-shapes of finite area

$$\lim_{H \to \pm\infty} (H - H_0)\, Y = 0 \tag{25}$$

The nth moment is given by

$$\langle H^n \rangle = \int_{-\infty}^{\infty} (H - H_0)^n Y dH \tag{26}$$

$$= -\frac{1}{n+1} \int_{-\infty}^{\infty} (H - H_0)^{n+1} Y' dH + (H - H_0)^{n+1} Y \Big|_{-\infty}^{\infty} \tag{27}$$

$$= -\frac{1}{n+1} \int_{-\infty}^{\infty} (H - H_0)^{n+1} Y' dH \tag{28}$$

which is valid if

$$\lim_{H \to \pm\infty} [(H - H_0)^{n+1} Y] = 0 \tag{29}$$

This condition (29) is satisfied by a Gaussian line-shape for all n, but not by a Lorentzian line-shape (except for $n = 0$).

There are limitations on the functional dependence of Y' for physically acceptable line-shapes. For example, from eq. (25), Y must vanish at $H \to \pm\infty$ if A is to be finite, and in addition,

$$\int_{-\infty}^{\infty} Y' dH = 0 \tag{30}$$

if A is to be physically meaningful.

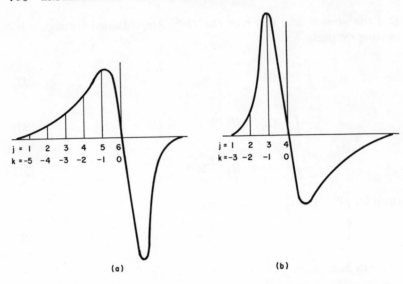

Fig. 20-4. Method of integrating an unsymmetrical absorption derivative line-shape: (a) on the low field side, and (b) on the high field side.

As mentioned above, the value of the nth moment is dependent on the choice of H_0, and to make this choice unambiguous one, may further require that

$$\int_{-\infty}^{\infty} (H - H_0)^2 Y' dH = 0 \qquad (31)$$

If these two requirements are not satisfied, then one may define correction factors B_3 and B_4 so that

$$\int_{-\infty}^{\infty} (Y' - B_3) dH = 0 \qquad (32)$$

$$\int_{-\infty}^{\infty} (H - H_0 - B_4)^2 (Y' - B_3) \, dH = 0 \qquad (33)$$

as was done in the summation case above [eqs. (8)–(13)]. In the ensuing discussion it will be assumed that the correction factors B_3 and B_4 are both zero.

Recall that a Gaussian line has the shape

$$^{G}Y(H) = y_m \exp\left[- \left(\frac{H - H_0}{\frac{1}{2}\Delta H_{1/2}} \right)^2 \ln 2 \right] \qquad (34)$$

and differentiation yields

$$^{G}Y'(H) = \frac{2y_m \ln 2}{\frac{1}{2}\Delta H_{1/2}} \left(\frac{H - H_0}{\frac{1}{2}\Delta H_{1/2}} \right) \exp\left[- \left(\frac{H - H_0}{\cdot\frac{1}{2}\Delta H_{1/2}} \right)^2 \ln 2 \right] \qquad (35)$$

Equation (16) gave the Gaussian line in terms of its maximum amplitude y_m' which occurs at

$$H - H_0 = \pm\tfrac{1}{2}\Delta H_{pp} \qquad (36)$$

and hence Y' has the form

$$^{G}Y'(H) = e^{1/2} y_m\left(\frac{H - H_0}{\frac{1}{2}\Delta H_{pp}} \right) \exp\left[- \frac{1}{2} \left(\frac{H - H_0}{\frac{1}{2}\Delta H_{pp}} \right)^2 \right] \qquad (35a)$$

Therefore the maximum absorption amplitude y_m and the maximum first derivative amplitude y_m' are related by the expression

$$y_m = e^{1/2} y_m'(\tfrac{1}{2}\Delta H_{pp}) \qquad (37)$$

where $e^{1/2} = 1.6487$. The Gaussian line-shape of eq. (16) may also be written in the form

$$^{G}Y'(H) = y_m'\left(\frac{H - H_0}{\frac{1}{2}\Delta H_{pp}} \right) \exp\left\{ - \frac{1}{2} \left[\left(\frac{H - H_0}{\frac{1}{2}\Delta H_{pp}} \right)^2 - 1 \right] \right\} \qquad (35b)$$

which is sometimes more convenient for calculations.

The integrations that are required for using the Gaussian first derivative line-shape to calculate the even moments are fairly easy using eqs. (20) and (21) of the last section, and they lead to the same results obtained with the absorption line itself, so they will not be repeated here. Since the line-shape in eq. (37) is in terms of ΔH_{pp} and y_m' rather than $\Delta H_{1/2}$ and y_m, the answers obtained in the derivative case have a slightly different form from those calculated with the absorption line $Y(H)$ itself. The characteristics of a Gaussian line-shape are summarized in the following expressions, and in Table 20–5:

$$\Delta H_{1/2} = (2 \ln 2)^{1/2} \, \Delta H_{pp} \tag{38}$$

$$A = (2\pi e)^{1/2}(\tfrac{1}{2}\Delta H_{pp})^2 \, y'_m \tag{39}$$

and

$$\langle H^n \rangle = (n - 1) \; !!(\tfrac{1}{2}\Delta H_{pp})^n \quad \text{(for even } n) \tag{40}$$

where $(n - 1) \; !! = (n - 1) \, (n - 3) \ldots (5) \, (3) \, (1)$. It is noteworthy that the nth even moment has such a simple relationship to $(\tfrac{1}{2}\Delta H_{pp})^n$.

TABLE 20–5

Comparison of Gaussian and Lorentzian Line-Shapes

Parameter	Gaussian shape	Lorentzian shape
$\Delta H_{1/2}/\Delta H_{pp}$	$(2 \ln 2)^{1/2} = 1.1776$	$3^{1/2} = 1.7321$
$y_m/(y_m'\Delta H_{pp})$	$e^{1/2}/2 = 0.8244$	$4/3 = 1.3333$
$y_m/(y_m''\Delta H_{pp}{}^2)$	$1/4 = 0.2500$	$3/8 = 0.3750$
$A/(y_m\Delta H_{1/2})$	$\tfrac{1}{2}(\pi/\ln 2)^{1/2} = 1.0643$	$\pi/2 = 1.5708$
$A/(y_m'\Delta H_{pp}{}^2)$	$\tfrac{1}{2}(\pi e/2)^{1/2} = 1.0332$	$2\pi/3^{1/2} = 3.6276$
$\langle H^2 \rangle/(\Delta H_{1/2})^2$	$1/(8 \ln 2) = 0.1803$	∞
$\langle H^4 \rangle/(\Delta H_{1/2})^4$	$3/[64(\ln 2)^2] = 0.0974$	∞
$\langle H^2 \rangle/(\Delta H_{pp})^2$	$1/4 = 0.2500$	∞
$\langle H^4 \rangle/(\Delta H_{pp})^4$	$3/16 = 0.1875$	∞
y_1''/y_2''	$\tfrac{1}{2}e^{3/2} = 2.2409$	$64^{1/3} = 4$
$H_1''/\Delta H_{pp}$	0.626	0.567
$H_2''/\Delta H_{pp}$	$3^{1/2} = 1.7321$	$3^{1/2} = 1.7321$
$H_3''/\Delta H_{pp}$	2.52	$81^{1/4} = 3$
$d'(0)/d'(3^{1/2}) = A/B$	$7/2 = 3.50$	$2^3 = 8$

For solid DPPH, $A/[y_m'(\Delta H_{pp})^2] = 2.2^*$

$\left. \begin{matrix} e = 2.718282 \\ \pi = 3.141593 \end{matrix} \right.$ $\left. \begin{matrix} \ln 2 \\ \log_e 2 \end{matrix} \right\} = 0.693147$

$2^{1/2} = 1.414214 \qquad \pi^{1/2} = 1.772454$

$3^{1/2} = 1.732051 \qquad (\ln 2)^{1/2} = 0.832555$

$e^{1/2} = 1.648722$

* J. S. Hyde, unpublished notes.

The Lorentzian derivative line-shape has the normalized form

$$^{L}Y'(H) = \frac{16y_m'\left(\frac{H - H_0}{\frac{1}{2}\Delta H_{pp}}\right)}{\left[3 + \left(\frac{H - H_0}{\frac{1}{2}\Delta H_{pp}}\right)^2\right]^2} \tag{41}$$

where

$$y_m = \frac{4}{3}(\Delta H_{pp})\, y_m' \tag{42}$$

It is straightforward to compute the following relations for this line-shape

$$A = \frac{2\pi}{3^{1/2}}\, y_m'(\Delta H_{pp})^2 \tag{43}$$

$$\Delta H_{1/2} = 3^{1/2}\, \Delta H_{pp} \tag{44}$$

The properties of the Lorentzian line-shape are given in Table 20–5.

The line-shape formulae are important to take into account when comparing the areas of different curves. For example, when a Lorentzian and a Gaussian spectrum have the same derivative amplitude y_m' and width ΔH_{pp}, the former corresponds to $(3.63/1.03) = 3.51$ times as many spins as the latter. This may be seen from the fifth entry of Table 20–5, where for this case,

$$\frac{\text{Lorentzian area}}{\text{Gaussian area}} = 4\left(\frac{2\pi}{3e}\right)^{1/2} = 3.51 \tag{45}$$

The corresponding figure for the ratio of the areas of a Lorentzian absorption line to a Gaussian one with the same amplitude y_m and width $\Delta H_{1/2}$ is $(1.57/1.06) = 1.48$.

In this and the preceding section we discussed the summation forms for computing the area and moments of spectral lines. These summations are readily adapted for computer calculations. The correction factors B, B_1, and B_2 are easily calculated by a computer before proceeding to the determination of A and the $\langle H^n \rangle$. Collins (1959) Lebedev, Chernikova, Tikhomirova, and Voevodskii (1963), Murthy (1963), and Young (1964) discuss such computer calculations. Tolkachev and Mikhailov (1964) describe a nomogram for the double integration of an ESR signal.

C. Area and Moments of a Second Derivative Absorption Curve

If the narrow band amplifier and lock-in detector are tuned to the second harmonic of the modulation frequency, then the recorded signal will be the second derivative of the resonance absorption. The second derivative may also be recorded with a double modulation arrangement. These second derivative signals are not customarily employed for computing areas and moments, and so this section will be confined to a discussion of the integral formulation of the line-shape

The second derivative of the line-shape Y'' is defined by

$$Y' = \int_{-\infty}^{H} Y'' dH \tag{1}$$

so that

$$A = \int_{-\infty}^{\infty} dH \int_{-\infty}^{H} dH' \int_{-\infty}^{H'} Y'' dH'' \tag{2}$$

$$= \frac{1}{2} \int_{-\infty}^{\infty} (H - H_0)^2 Y'' dH \tag{3}$$

and

$$\langle H^n \rangle = \frac{1}{(n+1)(n+2)} \int_{-\infty}^{\infty} (H - H_0)^{n+2} Y''(H) dH \tag{4}$$

where the formulae are derived by integrating by parts twice (cf. eqs. (21)–(29) of the last section).

The explicit form of Y'' for a normalized Gaussian line-shape may be obtained by differentiating eq. (16) or (35b) of the last section

$$^G Y''(H) = y_m'' \left[\left(\frac{H - H_0}{\frac{1}{2}\Delta H_{pp}} \right)^2 - 1 \right] \exp \left[-\frac{1}{2} \left(\frac{H - H_0}{\frac{1}{2}\Delta H_{pp}} \right)^2 \right] \tag{5}$$

where $y_m = y_m'' \, (\frac{1}{2}\Delta H_{pp})^2$ defines the normalization constant y_m''. The maxima may be found by differentiating $^G Y''$, and setting the result equal to zero

$$(d/dH) \, ^G Y''(H) = 0 \tag{6}$$

to obtain the expression

$$\frac{H - H_0}{\frac{1}{2}\Delta H_{pp}} \left[\left(\frac{H - H_0}{\frac{1}{2}\Delta H_{pp}} \right)^2 - 3 \right] \exp \left[-\frac{1}{2} \left(\frac{H - H_0}{\frac{1}{2}\Delta H_{pp}} \right)^2 \right] = 0 \tag{7}$$

which has the five solutions

$$(H - H_0)/\tfrac{1}{2}\Delta H_{pp} = 0, \pm 3^{1/2} \pm \infty \tag{8}$$

The quantities H_1'' and H_3'' shown in Fig. 20–5 correspond to the points where Y'' equals $\tfrac{1}{2}y_1''$ and $\tfrac{1}{2}y_2''$, respectively, and H_2'' is the separation of the peaks. For a Gaussian line-shape these parameters have the explicit values

$$H_1'' = 0.626\ \Delta H_{pp} \tag{9}$$

$$H_2'' = 3^{1/2}\ \Delta H_{pp} \tag{10}$$

$$H_3'' = 2.52\ \Delta H_{pp} \tag{11}$$

and the ratio y''_1/y''_2 is given by

$$y_1''/y_2'' = \tfrac{1}{2}e^{3/2} = 2.241 \tag{12}$$

For a normalized Lorentzian line $(y_m' = \tfrac{9}{32}y_m''\ \Delta H_{pp})$,

$$^L Y'' = 27y_m'' \left[\frac{1 - \left(\dfrac{H - H_0}{\tfrac{1}{2}\Delta H_{pp}} \right)^2}{\left[3 + \left(\dfrac{H - H_0}{\tfrac{1}{2}\Delta H_{pp}} \right)^2 \right]^3} \right] \tag{13}$$

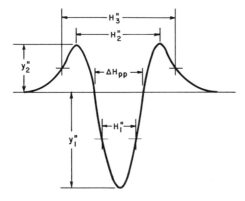

Fig. 20–5. Definitions of parameters used to characterize the second derivative of a resonant absorption line. The line-shape shown is Gaussian.

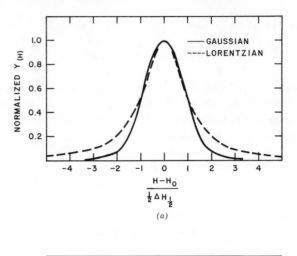

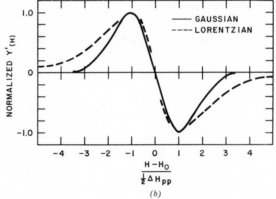

Fig. 20–6. (a) Lorentzian and Gaussian absorption curves with the same half amplitude line-width. (b) Lorentzian and Gaussian absorption first derivative curves with the same peak-to-peak line-width.

and its maxima are easily found to be at the same numerical values as in the Gaussian case

$$(H - H_0)/\tfrac{1}{2}\Delta H_{pp} = 0, \pm 3^{1/2}, \pm \infty \qquad (14)$$

As a result, for a Lorentzian line-shape we obtain

$$H''_1 = 0.567 \, \Delta H_{pp} \qquad (15)$$

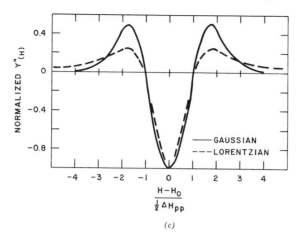

Fig. 20–6.   (c) Lorentzian and Gaussian absorption second derivative curves with the same peak-to-peak line-width.

$$H''_2 = 3^{1/2} \Delta H_{pp} \tag{16}$$

$$H''_3 = 3\Delta H_{pp} \tag{17}$$

$$y''_1/y''_2 = 4 \tag{18}$$

D. Comparison of Lorentzian and Gaussian Line-Shapes

The Lorentzian shape is slightly sharper in the center and decreases much more slowly in the wings beyond the half amplitude or first derivative points.   The two shape functions may be compared in the manner shown on Fig. 20–6, where the two absorption curves are drawn with the same half amplitude line-widths $\Delta H_{1/2}$, and the two first and second derivative curves are plotted with the same peak to peak line-widths ΔH_{pp}.   The line-shapes of experimental spectra are frequently compared to these two theoretical shapes by matching them at three points to the Lorentzian and Gaussian shapes in the manner shown in Fig. 20–7.

Figure 20–8 shows the dramatic difference between the two line-shapes when the absorption curves are matched at their inflection points, and when the first derivative curves are matched at the half amplitude points.

The difference between Lorentzian and Gaussian line-shapes is illustrated by the data in Tables 20–6 to 20–10. The dispersion line-shape is discussed in Sec. 20-G. Van Gerven and Van Itterbeek (1961) discuss Lorentzian and Gaussian line-shapes arising in weak magnetic field experiments.

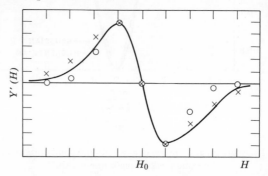

Fig. 20–7. An asymmetric experimental spectrum $Y'(H)$ matched to ($\times$) Lorentzian and (O) Gaussian shapes with the same amplitude y_m' and width ΔH_{pp}.

TABLE 20–6

Amplitudes of Gaussian and Lorentzian Absorption Line-Shapes at Multiples of $\tfrac{1}{2}\Delta H_{1/2}$ from the Center as Shown on Figure 20–6a Using Data Computed from Eqs. (9) and (23) of Sec. 20-A

$\left(\dfrac{H - H_0}{\tfrac{1}{2}\Delta H_{1/2}}\right)$	Amplitude $Y(H)$	
	Gaussian	Lorentzian[a]
0	1.0000	1.0000
0.5	0.8409	0.8000
1	0.5000	0.5000
1.5	0.2101	0.3077
2	0.0626	0.2000
3	0.00195	0.1000
4	1.5×10^{-5}	0.0588
5	—	0.0384
6	—	0.0270
7	—	0.0200
8	—	0.0154
9	—	0.0122
10	—	0.0099

[a] When $\left| H - H_0 \right| > 10\Delta H_{1/2}$, one may approximate $Y(H) \sim y_m \left[(H - H_0)/ \tfrac{1}{2}\Delta H_{1/2}\right]^{-2}$ for the Lorentzian shape.

The line-shape of an observed spectrum $Y'(H)$ may be deduced from its peak amplitude y_m' and line-width ΔH_{pp} by using the data of Table 20–7 to calculate the expected values for Lorentzian and Gaussian shapes. These points are placed on the experimental spectrum in the manner shown in Fig. 20–7. The illustrated spectrum has a shape between the two at low fields, and close to the former at high fields. Tables 20–6, 20–8, 20–9, and 20–10 may be used for checking other types of spectra. Marguardt, Bennett, and Burrell

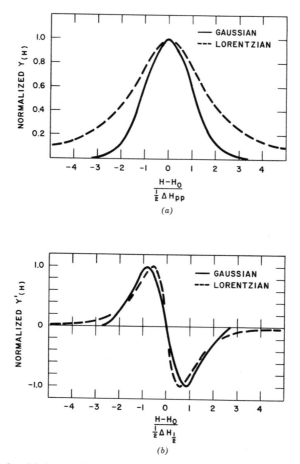

Fig. 20–8.   (a) Lorentzian and Gaussian absorption curves with the same peak-to-peak line-width ΔH_{pp}. (b) Lorentzian and Gaussian absorption first derivative curves with the same half amplitude line-width $\Delta H_{1/2}$.

TABLE 20-7

Amplitudes of Gaussian and Lorentzian Absorption First Derivative Line-Shapes at Multiples of $\frac{1}{2}\Delta H_{pp}$ from the Center, as Shown on Fig. 20–6b Using Data Computed from Eqs. (16) and (41) of Sec. 20-B

$\left(\dfrac{H - H_0}{\frac{1}{2}\Delta H_{pp}}\right)$	Amplitude $Y'(H)$	
	Gaussian[a]	Lorentzian[b]
0	0.0000	0.0000
0.5	0.7275	0.7574
1	1.0000	1.0000
1.5	0.8029	0.8701
2	0.4461	0.6531
3	0.0549	0.3333
4	0.0022	0.1773
5	3×10^{-5}	0.1020
6	1.5×10^{-7}	9.0631
7	—	0.0414
8	—	0.0285
9	—	0.0204
10	—	0.0151

[a] Note that $1.649\, xe^{-x^2/2} = xe^{-(x^2-1)/2}$ where $x = [(H - H_0)/(\frac{1}{2}\Delta H_{pp})]^2$.

[b] When $|H - H_0| > 10\Delta H_{pp}$, we may set $Y'(H) \sim 16 y_m'[(H - H_0)\frac{1}{2}\Delta H_{pp}]^{-3}$ for the Lorentzian shape.

(1961) and Ibers and Swalen (1962) describe how to obtain a least squares fit between a calculated and an observed spectrum, and Johnston and Hecht (1965) give a more recent treatment of this problem. One may use different techniques to subtract a known spectrum from an unknown to reveal hidden structure, as discussed in Sec. 14-K and illustrated in Fig. 14–40 [see also Smith and Pieroni (1964)].

Singer, Spry, and Smith (1957) and Tikhomirova and Voevodskii (1959) present graphical methods for determining whether or not an experimental spectrum is Gaussian or Lorentzian in shape. Young (1964) describes a Fortran II program for calculating and displaying Gaussian and Lorentzian absorption and derivative lines.

Swarup (1959) observed a gradual transformation of the ESR line-shape of Cr^{+3} in potassium cobalticyanide and potassium aluminum alum single crystals from Lorentzian to Gaussian as the

TABLE 20-8

Amplitudes of Gaussian and Lorentzian Absorption Second Derivative Line-Shapes at Multiples of $\frac{1}{2}\Delta H_{pp}$ from the Center as Shown on Figure 20-6c Using Data Computed from Eqs. (5) and (13) of Sec. 20-C[a]

$\left(\dfrac{H - H_0}{\frac{1}{2}\Delta H_{pp}}\right)$	Amplitude $Y''(H)$	
	Gaussian	Lorentzian
0	−1.0000	−1.0000
0.5	−0.6619	−0.5899
1	0.0000	0.0000
1.5	0.4058	0.2332
$3^{1/2}$	0.4463	0.2500
2	0.4060	0.2362
3	0.0889	0.1250
4	0.0050	0.0590
5	10^{-4}	0.0295
6	—	0.0159
7	—	0.0092
8	—	0.0057
9	—	0.0036
10	—	0.0025

[a] The maximum amplitude occurs at $(H - H_0)/\frac{1}{2}\Delta H_{pp} = 3^{1/2}$ for both line-shapes. It has the value $2e^{-3/2} = 0.44626$ for the Gaussian shape and $\frac{1}{4}$ for the Lorentzian shape.

[b] When $|H - H_0| > 10\Delta H_{pp}$, we may use the approximation $Y''(H) \sim 27 y_m''[(H - H_0)/\frac{1}{2}\Delta H_{pp}]^{-4}$ for Lorentzian lines.

chromium concentration changed. Grant and Strandberg (1964) developed a statistical theory of spin interactions, and showed that a resonance line is Lorentzian in the center, and Gaussian in the wings [see also, Anderson and Welling (1965)].

E. Cut-off Lorentzian Line-Shapes

The Lorentzian line-shape has an infinite second moment, as was mentioned above. One frequently encounters line-shapes which are Lorentzian near the center but which fall off faster than a Lorentzian in the wings, and consequently give a finite second moment. A simple line-shape of this type is the cut-off Lorentzian [Kittel and Abrahams (1953)]. It is assumed that the amplitude is identical to

TABLE 20-9

Amplitudes of Lorentzian Dispersion Line-Shape at Multiples of $\frac{1}{2}\Delta H_{1/2}$ from the Center Using Data Calculated from Eq. (1) of Sec. 20-G

$\left(\dfrac{H - H_0}{\frac{1}{2}\Delta H_{1/2}}\right)$	Amplitude, d[a]
0	0.0000
0.5	0.8000
1	1.0000
1.5	0.9231
2	0.8000
3	0.6000
4	0.4706
5	0.3846
6	0.3243
7	0.2800
8	0.2462
9	0.2195
10	0.1980

[a] When $|H - H_0|/\frac{1}{2}\Delta H_{1/2}$ exceeds 10 we may use the approximation $d \sim \Delta H_{1/2}/(H - H_0)$.

TABLE 20-10

Amplitudes of Lorentzian Dispersion First Derivative Line-Shape at Multiples of $\frac{1}{2}\Delta H_{pp}$ from the Center Using Data Calculated from Eq. (2) of Sec. 20-G

$\left(\dfrac{H - H_0}{\frac{1}{2}\Delta H_{pp}}\right)$	Amplitude, d'[a]
0	−1.0000
0.5	−0.7811
1	−0.3750
1.5	0.0816
$3^{1/2}$	0.0000
2	0.0612
3	0.1250
4	0.1080
5	0.0842
6	0.0651
7	0.0510
8	0.0408
9	0.0332
10	0.0274

[a] $d' \sim 3[(H - H_0)/\frac{1}{2}\Delta H_{pp}]^{-2}$ when $|H - H_0| > 10\Delta H_{pp}$.

that corresponding to a Lorentzian line from $-a \leq H \leq a$, and zero beyond these limits, as shown in Fig. 20–9. The first derivative curve is cut off at $H - H_0 = \pm a$ without taking account of the discontinuity there.

The area of a cut-off Lorentzian line is given by

$$A = y_m \int_{-a}^{a} \frac{dH}{1 + \left(\dfrac{H - H_0}{\frac{1}{2}\Delta H_{1/2}}\right)^2} \tag{1}$$

$$= y_m \Delta H_{1/2} \int_{0}^{\tan^{-1}(2a/\Delta H_{1/2})} d\theta \tag{2}$$

$$= y_m \Delta H_{1/2} [\pi/2 - \cot^{-1}(2a/\Delta H_{1/2})] \tag{3}$$

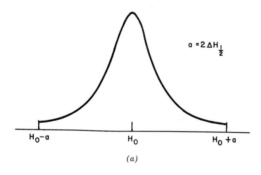

$a = 2\,\Delta H_{\frac{1}{2}}$

$H_0 - a$ H_0 $H_0 + a$

(a)

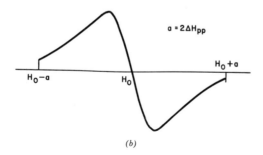

$a = 2\Delta H_{pp}$

$H_0 - a$ H_0 $H_0 + a$

(b)

Fig. 20–9.   Cut off Lorentzian line-shape: (a) absorption curve and (b) first derivative curve.

where $\tan \theta = 2(H - H_0)/\Delta H_{1/2}$. When

$$2a/\Delta H_{1/2} \gg 1 \qquad (4)$$

one may expand the arc cotangent in a power series, and neglect all but the first term, giving

$$\cot^{-1} (2a/\Delta H_{1/2}) \sim \Delta H_{1/2}/2a \qquad (5)$$

so that

$$A \sim y_m \Delta H_{1/2} (\pi/2 - \Delta H_{1/2}/2a) \qquad (6)$$

Thus the area of a Lorentzian line which is cut-off considerably beyond the half power point is equal to the area of the corresponding Lorentzian curve less a small correction term.   In terms of the first derivative line-shape one has, of course, (neglecting the discontinuity at $H = H_0 \pm a$)

$$A = (4/3^{1/2}) \, y_m'(\Delta H_{pp})^2 \, (\pi/2 - 3^{1/2}\Delta H_{pp}/2a) \qquad (7)$$

The second moment of a cut-off Lorentzian line-shape is given by

$$\langle H^2 \rangle = \frac{y_m}{A} \int_{-a}^{a} \frac{(H - H_0)^2 dH}{1 + \left(\dfrac{H - H_0}{\frac{1}{2}\Delta H_{1/2}}\right)^2} \qquad (8)$$

$$= \frac{\frac{1}{4}(\Delta H_{1/2})^3 y_m}{A} \int_{0}^{\tan^{-1} (2a/\Delta H_{1/2})} \tan^2 \theta \, d\theta \qquad (9)$$

$$= \frac{(\frac{1}{2}\Delta H_{1/2})^2 \left[\dfrac{2a}{\Delta H_{1/2}} - \dfrac{\pi}{2} + \cot^{-1} \dfrac{2a}{\Delta H_{1/2}}\right]}{[\pi/2 - \cot^{-1}(2a/\Delta H_{1/2})]} \qquad (10)$$

and when $a \gg \Delta H_{1/2}$, three of the terms may be neglected, giving

$$\langle H^2 \rangle \sim a\Delta H_{1/2}/\pi \qquad (11)$$

A similar integration provides the fourth moment in the same approximation $a \gg \Delta H_{1/2}$ [Kittel and Abrahams (1953)]

$$\langle H^4 \rangle \sim (1/3\pi) \, a^3 \Delta H_{1/2} \qquad (12)$$

The treatment presented in this section may also be applied to a cut-off Gaussian line-shape, and the results will be in terms of incomplete gamma functions.

F. The Voigt Line-Shape

When the spectral line is broadened independently by both Gaussian and Lorentzian effects, the absorption amplitude is given by [Posener (1959)]

$$Y_{(v,b)} = \frac{b}{\pi} \int_{-\infty}^{\infty} \frac{e^{-x^2} dx}{b^2 + (v - x)^2} \tag{1}$$

where b is a measure of the ratio of the Lorentzian line width $^L\Delta H_{1/2}$ to the Gaussian width $^G\Delta H_{1/2}$

$$b = (\ln 2)^{1/2} \, ^L\Delta H_{1/2}/^G\Delta H_{1/2} \tag{2}$$

and v is the distance from the line center H_0 in units of $^G\Delta H_{1/2}/2 \ln 2$, as follows

$$v = 2(\ln 2)^{1/2} (H - H_0)/^G\Delta H_{1/2} \tag{3}$$

This Voigt profile function (1) has been tabulated for various values of b and v. For a particular resonance line $^G\Delta H_{1/2}$ and $^L\Delta H_{1/2}$ will be constant, so that the shape Y becomes a function only of $(H - H_0)$

$$Y(H - H_0) = \frac{(\ln 2)^{1/2}}{\pi} \left(\frac{^L\Delta H_{1/2}}{^G\Delta H_{1/2}} \right)$$

$$\times \int_{-\infty}^{\infty} \frac{e^{-x^2} dx}{\left(\frac{^L\Delta H_{1/2}}{^G\Delta H_{1/2}} \right)^2 \ln 2 + \left(2(\ln 2)^{1/2} \frac{H - H_0}{^G\Delta H_{1/2}} - x \right)^2} \tag{4}$$

Unfortunately this cannot be integrated in closed form.

The Voigt line-shape is seldom encountered, so it will not be discussed further.

G. Dispersion Line-Shapes

A Lorentzian dispersion signal d has the form

$$d = \frac{2\left(\dfrac{H - H_0}{\frac{1}{2}\Delta H_{1/2}}\right)}{1 + \left(\dfrac{H - H_0}{\frac{1}{2}\Delta H_{1/2}}\right)^2} \tag{1}$$

and its first derivative d' is

$$d' = 3\frac{3 - \left(\dfrac{H - H_0}{\frac{1}{2}\Delta H_{pp}}\right)^2}{\left[3 + \left(\dfrac{H - H_0}{\frac{1}{2}\Delta H_{pp}}\right)^2\right]^2} \tag{2}$$

These two expressions are individually normalized so that each has a maximum amplitude of one, and as usual $\Delta H_{1/2} = 3^{1/2}\Delta H_{pp}$. The derivative d' vanishes at $H - H_0 = \pm\frac{1}{2}\Delta H_{1/2}$ and reaches extrema at

$$(H - H_0)/\tfrac{1}{2}\Delta H_{pp} = 0, \pm 3 \tag{3}$$

Numerical values for eqs. (1) and (2) are given in Tables 20–9 and 20–10. The ratio $d'(0)/d'(3^{1/2})$ equals 8 for a Lorentzian line and 7/2 for a Gaussian line. This ratio is called A/B in Sec. 14-A and corresponds to y_1''/y_2'' in Fig. 20–5 for the absorption derivative. Nagasawa (1965) discusses the variation of the ratio A/B and other dispersion-made parameters on the modulation frequency and relaxation time T_1.

Pake and Purcell (1948, 1949) analyzed the absorption χ' and dispersion χ'' of the magnetic resonance susceptibility χ

$$\chi = \chi' - i\chi'' \tag{4}$$

for both Lorentzian and Gaussian line-shapes. They used the simplified notation.

$$\chi' = \begin{cases} x/(1 + x^2) & \text{Lorentzian} \tag{5a} \\[2mm] \dfrac{2}{\pi^{1/2}}\, e^{-x^2/\pi} \displaystyle\int_0^{x/\pi^{1/2}} \exp y^2\, dy & \text{Gaussian} \tag{5b} \end{cases}$$

and

$$\chi'' = \begin{cases} 1/(1 + x^2) & \text{Lorentzian} \quad (6a) \\ e^{-x^2/\pi} & \text{Gaussian} \quad (6b) \end{cases}$$

where the dimensionless variable x corresponds to a normalized value of $(H - H_0)$, and their normalization constants differ from ours. Their line-shapes for the real and imaginary parts of the susceptibility χ are plotted in Fig. 20–10 and the corresponding first derivative line shapes are shown in Fig. 20–11.

When the ESR sample is held in a high-Q resonant cavity, the dispersion mode χ' corresponds to a change in frequency, and the absorption mode χ'' corresponds to a change in Q as one scans through the resonance condition.   When the klystron frequency is stabilized on the sample resonant cavity, the dispersion signal is "stabilized out" and only χ'' is observed.   When the klystron frequency is stabilized on an auxiliary cavity, then one observes either dispersion, absorption, or a mixture of the two, depending on the phase adjustment on the slide screw tuner or phase shifter in the microwave bridge.   If an experimental spectrum contains a mixture of χ' and χ'', then one may use the technique discussed at the end of Sec. 14-A, or that of Peter, Shaltiel, Wernick, Williams, Mock, and Sherwood (1962) to obtain the ratio of χ' to χ''.

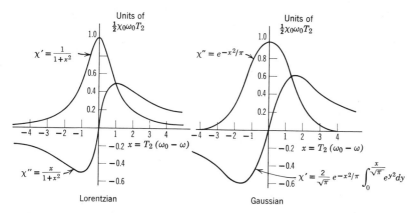

Fig. 20–10.   A comparison of the dispersion χ' and absorption χ'' curves for Lorentzian and Gaussian line-shapes [Pake and Purcell (1948, 1949)].

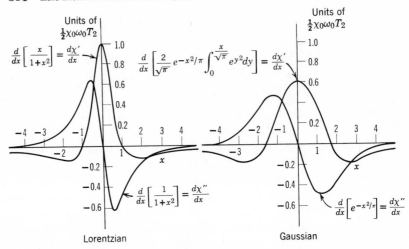

Fig. 20–11. A comparison of the dispersion $(d\chi'/dx)$ and absorption $(d\chi''/dx)$ derivatives for Lorentzian and Gaussian line-shapes [Pake and Purcell (1948, 1949)].

H. The Dysonian Line-Shape

The theory of the ESR line-shapes obtained from conduction electrons in metals was worked out by Dyson (1955) and confirmed experimentally by Feher and Kip (1955) in their extension of the original work of Griswold, Kip, and Kittel (1952) [see Cousins and Dupree (1965)]. Dyson showed that the line-shape depends upon the time T_D that it takes an electron to diffuse through the skin depth δ, the time T_T that it takes for the electron to traverse the sample, the electron spin lattice relaxation time T_1, and the electron spin-spin relaxation time T_2 (for metals $T_1 = T_2$). In the region of the normal skin depth where the electron mean free path Λ is small in comparison with the skin depth δ, Feher and Kip (1955) give the following formulae for the line-shape Y and its derivative Y' in the units of absorbed power P and power absorbed per unit angular frequency $Y_\omega' = dP/d\omega$ [or $Y'_H = dP/dH$].

(1) For $T_T \ll T_D$ one has

$$Y = \frac{\omega H_1^2}{4} (V) \, \omega_0 \chi_0 T_2 \frac{1}{1 + (\omega - \omega_0)^2 T_2^2} \tag{1}$$

$$Y'_\omega = -\frac{\omega H_1^2}{4} (V) \, \omega_0 \chi_0 T_2 \frac{2(\omega - \omega_0) \, T_2^2}{[1 + (\omega - \omega_0)^2 T_2^2]^2} \tag{2}$$

where V is the volume of the sample, H_1 is the rf magnetic field amplitude, χ_0 is the paramagnetic part of the static susceptibility, and $\omega_0 = g\beta H_0/\hbar$ is the resonant frequency. This is a Lorentzian line-shape which is independent of diffusion.

(2) For sufficiently thick samples one has $T_T \gg T_D$ and $T_T \gg T_2$; and for an arbitrary ratio of $T_D/T_2 = R^2$ the line-shape has the form

$$Y = -\left[\frac{\omega H_1^2}{4}(A\delta)\,\omega_0\chi_0 T_2\right]\left(\frac{T_D}{2T_2}\right)$$

$$\times \left\{ \frac{R^4(\chi^2 - 1) + 1 - 2R^2\chi}{[(R^2\chi - 1)^2 + R^4]^2}\left[\frac{2\xi}{R(1 + \chi^2)^{1/2}} + R^2(\chi + 1) - 3\right]\right.$$

$$\left. + \frac{2R^2(1 - \chi R^2)}{[(R^2\chi - 1)^2 + R^4]^2}\left[\frac{2\eta}{R(1 + \chi^2)^{1/2}} + R^2(\chi - 1) - 3\right]\right\} \quad (3)$$

where $\chi = (\omega - \omega_0)\,T_2$, $\xi = [(\omega - \omega_0)/(|\omega - \omega_0|)]\,[(1 + \chi^2)^{1/2} - 1]^{1/2}$, $\eta = [(1 + \chi^2)^{1/2} + 1]^{1/2}$, and $A = $ the surface area. Equation (3) is plotted in Fig. 20–12 and its graphically determined first derivative y' is shown in Fig. 20–13 for the cases $T_D/T_2 \ll 1$ and $T_D/T_2 \to \infty$. Equation (3) and its first derivative have simplified forms for the following two limiting cases:

(2a) In this case we have $T_T \gg T_2 \gg T_D$ which corresponds to metals of high conductivity (low temperature)

$$Y \cong \left[\frac{\omega H_1^2}{4}(A\delta)\,\omega_0\chi_0 T_2\right]$$

$$\times \left[\frac{\omega - \omega_0}{|\omega - \omega_0|}\left\{\frac{T_D}{T_2}\left[\frac{(1 + \chi^2)^{1/2} - 1}{1 + \chi^2}\right]^{1/2}\right\}^{1/2}\right] \quad (4)$$

$$Y'_\omega \cong -\left[\frac{\omega H_1^2}{4}(A\delta)\,\omega_0\chi_0 T_2^2\left(\frac{T_D}{T_2}\right)^{1/2}\right]$$

$$\times \left\{\frac{[2 - (1 + \chi^2)^{1/2}][1 + (1 + \chi^2)^{1/2}]^{1/2}}{2(1 + \chi^2)^{3/2}}\right.$$

$$\left. + \left(\frac{T_D}{T_2}\right)\left[\frac{(1 + \chi^2)^{1/2} - 1}{1 + \chi^2}\right]^{1/2}\right\} \quad (5)$$

When $T_D/T_2 \to 0$, the second term within the curly brackets becomes negligible relative to the first.

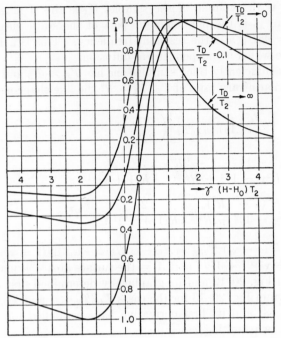

Fig. 20–12. Electron spin resonance power absorption $Y = P$ in thick metal films for different ratios of the diffusion time T_D to the spin-spin relaxation time T_2 [Feher and Kip (1955)].

(*2b*) Here we have $T_T \gg T_D \gg T_2$ corresponding to thick films with slowly diffusing magnetic dipoles. This condition applies to the case of paramagnetic impurities distributed throughout the volume of the metal. This condition also corresponds to the nuclear magnetic resonance of metals [Bloembergen (1952)] since the nuclei are almost completely stationary. The line-shapes are

$$Y = \left[\frac{\omega H_1^2}{4} (A\delta) \, \omega_0 \chi_0 T_2 \right] \left[\frac{1}{2} \frac{1 - T_2(\omega - \omega_0)}{1 + T_2{}^2(\omega - \omega_0)^2} \right] \tag{6}$$

$$Y'_\omega = \left[\frac{\omega H_1^2}{4} (A\delta) \, \omega_0 \chi_0 T_2 \right] \left[\frac{T_2}{4} \frac{T_2^2(\omega - \omega_0)^2 - 2T_2(\omega - \omega_0) - 1}{[1 + T_2{}^2(\omega - \omega_0)^2]^2} \right] \tag{7}$$

using Wagoner's (1960) correction for eq. (7).

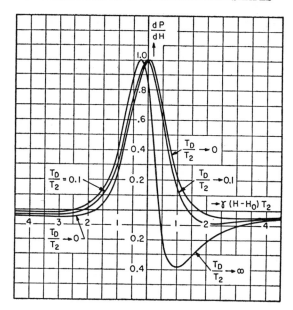

Fig. 20–13. Derivative of the ESR power absorption $Y' = dP/d\omega$ in thick metal plates for different ratios of the diffusion time T_D to the spin-spin relaxation time T_2 [Feher and Kip (1955)].

Equations (1)–(7) all omit terms in Dyson's formulae which replace $(\omega - \omega_0)$ by $(\omega + \omega_0)$, since near resonance, the latter terms are negligible for sufficiently narrow lines. The above expressions also neglect the effect of surface relaxations which are important whenever there exist strong spin-dependent forces during a collision of the electron with the surface. Surface relaxation effects are more important in the cases of thin films and small particles than they are in the thick cases. Dyson's original paper (1955) should be consulted for further details.

Figures 20–14 and 20–15 show the dependence of two line-shape parameters on the ratio $(T_D/T_2)^{1/2}$. They may be employed to determine values of T_2 and the g factor. Figures 20–16 and 20–17 reveal how the asymmetry of the line varies with the ratio $(T_D/T_2)^{1/2}$. Feher and Kip (1955) discuss the physical significance of the ratio A/B. Wagoner (1960) applied these figures to graphite.

Feher and Kip (1955) found satisfactory agreement between Dyson's theory and their experimental results. They assumed that

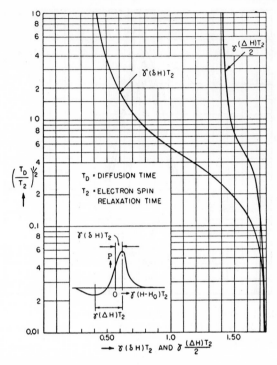

Fig. 20–14. Plots of $(T_D/T_2)^{1/2}$ vs. $\gamma(\delta H)T_2$ and $\gamma\Delta HT_2/2$ for the ESR power absorption in thick metal films [Feher and Kip (1955)].

the mean free path Λ is small compared to the skin depth δ, and that all of the electrons have the velocity v in accordance with the expression

$$T_D = 3(\delta^2/v\Lambda)/2 \qquad (8)$$

One may use the well-known conductivity formula

$$\sigma = Ne^2\Lambda/m^*v \qquad (9)$$

where N is the number of electrons per cm^3 and m^* is the effective mass to obtain

$$T_D = \tfrac{3}{2}\,(\delta^2 Ne^2/\sigma m^* v^2) \qquad (10)$$

When the electron mean free path Λ exceeds the skin depth δ, then the skin effect is anomalous, and the exact theory of Reuter and

Sondheimer (1948) must be utilized. Kittel extended the Dyson theory to the case of the anomalous skin effect $\delta < \Lambda$ under the assumption that the diffusion time T_D is short in relation to the relaxation time. The line-shape in terms of the complex impedance $Z = A + iB$ is

$$
Y = \left[\frac{\omega H_1^2}{4} (\Lambda A) \, \omega_0 \chi_0 \left(\frac{c^2}{4\pi\omega\Lambda} \right)^2 (6T_2\tau)^{1/2} \right]
$$
$$
\times \left\{ (B^2 - A^2) \left[\frac{(1+\chi^2)^{1/2} + 1}{1 + \chi^2} \right]^{1/2} \right.
$$
$$
\left. + 2AB \frac{\omega - \omega_0}{|\omega - \omega_0|} \left[\frac{(1+\chi^2)^{1/2} - 1}{1 + \chi^2} \right]^{1/2} \right\} \quad (11)
$$

$$
Y'_H = \left[\frac{\omega H_1^2 \gamma T_2}{4} (\Lambda A) \, \omega_0 \chi_0 \left(\frac{c^2}{4\pi\omega\Lambda} \right)^2 (6T_2\tau)^{1/2} \right]
$$
$$
\times \left\{ \frac{B^2 - A^2}{2} \left(\frac{2 + (1+\chi^2)^{1/2}}{1 + \chi^2} \right) \left[\frac{(1+\chi^2)^{1/2} - 1}{1 + \chi^2} \right]^{1/2} \right.
$$
$$
\times \left(\frac{\omega - \omega_0}{|\omega - \omega_0|} \right) + AB \, \frac{[(1+\chi^2)^{1/2} - 2][(1+\chi^2)^{1/2} + 1]}{(1+\chi^2)^{3/2}} \right\}
$$
$$
(12)
$$

The ratio B/A may be obtained from Fig. 1 of Reuter and Sondheimer (1948). Equations (11) and (12) are plotted in Fig. 20–18 for the region of the completely anomalous skin effect where $\delta \ll \Lambda$ and $B/A = 3^{1/2}$.

Dresselhaus, Kip, and Kittel (1955) give expressions for the line-shape obtained from plasma resonance in crystals in terms of the parameters ν and ν' which are defined by $(\omega\tau = \nu)$

$$
\nu_c = \omega_c\tau = (eH/m^*c)\tau \quad (13)
$$

$$
\nu' = \omega'\tau = \nu - \nu_p^2/\nu \quad (14)
$$

$$
\nu_p = \omega_p\tau = \tau(L_iNe^2/m^*)^{1/2} \quad (15)
$$

where H is the applied magnetic field, L_i is the depolarization factor, N is the conduction electron concentration, ω is the applied frequency, ω_c is the cyclotron frequency, ω_p is the plasma frequency,

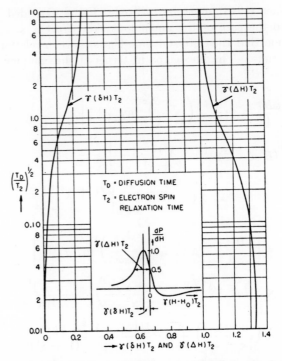

Fig. 20–15.   Plots of $(T_D/T_2)^{1/2}$ vs. $\gamma(\delta H)T_2$ and $\gamma(\Delta H)T_2$ for the derivative of the ESR power absorption in thick metal films [Feher and Kip (1955)].

and τ is the relaxation time.   The theoretical line-shape is shown in Figs. 20–19 and 20–20 for two types of modulation in the limiting case $\nu \ll \nu'$ so that $\nu' = -\nu_p^2/\nu$.   Rukhadze and Silin (1962) discuss cyclotron resonance line-shapes in nonrelativistic plasmas.

I. Dipole-Dipole Broadening of Small Clusters

The local magnetic field $\mathbf{H}$ produced by a magnetic dipole of spin $\mathbf{S}_1$ at a distance $\mathbf{r}$ from its center is given by

$$\mathbf{H} = (g\beta/r^3)\,[\mathbf{S}_1 - 3\mathbf{r}(\mathbf{r}\cdot\mathbf{S}_1/r^2)] \tag{1}$$

This local magnetic field alters the total value of $\mathbf{H}$ at the positions of neighboring unpaired spins, and thereby broadens their resonant

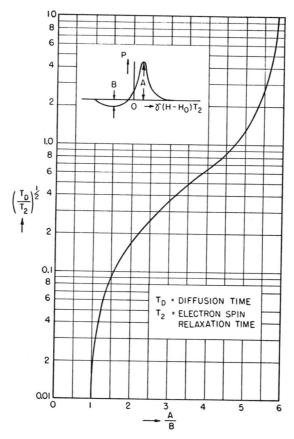

Fig. 20–16.   The ratio $(T_D/T_2)^{1/2}$ vs. A/B for the ESR power absorption in thick metal plates [Feher and Kip (1955)].

lines.   The dipolar interaction energy $\mathcal{H}_{dd}$ between $\mathbf{S}_1$ and an identical magnetic moment with spin $\mathbf{S}_2$ is given by

$$\mathcal{H}_{dd} = (g^2\beta^2/r^3)\ [\mathbf{S}_1\cdot\mathbf{S}_2 - 3(\mathbf{r}\cdot\mathbf{S}_1)(\mathbf{r}\cdot\mathbf{S}_2)/r^2] \tag{2}$$

In a strong applied magnetic field $\mathbf{H}_0$ oriented at an angle relative to the vector $\mathbf{r}$, the two spins will be quantized along H_0, and for like spins $S_1 = S_2$, eq. (2) becomes

$$\mathcal{H}_{dd} = S(S + 1)\ (g^2\beta^2/r^3)\ (1 - 3\cos^2\theta) \tag{3}$$

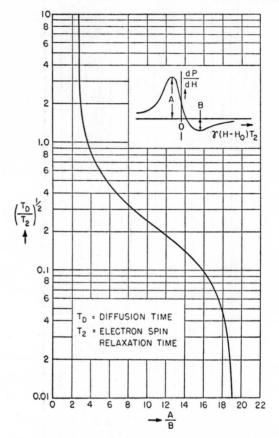

Fig. 20–17.   The ratio $(T_D/T_2)^{1/2}$ vs. A/B for the derivative of the ESR power absorption in thick metal plates [Feher and Kip (1955)].

If the spins are not identical, then $\mathcal{H}_{dd}$ is reduced by the factor 2/3. In other words, a like neighbor is 3/2 as effective in broadening a line as an unlike neighbor.

By averaging the dipolar interaction over all angles corresponding to a random distribution of directions **r**, the line-shape for a pair of interacting dipoles was found by Pake (1948) to have the form shown in Fig. 20–21c. This line-shape was observed experimentally by Pake (1948) and by Gutowsky, Kistiakowsky, Pake, and Purcell (1949).   The line-shape collapses to half its width when the nuclei rotate rapidly about a line perpendicular to the internuclear axis.

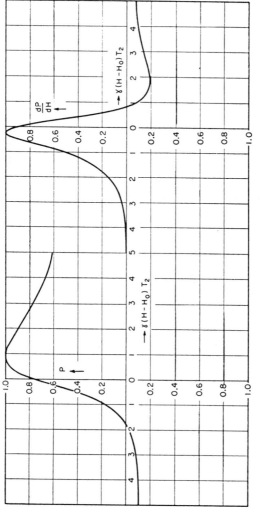

Fig. 20–18.   Theoretical curves for the ESR absorption $Y = P$ and its derivative $Y'_H = dY/dH$ in the region of the completely anomalous skin effect [Feher and Kip (1955)].

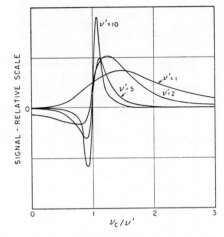

Fig. 20-19. The theoretical line-shape in plasma resonance absorption when the carrier concentration is modulated [Dresselhaus, Kip, and Kittel (1955)].

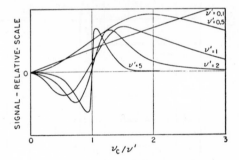

Fig. 20-20. The theoretical line-shape in plasma resonance when the magnetic field is modulated [Dresselhaus, Kip, and Kittel (1955)].

The treatment just discussed has been generalized to three magnetic moments forming the apices of an equilateral triangle by Andrew and Bersohn (1950), and observed experimentally by Richards and Smith (1951), and by Kakiuchi, Shono, Komatsu, and Kigoshi (1951, 1952). The powder pattern line-shape has nine points which "blow up" to infinity, as shown on Fig. 20-21. In practice these infinities are rendered finite by other broadening mechanisms [see Andrew (1953), p. 157]. When this three-spin system rotates about the threefold symmetry axis normal to its

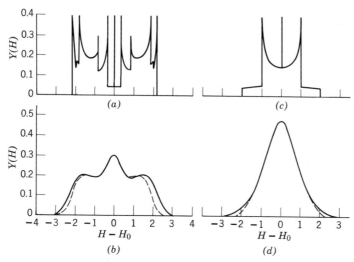

Fig. 20–21. Powder pattern line-shapes obtained for (a) three nuclei of spin ½ at the apices of an equilateral triangle and (c) two nuclei when the component (or single crystal) line-width in each case is a delta function. When the component lines have a finite width the observed line-shapes change from (a) and (c) to the solid lines of (b) and (d), respectively. The dashed lines of (b) and (d) correspond to experimental data. [Andrew and Bersohn (1950)]. The abscissa is in the units $3\mu/2R^3$ where μ is the magnetic moment and R is the distance between the nuclei.

plane, it produces the same line-shape as two coupled spins [Fig. 20–21(c) and (d); Andrew and Bersohn (1950)]. The case of a three-spin system with one nucleus between a pair of another species was analyzed by Waugh, Humphrey, and Yost (1953). Blinc, Trontelj, and Volavšek analyzed a nearly linear five-spin system.

Line broadening by the pseudodipolar coupling mechanism is seldom appreciable, and will not be discussed [see Van Vleck (1937); White (1959); Abragam (1961); Seiden (1965)].

J. Line-Shapes for Anisotropic g Factors

Many paramagnetic single crystals have electron spin resonance absorptions which occur at magnetic field strengths that depend on the orientation of the crystal with respect to the magnetic field direction [Kikuchi and Cohen (1954); Bowers and Owen (1955);

Van Roggen, Van Roggen, and Gordy (1957)]. This phenomenon can be explained by noting that for paramagnetic substances the fine structure Hamiltonian $\mathfrak{K}$, omitting the terms which depend on the nuclear spin is given by [see p. 18 and Pryce (1950)].

$$\mathfrak{K} = \mathbf{S} \cdot \mathbf{D} \cdot \mathbf{S} + \beta \mathbf{S} \cdot \mathbf{g} \cdot \mathbf{H}$$

where $\mathbf{D}$ and $\mathbf{g}$ are tensors which are constants for a given orbital state, β is the Bohr megneton, and $\mathbf{H}$ is the strength of the applied magnetic field. If the total electronic spin S is $\frac{1}{2}$, the first term, which represents the zero field splitting, vanishes [Kramers' degeneracy, Kramers (1930)]. Then the resonance magnetic field H' is

$$H' = \hbar\nu/g'\beta \tag{1}$$

where the value of H' depends on the orientation of the crystal in accordance with the expression

$$g' = (g_1{}^2 \cos^2 \theta_1 + g_2{}^2 \cos^2 \theta_2 + g_3{}^2 \cos^2 \theta_3)^{1/2} \tag{2}$$

Here the θ_i are the angles between the direction of the magnetic field and the coordinate axes in which the $\mathbf{g}$ tensor is diagonal, and the g_i are the diagonal components of $\mathbf{g}$. This coordinate system need not be the same as the symmetry axes of the crystal, but it corresponds to the symmetry axes for the local internal electric field.

When the paramagnetic substance is in the form of a powder or is suspended in an amorphous solid, the absorption line-shape will, in general, be asymmetric because of the random orientations of the molecules in the substance. Sands (1955) obtained a resonance line-shape by assuming a random distribution of orientations, and then averaging the resonance magnetic field over all orientations. However, Sands assumed that the crystalline electric field has at, least tetragonal symmetry, and hence sets $g_2 = g_3 = g_\perp$. This section will derive the line-shape by a similar method assuming three unequal $\mathbf{g}$ tensor components $g_1 \geq g_2 \geq g_3$ [Bloembergen and Rowland (1953); Kohin and Poole (1958); Kneubühl (1960)]. A more accurate calculation would take into account the variation of the transition probability with the g factor [Bleaney (1960)] as was done in many of the more recent articles listed in Table 20–11.

The orientation of a particular molecule in the sample may be specified by the two angles θ_1 and θ_2 since all the θ_i are not independent. It is more convenient, however, to choose an alternate pair of independent variables u and ψ to specify the orientation. These are defined by

$$u = \cos \theta_1$$

$$\cos^2 \theta_2 = (1 - u^2) \sin^2 \psi \tag{3}$$

where θ and ψ are two of the Euler angles describing the orientation of the molecular axes. Specification of the third Euler angle ϕ is unnecessary since rotations about the direction of the applied magnetic field are immaterial. These parameters are illustrated in Fig. 20–22. We then obtain

$$g' = [(g_1{}^2 - g_3{}^2) u^2 + (g_2{}^2 - g_3{}^2)(1 - u^2) \sin^2 \psi + g_3{}^2]^{1/2} \tag{4}$$

We now calculate the probability $p(u_1, \psi_1)$ that a molecule will assume an orientation u_1, ψ_1 such that $u \leq u_1 \leq u + du$ and $\psi \leq \psi_1 \leq \psi + d\psi$. Let $p(u_1, \psi_1) = p(u_1) \, p(u_1|\psi_1)$, where $p(u_1)$ is the probability that $u \leq u_1 \leq u + du$ and $p(u_1|\psi_1)$ is the probability that, for a given $u_1, \psi \leq \psi_1 \leq \psi + d\psi$. Assuming a random orienta-

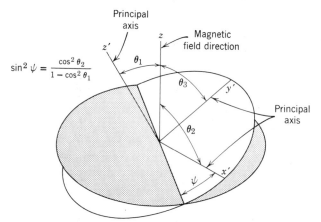

Fig. 20–22. Illustration of the angles used to specify the orientation of a crystal [Kohin and Poole (1958)].

tion, both $p(u_1)$ and $p(u_1|\psi_1)$ are constants times du and $d\psi$, respectively. Then the normalized probability is

$$4\pi p(u, \psi) = du d\psi \tag{5}$$

It is now necessary to integrate this probability distribution over the line-shape of the component lines. We take $Y(H - H')$ to be the line-shape factor for the absorption in a single crystal, where H is the applied magnetic field and $H' = H'(u,\psi)$ is the field for the resonance maximum of the single crystal as given by eqs. (1) and (2). Here Y is assumed not to depend explicitly on the orientation [see Livingston and Zeldes (1956)]. It is normalized such that

$$\int_{-\infty}^{\infty} Y(H - H')\, dH = 1.$$

Then, for a randomly oriented group of crystals, the normalized intensity $I(H)$ is given by

$$
\begin{aligned}
I_{(H)} &= \frac{1}{4\pi} \int_{-1}^{1} \int_{0}^{2\pi} Y(H - H')\, du d\psi \\
&= \frac{2}{\pi} \int_{0}^{1} \int_{0}^{\pi/2} Y(H - H')\, du d\psi
\end{aligned}
\tag{6}
$$

To perform this integration we will use eq. (4) to change the independent variables from u,ψ to u,g', and we will then integrate first over the variable u. This may be accomplished by putting $d\psi = (\partial\psi/\partial g)\, dg$. For a fixed value of g', the limits of integration for u may be evaluated by mapping the area of integration onto the u,g' plane (Fig. 20–23). The integral thereby decomposes into two integrals depending on whether g' is less than or greater than g_2. We write

$$I_A(g') = (1/g')\, (\partial\psi/\partial g')\, du \text{ for } g_2 \le g' \le g_1$$

and

$$I_B(g') = (1/g')\, (\partial\psi/\partial g')\, du \text{ for } g_3 \le g' \le g_2$$

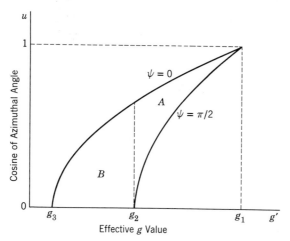

Fig. 20–23.   Mapping of the u,g' plane showing regions A and B over which the integration for the intensity is to be performed [Kohin and Poole (1958)].

Then in region A, $u_{(\psi=\pi/2)} \leq u \leq u_{(\psi=0)}$, and in region B, $0 \leq u \leq u_{(\psi=0)}$. By means of suitable transformations both of these integrals may be converted to complete ellipitic integrals of the first kind K [see Jahnke and Emde (1945)].   We then obtain

$$I_A(g') = (1/a_g \, K) \, (b_g/a_g) \tag{7a}$$

$$I_B(g') = (1/b_g \, K) \, (a_g/b_g) \tag{7b}$$

where

$$a_g = [(g_2{}^2 - g_3{}^2) \, (g_1{}^2 - g^2)]^{1/2} \tag{8a}$$

$$b_g = [(g_1{}^2 - g_2{}^2) \, (g^2 - g_3{}^2)]^{1/2} \tag{8b}$$

Equation (7) can be used to obtain the probability distribution as a function of g.

If we replace all g values in eq. (7) by the appropriate H-values, the normalized intensity is given by

$$I(H) = \frac{2H_1 H_2 H_3}{\pi} \left\{ \int_{H_1}^{H_2} \frac{I_A(H')}{(H')^2} \, Y(H - H') \, dH' \right.$$

$$\left. + \int_{H_2}^{H_3} \frac{I_B(H')}{(H')^2} \, Y(H - H') \, dH' \right\} \tag{9}$$

where the factor $H_1H_2H_3/(H')^2$ appears after making this replacement. Now if we assume that the component lines are extremely narrow, we can put $Y(H - H') = \delta(H - H')$ where $\delta(H - H')$ is the Dirac delta function. Then

$$I(H) = \frac{2H_1H_2H_3}{\pi H^2} \begin{cases} \dfrac{1}{a_H} K(a_H/b_H) & H_1 \leqslant H \leqslant H_2 \\ \dfrac{1}{b_H} K(b_H/a_H) & H_2 \leqslant H \leqslant H_3 \\ 0 & \text{otherwise} \end{cases} \quad (10)$$

where

$$a_H = [(H_3{}^2 - H_2{}^2)(H^2 - H_1{}^2)]^{1/2} \tag{11a}$$

$$b_H = [(H_2{}^2 - H_1{}^2)(H_3{}^2 - H^2)]^{1/2} \tag{11b}$$

This line-shape has been plotted in Fig. 20–24 taking carbazyl (N-picryl-9-amino-carbazyl) as an example. The values assumed for the parameters are taken from Kikuchi and Cohen (1954). The three g factors g_1, g_2, and g_3 are related to the magnetic field strengths H_1, H_2, and H_3 by the relation

$$H_1 = h\nu/g_1\beta \tag{12a}$$

$$H_2 = h\nu/g_2\beta \tag{12b}$$

$$H_3 = h\nu/g_3\beta \tag{12c}$$

where $h\nu$ is the quantum of microwave energy. These relations may be used to deduce g factors from powder pattern spectra. Bloembergen and Rowland (1953) calculated a similar line-shape using the approximation $(g_1 + g_2)/(g_2 + g_3) = 1$.

If the component line-shape cannot be assumed to be extremely narrow, then the integrals in eq. (9) may be evaluated numerically without difficulty. The infinite peak is so narrow that the area lost by cutting it off after $K = \pi$ is negligible. The general effect of integrating over a line of nonzero width is to lower and widen the peak, and to round off the shoulders. This is illustrated in Fig. 20–24 for carbazyl, where a Gaussian line-shape having a width of 0.5 G is assumed.

This description of the line-shape for a paramagnetic substance is particularly useful for the determination of the principle g values of a substance when it is impossible to prepare the substance in the form of a single crystal.   This is also true in the case of many free radicals formed directly in solids by ultra-violet rays, x-rays, or gamma rays, or condensed in solids after their formation in an electric discharge. In either case, the free radicals would be expected to see randomly oriented crystalline fields.   The three g tensor components can be most easily obtained by examining the derivative of the absorption, as is normally done in electron spin resonance spectrometers (Fig. 20–25).   If the component line-width is smaller than the separation between the g tensor components, the derivative will have maxima very near to g_1 and g_3, and will cross the axis sharply very close to g_2. The g tensor components may then be obtained quite accurately.   As the component line-width becomes wider, however, the peaks at g_1

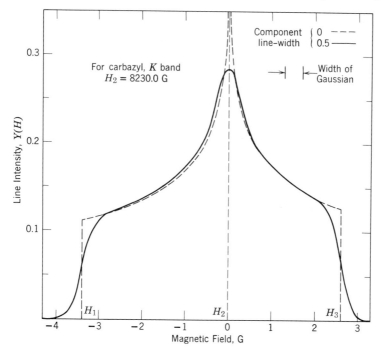

Fig. 20–24.   Calculated powder pattern line-shape for carbazyl assuming both zero and nonzero component line-widths [Kohin and Poole (1958)].

and g_3 tend to become obscured, as shown in Fig. 20–26 for the case of axial symmetry where $g_1 = g_2 = g_\perp$ and $g_3 = g_\parallel$.

If the anisotropic molecule rotates about randomly with a correlation time which is much shorter than the reciprocal of the spread of the spectrum in frequency units $\hbar/(|g_1 - g_3|\beta H)$, then a single resonant line is obtained at the average g factor g_0 given by

$$g_0 = \tfrac{1}{3}(g_1 + g_2 + g_3) \tag{13}$$

The correlation time is the average time that it takes a molecule to move through an angle of one radian or a distance equal to its diameter.

If there is an axis of magnetic symmetry, then the spin will be characterized by $g_\parallel$ along the axis and $g_\perp$ at right angles to the axis. With axial symmetry the three g factors of the general case may be related to $g_\parallel$ and $g_\perp$ as follows

$$\left.\begin{aligned} g_1 &= g_\parallel \\ g_2 &= g_3 = g_\perp \end{aligned}\right\} g_\perp < g_\parallel \tag{14a}$$

$$\left.\begin{aligned} g_1 &= g_2 = g_\perp \\ g_3 &= g_\parallel \end{aligned}\right\} g_\parallel < g_\perp \tag{14b}$$

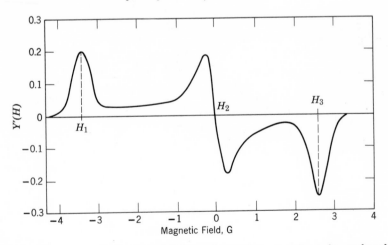

Fig. 20–25. Derivative of the ESR powder pattern line-shape for carbazyl [Kohin and Poole (1958)].

The two cases arise because of our assumption that $g_1 \geq g_2 \geq g_3$. The line-shape for $g_\parallel \ll g_\perp$ has the form shown on Fig. 20–27. Mathematically it corresponds to the merging of the infinity found at g_2 in Fig. 20–24 with the discontinuity at the edge of the line-shape.

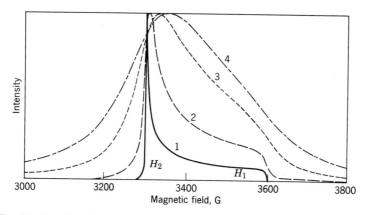

Fig. 20–26. The effect of increasing the component line-width on the calculated spectrum for an axially symmetric powder pattern. Lorentzian linewidths: (1) 1 G; (2) 10 G; (3) 50 G; (4) 100 G [Ibers and Swalen (1962)].

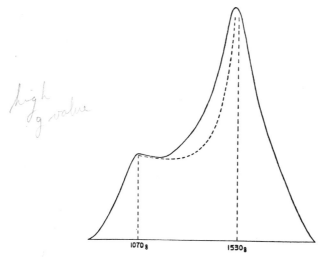

Fig. 20–27. (– –) The delta function line-shape for an axially symmetric g factor compared to (—) an experimental spectrum for a glass sample [Sands (1955)].

The case of axial symmetry is frequently met in practice. Again, rapid rotation will reduce the spectrum to a symmetrical resonance centered at g_0

$$g_0 = \tfrac{1}{3}(g_\parallel + 2g_\perp) \tag{15}$$

The effect of axially symmetric hyperfine structure on the line-shape of a sample with an axially symmetric g factor was solved by O'Reilly (1958) with the aid of the Hamiltonian $\mathcal{3C}$

$$(1/\beta)\,\mathcal{3C} = g_\parallel H_z S_z + g_\perp (H_x S_x + H_y S_y) + A I_z S_z$$
$$+ B(I_x S_x + I_y S_y) \tag{16}$$

where I is the nuclear spin, and the hyperfine constants A and B are in gauss. Each hyperfine component is characterized by its projection M_I along the z axis which lies in the magnetic field direction. There are components corresponding to M_I which assume integer or half integer values ranging from I to $-I$. As shown on Fig. 20–28 each component hyperfine line will stretch from $(H_0 g_0 - B m_I)/g_\perp$ to $(H_0 g_0 - A m_I)/g_\parallel$ on the magnetic field scale, where $H_0 = h\nu/g_0\beta$, and g_0 is defined by eq. (15). One often finds experimentally that the powder patterns of the various hyperfine components overlap each other.

A number of investigators have performed calculations and obtained theoretical line-shape functions for polycrystalline substances. These calculations are summarized in Table 20–11. A shorter form

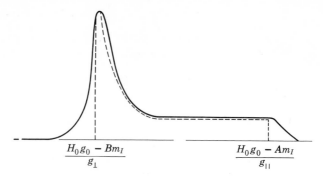

Fig. 20–28. Powder pattern line-shape for one hyperfine component m_I when $g_0 H_0 \gg A, B$ [O'Reilly (1958)].

of this table is found in the article by Ibers and Swalen (1962). Draghicescu (1963) has reviewed anisotropy in ESR studies, but the contents of his paper are not readily available linguistically. Hughes and Rowland (1964) present numerical integrations of anisotropic Gaussian line-shapes. Lefebvre and Maruani (1965) developed a

TABLE 20-11

Summary of Line-Shape Calculations with Anistropic g Factors

g tensor	Hfs	Crystallite line-shape	Ref.
Axial	None	Delta	Bleaney (1950, 1951, 1960)
Asymmetric	None	Delta	Bloembergen and Rowland (1953)
Axial	None	Delta	Sands (1955)
Isotropic	None	Delta	Singer (1955)[a]
Asymmetric	None	Delta	Kohin and Poole (1958)
Axial	Axial	Delta	O'Reilly (1958)
Axial	None	Lorentzian and Gaussian	Searl, Smith, and Wyard (1959, 1960, 1961)[b]
Asymmetric	None	Delta	Kneubühl (1960)
Isotropic	Asymmetric	Delta and Gaussian	Blinder (1960)
Isotropic	Asymmetric	Gaussian	Lefebvre (1960)
Isotropic	Asymmetric	Delta	Sternlicht (1960)
Asymmetric	None	Lorentzian	Chirkov and Kokin (1960)
Axial	Axial	Delta	Neiman and Kivelson (1961)
Asymmetric	—	Gaussian	Lefebvre (1961)
Axial	—	—	Kneubühl and Natterer (1961)
Axial	None	Lorentzian	Ibers and Swalen (1962)
Axial	None	—	Heuer (1961)
Axial	None	Delta	Gersmann and Swalen (1962)
Axial	Axial	Lorentzian and Gaussian	Vänngård and Aasa (1963)
Axial	Axial	Gaussian	Hughes and Rowland (1964)
Axial	None	Arbitrary	Korolkov and Potapovich (1964)
Asymmetric	None	—	Johnston and Hecht (1965)
Axial	Axial	Lorentzian and Gaussian	Malley (1965)[b]
Asymmetric	None	Lorentzian	Schoffa and Bürk (1965)

[a] Zero field $S = 3/2$ term included.
[b] Valid only for small anisotropy.

computer program for interpreting the ESR spectra of dilute free radicals in amorphous solids.   Aasa and Vänngård (1964) obtained a correction factor which may be used to convert integrated areas to spin concentrations by taking into account the dependence of the transition probability on the g factor [Bleaney (1960)].

Burns (1961) and Weil and Hecht (1963) discuss the experimental determination of anisotropic g factors and zero field splitting parameters from powdered samples.   Weil and Anderson (1958) show how to evaluate completely anisotropic g factors from ESR data obtained at a series of orientations in the magnetic field.   Scheffler and Stegmann (1963) determined g factors to a precision of ca. 5×10^{-6} [see also Bronstein and Volterra (1965)].   Kneubühl and Natterer (1961) discuss the complex ESR line-shapes in anisotropic substances with fine structure ($S > \frac{1}{2}$, $D \neq 0$).   Kottis and Lefebvre (1963) calculated the line-shape for randomly oriented molecules in a triplet state [see also, Hudson and McLachlan (1965)].

Shaltiel and Low (1961) discuss the effects of mosaic structure on anisotropic broadening in dilute single crystals.   This broadening results from the various crystallites of the single crystal making slightly different angles with respect to the applied magnetic field direction.   Shaltiel and Low derived a general formula for the line-shape and width, and estimated the average deviation of the crystallites from the crystal symmetry axis.   See also Curtis, Kirkby, and Thorp (1965).   Lünd and Vänngård (1965) show how to evaluate fine and hyperfine constants in a single crystal with hyperfine structure and several molecules per unit cell.   Schonland (1959) used a similar method to determine principal g values.   Scott, Stapleton, and Wainstein (1965) present a study of rare earth double nitrates whose line widths are strongly orientation dependent.   Erdös (1964) published a theoretical discussion of anisotropic g factors.

K. Origin of the Moments of Spectral Lines

The first few sections of this chapter explained how to determine the moments of experimentally observed resonance lines.   This section will explain how to compute moments from the positions of paramagnetic centers and nuclei in the crystal lattice for comparison with the measured values.   Judeikis (1964) analyzed the errors that result from neglecting the "wings" of the line in calculating moments from observed spectra.

The basic article on this subject was written by Van Vleck (1948). A system of electron spins S_j interacting with an applied magnetic field H (Zeeman energy) produces a resonance line whose width is determined by the dipolar interaction [Luttinger and Tisza (1946)] and the exchange interaction [Van Vleck (1932)] with other spins in accordance with the Hamiltonian

$$\mathcal{3C} = g\beta H \underbrace{\sum_j S_{zj}}_{\text{Zeeman energy}} + \underbrace{\sum_{k>j} \tilde{A}_{jk} \mathbf{S}_j \cdot \mathbf{S}_k}_{\text{Exchange energy}}$$

$$+ g^2\beta^2 \sum_{k>j} \underbrace{\left[\frac{\mathbf{S}_j \cdot \mathbf{S}_k}{r_{jk}{}^3} - 3\frac{(\mathbf{r}_{jk} \cdot \mathbf{S}_j)(\mathbf{r}_{jk} \cdot \mathbf{S}_k)}{r_{jk}{}^5} \right]}_{\text{Dipole-dipole (dipolar) energy}} \quad (1)$$

where r_{jk} is the distance between the jth and kth spins, and A_{jk} is proportional to the exchange integral J_{jk}. One should note that the first term in the dipolar energy is of the same form as the exchange interaction [Van Vleck (1948)].

When a single crystal is considered, the various moments of the spectral line depend upon the direction cosines of the applied magnetic field H relative to the crystalline axes as a result of the scalar products $(\mathbf{r}_{jk} \cdot \mathbf{S}_j)$. For example, an array of spins arranged on a simple cubic lattice has a second moment $\langle H^2 \rangle$ given by

$$\langle H^2 \rangle = (36.8/d^6)\, g^2\beta^2 [\tfrac{1}{3}S(S+1)]$$

$$[(\lambda_1{}^4 + \lambda_2{}^4 + \lambda_3{}^4) - 0.187] \quad (2)$$

where λ_1, λ_2, and λ_3 are the direction cosines of the applied magnetic field H relative to the principal cubic axes, and d is the lattice constant or nearest neighbor spin-spin separation. For a powder sample with cubic symmetry, the second moment is averaged over a sphere to give

$$\langle H^2 \rangle = \frac{3}{5}\, g^2\beta^2 S(S+1) \sum_j \left(\frac{1}{r_{jk}}\right)^6 \quad (3)$$

where of course the term $j = k$ is excluded from the summation. It should be emphasized that eq. (3) is for a general type of cubic symmetry, while eq. (2) is for the more particular simple cubic structure. These two expressions are for identical spins. If one type of spin is broadened by another type (e.g., a free radical electron spin broadened by protons), the second moment is decreased by the factor 4/9 to give

$$\langle H^2 \rangle = \frac{4}{15} g^2 \beta^2 S(S + 1) \sum_j \left(\frac{1}{r_{jk}} \right)^6 \tag{4}$$

In these formulae the g factor corresponds to the spin which causes the broadening, not the one being measured. Van Vleck (1948) also gives formulae for fourth moments, and Glebashev (1957) computed 6th moments by the Van Vleck method. The two eqs. (3) and (4) do not include subsidiary lines at ~ 0, $2g\beta H$, and $3g\beta H$ in the moment calculation since they are not observed at high fields. They were removed by truncating the Hamiltonian. Their inclusion would increase $\langle H^2 \rangle$ by the factor 10/3 [for the "10/3 effect," see Van Vleck (1948)].

The exchange interaction does not influence the second moment, but it does affect the fourth moment. In the absence of exchange, dipolar broadening produces a Gaussian shaped absorption curve. The exchange interaction between like spins causes the absorption line to be more peaked in the center, and to taper more gradually in the wings, and thereby renders the line-shape closer to Lorentzian than Gaussian. On the other hand, the exchange interaction between unlike spins tends to broaden absorption lines, but in practice this effect is much less prevalent than exchange narrowing by like spins. Kittel and Abrahams (1953) showed that in the case of magnetically dilute crystals dipolar broadening produces a Lorentzian shape [see also McMillan and Opechowski (1960); Grant and Strandberg (1964); Wyard (1965)]. Dipolar broadening due to solvent segregation in frozen aqueous solutions is discussed by Ross (1965).

When the exchange interaction energy is very large compared to the dipolar energy, the line-width ΔH is proportional to the square of the line-width ΔH_{dd} that arises from dipole-dipole broadening divided by the rate of exchange ω_e expressed in frequency units [Anderson and Weiss (1953); Van Vleck (1948)]

$$\Delta H \approx \gamma (\Delta H_{dd})^2 / \omega_e \tag{5}$$

$$\approx (\Delta H_{dd})^2 / H_e \tag{6}$$

The contributions from the exchange H_e and the dipolar H_{dd} interactions are given by

$$H_e = (1.7J/g\beta) \, [S(S + 1)]^{1/2} \tag{7}$$

$$\Delta H_{dd} = 2.3(g\beta\rho) \, [S(S + 1)]^{1/2} \tag{8}$$

where S is the spin, J is the exchange integral, and ρ is the density of spins per cubic centimeter. The last two equations are for a simple cubic lattice, and are given by Anderson and Weiss (1953) to illustrate the use of eqs. (5) and (6) for extreme exchange narrowing. The NMR of chemically exchanging nuclei has been discussed by a number of authors, such as Gutowsky, McCall, and Slichter (1953); Gutowsky and Saika (1953), Solomon and Bloembergen (1956), Kaplan (1958), McConnell (1958), and O'Reilly and Poole (1963).

Molecular rotation has the effect of narrowing a magnetic resonance line. Several authors [Andrew (1959); Andrew, Bradbury, and Eades (1958); Andrew and Newing (1958)] showed that molecular rotation produces weak sidebands or satellite lines which are difficult to observe, but which contribute to the overall second moment in such a way that the second moment remains invariant in magnitude. Bloch (1958) and Sarles and Cotts (1958) discuss line narrowing by double frequency irradiation. Köhler (1965) treats the line-shape and second moment with superimposed Overhauser and solid state effects. Tumanov (1962) and Grant (1964) discuss cross relaxation and moments.

Kambe and Ollom (1956) modified Van Vleck's theory to include quadrupole coupling or the crystalline field effect [see Volkoff (1953)]. Kopvillem (1958) extended the work of Van Vleck (1948) to the case where the g factor is a tensor. Yokota (1952) showed that Van Vleck's moment method is equivalent to the Fourier transform technique which is often used in the theory of pressure broadening. O'Reilly and Tsang (1962, 1963) employed lattice harmonics of the appropriate crystal field group to compute second and fourth moments, and to make vibrational corrections to moments. McMillan and Opechowski (1960, 1961) discuss the temperature dependence of moments. Korst, Savel'ev, and Sokolov (1962) averaged Van Vleck's moment formulae over the zero point vibrations in solids. Murthy (1963) presents a method for calculating moments by means of an analog computer. Verdier, Whipple, and Schomaker (1961) used a generalized convolution transform to analyze moments.

One may deduce from eqs. (3) and (4) that the calculation of moments requires the computation of lattice sums such as those which Mayer (1933), Gutowsky and McGarvey (1952), Kaplan (1961), and Chang (1961) evaluated for several lattices.

Divers articles such as Hervé (1957, 1960), Kopvillem (1960), Koloskova and Kopvillem (1960), and Vincow and Johnson (1963) may be consulted for experimental measurements of moments. Vincow and Johnson (1963) derived expressions for the effects of finite line-width, satellite lines, carbon-13 in natural abundance, g factor anisotropy, and π electron spin density on the second moments of π electron radicals. Lefebvre (1961) computed the NMR line-shape for protons in a polycrystalline aromatic radical. Abragam and Kambe (1953) applied the Van Vleck method to quadrupole resonance. Tjon (1966) discusses the line-shape for free induction decays in a rigid lattice. This method is used routinely to interpret the NMR spectra of solids, liquids, and gases, and books on NMR such as Andrew (1956), Pople, Schneider, and Bernstein (1959), Lösche (1957), Abragam (1961), etc., may be consulted for further details. Loudon (1960), Stoneham (1965), and Mayer, Bennett, Donohu, and Daniel (1966) discuss the relationship between line-shapes obtained during ordinary ESR studies and those obtained in acoustic resonant absorption experiments.

Most of the theories of resonance line-widths and line-shapes, such as those discussed in this chapter, are only valid for cases in which the line-width in gauss is small compared to the applied magnetic field. Garstens (1954) modified the original Bloch theory (1946) for the case in which this assumption is not valid, and Garstens, Singer and Ryan (1954) and Garstens and Kaplan (1955) obtained experimental data at low magnetic fields and low resonant frequencies ($f_0 < 15$ Mc) on DPPH that agreed with their modified theory. Rogers, Anderson, and Pake (1959) explain the narrowing of the line-width of solid DPPH in low fields by the 10/3 effect discussed earlier in this section, and Tchao (1960) attributes the residual width of 2.1 G at zero field to anisotropic diamagnetism of the benzene rings (see also Walter, Codrington, D'Adamo, and Torrey (1956)]. Henderson and Rogers (1966) observed the 10/3 effect in the ESR of two copper salts.

We shall conclude this section with some parenthetical remarks about summations. Suppose a set of four spins has the simplified (but unrealistic) Hamiltonian $\mathcal{3C}$

$$\mathcal{3C} = g\beta H \sum_j S_{zj} + g^2\beta^2(1 - 3\cos^2\theta) \sum_{k>j} \left(\frac{1}{r_{jk}}\right)^3 \qquad (9)$$

One may write the righthand side explicitly as follows:

$$\mathcal{3C} = g\beta H \left[S_{z1} + S_{z2} + S_{z3} + S_{z4}\right] + g^2\beta^2(1 - 3\cos^2\theta)$$

$$\times \left[\left(\frac{1}{r_{12}}\right)^3 + \left(\frac{1}{r_{13}}\right)^3 + \left(\frac{1}{r_{14}}\right)^3 + \left(\frac{1}{r_{23}}\right)^3 + \left(\frac{1}{r_{24}}\right)^3 + \left(\frac{1}{r_{34}}\right)^3\right] \qquad (10)$$

This is expected because the interaction energy term $g^2\beta^2(1 - 3\cos^2\theta)/r_{ij}^3$ should only be counted once for each pair of spins. The summation

$$\sum_{k\neq j} \left(\frac{1}{r_{jk}}\right)^3 = \left[\left(\frac{1}{r_{12}}\right)^3 + \left(\frac{1}{r_{13}}\right)^3 + \left(\frac{1}{r_{14}}\right)^3 + \left(\frac{1}{r_{21}}\right)^3 + \left(\frac{1}{r_{23}}\right)^3 + \left(\frac{1}{r_{24}}\right)^3\right.$$

$$\left. + \left(\frac{1}{r_{31}}\right)^3 + \left(\frac{1}{r_{32}}\right)^3 + \left(\frac{1}{r_{34}}\right)^3 + \left(\frac{1}{r_{41}}\right)^3 + \left(\frac{1}{r_{42}}\right)^3 + \left(\frac{1}{r_{43}}\right)^3\right] \qquad (11)$$

has twice as many terms as $\sum_{k>j} r_{gh}^{-3}$ so that

$$\sum_{k>j} \left(\frac{1}{r_{jk}}\right)^3 = \frac{1}{2} \sum_{k\neq j} \left(\frac{1}{r_{jk}}\right)^3 \qquad (12)$$

since of course $r_{jk} = r_{kj}$. Some authors use the summation on the righthand side of eq. (12) instead of that on the lefthand side.

In the second moment calculation, we select a typical spin and calculate the broadening interaction with all of the others in the sample. To illustrate the method by our four-spin case, we choose $k = 2$, and assume (erroneously) that eq. (3) is valid for such a small cluster. Ergo,

$$\langle H^2 \rangle = \frac{3}{5} g^2\beta^2 S(S + 1) \left[\left(\frac{1}{r_{12}}\right)^6 + \left(\frac{1}{r_{32}}\right)^6 + \left(\frac{1}{r_{42}}\right)^6\right] \qquad (13)$$

In practice, the second moment sum is over about 10^{24} atoms, but only the nearby ones make an appreciable contribution to the result.

One may approximate the second moment by summing directly over the nearest neighbors (nn), and then integrating over the remaining spins in the sample. If the density or number of spins per unit volume is ρ, then the average number in a thin spherical layer of thickness dr at a distance r from the origin will be $4\pi r^2 \rho dr$. Therefore

$$\langle H^2 \rangle \approx \frac{3}{5} g^2 \beta^2 S(S+1) \left[\sum_{nn} \left(\frac{1}{r_{jk}}\right)^6 + 4\pi\rho \int_{a_0}^{\infty} \frac{r^2 dr}{r^6} \right] \quad (14)$$

$$\approx \frac{3}{5} g^2 \beta^2 S(S+1) \left[\sum_{nn} \left(\frac{1}{r_{jk}}\right)^6 + \frac{4}{3}\pi\rho \left(\frac{1}{a_0}\right)^3 \right] \quad (15)$$

where a_0 is the distance to the nearest spin that is not included in the summation. The same units of length must be used for a_0, r_{jk}, and ρ, e.g., ρ might be the number of spins per cubic angstrom unit. For this approximation to be valid, the magnitude of the summation term much greatly exceed that of the integral term. If there are several species of spins in the sample, then each type will contribute to the moments, and should be summed separately. The numerical factor of $3/5$ in eqs. (14) and (15) for like spins must be changed to $4/15$ for unlike spins, as explained above in this section.

Van Vleck's theory (1948) of moments is a high temperature approximation which is valid in most experimental arrangements. Below liquid helium temperature and at high frequencies one often attains the low temperature condition $g\beta H > kT$ (cf. Sec. 14-E, especially Figs. 14–9 and 14–10). In this region the theory of moments must be modified by weighting the spin levels with their proper Boltzmann factors, as discussed by Pryce and Stevens (1950), Kambe and Usui (1952), McMillan and Opechowski (1960, 1961), Svare and Seidel (1964), and Svare (1965.)

Grant (1964) discusses moment theory from a mathematical viewpoint. He asserts that "A knowledge of any finite number of moments, alone, yields no information about the [line-shape] function within any finite interval" of a magnet scan. Those of us who are not mathematicians should remain aloof from such philosophical subtilties, and reaffirm our credo in the preceding mathematical formalism.

L. Overlapping Resonances

The line-shapes that result from the overlapping of two to six hyperfine components with a Gaussian line-shape and Gaussian intensity distributions were reconstructed manually by Poole and Anderson (1959), and are shown on Fig. 1–5. A more extensive set of overlapping spectra were worked out on a computer and published in the book by Lebedev and Voevodksii (1963) [see also Rotaru, Valeriu, and Weiner (1964)]. Kummer (1963) discusses whether or not more than one set of parameters (coupling constants) is compatible with an experimental spectrum. Garrett, Hinckley, and Morgan (1966) synthesized unresolved Mn II structure.

First derivative spectral lines are narrower and more resolved than the absorption spectrum itself, and second derivative spectra are even better in this respect. A glance at Fig. 14–38 and a careful comparison of the curves in Figs. 20–6 and 20–7 will convince one of this fact. The difficulty with second derivative presentation is that the peaks shown in Fig. 20–6c at $H - H_0 = \pm 3^{1/2}\Delta H_{pp}$ above the baseline tend to interfere with the adjacent hyperfine components to produce misleading spectra. This liability is considerably more pronounced with Gaussian than it is with Lorentzian shapes. Johnson and Chang (1965) recorded third derivative spectra for even greater resolution.

Ageno and Frontali (1963) give a graphical method for separating overlapping Gaussian curves, and Allen (1962) discusses several methods for unravelling complex spectra. Allen, Gladney, and Glarum (1964) and Glarum (1965) show how to enhance considerably the resolving power of an ESR spectrometer [cf. Sec. 14-I]. Kaplan (1965) discusses line-widths of inhomogeneously broadened lines.

It is possible to synthetically produce a complex resonance line on an oscilloscope by means of electronic Gaussian or Lorentzian function generators. This may be compared to an observed spectrum, and the hyperfine intensity ratio deduced from the individual output of each function generator [Giardino and Wisert (1965)].

The electron spin resonance spectra of free radicals in solution frequently contain many resolved hyperfine components. The original analysis of magnetic resonance line-widths [Bloembergen, Purcell, and Pound (1948)] was not sufficiently general to account for these experimental observations. The general theory of Kubo and Tomita (1954) was extended by Kivelson (1957, 1960) to explain the observed widths [Schreurs, Blomgren, and Fraenkel (1960); Shreurs and Fraenkel (1961); Rogers and Pake (1960); Kivelson and Collins (1963)] and saturation behavior [Lloyd and Pake (1954); Stephen and Fraenkel (1960); Stephen (1961)]. Some spectra of free radicals exhibit hyperfine structure with lines which alternate in width from one hyperfine component to the next [e.g., see Bolton and Carrington (1962); Freed, Rieger and Fraenkel (1962); Freed and Fraenkel (1962, 1963, 1964); Barton and Fraenkel (1964); Bolton and Fraenkel (1964); Gendell, Freed, and Fraenkel (1964)]. The Kivelson theory was revised and extended by Freed and Fraenkel (1963, 1964) to explain these alternating line-widths, and a new method was developed for determining the relative signs of isotropic hyperfine splittings.

References

R. Aasa and T. Vänngård, Z. Naturforsch, 19A, 1425 (1964).

A. Abragam, The Principles of Nuclear Magnetism, Clarendon, Oxford, 1961.

A. Abragam and K. Kambe, Phys. Rev., 91, 894 (1953).

M. Ageno and C. Frontali, Nature, 198, 1294 (1963).

L. C. Allen, Nature, 196, 663 (1962).

L. C. Allen, H. M. Gladney, and S. H. Glarum, J. Chem. Phys., 40, 3135 (1964).

H. G. Anderson and H. Welling, Phys. Rev., 139, A321 (1965).

P. W. Anderson and P. R. Weiss, Rev. Mod. Phys., 25, 269 (1953).

E. R. Andrew, Nuclear Magnetic Resonance, Cambridge University Press, Oxford, 1956.

E. R. Andrew, Phys. Rev., 91, 425 (1953); Bulletin du Groupement Ampère, 8th Colloque Ampère, 1959, p. 103.

E. R. Andrew and R. Bersohn, J. Chem. Phys., 18, 159 (1950).

E. R. Andrew, A. Bradbury, and R. G. Eades, Arch. Sci. Spec. Publ., 11, 223 (1958).

E. R. Andrew and R. A. Newing, Proc. Phys. Soc., 72, 959 (1958).

C. A. Barth, A. F. Hildebrandt, and M. Patapoff, Discussions Faraday Soc., 33, 162 (1962); Nature, 182, 1659 (1958).

B. L. Barton and G. K. Fraenkel, J. Chem. Phys., 41, 695 (1964).

A. Ben-Reuven, Phys. Rev. Letters, 14, 349 (1965).

B. Bleaney, Proc. Phys. Soc., A63, 407 (1950); 75, 621 (1960); Phil. Mag., 42, 441 (1951).

R. Blinc, Z. Trontelj, and B. Volavšek, J. Chem. Phys., 44, 1028 (1966).

S. M. Blinder, J. Chem. Phys., 33, 748 (1960).

F. Bloch, Phys. Rev., 70, 460 (1946); ibid., 111, 841 (1958).

N. Bloembergen, J. Appl. Phys., 23, 1383 (1952).

N. Bloembergen, E. M. Purcell, and R. V. Pound, Phys. Rev., 73, 679 (1948).

N. Bloembergen and T. J. Rowland, *Acta Met.*, **1**, 731 (1953); *Phys. Rev.*, **97**, 1679 (1955).

J. R. Bolton and A. Carrington, *Mol. Phys.*, **5**, 161 (1962).

J. R. Bolton and G. K. Fraenkel, *J. Chem. Phys.*, **41**, 944 (1964).

K. D. Bowers and J. Owen, *Rept. Progr. Phys.*, **18**, 304 (1955).

R. G. Breene, Jr., *The Shift and Shape of Spectral Lines*, Pergamon, N. Y., 1961.

J. Bronstein and V. Volterra, *Phys. Letters*, **16**, 211 (1965).

G. Burns, *J. Appl. Phys.*, **32**, 2048 (1961).

A. Charlier, H. Danan, and P. Taglang, *J. Phys. (France)*, **25**, Suppl. 11, 183A (1964).

H. Cheng, *Phys. Rev.*, **124**, 1359 (1961).

A. K. Chirkov and A. A. Kokin, *Zh. Eksper. Teor. Fiz.*, **39**, 1381 (964) (1960).

R. C. Collins, *RSI*, **30**, 492 (1959).

J. E. Cousins and R. Dupree, *Phys. Letters*, **14**, 177 (1965).

D. A. Curtis, C. J. Kirkby, and J. S. Thorp, *Brit. J. Appl. Phys.*, **16**, 1681 (1965).

P. Dräghicescu, *Stud. Cercetari Fiz. (Rumania)*, **14**, 201 (1963).

G. Dresselhaus, A. F. Kip, and C. Kittel, *Phys. Rev.*, **100**, 618 (1955).

F. J. Dyson, *Phys. Rev.*, **98**, 349 (1955).

P. Erdös, *Helv. Phys. Acta*, **37**, 493 (1964).

G. Feher and A. Kip, *Phys. Rev.*, **98**, 337 (1955).

C. D. Flynn and E. F. W. Seymour, *Proc. Phys. Soc.*, **75**, 337 (1960).

J. H. Freed and G. K. Fraenkel, *J. Chem. Phys.*, **37**, 1156 (1962); **39**, 326 (1963); **40**, 1815 (1964); **41**, 699, 2077, 3623 (1964).

J. H. Freed, P. H. Rieger, and G. K. Fraenkel. *J. Chem. Phys.*, **37**, 1881 (1962).

B. B. Garrett and L. O. Morgan, *J. Chem. Phys.*, **44**, 890 (1966); C. C. Hinckley and L. O. Morgan, *ibid.*, 898 (1966).

M. A. Garstens, *Phys. Rev.*, **93**, 1228 (1954).

M. A. Garstens, L. S. Singer, and A. H. Ryan, *Phys. Rev.*, **96**, 53 (1954).

M. A. Garstens and J. I. Kaplan, *Phys. Rev.*, **99**, 459 (1955).

J. Gendell, J. H. Freed, and G. K. Fraenkel, *J. Chem. Phys.*, **41**, 949 (1964).

H. R. Gersmann and J. D. Swalen, *J. Chem. Phys.*, **36**, 3221 (1962).

D. A. Giardino and C. O. Wisert, 1965, private communication.

S. H. Glarum, *RSI*, **36**, 771 (1965).

G. Ya. Glebashev, *Zh. Eksper. Teor. Fiz.*, **32**, 82 (1957).

W. J. C. Grant, *Physica*, **30**, 1433 (1964); *Phys. Rev.*, **134**, A1554, A1564, A1574 (1964), **135**, A1265 (1964).

W. J. C. Grant and M. W. P. Strandberg, *Phys. Rev.*, **135**, A715, A727 (1964).

T. W. Griswold, A. F. Kip, and C. Kittel, *Phys. Rev.*, **88**, 951 (1952).

H. S. Gutowsky, G. B. Kistiakowsky, G. E. Pake, and E. M. Purcell, *J. Chem. Phys.*, **17**, 972 (1949).

H. S. Gutowsky, D. W. McCall, and C. P. Slichter, *J. Chem. Phys.*, **21**, 279 (1953).

H. S. Gutowsky and B. R. McGarvey, *J. Chem. Phys.*, **21**, 1423 (1952).

H. S. Gutowsky and A. Saika, *J. Chem. Phys.*, **21**, 1688 (1953).

A. J. Henderson and R. N. Rogers, *Bull. Am. Phys. Soc.*, **11**, 204 (1966).

J. Hervé, *C. R. Acad. Sci.*, **244**, 1182 (1957); **245**, 653 (1957); *Ann. Phys. (Paris)*, **5**, 321 (1960).

K. Heuer, *Jenaer. Jahrbuch*, **I**, 233 (1961).

A. Hudson and A. D. McLachlan, *J. Chem. Phys.*, **43**, 1518 (1965).

D. G. Hughes and T. J. Rowland, *Can. J. Phys.*, **42**, 209 (1964).

J. A. Ibers and J. D. Swalen, *Phys. Rev.*, **127**, 1914 (1962).

E. Jahnke and F. Emde, *Tables of Functions*, Dover, N. Y., 1945, p. 73.

The integral is defined by

$$K(k) = \int_0^1 \frac{dx}{(1 - x^2)^{1/2}(1 - k^2 x^2)^{1/2}}$$

The transformations are to let $v = (1 - \alpha^2 u^2)^{1/2}$ in I_B and $v = \gamma(1 - \alpha^2 u^2)^{1/2}/$ $(\gamma^2 - 1)^{1/2}$ in I_A where $\alpha = [(g_1{}^2 - g_3{}^2)/(g'^2 - g_3{}^2)]^{1/2}$ and $\gamma = (1/\alpha)[(g_2{}^2 - g_1{}^2)/ (g_2{}^2 - g'^2)]^{1/2}$.

C. S. Johnson, Jr. and R. Chang, *J. Chem. Phys.*, **43**, 3183 (1965).

T. S. Johnston and H. G. Hecht, *J. Mol. Spectry.*, **17**, 98 (1965).

Y. Kakiuchi, H. Shono, H. Komatsu, and K. Kigoshi, *J. Chem. Phys.*, **19**, 1069 (1951), *J. Phys. Soc. Japan*, **7**, 102 (1952).

H. S. Judeikis, *J. Appl. Phys.*, **35**, 2615 (1964).

K. Kambe and J. F. Ollom, *J. Phys. Soc. Japan*, **11**, 50 (1956).

K. Kambe and T. Usui, *Progr. Theor. Phys.*, **8**, 302 (1952).

J. I. Kaplan, *J. Chem. Phys.*, **28**, 278 (1958); **34**, 2205 (1961); **42**, 3789 (1965); *J. Phys. Soc. Japan*, **19**, 1994 (1964).

A. Kiel, *Paramagnetic Resonance, Phys. Rev.*, **126**, 1292 (1962); **2**, 525 (1963).

C. Kikuchi and W. V. Cohen, *Phys. Rev.*, **93**, 394 (1954).

C. Kittel and E. Abrahams, *Phys. Rev.*, **90**, 238 (1953).

D. Kivelson, *J. Chem. Phys.*, **27**, 1087 (1957); **33**, 1094 (1960).

D. Kivelson and G. Collins, *Paramagnetic Resonance*, **2**, 496 (1963).

F. K. Kneubühl, *J. Chem. Phys.*, **33**, 1074 (1960); *Helv. Phys. Acta*, **35**, 259 (1962).

F. K. Kneubühl and B. Natterer, *Helv. Phys. Acta*, **34**, 710 (1961).

R. P. Kohin and C. P. Poole, Jr., *Bull. Am. Phys. Soc. II*, **3**, 8 (1958).

R. Köhler, *Ann. Phys. (Germany)*, **15**, 389 (1965).

N. G. Koloskova and U. Kh. Kopvillem, *Fiz. Tverd. Tela*, **2**, 1368 (1960).

U. Kh. Kopvillem, *Zh. Eksper. Teor. Fiz.*, **34**, 1040 (719) (1958); *ibid.*, **38**, 151 (109) (1960).

N. N. Korst, V. A. Savel'ev, and N. D. Sokolov, *Dokl. Akad. Nauk.*, **147**, 594 (1962); trans. *Soviet Phys. Dokl.*, **7**, 1037 (1963).

P. Kottis and R. Lefebvre, *J. Chem. Phys.*, **39**, 393 (1963); **41**, 379, 3660 (1964).

H. A. Kramers, *Proc. Amsterdam Acad. Sci.*, **33**, 959 (1930).

R. Kubo and K. Tomita, *J. Phys. Soc. Japan*, **9**, 888 (1954).

V. S. Korolkov and A. K. Potapovich, *Optika i Sepkt.*, **16**, 461 (251) (1964).

H. Kummer, *Helv. Phys. Acta*, **36**, 901 (1963).

Ya. S. Lebedev, D. M. Chernikova, N. N. Tikhomirova, and V. V. Voevodskii, *Atlas of Electron Spin Resonance Spectra*, Consultants Bureau, N. Y., 1963.

R. Lefebvre, *J. Chem. Phys.*, **33**, 1826 (1960); **34**, 2035 (1961); **35**, 762 (1961).

R. Lefebvre and J. Maruani, *J. Chem. Phys.*, **42**, 1480 (1965); see also J. Maruani, *Proc. 12th Colloque Ampère*, Bordeaux, 1963, p. 303.

R. Livingston and H. Zeldes, *J. Chem. Phys.*, **24**, 170 (1956).

J. P. Lloyd and G. E. Pake, *Phys. Rev.*, **94**, 579 (1954).

A. Lösche, *Kerninduktion*, Veb. Deutscher Verlag. der Wissenschaften, Berlin, East Germany, 1957.

R. Loudon, *Phys. Rev.*, **119**, 919 (1960).

A. Lund and T. Vänngård, *J. Chem. Phys.*, **42**, 2979 (1965).

J. M. Luttinger and L. Tisza, *Phys. Rev.*, **70**, 954 (1946).

M. M. Malley, *J. Molecular Spectry.*, **17**, 210 (1965).

H. M. McConnell, *J. Chem. Phys.*, **28**, 430 (1958).

M. McMillan and W. Opechowski, *Can. J. Phys.*, **38**, 1168 (1960); **39**, 1369 (1961).

D. W. Marguardt, R. G. Bennett, and E. J. Burrell, *J. Mol. Spectry.*, **7**, 269 (1961).

J. E. Mayer, *J. Chem. Phys.*, **1**, 270, 327 (1933).

H. C. Meyer, J. S. Bennett, P. L. Donoho, and A. C. Daniel, *Bull. Am. Phys. Soc.*, **11**, 202 (1966).

S. V. Murthy, *RSI*, **34**, 106 (1963).

H. Nagasawa, *J. Phys. Soc. Japan*, **20**, 1808 (1965).

R. Neiman and D. Kivelson, *J. Chem. Phys.*, **35**, 156 (1961).

D. E. O'Reilly, *J. Chem. Phys.*, **29**, 1188 (1958).

D. E. O'Reilly, and C. P. Poole, Jr., *J. Phys. Chem.*, **67**, 1762 (1963).

D. E. O'Reilly and T. Tsang, *Phys. Rev.*, **128**, 2639 (1962); **131**, 2522 (1963).

G. E. Pake, *J. Chem. Phys.*, **16**, 327 (1948).

G. E. Pake and E. M. Purcell, *Phys. Rev.*, **74**, 1184 (1948); **75**, 534 (1949).

M. Peter, D. Shaltiel, J. H. Wernick, H. J. Williams, J. B. Mock, and R. C. Sherwood, *Phys. Rev.*, **126**, 1395 (1962).

C. P. Poole, Jr., and R. S. Anderson, *J. Chem. Phys.*, **31**, 346 (1959).

J. A. Pople, W. G. Schneider, and H. J. Bernstein, *High Resolution Nuclear Magnetic Resonance*, McGraw-Hill, N. Y., 1959.

D. W. Posener, *Australian J. Phys.*, **12**, 184 (1959).

M. H. L. Pryce, *Proc. Phys. Soc.*, **A63**, 25 (1950).

M. H. L. Pryce and K. W. H. Stevens, *Proc. Phys. Soc.*, **A63**, 36 (1950).

G. E. H. Reuter and E. H. Sondheimer, *Proc. Roy. Soc.*, **A195**, 336 (1948).

R. E. Richards and J. A. S. Smith, *Trans. Faraday Soc.*, **47**, 1261 (1951).

E. A. Rinehart, R. L. Legan, and C. C. Lin, *RSI*, **36**, 511 (1965); see also E. A. Rinehart, R. H. Kleen, and C. C. Lin, *J. Mol. Spectry.*, **5**, 458 (1960).

R. N. Rogers, M. E. Anderson, and G. E. Pake, *Bull. Am. Phys. Soc.*, **4**, 261 (1959).

R. N. Rogers and G. E. Pake, *J. Chem. Phys.*, **33**, 1107 (1960).

R. T. Ross, *J. Chem. Phys.*, **42**, 3919 (1965).

M. Rotaru, A. Valeriu, and M. Weiner, *Rev. Roumaine Phys.*, **9**, 269 (1964).

A. A. Rukhadze and V. P. Silin, *Zh. Tekh. Fiz.*, **32**, 423 (307) (1962).

R. H. Sands, *Phys. Rev.*, **99**, 1222 (1955).

L. R. Sarles and R. M. Cotts, *Phys. Rev.*, **111**, 853 (1958).

K. Scheffler and H. B. Stegmann, *Ber. Bunsengesell. Phys. Chem.*, **67**, 864 (1963).

G. Schoffa and G. Bürk, *Phys. Status Solid.*, **8**, 557 (1965).

D. S. Schonland, *Proc. Phys. Soc.*, **73**, 788 (1959).

J. W. H. Schreurs, G. E. Blomgren, and G. K. Fraenkel, *J. Chem. Phys.*, **32**, 1861 (1960).

J. W. H. Schreurs and G. K. Fraenkel, *J. Chem. Phys.*, **34**, 756 (1961).

P. L. Scott, H. J. Stapleton, and C. Wainstein, *Phys. Rev.*, **137**, A71 (1965).

J. W. Searl, R. C. Smith, and S. J. Wyard, *Proc. Phys. Soc.*, **74**, 491 (1959); **78**, 1174 (1961); *Arch. Sci. Fasc. Spec.*, **13**, 236 (1960) (9th Colloque Ampère).

P. E. Seiden, *Phys. Rev. Letters*, **14**, 370 (1965).

D. Shaltiel and W. Low, *Phys. Rev.*, **124**, 1062 (1961).

L. S. Singer, *J. Chem. Phys.*, **23**, 379 (1955).

L. S. Singer, W. J. Spry, and W. H. Smith, *Proc. 1957 Conf. on Carbon*, Pergamon, N. Y., 1957, p. 121.

D. R. Smith and J. J. Pieroni, *Can. J. Chem.*, **42**, 2209 (1964).

I. Solomon and N. Bloembergen, *J. Chem. Phys.*, **25**, 261 (1956).

M. J. Stephen, *J. Chem. Phys.*, **34**, 484 (1961).

M. J. Stephen and G. K. Fraenkel, *J. Chem. Phys.*, **32**, 1435 (1960).

H. Sternlicht, *J. Chem. Phys.*, **33**, 1128 (1960); see *ibid.*, **42**, 2250 (1965) for applications to NMR relaxation.

A. M. Stoneham, *Phys. Letters*, **14**, 297 (1965).

O. Štirand, *ETP*, **10**, 313 (1962).

I. Svare, *Phys. Rev.*, **138**, A1718 (1965).

I. Svare and G. Seidel, *Phys. Rev.*, **134**, A172 (1964).

P. Swarup, *Can. J. Phys.*, **37**, 848 (1959).

Y. H. Tchao, *C. R. Acad. Sci.*, **251**, 668 (1960).

N. N. Tikhomirova and V. V. Voevodskii, *Optica i Spectrosk.*, **7**, 829 (486) (1959).

J. A. Tjon, *Phys. Rev.*, **143**, 259 (1966).

H. J. Tobler, A. Bauder, and H. H. Günthard, *JSI*, **42**, 236 (1965).

V. A. Tolkachev and A. J. Mikhailov, *PTE*, **6**, 95 (1242) (1964).

C. H. Townes and A. L. Schawlow, *Microwave Spectroscopy*, McGraw-Hill, N. Y., 1955, Chap. 13.

V. S. Tumanov, *Fiz. Tverd. Tela*, **4**, 2419 (1773) 1962).

L. Van Gerven and A. Van Itterbeek, *Arch. Sci., Spec. No.*, **14**, 117 (1961) (10th Colloque Ampère).

T. Vänngård and R. Aasa, *Paramagnetic Resonance*, **2**, 509 (1963).

A. Van Roggen, L. Van Roggen, and W. Gordy, *Phys. Rev.*, **105**, 50 (1957).

J. H. Van Vleck, *The Theory of Electric and Magnetic Susceptibilities*, Oxford University Press, Oxford, 1932.

J. H. Van Vleck, *Phys. Rev.*, **52**, 1178 (1937); *ibid.*, **74**, 1168 (1948); *Nuovo Cimento Suppl.*, **6**, No. 3, 993 (1957).

J. H. Van Vleck and V. F. Weisskopf, *Rev. Mod. Phys.*, **17**, 227 (1945).

P. H. Verdier, E. B. Whipple, and V. Schomaker, *J. Chem. Phys.*, **34**, 118 (1961).

G. Vincow and P. M. Johnson, *J. Chem. Phys.*, **39**, 1143 (1963).

G. N. Volkoff, *Can. J. Phys.*, **31**, 820 (1953).

S. Vonsovskii, Ed., *Ferromagnetic Resonance*, Trans. from Russian, Pergamon, London, 1965.

G. Wagoner, *Phys. Rev.*, **118**, 647 (1960).

R. L. Walter, R. S. Codrington, A. F. D'Adamo, Jr., and H. C. Torrey, *J. Chem. Phys.*, **25**, 319 (1956).

J. S. Waugh, F. B. Humphrey, and D. M. Yost, *J. Phys. Chem.*, **57**, 486 (1953).

J. A. Weil and J. H. Anderson, *J. Chem. Phys.*, **28**, 864 (1958).
J. A. Weil and H. G. Hecht, *J. Chem. Phys.*, **38**, 281 (1963).
R. L. White, *Phys. Rev.*, **115**, 1519 (1959).
S. J. Wyard, *Proc. Phys. Soc.*, **86**, 587 (1965).
I. Yokota, *Prog., Theoret. Phys.*, **8**, 380 (1952).
W. A. Young, *J. Appl. Phys.*, **35**, 460 (1964).

CHAPTER 21

Summary of Spectrometer Operation

The preceding chapters have dealt with a large number of topics under the general categories of background material, information that is useful for designing equipment, and information that aids in the operation of electron spin resonance spectrometers. The present chapter will present a summary of the third category. The discussion in much of this chapter presupposes the use of a magnetic field modulated spectrometer of standard design. Such spectrometers are available commercially. No references will be included in this chapter, since other sections of the book may be consulted for further details.

A. Microwave Frequency

For routine studies with the ESR spectrometer, it is most convenient to employ X band ($\sim$9.5 Gc). If more information is desired than can be obtained from X band, then one may make measurements at R band (35 Gc), at K band ($\sim$25 Gc), or at S band ($\sim$3 Gc). R band is often preferable since the resolution increases with the frequency.

The principal object of varying the frequency is to sort out the frequency-dependent and the frequency-independent terms in the Hamiltonian. Hyperfine structure intervals will be independent of frequency, and anisotropic g factors will produce separations which vary linearly with the frequency. When zero field splittings (e.g., D and E) are either much greater or much less than the microwave energy $g\mu_B \mathbf{H} \cdot \mathbf{S}$, their influence on the spectrum will be almost independent of the frequency, while in the intermediate region where the zero field splitting is close to the Zeeman energy, there will be a complex variation of the observed spectrum with frequency. In general, second order effects calculated from perturbation theory frequently exhibit a complex dependence on the microwave frequency. Separate resonances which are partially superimposed will

851

separate out and be resolved at higher frequencies since their separation in gauss is proportional to the microwave frequency.

Another reason for varying the microwave frequency is to ascertain the principal line-broadening mechanisms. If the line-width is due to dipole-dipole broadening, exchange narrowing, or unresolved hyperfine structure, then it will not change with frequency, while if it is due to unresolved g factor anisotropy it will increase with increasing frequency.

The foregoing discussion demonstrates that it is much easier to interpret an ESR spectrum that is measured at two or more microwave frequencies instead of merely at one.

B. Temperature

Most of the terms in the Hamiltonian are independent of temperature, while the line-width and relaxation times are often strongly dependent on the temperature. For a rigid lattice, the dipole-dipole broadening, exchange interaction, and g factor anisotropy mechanisms do not change with the temperature. If any of the electron spins or nuclei which are responsible for the line broadening mechanism undergo changes in their translational, rotational, or vibrational motion with temperature, then such changes will produce strongly temperature-dependent line-widths and relaxation times. In general, rapid motion can average out the other line broadening mechanisms, and narrow an ESR resonance absorption line. As a result, solids ordinarily have much broader lines than fluids, and highly viscous liquids and glasses are intermediate between these two. Sometimes variable temperature studies can sort out the range where certain groups such as methyl groups stop rotating.

Variable temperature studies supply detailed information about crystallographic phase transitions, and about such magnetic phenomena as the onset of paramagnetism, ferromagnetism, and antiferromagnetism.

Low temperature relaxation time measurements often reveal a strong dependence of the spin lattice relaxation time T_1 on the temperature (e.g., $T_1 \propto 1/T$ or $T_1 \propto T^{-7}$). Such information allows one to deduce the principal relaxation process (e.g., the direct process or the Raman scattering process). Some spin systems are only detectable at very low temperatures.

The intensity of ordinary ESR spectra depends inversely on the temperature when $g\beta H \ll kT$, and exponentially on $1/T$ otherwise. Triplet states and systems with zero field splittings will exhibit a more complex behavior.

C. Microwave Power

When the microwave power is gradually increased, the signal from a typical paramagnetic spin system will at first increase in amplitude, then it will reach a maximum, and finally greater power levels will cause a decrease in the ESR amplitude. The latter phenomenon is referred to as saturation. The onset of saturation is accompanied by a gradual broadening and distortion of the resonant line, and so in general, it is best to study spin systems below saturation. The relaxation times may be determined by obtaining the power dependence of the ESR amplitude from below saturation to considerably into the saturated region.

In order to obtain an accurate line-shape, it is necessary to work well below saturation, while the best sensitivity (maximum amplitude) is obtained when the spin system is partially saturated. Accurate spin concentrations can only be determined below saturation.

When studies are made at liquid helium temperature, it is frequently necessary to work at very low powers of the order of microwatts. This entails the use of a low-power bridge.

D. Choice of Modulation Frequency and Amplitude

It is important to employ a modulation frequency f_m which is much less than the line-width ΔH_{pp} expressed in frequency units Δf_{pp}

$$f_m \ll \Delta f_{pp} = (\gamma/2\pi)\, \Delta H_{pp} = (g\beta/h)\, \Delta H_{pp} \qquad (1)$$

A modulation frequency of 100 kc may be employed for line-widths as narrow as $1/10$ G, but the same modulation frequency will appreciably distort lines less than this width.

As the modulation amplitude H_m is gradually increased, the observed line-width will be unchanged as long as H_m is much less than the line-width ΔH_{pp}. When H_m becomes close to ΔH_{pp}, then the observed line will begin to broaden and distort. When $H_m \ll \Delta H_{pp}$, the amplitude of the ESR signal will increase linearly with the modulation amplitude, while after H_m exceeds ΔH_{pp}, the amplitude will begin to decrease with increasing H_m. The ESR signal will reach a maximum near the point $H_m \sim 3\Delta H_{pp}$. In order to determine ESR spin concentrations and line-shapes, it is best to have $H_m \ll \Delta H_{pp}$, and a practical criterion is to keep $H_m \leq \Delta H_{pp}/5$. When one attempts to detect very weak signals, then one may set $H_m \sim 3\Delta H_{pp}$ for maximum sensitivity.

A practical technique to use in determining the desired value of H_m is to record the ESR signal with successively doubling modulation amplitudes. One may obtain a reasonably undistorted spectrum by using $1/4$ of the lowest value of H_m that does not produce a doubling of the ESR signal amplitude. Maximum sensitivity, of course, corresponds to the H_m which furnishes the greatest ESR signal amplitude, and this point may also be determined by successively doubling the modulation amplitude.

E. Magnet Scan

An ESR spectrum can either be spread out over several thousand gauss or confined to a small fraction of a gauss, and in searching for unknown resonances one must "guess" at the line-width, and set the scan accordingly. Sometimes it will be advantageous to make several scans covering different ranges of gauss, and perhaps centered at different field values. If a narrow scan is employed to record a very broad line, then the resonance will manifest itself as a sloping baseline, and if a broad scan is used to record a very narrow resonance, the absorption will be unusually weak and distorted. The use of too broad a scan with a weak, sharp resonance may even render it undetectable.

Once the overall features of a complex resonance are known, it may be necessary to use specially selected narrow scans to resolve particular features of the spectrum. Even when a narrow resonance is properly recorded, it is often worthwhile to make a broad scan (e.g., over a range of 1000 G) to insure that one has not overlooked an additional broad background resonance.

F. Scanning Rate and Response Time

The scanning rate dH/dt is the rate at which one varies the magnetic field, and it is conveniently expressed as the number of gauss per minute (G/min). The response time or time constant τ is a measure of the inability of the narrow band detector to pass without distortion ESR signals which are scanned through in a time shorter than τ. For an undistorted signal it is required that τ be less than one-tenth the time that it takes to scan between the two first derivative peaks of the resonant line. If the time constant τ is too long, then the observed line-shape will be distorted.

The amplitude of the noise on the recorder decreases as the response time increases, so from the viewpoint of noise it is always desirable to increase τ. As a rule of thumb, one may say that the strongest undistorted line is obtained when the peak-to-peak scanning time is ten times τ, while the best signal-to-noise ratio occurs when the peak-to-peak scanning time equals τ. The former should be employed routinely for most applications, while the latter may be resorted to for signals that are close to the limit of detectability where one does not mind obtaining a distorted line-shape. The signal-to-noise enhancement technique may be employed if sensitivity is a problem.

An observed spectrum may be tested for the proper response time by recording it with successively increasing response times until one reaches the value of τ where the amplitude decreases. The next lower time constant may be used for recording undistorted line-shapes with high sensitivity.

It should be emphasized that the important parameter that requires adjustment is the ratio of dH/dt to τ, and when one of these is doubled, the other should be doubled also. It is possible to predetermine the time constant and then test the observed spectrum for the proper value of dH/dt. However, the most convenient experimental procedure is to select the desired scan and scanning rate beforehand, and then use the value of τ which corresponds to the above criterion.

When one studies a complex spectrum containing both broad and narrow absorption lines, it may be desirable to use several scans with different time constants in order to resolve properly all of the component resonances.

G. Standard Samples and Routine Maintenance

It is advisable to have one or more standard samples to examine from time to time in order to test the spectrometer. A strong resonance may be employed to set the lock-in detector phase, and several samples of gradually decreasing spin concentration are convenient for checking the spectrometer sensitivity. An unusual change in the appearance of either the signal or the noise is a sign of trouble. A sample with a broad resonant line and another with a narrow width may be used to check scans, modulation amplitudes, and magnet settings.

One should periodically check several test voltages to insure that they give the proper dc value and ac ripple or signal. Every time the klystron is turned on, the meter readings for the klystron filament voltage, beam current, and reflector voltage should be noted.

Care should be exercised to perform certain routine maintenance chores on a regular schedule such as changing the water filter on the magnet and charging storage batteries.

Appendix A

Engineers are accustomed to using MKS units (meter-kilometer-second) and chemists ordinarily employ CGS units (centimeter-gram-second) while physicists are divided in their loyalties. This book has tried to use MKS units for electromagnetism and a somewhat mixed system otherwise, while most of the magnetic resonance literature is written in the CGS system. For comparison purposes, we hereby present (pp. 858–859) some of the important formulae in both systems. Section 9-J, p. 382, also gives a brief discussion of units.

MKS System	Page	CGS System

Maxwell's Equations

MKS System	Page	CGS System
$\nabla \cdot \mathbf{D} = \rho$	51	$\nabla \cdot \mathbf{D} = 4\pi\rho$
$\nabla \cdot \mathbf{B} = 0$	51	$\nabla \cdot \mathbf{B} = 0$
$\nabla \times \mathbf{E} = -\partial \mathbf{B}/\partial t$	51	$\nabla \times \mathbf{E} = -(1/c)(\partial \mathbf{B}/\partial t)$
$\nabla \times \mathbf{H} = \partial \mathbf{D}/\partial t + \mathbf{J}$	51	$\nabla \times \mathbf{H} = (1/c)(\partial \mathbf{D}/\partial t) + (4\pi/c)\mathbf{J}$
$\mathbf{E} = -\nabla\phi - \partial \mathbf{A}/\partial t$	62	$\mathbf{E} = -\nabla\phi - (1/c)(\partial \mathbf{A}/\partial t)$
$\mathbf{B} = \nabla \times \mathbf{A}$		$\mathbf{B} = \nabla \times \mathbf{A}$

Wave Equations and Lorentz Condition

MKS System	Page	CGS System
$\nabla^2 \mathbf{A} - \mu\epsilon(\partial^2 \mathbf{A}/\partial t^2) = -\mu\mathbf{J}$	62	$\nabla^2 \mathbf{A} - (\epsilon\mu/c^2)(\partial^2 \mathbf{A}/\partial t^2) = -4\pi\mu\mathbf{J}/c$
$\nabla^2\phi - \mu\epsilon(\partial^2\phi/\partial t^2) = -\rho/\epsilon$	62	$\nabla^2\phi - (\epsilon\mu/c^2)(\partial^2\phi/\partial t^2) = -4\pi\rho/\epsilon$
$\nabla^2 \mathbf{H} - \mu\epsilon(\partial^2 \mathbf{H}/\partial t^2) = -\nabla \times \mathbf{J}$	63	$\nabla^2 \mathbf{H} - (\epsilon\mu/c^2)(\partial^2 \mathbf{H}/\partial t^2) = -4\pi/c\, \nabla \times \mathbf{J}$
$\nabla^2 \mathbf{E} - \mu\epsilon(\partial^2 \mathbf{E}/\partial t^2) = (1/\epsilon)\nabla\rho + \mu(\partial \mathbf{J}/\partial t)$	63	$\nabla^2 \mathbf{E} - (\epsilon\mu/c^2)(\partial^2 \mathbf{E}/\partial t^2) = (4\pi/\epsilon)\nabla\rho + 4\pi\mu/c^2(\partial \mathbf{J}/\partial t)$
$\nabla \cdot \mathbf{A} + \mu\epsilon(\partial\phi/\partial t) = 0$	62	$\nabla \cdot \mathbf{A} + (\mu\epsilon/c)(\partial\phi/\partial t) = 0$

Constitutive Relations

MKS System	Page	CGS System
$\mathbf{B} = \mu\mathbf{H} = \mu_0(1 + \chi)\mathbf{H} = \mu_0(\mathbf{H} + \mathbf{M})$	55	$\mathbf{B} = \mu\mathbf{H} = (1 + 4\pi\chi)\mathbf{H} = \mathbf{H} + 4\pi\mathbf{M}$
$\mathbf{D} = \epsilon\mathbf{E} = \epsilon_0(1 + \chi_e)\mathbf{E} = \epsilon_0\mathbf{E} + \mathbf{P}$	56	$\mathbf{D} = \epsilon\mathbf{E} = (1 + 4\pi\chi_e)\mathbf{E} = \mathbf{E} + 4\pi\mathbf{P}$

Parameters for Free Space

$\mu_0 = 4\pi \times 10^{-7} H/M = 4\pi \times 10^{-7} W/AtM^2$	55	$\mu_0 = 1$
$\epsilon_0 = 10^{-9}/36\pi\ F/M$		$\epsilon_0 = 1$
$Z_0 = (\mu_0/\epsilon_0)^{1/2} = 120\pi\Omega$	78	
$c = (\mu_0\epsilon_0)^{-1/2} = 2.998 \times 10^8\ M/sec$	80	$c = 2.998 \times 10^{10}\ cm/sec$
$\mathbf{B_1} = -(\mu_0/4\pi)g_1\beta\{(\mathbf{S_1}/r^3) - 3[(\mathbf{S_1}\cdot\mathbf{r})\mathbf{r}/r^5]\}$	820	$\mathbf{B_1} = -g_1\beta\{(\mathbf{S_1}/r^3) - 3[(\mathbf{S_1}\cdot\mathbf{r})\mathbf{r}/r^5]\}$
$E_{dd} = -g_2\beta\mathbf{S_2}\cdot\mathbf{B_1}$		$E_{dd} = -g_2\beta\mathbf{S_2}\cdot\mathbf{B_1}$
$= (\mu_0/4\pi)g_1g_2\beta^2\left[\dfrac{\mathbf{S_1}\cdot\mathbf{S_2}}{r^3} - 3\dfrac{(\mathbf{S_1}\cdot\mathbf{r})(\mathbf{S_2}\cdot\mathbf{r})}{r^5}\right]$	821, 837	$= g_1g_2\beta^2\left[\dfrac{\mathbf{S_1}\cdot\mathbf{S_2}}{r^3} - 3\dfrac{(\mathbf{S_1}\cdot\mathbf{r})(\mathbf{S_2}\cdot\mathbf{r})}{r^5}\right]$
$= (\mu_0/4\pi)g_1g_2\beta^2 S(S+1)(1 - 3\cos^2\theta)(1/r^3)$	821, 841	$= g_1g_2\beta^2 S(S+1)(1 - 3\cos^2\theta)(1/r^3)$
$H = NI/L$	361	$H = 4\pi NI/L$
$E_{Zee} = g\beta\mathbf{S}\cdot\mathbf{B_0}$	18	$E_{Zee} = g\beta\mathbf{S}\cdot\mathbf{H}$
$\beta = e\hbar/2m$	15	$\beta = e\hbar/2mc$

Appendix B

The Growth of Single Crystals

A large percentage of the electron spin resonance literature is devoted to the study of single crystals. These crystals are ordinarily diamagnetic host lattices such as CaF_2, MgO, or Al_2O_3 doped with a small percentage of a transition metal ion, although other systems such as irradiated organic single crystals have also been studied. Before concluding this book, a few words will be said about methods of growing single crystals. The books listed at the end of this appendix may be consulted for further details.

The easiest way to obtain a single crystal is to select a type which can be grown from aqueous solution near room temperature. A thermostatically controlled constant temperature bath may be set up in a location which is free from disturbances. The bath is filled with a saturated solution of the substance to be crystallized, and a very small crystal or "seed crystal" may be introduced to form a nucleus for the growth. The use of a cover plate will slow down the rate of evaporation, and thereby improve the perfection of the resulting crystal. This method may also be used with solvents other than water (e.g. benzene). Organic crystals are often grown in this manner.

Crystals of transition elements in diamagnetic hosts are often grown from the melt in a high temperature oven (e.g., in the range 1000–2000°C). It is important to regulate the temperature accurately so that the somewhat supercooled melt is slowly cooled down through the neighborhood of the freezing point. A number of experimental arrangements such as the Verneuil method have been devised for growing large crystals, and they are described in the references [e.g., see Buckley (1951) or Gilman (1963)].

References

H. E. Buckley, *Crystal Growth*, Wiley, N. Y., 1951.

R. H. Doremus, B. W. Roberts, and D. J. Turnbull, Eds., *Growth and Perfection of Crystals*, Wiley, N. Y., 1958.

J. J. Gilman, Ed., *The Art and Science of Growing Crystals*, Wiley, N. Y., 1963.

A. Holden and P. Singer, *Crystals and Crystal Growing*, Doubleday, N. Y., 1960.

A. V. Shubnikov and N. N. Sheftal, *Growth of Crystals*, Consultants Bureau, N. Y., 1959.

A. R. Verma, *Crystal Growth and Perfection*, Academic Press, N. Y., 1953.

Selected Bibliography

Colloques Ampères (Ampère Colloquia)

Sponsored by Groupement Ampère (Atoms et Molécules
pour Etudes Radio-électriques)

1. Genève, 1952, *Colloques Internationaux du Centre National de la Recherche Scientifique*, unpublished.
2. Grenoble, 1953, *Annales del' Institut Polytechnique de Grenoble, Spec. No.*, 1953.
3. Paris, 1954, *Onde Electrique*, **35**, 437–505 (1955).
4. Paris, 1955, *Cahiers Phys.*, **5**, 60, 62 (1955).
5. Geneva, 1956, *Archives des Sciences, Fascicule Spec.*, Vol. 9, 1956.
6. Rennes-St. Malo, April 1957, *Archives des Sciences, Fascicule Spec.*, Vol. 10, 1957.
7. Paris, 1958, *Archives des Sciences, Fascicule Spec.*, Vol. 11, 1958.
8. London, 1959 (Maxwell-Ampère Conference), *Bulletin du Groupement Ampère, Fascicule Spec.*, Archives des Sciences, **12**, 251 pp. (1959).
9. Pisa, Sept. 1960, *Bulletin du Groupement Ampère*, Institut de Physique de l'Universite de Geneva, Switzerland, 1960; *Arch. Sci., Spec. No.*, **13**, (1960).
10. Leipzig, Sept. 1961, *Bulletin du Groupement Ampère*, Institut de Physique de l'Université de Geneva, Switzerland, 1961; *Spectroscopy and Relaxation at Radiofrequencies*, Amsterdam, 1962; *Arch. Sci., Spec. No.*, **14**, (1961).
11. Eindhoven, July 1962, *Magnetic and Electric Resonance and Relaxation*, J. Smidt, Ed., Wiley, N. Y., 1963.
12. Bordeaux, Sept. 1963, *Electronic Magnetic Resonance and Solid Dielectrics*, R. Servant, and A. Charru, Eds., North Holland, Amsterdam, 1964.
13. Leuven, 1964, *Koninlijke Vlaamse Academie Voor Wetenschappen*, Brussels, 1964; North Holland, Amsterdam, 1965.
14. Ljubljana, 1966.

DPPH (α,α'-Diphenyl-β-Picryl Hydrazyl)

J. Q. Adams and J. R. Thomas, "Electron Paramagnetic Resonance of a Hydrazine Radical Ion," *J. Chem. Phys.*, **39**, 1904 (1963).

M. E. Anderson, G. E. Pake, and T. R. Tuttle, Jr., "Proton Resonance in Diphenyl Picryl Hydrazyl," *J. Chem. Phys.*, **33**, 1581 (1960).

H. G. Beljers, L. van der Kint, and J. S. van Wieringen, "The Overhauser Effect in a Free Radical," *Phys. Rev.*, **95**, 1683 (1954).

R. G. Bennett and A. Henglein, "E.S.R. Line Widths of Some DPPH Derivatives," *J. Chem. Phys.*, **30**, 1117 (1959).

J. E. Bennett and E. J. H. Morgan, "Effect of Oxygen on ESR of DPPH," *Nature*, **182**, 199 (1958).

G. Berthet, "Electron Spin Resonance and the Structure of Some Stable Organic Free Radicals," *Ann. Phys. (Paris)*, **3**, 629 (1958).

G. Berthet, "Improved ESR Spectrometer (DPPH)," *C. R. Acad. Sci.*, **241**, 1730 (1955).

G. Berthet and Gene He, "ESR Spectrometer, DPPH in Methyl Cyclehexane and Benzene," *C. R. Acad. Sci.*, **241**, 1730 (1955).

F. Bruin and M. Bruin, "Some Measurements on the Spectral Line Shape and Width of a Paramagnetic Resonance Absorption Line," *Physica*, **22**, 129 (1956).

J. Burget, M. Odehnal, V. Petříček, J. Šácha, and L. Trlifaj, "Double Quantum Transitions in Free Radicals," *Czech. J. Phys.*, **11**, 719 (1961).

A. Chapiro, J. W. Boag, M. Ebert, and L. H. Gray, "Radiolysis of Dilute Solutions of DPPH in Organic Solvents, Part I," *J. Chim. Phys.*, **50**, 468 (1953); *Part II, ibid.*, **51**, 165 (1954); *Part III, ibid.*, **52**, 645 (1955).

A. K. Chirkov and A. A. Kokin, "Paramagnetic Resonance of Free Radicals in Weak Fields," *Zh. Eksper. Teor. Fiz.*, **35**, 50 (36) (1958).

I. S. Ciccarello, T. Garofano, and M. Santangelo, "Nuclear Hyperfine Structure of a Hydrazinic Free Radical," *Nuovo Cimento*, **12**, 389 (1959).

I. S. Ciccarello, T. Garofano, and M. Santangelo, "Further Investigations on the Electronic Structure of Free Radicals," *Arch. Sci. (Switzerland)*, **13**, 256 (1960).

I. S. Ciccarello, T. Garofano, and M. Santangelo, "Nuclear Hyperfine Structure of Hydrazylic Free Radicals," *Nuovo Cimento*, **17**, 881 (1960).

V. W. Cohen, C. Kikuchi, and J. Turkevich, "Anisotropy in Paramagnetic Resonance Absorption of Picryl-n-Amino Carbazyl," *Phys. Rev.*, **85**, 379 (1952).

P. Cornaz and J. P. Borel, "Study of the Paramagnetic Resonance of Picryl-Amino-Carbazyl as a Function of the Temperature," *Helv. Phys. Acta*, **34**, 407 (1961).

M. R. Das, A. V. Patankar, and B. Venkataraman, "Electron Spin Resonance Studies of the Free Radicals Derived from Tetraphenyl-Hydrazine," *Arch. Sci.*, **13**, 259 (1960).

R. M. Deal and W. S. Koski, "Inequality of the Coupling Constants of the Hydrazyl Nitrogens in DPPH," *J. Chem. Phys.*, **31**, 1138 (1959).

Y. Deguchi, "Proton Hyperfine Spectra of Diphenyl Picryl Hydrazyl," *J. Chem. Phys.*, **32**, 1584 (1960).

H. W. DeWijn and J. C. M. Henning, "Determination of the g-Tensor Anisotrophy of Triclinic DPPH at 4.5 mm Wavelength," *Physica*, **28**, 592 (1962).

H. E. Doorenbos and B. R. Loy, "E.S.R. of the N_2F_4-NF_2 Equilibrium," *J. Chem. Phys.*, **39**, 2393 (1963).

G. Eia and J. J. Lothe, "DPPH as a Standard in ESR," *Acta Chem. Scand.*, **12**, 1535 (1958).

R. Gabillard and J. A. Martin, "Measurement of the Relaxation Times T_1 and T_2 of the Free Radical Diphenyl Picryl Hydrazyl," *C. R. Acad. Sci.*, **238**, 2307 (1954).

R. Gabillard and B. Ponchel, "Application of Lateral Frequency-Modulation to a New Measurement Procedure for the Relaxation Time T_2," *11-th Ampère Colloquium*, Eindhoven, 1962, p. 749.

M. A. Garstens, L. S. Singer, and A. H. Ryan, "Magnetic Resonance Absorption of Diphenyl Picryl Hydrazyl at Low Magnetic Fields," *Phys. Rev.*, **96**, 53 (1954).

H. J. Gerritsen, R. Okkes, H. M. Gijsman, and J. van den Handel, "Some Magnetic Properties of Diphenyl Trinitrophenyl Hydrazyl at Low Temperatures," *Physica*, **20**, 13 (1954).

E. M. Gasanov, A. M. Prokhorov, and V. B. Fedorov, "Paramagnetic Relaxation in Systems with Strong Exchange Interactions at Low Temperatures," *Fiz. Tverd. Tela*, **6**, 193 (153) (1964).

J. P. Goldsborough, M. Mandel, and G. E. Pake, "Influence of Exchange Interaction on Paramagnetic Relaxation Times," *Phys. Rev. Letters*, **4**, 13 (1960).

R. B. Griffiths, "Theory of Magnetic Exchange-Lattice Relaxation in Two Organic Free Radicals," *Phys. Rev.*, **124**, 1023 (1961).

H. S. Gutowsky, H. Kusumoto, T. H. Brown, and D. H. Anderson, "Proton Magnetic Resonance and Electron Spin Densities of Hydrazyl," *J. Chem. Phys.*, **30**, 860 (1959).

P. Hedvig, "The Paramagnetic Cotton Mouton Effect in DPPH," *Acta Phys., Hung.*, **6**, 489 (1957).

J. Hervé, R. Reimann, and R. D. Spence, "Proton Magnetic Resonance in DPPH at Low Temperature," *Arch. Sci.*, **13**, 396 (1960).

R. W. Holmberg, R. Livingston, and W. T. Smith, Jr., "Paramagnetic Resonance Study of Hyperfine Interactions in Single Crystals Containing α,α' Diphenyl β-Picryl Hydrazyl," *J. Chem. Phys.*, **33**, 541 (1960).

C. A. Hutchison, Jr., R. C. Pastor, and A. G. Kowalski, "ESR in Organic Free Radicals; Fine Structure," *J. Chem. Phys.*, **20**, 534 (1952).

A. V. Il'yasov, N. S. Garif'yanov, and R. Kh. Timerov, "On the Nature of Spin Lattice Relaxation in Magnetically Diluted Free Radicals," *Dokl. Akad. Nauk. SSSR*, **150**, 588 (1963).

H. S. Jarrett, "Paramagnetic Resonance Absorption: Hyperfine Structure in Dilute Solutions of Hydrazyl Compounds," *J. Chem. Phys.*, **21**, 761 (1953).

P. Jung, J. Van Cakenberghe, and J. Uebersfeld, "Paramagnetic Resonance along the Direction of the Polarizing Field," *Physica*, **26**, 52 (1960).

Yu. S. Karimov and I. F. Shchegolev, "Hyperfine Interaction in the Diphenyl Picrylhydrazyl Molecule," *Zh. Eksper. Teor. Fiz.*, **40**, 3 (1) (1961).

C. Kikuchi and V. W. Cohen, "Paramagnetic Resonance Absorption of Carbazyl and Hydrazyl," *Phys. Rev.*, **93**, 394 (1954).

Y. W. Kim and P. W. France, "Electron Paramagnetic Resonance Absorption Studies of Neutron-Irradiated DPPH," *J. Chem. Phys.*, **38**, 1453 (1963).

B. M. Kozyrev, Yu. V. Yablokov, R. O. Matevosyan, M. A. Ikrina, A. V. Il'yasov, Yu. M. Ryzhmanov, L. I. Stashkov, and L. F. Shatrukov, "Electron Paramagnetic Resonance of Substituted DPPH," *Opt. i Spektroskopiya*, **15**, 625 (340) (1963).

Krishnaji and B. N. Misra, "Electron Spin Resonance Absorption in Recrystallized Free Radicals at low fields," *J. Chem. Phys.*, **41**, 1027 (1964).

Krishnaji and B. N. Misra, "Spin-Lattice Relaxation in Free-Radical Complexes," *Phys. Rev.*, **135**, A1068 (1964).

A. V. Kubarev and Yu. A. Mezenev, "Apparent Change of Gyromagnetic Ratio in a Weak Magnetic Field," *PTE*, **6**, 52 (909) (1960).

R. Lefebvre, J. Maruani, and R. Marx, "Electron Spin Resonance Evidence of a Distortion of DPPH in a Crystalline Medium," *J. Chem. Phys.*, **41**, 585 (1964).

R. Livingston and H. Zeldes, "Paramagnetic Resonance Absorption in Diphenyl-Picrylhydrazyl," *J. Chem. Phys.*, **24**, 170 (1956).

G. S. Lomkatsi, "Polarization of Hydrogen Nuclei in a Free Radical," *Zh. Eksper. Teor. Fiz.*, **38**, 635 (455) (1960).

N. W. Lord and S. M. Blinder, "Isotropic and Anisotropic Hyperfine Interactions in Hydrazyl and Carbazyl," *J. Chem. Phys.*, **34**, 1693 (1961).

K. Masuda and J. Yamaguchi, "Electric Conduction of DPPH in Benzene," *J. Phys. Soc., Japan*, **19**, 1190 (1964).

K. Möbius and F. Schneider, "Electron Spin Resonance Study of DPPH-Hydroperoxide Solutions," *Z. Naturforsch.*, **18a**, 428 (1963).

A. K. Morocha, "Theory of the Spin-Lattice Relaxation in Paramagnetics with Strong Exchange Interactions," *Fiz. Tverd. Tela.*, **4**, 2297 (1683) (1962).

A. M. Prokhorov and V. B. Fedorov, "Antiferromagnetism of Free Radicals," *Zh. Eksper. Teor. Fiz. USSR*, **43**, 2105 (1489) (1962).

R. Reimann, "Structure of the Proton Magnetic Resonance Line in DPPH at Low Temperatures," *Arch. Sci.*, **14**, 17 (1961).

R. Roest and N. J. Poulis, "The Spin-Spin Relaxation Time of Diphenyl Picryl Hydrazyl in Weak Fields," *Physica*, **25**, 1253 (1959).

K. V. Sane and J. A. Weil, "Paramagnetic Resonance of Hydrazyl-type Radicals in Viscous Media," *11-th Ampère Colloquium, Eindhoven*, 1962, p. 431.

L. S. Singer, "Exchange Narrowed ESR Absorption Lines at Low Intermediate Frequencies," *Paramagnetic Resonance*, **2**, 577 (1963).

L. S. Singer and C. Kikuchi, "Paramagnetic Resonance Absorption in Single Crystals of DPPH at Low Temperatures," *J. Chem. Phys.*, **23**, 1738 (1955).

L. S. Singer and E. G. Spencer, "Temperature Variation of the Paramagnetic Resonance Absorption of Two Free Radicals," *J. Chem. Phys.*, **21**, 939 (1953).

P. Swarup and B. N. Misra, "A Note on the Paramagnetic Resonance of a Free Radical," *Z. Phys.*, **159**, 384 (1960).

Y. Tchao, "Dynamic Proton Polarization in Solid DPPH and in Its Solutions," *Arch. Sci.*, **14**, 479 (1961).

Y. Tchao, "Study of the Dynamic Polarization of Protons in Powdered DPPH by Saturation of the Electronic Resonance in Weak Fields," *C. R. Acad. Sci.*, **252**, 1765 (1961).

H. Ueda, Z. Kuri, and S. Shida, "Electron Spin Resonance Studies of DPPH Solutions," *J. Chem. Phys.*, **36**, 1676 (1962).

L. Van Gerven, A. van Itterbeek, and E. de Wolf, "The Transverse Relaxation Time of Paramagnetic Electron Resonance in DPPH between 1.5°K and 300°K," *J. Phys. Rad.*, **18**, 417 (1957).

A. van Itterbeek and M. Labro, "Static Magnetic Susceptibility of DPPH between 294°K and 1.2°K," *Physica*, **30**, 157 (1964).

J. C. Verstelle, "Paramagnetic Resonance Line Forms in DPPH at Radio Frequencies," *Physica (Suppl.)*, **24**, S159 (1958).

J. C. Verstelle, G. W. J. Drewes, and C. J. Gorter, "The Spin-Spin Relaxation of DPPH in Parallel Fields," *Physica*, **26**, 520 (1960).

J. E. Wertz, C. F. Koelsch, and J. L. Vivo, "Re-Examination of Two Free Radicals," *J. Chem. Phys.*, **23**, 2194 (1955).

P. P. Yodzis and W. S. Koski, "g-Tensor Anisotrophy in Polycrystalline Diphenyl Picryl Hydrazyl," *J. Chem. Phys.*, **38**, 2313 (1963).

ESR and General Magnetic Resonance, Review Articles

R. S. Anderson, "Electron Spin Resonance," Sec. 4.2, p. 441, *Methods of Experimental Physics*, Vol. 3, D. Williams, Ed., Academic Press, N. Y., 1962.

H. M. Assenheim, "The Interpretation of Spectra in Electron Spin Resonance Investigations," *Res. Develop.*, 22 (June 1963).

D. M. S. Bagguley and J. Owen, "Microwave Properties of Solids," *Rept. Prog. Phys.*, **20**, 304 (1957).

G. Berthet, "Paramagnetic Electron Resonance," *Cahiers Phys.*, **67**, 6 (1956).

B. Bleaney and K. W. H. Stevens, "Paramagnetic Resonance," *Rept. Prog. Phys.*, **16**, 108 (1953).

B. Bölger, "On the Power Transfer between Paramagnetic Spins and the Crystal Lattice," *Proc. Korinkl. Ned. Akad. Wetenschop. B. No. 5*, **62**, 315 (1959); see *Phys. Abstr.*, 1960, No. 4519, 4520, 11932–11936 for other papers in this series.

K. D. Bowers and J. Owen, "Paramagnetic Resonance II," *Rept. Prog. Phys.*, **18**, 304 (1955).

K. W. Bowers, "Electron Spin Resonance of Radical Ions," *Advances in Magnetic Resonance*, Vol. 1, J. S. Waugh, Ed., Academic Press, N. Y., 1966, p. 317.

Collected Articles, *Nuovo Cimento Suppl.*, **6**, Ser. 10, 808 (1957).

G. Feher, "Electron Nuclear Double Resonance (ENDOR) Experiments," *Physica*, **24**, S80 (1958).

G. Feher, "Review of Electron Spin Resonance Experiments in Semiconductors," *Paramagnetic Resonance*, Vol. 2, Academic Press, N. Y., 1963, p. 715.

D. Fox, M. M. Labes, and A. Weissberger, Eds., *Physics and Chemistry of the Organic Solid State*, Wiley, N. Y., Vol. I, 1963, 1965.

G. K., Fraenkel, "Paramagnetic Resonance Absorption" in *Technique of Organic Chemistry*, Vol. 1, A. Weissberger, Ed., Interscience, N. Y., 1960, p. 2801.

W. Gordy, "Microwave Spectroscopy," *Rev. Mod. Phys.*, **20**, 668 (1948).

C. J. Gorter, "Applications of Electron Spin Resonance," *Mem. Acad. Roy. Belgique Cl. Sci.*, **33**, 9 (1961).

G. G. Hall and A. T. Amos, "Molecular Orbital Theory of the Spin Properties of Conjugated Molecules," *Advances in Atomic Molecular Physics*, Vol. 1, Academic Press, N. Y., 1965, p. 1.

L. C. Hebel, Jr., "Spin Temperature and Nuclear Relaxation in Solids," *Solid State Phys.*, **15**, 409 (1963).

D. J. E. Ingram, "Electron Spin Resonance Underlying Principles and Practical Applications," *Res. Develop.*, **5**, 58 (1962).

D. J. E. Ingram, "From Radar to Spectroscopy: New Regions of the Spectrum," *Nature*, **191**, 1146 (1961).

H. S. Jarrett, "Electron Spin Resonance Spectroscopy in Molecular Solids," *Solid State Phys.*, **14**, 215 (1963).

R. A. Kamper, "Paramagnetic Resonance," *Am. J. Phys.*, **28**, 249 (1960).

A. Kastler, "The Methods of Paramagnetic Resonance," *Cahiers Phys.*, **65**, 1 (1956).

G. R. Khutsishvili, "The Overhauser Effect and Related Phenomena," *Soviet Phys. Usp.*, **3**, 285 (1960).

G. R. Khutsishvili, "Relaxation and Orientation of Nuclei," *Akad. Nauk. Gruzinskoi SSR*, [Trudi (works) of the Institute of Physics], **4**, 3 (1956).

C. Kikuchi and R. D. Spence, "Microwave Methods in Physics I Microwave Spectroscopy," *Am. J. Phys.*, **17**, 288 (1949).

C. Kikuchi and R. D. Spence, "Microwave Methods in Physics II Microwave Absorption in Paramagnetic Substances," *Am. J. Phys.*, **18**, 167 (1950).

D. Kivelson and C. Thomson, "Electron Spin Resonance," *Ann. Rev. Phys. Chem.*, **15**, 197 (1964).

A. Kowalsky and M. Cohn, "Application of NMR in Biochemistry," *Ann. Rev. Biochem.*, **33**, 481 (1964).

G. W. Ludwig and H. H. Woodbury, "Electron Spin Resonance in Semiconductors," *Solid State Phys.*, **13**, 223 (1962).

J. R. Morton, "Electron Spin Resonance Spectra of Oriented Free Radicals," *Chem. Rev.*, **64**, 453 (1964).

D. E. O'Reilly, "Magnetic Resonance Techniques in Catalytic Research," *Advan. Catalysis*, **12**, 31 (1960).

J. W. Orton, "Paramagnetic Resonance Data," *Rept. Progr. Phys.*, **22**, 204 (1959).

J. W. Orton, *The Application of Paramagnetic Resonance to Non-Destructive Testing Progress in Non-Destructive testing*, Vol. 2, Heywood, London, 1960, p. 223.

G. E. Pake, "Radiofrequency and Microwave Spectroscopy of Nuclei," *Ann. Rev. Nucl. Sci.*, **4**, 33 (1954).

J. G. Powles, "Nuclear Magnetism in Pure Liquids," *Rept. Progr. Phys.*, **22**, 433 (1959).

F. Schneider, "Instruments and Measuring Techniques in Electron Spin Resonance Spectroscopy I and II" *Z. Instr.*, **71**, 315 (1963); **72**, 11 (1964).

A. G. Semenov, "Electron Paramagnetic Resonance Spectrometers," *PTE*, **5**, 5 (875) (1962).

J. N. Shoolery and H. E. Weaver, "Nuclear and Paramagnetic Resonance," *Ann. Rev. Phys. Chem.*, **6**, 433 (1955).

R. G. Shulman, "Electron and Nuclear Spin Resonance," *Ann. Rev. Phys. Chem.*, **13**, 325 (1962).

J. A. S. Smith, "Radiofrequency Spectroscopy at High Pressures," *High Pressure Physics and Chemistry*, Vol. 2, Academic, N. Y., 1963, p. 293.

M. C. R. Symons, "The Identification of Organic Free Radicals by ESR," *Ann. Rept. Chem. Soc.*, **59**, 45 (1962); "Electron Spin Resonance," *Advan. Phys. Org. Chem.*, **1**, 284 (1963).

S. Walker and H. Straw, "Spectroscopy," *Atomic, Microwave and Radiofrequency Spectroscopy*, Vol. 1, Chapman & Hall, London, 1961.

M. Weger, "Passage Effects in Paramagnetic Resonance Experiments," *Bell System Tech. J.*, **39**, 1013 (1960).

G. A. Woonton, "Relaxation in Diluted Paramagnetic Salts at Very Low Temperatures," *Advan. Electronics Electron. Phys.*, **15**, 163 (1961).

ESR and Magnetic Resonance, Elementary Treatments*

H. M. Assenheim, "The Interpretation of Spectra in Electron Spin Resonance Investigations," *Res. Develop.*, 22 (June 1963).

H. M. Assenheim, "A Modern Electron Spin Resonance Spectrometer," *Lab. Prac.*, (Nov. 1964).

H. M. Assenheim, "Electron Spin Resonance," *Chem. Prod.*, **25**, 339 (1962).

G. Bemski, "Studies in Electronic Structure of Covalent Semiconductors by EPR," *Am. J. Phys.*, **30**, 902 (1962).

D. I. Bolef, "Acoustic Techniques in Magnetic Resonance," *Science*, **136**, 359 (1962).

A. Carrington, "The Principles of ESR," *Endeavour*, **21**, No. 81, 51 (1962).

J. A. Cowen and W. H. Tanttila, "Versatile Magnetic Resonance Spectrometer," *Am. J. Phys.*, **26**, 381 (1958).

E. A. Faulkner, "Microwave Circuit Design for E.S.R. Spectrometers," *Lab. Prac.*, (Nov. 1964).

R. A. Fowler and H. S. Story, "Mechanical Analog of Magnetic Resonance," *Am. J. Phys.*, **29**, 709 (1961).

E. S. Gravlin and J. A. Cowen, "Simple Microwave Resonance Spectrometer," *Am. J. Phys.*, **27**, 566 (1959).

A. B. Grossberg, "Simple ESR Experiment at Low Magnetic Fields," *Am. J. Phys.*, **30**, 927 (1962).

J. P. Heller, "An Unmixing Demonstration," *Am. J. Phys.*, **28**, 348 (1960).

J. J. Hill, "A Magnetic Resonance Demonstration Model," *Am. J. Phys.*, **31**, 446 (1963).

D. J. E. Ingram, "Electron Spin Resonance, An Introductory Survey," *Lab. Prac.*, 1056 (1964).

D. J. E. Ingram, "ESR Underlying Principles and Practical Applications," *Res. Develop.*, **5**, 58 (Jan. 1962).

J. I. Kaplan, "Correlation Times, Line Widths, and Cross Relaxation of Spin Systems in Solids," *Am. J. Phys.*, **28**, 491 (1960).

C. Kikuchi and R. D. Spence, "Microwave Methods in Physics II, Microwave Absorption in Paramagnetic Substances," *Am. J. Phys.*, **18**, 167 (1950).

P. J. Limon and R. H. Webb, "A Magnetic Resonance Experiment for the Under graduate Laboratory," *Am. J. Phys.*, **32**, 361 (1964).

R. G. Marcley, "Apparatus for EPR at Low Fields," *Am. J. Phys.*, **29**, 492 (1961).

* See the resource letter NMR-EPR by R. E. Norberg, *Am. J. Phys.*, **33**, 71 (1965).

R. G. Marcley, "NMR Absorption Apparatus," *Am. J. Phys.*, **29**, 451 (1961).

G. E. Pake, "Magnetic Resonance," *Sci. Am.*, **199**, 58 (1958).

J. Rothstein, "Nuclear Spin Echo Experiments and the Foundations of Statistical Mechanics," *Am. J. Phys.*, **25**, 510 (1957).

R. H. Webb, "Steady State Polarizations via Electronic Transitions," *Am. J. Phys.*, **29**, 428 (1961).

ESR and Related Fields, Books

S. A. Al'tshuler and B. M. Kozyrev, *Electron Paramagnetic Resonance*, Transl. Scripta Technica, C. P. Poole, Jr., Ed., Academic, N. Y., 1964.

G. B. Benedek, *Magnetic Resonance at High Pressure*, Interscience, N. Y., 1963.

B. H. J. Bielski and J. M. Gebicki, *Atlas of Electron Spin Resonance Spectra*, Academic Press, N. Y., 1966, in press.

W. J. Caspers, *Theory of Spin Relaxation*, Interscience, N. Y., 1964.

W. Gordy, W. V. Smith, and R. F. Trambarulo, *Microwave Spectroscopy*, Wiley, N. Y., 1953.

C. J. Gorter, *Paramagnetic Relaxation*, Elsevier, Amsterdam, 1947.

H. M. Hershenshon, *NMR and ESR Spectra* (Index 1958–1963), Academic, N. Y. 1965.

D. J. E. Ingram, *Spectroscopy at Radio and Microwave Frequencies*, Butterworths, London, 1955.

D. J. E. Ingram, *Free Radicals as Studied by Electron Spin Resonance*, Butterworths, London, 1958.

C. D. Jeffries, *Dynamic Nuclear Orientation*, Interscience, N. Y., 1963.

Ya. S. Lebedev et al., *Atlas of ESR Spectra*, Consultants Bureau, N. Y., 1963.

William Low, "Paramagnetic Resonance in Solids," *Solid State Phys.*, Suppl. 2, Seitz and Turnbull, Eds., Academic Press, N. Y., 1960.

G. Pake, *Paramagnetic Resonance*, Benjamin, N. Y., 1962.

T. L. Squires, *An Introduction to Electron Spin Resonance*, Academic, N. Y., 1964.

M. W. P. Strandberg, *Microwave Spectroscopy*, Wiley, N. Y., 1954.

S. V. Vonsovskii, Ed., *Ferromagnetic Resonance*, U. S. Dept. of Commerce, Washington, 1964.

Low Temperature ESR and Nuclear Orientation

A. Abragam and M. Borghini, "Dynamic Polarization of Nuclear Targets," *Progress in Low Temperature Physics*, Vol. 4, North-Holland, Amsterdam, 1964, p. 384.

E. Ambler, "Methods of Nuclear Orientation," *Progress in Cryogenics*, **235**, 233 (1960).

C. DeWitt, B. Dreyfus, and P. G. de Gennes, Eds., *Low Temperature Physics*, (Les Houches Lectures, Univ. Grenoble, 1961) Gorden & Breach, N. Y., 1962.

C. J. Gorter, Ed., *Progress in Low Temperature Physics*, Annual series, Interscience, N. Y., begins in 1957.

C. D. Jeffries, "Dynamic Orientation of Nuclei," *Ann. Rev. Nucl. Sci.*, **14**, 101 (1964).

C. D. Jeffries, "Dynamic Nuclear Orientation," *Progr. Cryogenics*, **3**, 131 (1961).

International Conference on Low Temperature Physics and Chemistry, Univ. Wisconsin Press, Madison, Wisc., 1959.

Magnetic Resonance Conferences

(See also list of Colloques Amperes)

"Application of Radiofrequency Spectroscopy to Biochemistry and Chemical Structure." *Mem. Acad. Roy. Belgique Cl. Sci.*, **33**, No. 3, 363 pp. (1961).

Colloques Internationaux du Centre National de la Recherche Scientifique (CNRS) No. 27 Ferromagnetism et Antiferromagnetisme, Grenoble, July 1950 (13 Quai Anatole France, Paris 7e).

Defects in Crystalline Solids, conference held at H. H. Wills Physical Lab., University of Bristol, July 1954, The Physical Society, London, 1955.

"Ferromagnetism and Ferroelectricity Symposium," Leningrad, 1963, *Bull. Acad. Sci. USSR*, **28**, No. 3 and 4 (1965), p. 321.

"Fourteenth Spectroscopy Conference Gorkii 1961," *Bull. Acad. Sci. USSR, Phys. Ser.*, **27**, No. 1, 1 (1963).

A. Gozzini, Ed., *Topics in Radiofrequency Spectroscopy* (Scuola Internationale di Fisica, Corso 17), Academic, N. Y., 1962.

"Ions of the Transition Elements," *Disc. Faraday Soc.*, No. 26 (1958).

E. R. Lippincott and M. Margoshes, Eds., *Proc. Xth Colloquium Spectroscopicium Internationale*, University of Maryland, 1962, Spartan Books, Washington, D. C., 1963.

W. Low, Ed., *Paramagnetic Resonance*, Vols. 1 and 2, Academic Press, N. Y., 1963.

D. Ter Haar, Ed., *Fluctuation, Relaxation and Resonance in Magnetic Systems*, Scottish Universities' 2nd Summer School, (1961), Oliver & Boyd, Edinburgh, 1962.

"Unstable Chemical Species: Free Radicals, Ions and Excited Molecules," *Annals. N. Y., Acad. Sci.*, **67**, 447 (1957).

"Varenna Conference on Magnetism," *Nuovo Cimento*, **6** (Suppl., Ser. 10), 805–1233 (1957) (1956 lectura).

"Washington Conference on Magnetism," University of Maryland, September 1952, *Rev. Mod. Phys.*, **25**, No. 1, p. 1 (1953).

O. V. St. Whitelock, Ed., "Nuclear Magnetic Resonance," *Ann. N. Y. Acad. Sci.*, **70**, 763 (1958).

Magnetism

S. Chikazumi, *Physics of Magnetism*, Wiley, N. Y., 1964.

I. S. Jacobs and E. G. Spencer, Eds., "Proceedings of the Tenth Conference on Magnetism and Magnetic Materials," *J. Appl. Phys.*, **36**, 877 (1965).

B. Lax and K. J. Button, *Microwave Ferrites and Ferrimagnetics*, McGraw-Hill, N. Y., 1962.

A. H. Morrish, R. J. Prosen, and S. M. Rubens, Eds., *Magnetic Materials Digest 1964*, M. W. Lads, Philadelphia, 1964, 260 pp.

Proceedings of the International Conference on Magnetism (Nottingham, 1964), Institute of Physics and the Physical Society, 1965, London.

Proceedings of the Symposium on Magnetism and Magnetic Materials, (with many ESR articles) published annually in *J. Appl. Phys.*, March issue.

G. T. Rado and H. Suhl, Eds., *Magnetism* Vol. 1, "Magnetic Ions in Insulators, Their Interactions, Resonances and Optical Properties," 1963; Vol. 2a "Statistical Models, Magnetic Symmetry, Hyperfine Interactions, and Metals," 1965; Vol. 3, "Spin Arrangements and Crystal Structure Domains and Micromagnetics," 1963; Vol. 4, "Exchange Interactions Among Itinerant Electrons," Academic Press, N. Y., 1966.

T. D. Rossing, Ferromagnetic Resonance and Relaxation, *Magnetic Materials Digest 1964*, M. W. Lads, Philadelphia, 1964, p. 218.

E. A. Turov, *Physical Properties of Magnetically Ordered Crystals*, Academic Press, N. Y., 1965.

Miscellaneous Books

M. Abramowitz and I. A. Stegun, Eds., *Handbook of Mathematical Functions*, Dover, N. Y., 1965.

A. M. Bass and H. P. Broida, Eds., *Formation and Trapping of Free Radicals*, Academic Press, N. Y., 1960.

Ya. G. Dorfman, *Diamagnetism and the Chemical Bond*, Transl. Scripta Technica, C. P. Poole, Jr., Ed., Arnold, London, 1965.

J. S. Griffith, *The Theory of Transition-Metal Ions*, Cambridge University Press, Cambridge, 1961.

B. R. Judd, *Operator Techniques in Atomic Spectroscopy*, McGraw-Hill, N. Y., 1963.

I. S. Longmuir, *Advances in Polarography*, Pergamon, N. Y., 1960.

W. Paul and D. M. Worschauer, *Solids Under Pressure*, McGraw-Hill, N. Y., 1963.

N. F. Ramsey, *Nuclear Moments*, Wiley, N. Y., 1953.

N. F. Ramsey, *Molecular Beams*, Clarendon, Oxford, 1956.

Nuclear Magnetic Resonance
Articles and Reviews

E. R. Andrew, "Nuclear Magnetic Resonance Investigation of Solids," *Ber. Bunsengesell. Phys. Chem.*, **67**, 295 (1963).

L. E. Drain, "Nuclear Magnetic Resonance and its Application to the Testing of Materials," *Progress in Non-Destructive Testing.* **1**, 227 (1958).

H. S. Gutowsky, "Nuclear Magnetic Resonance," *Ann. Rev. Phys. Chem.*, **5**, 333 (1954).

D. M. Grant, "High Resolution Nuclear Magnetic Resonance," *Ann. Rev. Phys. Chem.*, **15**, 489 (1964).

R. A. Y. Jones, "Nuclear Magnetic Resonance," *Sci. Progr.*, **51**, 198 (1963).

G. R. Khutsishvili, "Relaxation and the Orientation of Nuclei," *Tr. Inst. Fiz.* (*Acad. Sci. USSR*), **4**, 3 (1956).

W. D. Knight, "Electron Paramagnetism and NMR in Metals," *Solid State Phys.*, **2**, 91 (1956).

A. Kowalsky and M. Cohn, "Applications of NMR in Biochemistry," *Ann. Rev. Biochem.*, **33**, 481 (1964).

F. Koch, "Some Experiments with Models Illustrating Free Precession and Emission in Nuclear Magnetic Resonance," *Arch. Sci.*, **14**, 271 (1961).

D. J. Kroon, "Nuclear Magnetic Resonance," *Philips Tech. Rev.*, **21**, 286 (1960).

D. J. Kroon, "Line Shape of Proton Magnetic Resonance in Paramagnetic Solids," *Philips Res. Rept.*, **15**, 501 (1960).

G. Lindström, "Nuclear Resonance Absorption Applied to Precise Measurements of Nuclear Magnetic Moments and the Establishment of an Absolute Energy Scale in β-Spectroscopy," *Arkiv. Fysik.*, **4**, 1 (1951).

D. W. McCall and R. W. Hamming, "Nuclear Magnetic Resonance in Crystals," *Acta Cryst.*, **12**, 31 (1959).

G. E. Pake, "Fundamentals of Nuclear Magnetic Resonance Adsorption I and II," *Am. J. Phys.*, **18**, 438, 473 (1950).

G. E. Pake, "Nuclear Magnetic Resonance," *Solid State Phys.*, **2**, 1 (1956).

R. V. Pound, "Nuclear Paramagnetic Resonance," *Progr. Nucl. Phys.*, **2**, 21 (1952).

T. J. Rowland, "Nuclear Magnetic Resonance in Metals," *Progr. Mater. Sci.*, **9**, 1 (1961).

J. N. Shoolery, "Some New Structural and Analytical Applications of High-Resolution NMR," *Arch. Sci.*, **13**, 495 (1960).

H. Strehlow, "Bases and Applications of Nuclear Magnetic Resonance in Physical Chemistry," *Ber. Bunsengesell. Phys. Chem.*, **67**, 250 (1963).

M. Weger, "Passage Effects in Paramagnetic Resonance Experiments," *Bell Syst. Tech. J.*, **39**, 1013 (1960).

Nuclear Magnetic Resonance

Books

A. Abragam, *The Principles of Nuclear Magnetism*, Clarendon, Oxford, 1961.

I. V. Aleksandrov, *Theory of Nuclear Magnetic Resonance*, Transl. Scripta Technica, C. P. Poole, Jr., Ed., Academic, N. Y., 1966.

E. R. Andrew, *Nuclear Magnetic Resonance*, Cambridge University Press, Cambridge, 1955.

R. J. Blin-Stoyle, *Theories of Nuclear Moments*, Oxford Univ. Press, Oxford, 1957.

N. Bloembergen, *Nuclear Magnetic Relaxation*, Benjamin, N. Y., 1961.

J. W. Emsley, J. Feeney, and L. H. Sutcliffe, *High Resolution Nuclear Magnetic Resonance Spectroscopy*, Vol. 1, Pergamon, N. Y., 1965.

M. G. Howell, A. S. Kende, and J. S. Webb, Eds., *Formula Index to NMR Data*, Vols. 1 and 2, Plenum Press, N. Y., 1965.

L. M. Jackman, *Applications of Nuclear Magnetic Resonance Spectroscopy in Organic Chemistry*, Pergamon, N. Y., 1959.

A. Lösche, *Kerninduktion*, Deutscher Verlag der Wissenschaften, Berlin, 1957.

K. Nakanishi, L. Durham, and M. C. Woods, *A Guide to the Interpretation of NMR Spectra,"* Holden Day, 1966.

J. A. Pople, W. G. Schneider, and H. J. Bernstein, *High Resolution Nuclear Magnetic Resonance,* McGraw-Hill, N. Y., 1959.

J. D. Roberts, *Nuclear Magnetic Resonance,* McGraw-Hill, N. Y., 1959.

A. K. Saha and T. P. Das, *Theory and Applications of Nuclear Induction,* Saha Institute of Nuclear Physics, Calcutta, India, 1957.

H. Strehlow, *Magnetische Kernresonanz and Chemische Struktur,* D. Steinkopff, Ed., Darmstadt, 1962.

K. B. Wiberg, *The Interpretation of NMR Spectra,* W. A. Benjamin, N. Y., 1962.

A. I. Zhernovoi and G. D. Latyshev, *NMR in a Flowing Liquid,* Consultants Bureau, N. Y., 1965.

Nuclear Magnetic Resonance

Elementary Articles

F. Bloch, "The Principle of Nuclear Induction," *Science,* **118**, 425 (1953).

B. L. Donnally and E. Bernal, "Some Experiments on Nuclear Magnetic Resonance," *Am. J. Phys.,* **31**, 779 (1963).

E. L. Hahn, "Free Nuclear Induction," *Phys. Today,* **6**, 4 (Nov. 1953).

D. J. E. Ingram, "Nuclear Magnetic Resonance (Part I)," *Contemp. Phys.,* **7**, 13, (1965); Part II, *ibid.,* **7**, 1031 (1965).

E. M. Purcell, "Research in Nuclear Magnetism," *Science,* **118**, 431 (1953).

E. M. Purcell, "Nuclear Magnetism," *Am. J. Phys.,* **22**, 1 (1954).

S. Walker and H. Straw, *Spectroscopy,* Chapman & Hall, London, 1961, Chap. 5.

Nuclear Quadrupole Resonance (NQR)

A. D. Buckingham, "Molecular Quadrupole Moments," *Quart. Rev.,* **13**, 183 (1959).

M. H. Cohen and F. Reif, "Quadrupole Effects in NMR Studies of Solids," *Solid State Phys.,* **5**, 322 (1957).

M. H. Cohen and F. Reif, *NMR Studies of Defects in Ionic Crystals,* Public. Phys. Soc., London, 1955, p. 48.

T. P. Das and E. L. Hahn, "Nuclear Quadrupole Resonance Spectroscopy," *Solid State Physics,* Suppl. 1, Seitz and Turnbull, Eds., Academic Press, N. Y., 1958.

H. G. Dehmelt, "Nuclear Quadrupole Resonance," *Am. J. Phys.,* **22**, 110 (1954); *ibid.,* **22**, *erratum,* p. 317.

V. S. Grechishkin, "Nuclear Quadrupole Resonance," *Usp. Fiz. Nauk.,* **69**, 189 (699) (1959).

P. Grivet and A. Bassompierre, "Nuclear Quadrupole Resonance," *Mem. Acad. Roy. Belgique Cl. Sci.,* **33**, 219 (1962).

O. Nagai and T. Nakamura, "Quadrupole Interaction in Crystals," *Progr. Theor. Phys. (Japan),* **24**, 432 (1960).

J. C. Raich and R. H. Good, Jr., "Discussion of Quadrupole Precession," *Am. J. Phys.,* **31**, 356 (1963).

Author Index*

A

Aasa, R., 591, *595*, 835, 836, *844*, 848

Abkowitz, M., 625, *659*

Abragam, A., 18, *33*, *334*, 530, *595*, 698, 717, *730*, 735, 736, 738, 742, 744, 747, 749, 750, *768*, *769*, *773*, 825, 840, *844*, *870*, *873*

Abraham, M., 747, *769*

Abraham, R. J., 369, *383*, 478, *518*

Abrahams, E., 807, 810, 838, *846*

Abramowitz, M., *872*

Ackermann, P., 758, *769*

Acrivos, J. V., 418, *423*

Adair, T. W. III, 367, *383*

Adams, F. C., 621, 624, *633*

Adams, J. Q., *863*

Adams, M., 620, 621, *633*

Adams, N. L., Jr., 365, *384*

Adams, R. N., 625, *634*

Adkins, C. J., 652, *659*

Adler, F., 327, *334*

Agdur, B., 263, *334*

Ageno, M., 843, *844*

Ager, R., 285, 321, *334*, *336*, 756, *771*

Akhmanov, S. A., 478, *518*

Alaeva, T. I., 262, *334*

Albold, E., 478, *518*

Aleksandrov, I. V., *873*

Alexeff, I., 456, *472*

Alger, R. S., 683, *692*

Allen, G., 643, *659*

Allen, L. C., 579, 581–584, *595*, 843, *844*

Alsop, L. E., 728, 729, *731*

Altschuler, H. M., 303, *334*

Al'tshuler, S. A., 29, *33*, 475, *518*, 590, *595*, 602, *633*, 727, *730*, 735, 749, 763, *769*, *870*

Ambler, E., 643, 645, 646, *659*, *870*

Ambrasas, V., 369, *384*

Amos, A. T., *867*

Anderegg, M., *208*, 482, *518*

Anderson, C. T., 208, *208*

Anderson, D. H., *863*, *865*

Anderson, H. G., 807, *844*

Anderson, J. H., 684, 686, *692*, 836, *849*

Anderson, J. M., 748, *769*

Anderson, M. E., 840, *847*

Anderson, P. W., 705, 728, *730*, *731*, 838, 839, *844*

Anderson, R. A., 577, 579, *595*

Anderson, R. S., 23, *34*, 192, 193, 269, *337*, 843, *847*, *867*

Anderson, T. H., 683, *692*

Anderson, W. A., 365, *383*, *596*

Andresen, S. G., 321, *334*

Andrew, E. R., 365, *383*, 412, *423*, 716, 717, *730*, 759, *769*, 824, 825, 839, 840, *844*, *872*, *873*

Andrews, G. B., 435, *445*

Ankorn, V. J., 601, 608, 612, *633*

Antonenko, I. O., 376, *383*

Arams, F. R., 237, *255*, 572, *598*

Arbuzov, A. Ye, 590, *595*

Armbruste, R., 374, *384*

Arnal, R., 456, *472*

Arndt, R., 398, 411, *423*, 686, *692*

Arp, V. D., 645, *659*

Artman, J. O., 318, 325, *334*, 393, *423*, 476, *518*, 696, *730*

Assenheim, H. M., 482, *518*, *867*, *869*

Atsarkin, V. A., 480, *518*, 544, *595*

Aubrun, J. N., 579, *595*

Auld, B. A., 186, *208*, 314, *334*

Ault, L. A., 314, *338*

Austen, D. E. G., 621, *633*

Autler, S. H., 367, *383*

* *Italic* numbers refer to reference pages.

875

Bjorken, J. D., 365, *383*
Black, H. S., 458, *472*
Blackburn, J. F., *124*
Blackwell, J. H., 213, *256*
Blake, C. B., 646, 653, *659*
Blanpain, R., 647, *659*
Blatt, J. M., 12, *39*
Bleaney, B., 2, 18, 33, *33*, 738, *769*, 826, 835, 836, *844*, *867*
Blears, D. J., 643, *659*
Blentzinger, P., 456, *472*
Blinder, S. M., 835, *844*, *866*
Bline, R., 825, *844*
Blin-Stoyle, R. J., 743, *769*, *874*
Bloch, F., 2, *33*, 514, *519*, 705, 717, *730*, 736, 737, 750, *769*, 839, *844*, *874*
Bloembergen, N., 2, *34*, 318, 330, 332, *334*, *339*, 589, *596*, 654, 655, *661*, *662*, 696, 698, 699, 705, 714, 717, 718, *730*, 759, 763, *769*, *773*, 816, 826, 830, 835, 839, 843–845, 848, *873*
Blois, M. S., 620, 621, *633*
Blomfield, D. L. H., *445*
Blomgren, G. E., 844, *847*
Bloom, M., 412, *424*
Blum, H., 329, 330, *336*, 480, *520*, 757, *770*
Blumberg, W. E., 17, *34*, *338*, *424*, 515, *521*, 750, *769*
Blume, R. J., 389, *423*
Blume, S., 570, *596*
Boag, J. W., *864*
Bodi, A., 596, *596*
Bogle, G. S., 478, 508, *519*
Bohm, H. V., 653, *660*
Bohr, A., 749, *769*
Bolef, D. I., 263, *335*, 480, *519*, 727, *730*, 763, 767–769, *771*, *869*
Bölger, B., 727, *730*, *867*
Bolt, R. H., 767, *771*
Bolton, H. C., 530, *596*
Bolton, J. R., 29 ,*33*, 624, 627, *633*, 844, *845*
Bömmel, H. E., 263, *335*, 763, *769*
Bonhomme, H. J., 376, *383*
Bonnet, G., 375, *383*, 535, *596*
Booman, K. A., 642, *661*

Borel, J. P., *208*, 482, *518*, *864*
Borg, D. C., 633, *633*
Borghini, M., 748, *769*, *870*
Bosch, B. G., 435, *445*, 569, *596*
Bösnecker, D., 456, *472*, 478, *519*
Bott, I. B., 187, 209
Bottreau, A., 250, *255*
Boudouris, G., 299, 316, *335*
Bouthinon, M., 208, *209*
Bowers, K. D., 29, *33*, 318, *335*, 342, *383*, 420, *423*, 478, 499, 500, *519*, 724, 728, *730*, *731*, 760, *769*, 825, *845*
Bowers, K. W., 621, 626, 628, *633*, *867*
Bowers, V. A., 27, *33*, 649, *660*, 679, 680, *693*
Boyd, G. D., 262, 318, *335*
Bozorth, R. M., 355–358, 383
Brackett, E. B., 120, *123*
Bradbury, A., 369, *383*, 839, *844*
Bradley, R. S., 653, *659*
Brainerd, J. C., *123*
Brannen, E., 186, *209*
Braude, E. A., 673, *692*
Brault, A. L., 440, *445*
Braunschweiger, P. G., 208, *210*, 277, *338*
Breit, G., 738, *769*
Bresler, S. E., 478, *519*, 544, *596*
Brewer, D. F., 645, *659*
Brickwedde, F. G., 645, *659*
Bridgman, P. W., 655, *659*
Brodwin, M. E., 316, *335*, 482, 514, *519*, 542, *596*
Broekaert, P., 698, 731
Brogden, T. W. P., 523, *596*
Broida, H. P., 644, *662*, 679, 680, *692*, *693*, *872*
Bromberg, N. S., 576, 597
Bronstein, J., 836, *845*
Bronwell, A. R., *123*
Brooks, G. H., 334, *338*
Brophy, J. J., 448, *472*
Brovetto, P., 749, *769*
Brown, G., 484, *519*
Brown, H. H., 365, *383*
Brown, H. W., *336*, 415, 416, *423*, 634
Brown, M. R., 189, *209*

Frederick, N. V., 518, *519*
Freed, J. H., *633*, 844, *845*
Freethey, F. E., 316, 321, *338*
French, A. P., 15, *33*
Fric, C., 279, *335*
Friedberg, S. A., 647, *660*
Fritz, J. J., *660*
Froelich, H. C., 186, *209*, 643, *660*
From, W. H., 576, *597*
Fröman, P. O., 686, *692*
Frömel, W., 673, *693*
Frontali, C., 843, *844*
Froome, K. D., 186, *209*
Fujisawa, K., 187, *209*
Fukuda, K., 680, *692*
Fulford, J. A., 213, *256*
Fulk, M. M., 644, *660*
Fuller, C. S., 738, *770*
Furth, H. P., 372, *383*
Fuschillo, N., 652, *660*

G

Gaara, P., 590, *596*
Gabillard, R., 380, *383*, 415, *423*, 579, *596*, *597*, *864*
Galkin, A. A., 478, *519*, 621, *633*
Gambling, W. A., 44, *50*, 174, 208, *209*, 257, *339*, 435, *445*, 482, 502, *519*, 544, 564–569, 572, 573, *596*, *597*, *600*
Gamo, H., 263, *336*
Ganapolskii, E. M., 768, *770*
Gannus, V. K., 643, *661*
Ganssen, A., 174, 208, *211*, 257, 318, *336*, *338*, 567, *599*
Garcia de Quevado, J. L., 422, *425*
Gardner, F. G., 144, *167*
Gardner, J. H., 655, 657, 658, *660*
Garif'yanov, N. S., 415, *423*, 590, *595*, *865*
Garofano, T., *864*
Garrett, B. B., 843, *845*
Garrett, W., 761, *770*
Garscadden, A., 456, *472*
Garstens, M. A., 318, *336*, 840, *845*, *865*
Garwin, R. C., 376, *383*

Gasanov, E. M., *865*
Gaballe, T. H., 647, *660*, *661*
Gebicki, J. M., *870*
Geiszler, T. D., 252, *256*
Gendell, J., 844, *845*
Genzel, L., 188, *209*, 262, *339*
Gerasimenko, V. L., 736, *769*
Gere, E. A., 738, 751, *770*
Germain, C., 380, *383*
Gerritsen, H. J., *865*
Gersmann, H. R., 835, 845
Geschwind, S., 650, 651, *660*
Geske, D. H., 621, 622, *633*
Gevers, M., 181, *211*, 213, *256*
Gheorghiu, D., 452, *472*
Gheorghiu, O. C., 312, *336*
Ghosh, U. S., 482, *519*
Giardino, D. A., 843, *845*
Giauque, W. F., *383*, 647, 653, *660*
Gibson, J. F., 678, *692*
Gibson, L. E., 577, *595*
Gijsman, H. M., *865*
Gilchrist, A., 642, *660*
Gill, J. C., 705, *731*
Gilliam, O. R., 184, *209*, 255, *256*
Gilman, J. J., 861, *862*
Gilvarry, J. J., 369, *383*
Ginzton, E. L., 43, *50*, *123*, 171, *209*, 299, *336*
Giordmaine, J. A., 728, 729, *731*
Giori, D. C., 327, *335*
Girard, B., 374, *385*
Gittins, J. F., 174, *209*
Giulotto, L., 730, *731*
Given, P. H., 621, *633*
Gladney, H. M., 579, 581–584, *595*, 843, *844*
Glarum, S. H., 418, *423*, 579, 581–585, *595*, *597*, 843, *844*, *845*
Glauche, E., 482, *519*
Glebashev, G. Ya., *845*
Glicksman, M., *123*
Golay, M. J. E., 365, *383*
Goldman, M., 398, *423*, 746, 747, 749, *770*
Goldsborough, J. P., 482, *519*, 544, *597*, 680, *692*, *865*

Ramo, S., 35, 39, *50*, 54, 74, *76*, 88, 100, 107, 116–118, 120, *123*, 131, 132, *167*, 315, *337*
Ramsey, N. F., 680, *693*, *872*
Randall, E. W., 748, *769*
Randolph, M. L., 467, *472*, 591, 592, 593, *598*
Raoult, G., 279, *337*, 514, *521*
Rauch, W. G., 688, *692*
Redfield, A. G., 716, *732*
Redhardt, A., 206, *210*, 334, *337*
Reed, E. D., 316, *337*
Reed, R., 262, *337*
Reeves, R. A., 591, *596*
Reich, H. A., 683, *692*
Reich, H. J., *123*
Reichert, J. F., 263, 332, 333, *337*, 763, *772*
Reif, F., 29, *33*, *874*
Reimann, R., *865*, *866*
Reinhold, F., 257, *336*, 748, 752, 754, *770*
Reinhold, R., 570, *597*
Reinmuth, W. H., 624, *634*
Reinov, N. M., 644, *660*
Reintjes, J. F., 104–106, 114, *124*, 171, *210*, 277, 286, *337*
Renk, K. F., 262, *339*
Renn, K., 589, *597*
Rensen, J. G., 639, *662*
Retherford, R. C., 683, *693*
Reuter, G. E. H., 818, *847*
Rexroad, H. N., 602, *634*, 730, *732*
Reynolds, J. F., 334, *337*, 683, *693*
Rhinehart, W. A., 464, *472*
Richards, R. E., 484, *520*, *521*, 570, *597*, 735, 753, *771*, *772*, 824, *847*
Richter, G., 704, *732*
Ridenour, L. N., *124*
Rieckhoff, K. E., 276, *338*, 644, *661*, 679, *693*
Rieger, P. H., 624, *634*, 844, *845*
Rinehart, E. A., 392, 393, 418, 423, *424*, 775, *847*
Risley, A. S., 186, *210*
Ristau, O., 478, *521*
Rivers, W. K., 439, *445*

RLS-1, *124*
RLS-2, *124*
RLS-3, *124*
RLS-4, *124*
RLS-5, *124*
RLS-6, *124*, 172, *210*, *598*
RLS-7, *124*, 171, 174, 179, 180, *210*, 533, *598*
RLS-8, 39, 46, *50*, 97, 103, 108, 109, *124*, 129, 135, 138–141, 145, 147, 148, 150, 153, 159–161, 164, 165, *167*, 224, 228, 229, 233, 237–240, 244, 248, 281, 283, 314, *338*
RLS-9, 75, *76*, 87, 95, 97, *124*, 135, *167*, 213, 237, 238, 239, 243, 248, 249, 252, 253, 255, 281, 303, 312, *338*
RLS-10, 96, 111, 117–119, *124*, 213, 228, 229, 243, 282, *338*
RLS-11, 44, *50*, *124*, 175, 177, 178, 180, 195–200, *210*, 213, 216–219, 225–229, 232, 233, 241, 242, 245, 247, 249, 250, 252, 254, *256*, 262, 271, 273–278, 283, 287, 288, *338*, 533, *598*
RLS-12, 11, *34*, *124*, 213, 242, 250, 251, *256*
RLS-13, *124*, 530, *598*
RLS-14, *124*, 213, 231–234, 237, 249, *256*, 280, 281, 285, 286, *338*
RLS-15, *124*, 184, *210*, 431–436, 438, 444, *445*
RLS-16, *124*, 432, 436, 439, 440, 443, 444, *445*, 532, 535, *598*
RLS-17, 95, *124*
RLS-18, *124*, 444, *445*
RLS-19, *124*, 456, *472*
RLS-20, *124*
RLS-21, *124*
RLS-22, *124*, *598*
RLS-23, *124*, 444, *445*, 571, *598*
RLS-24, *124*, 532, 533, *598*
RLS-25, *124*
RLS-26, *124*
RLS-27, *124*
RLS-28, *124*
Roberts, A., *124*
Roberts, C. A., *337*
Roberts, G., 316, *338*, 589, *598*

Van Hiep, T., 579, *595*
Vanier, J., 480, *520*, 680, *693*, 720, *731*
van Iperen, B. B., *211*
van Itterbeek, A., 456, *473*, 730, *733*, 804, *848*, *866*
van Ladesteyn, D., 195, *209*, 411, *423*
Vänngård, T., 591, *595*, 686, *692*, 835, 836, *844*, *847*, *848*
Van Overbeek, J., 467, *472*
Van Roggen, A., 826, *848*
Van Roggen, L., 826, *848*
Van Soest, P. C., 758, *770*
Van Steenwinkel, R., 752, *773*
Van Till, H., 652, *659*
Van Vleck, J. H., 725, 727, 728, *733*, 750, *773*, 775, 825, 836, 838, 839, 842, *848*
Van Voorhis, S. N., *124*
van Wieringen, J. J., 639, *662*, 686, *694*, 759, *769*, *863*
Vanwormhoudt, M. C., 315, *335*
Varacca, V., 327, *335*
Vartanian, P. H., 186, *208*, 224, *256*
Veazey, S. E., 641, *662*
Veigele, W. J., 653, *662*
Veillet, P., 579, *595*
Venkataraman, B., 620, *635*, *864*
Verdier, P. H., 257, *339*, 412, *425*, 595, *599*, 839, *848*
Verein, N. V., 307, *337*, 423, *424*, 544, *598*
Verkin, B. I., 262, *339*
Verma, A. R., *862*
Verma, G. S., 727, *733*, 763, *773*
Verstelle, J. C., *867*
Verweel, J., 328, *339*
Vessot, R. F. C., 680, *693*
Vetchinkin, A. N., 653, *662*
Vetter, M. J., 263, 328, *339*
Viet, N. T., 262, *339*
Villeneuve, A. T., 314, *339*
Vinal, G. W., 368, *385*
Vincent, C. H., 369, 373, *385*, 457, *473*
Vincow, G., 840, *848*
Visweswarmurthy, S., *385*, 412, *425*, 579, *599*
Vitolin, A., 376, *385*

Vivo, J. L., *867*
Voevodskii, V. V., 23, *33*, 686, *693*, 799, 806, 843, *846*, *848*
Vogel, S., 263, *337*
Voigt, F., 482, *519*
Volavšek, B., 825, *844*
Volkoff, G. M., 839, *848*
Volpicelli, R. J., 369, *384*
Volterra, V., 836, *845*
Vonbun, F. O., 321, *339*
Vonsovskii, S., *848*, *870*
Vrščaj, S., 369, *385*

W

Wagner, P. E., 321, *335*
Wagner, W. G., 262, 318, *339*
Wagoner, G., 320, *338*, 590, *599*, 639–641, *662*, 715, *733*, 816, 817, *848*
Wahlquist, H., 398, 401, 402, 408, 411, *425*
Wainstein, C., 836, *848*
Wait, D. F., 658, *659*
Walker, S., *869*, *874*
Walling, C., 672, *694*
Wallman, H., *124*
Walsh, W. M., 331, 332, *339*, 654–656, *662*
Walter, J., 530, 570, *599*
Walter, R. L., 840, *848*
Waltz, M. C., 533, *597*
Wamser, C. A., 620, *635*
Wang, S., 589, *596*, 714, 717, 718, *730*
Wang, T. C., 573, *599*
Waniek, R. W., 372, *383*
Ward, R. L., 621, *635*
Waring, R. K., 207, *211*
Warren, R. F., 643, *659*
Wartewig, S., 649, *663*
Waters, D. M., 316, 321, *338*
Watkins, G. D., 376, 385, 637, 659, *663*, 757, 758, *773*
Waugh, J. S., 415, *424*, 590, *599*, 825, *848*
Weaver, H. E., 372, *384*, *868*
Webb, J. S., *873*

Subject Index

A

Absorption, 414, 463, 514, 523, 534, 542, 551, 567, 570, 701, 702, 705, 716, 719
    comparison with dispersion, 813
Absorption coefficient, 678, 691
    mass, 691
Absorption derivative, 777, 784
Acenaphthenequinone, 631
A center, 689
Acetaldehyde, 673
Acetone, 571, 673, 683
Acetophenone, 630, 632
Acetylpyridine, 631
Acoustic ESR, 2, 763ff, 840
Acrilonitrile, 624, 632
Address, 579
Adiabatic condition, 700, 738
Adiabatic demagnetization, 643, 644, 652
Adiabatic fast passage ,737, 738
Admittance, characteristic, 441
Admittance matrix, 127, 223
Alignment, nuclear, 744
Alkali halide, 688, 689
Alkali metal, 620
Alpha particle, 665, 667–669
Alumina, 71, 231, 285, 655
Ammonia, 1, 2, 30, 344, 621, 624
Ammoniumiodide, tetramethyl (TMAI), 632
Ammonium perchlorate, tetra n-propyl (TNPAP), 624, 632
Ampère's law, 59
Amplifier, 174, 195, 576
    dc, 192, 198, 199, 246, 390, 573
    difference, 206
    i.f., 444
    microwave, 571
    modulation coil, 420
    narrow band, 1, 246, 448, 546, 559. 560, 800
    push–pull, 198, 420, 449
    reactance, 574
    triode, 171
    tuned, 202, 203, 449
    twin T, 450
    variable resistance. *See* Parametric amplifier.
Analyzer, pulse height, 577
Angular momentum, 11
Aniline, 673
Anion, 620
Annealing, 685
Antenna, 1, 7, 570, 765
    linear array, 250
    loop, 246
    microwave, 250
    parabolic, 250
    rotating, 252
    waveguide, 217
Anthracene, 620, 632, 673
Antibonding energy level, 673, 677
Antiferromagnetism, 30, 32, 33, 56, 637, 852
Antimony, 31, 738, 739, 742
Aquadag, 217
Aqueous sample, 269
Aqueous solution cell, 294, 624
Areal density, 691
Area lineshape, 776, 784
Arsenic, 31
Atomic beam, 683
Atoms
    ESR, 488
    trapping, 652
ATR tube, 213
Attenuated total reflectance (ATR), 69
Attenuating materials, 217

903

narrowing, 590, 852
  rate of, 838
Extinction coefficient, 678, 691

F

Fabry-Perot. *See* Interferometer.
Faraday rotation, 220, 221, 318, 393, 509
Faraday's law, 59
Fast passage effect, 737
F centers, 31, 602, 666, 689, 690, 701
Feedback, 389, 451, 457, 576
Fermi contact interaction, 735
Fermi levels, 736
Ferrimagnetism, 30
Ferrite, 130, 186, 220, 221, 236, 312, 579
Ferromagnetic insulator, 726
Ferromagnetic resonance, 2, 725, 726
Ferromagnetism, 30, 32, 350ff, 639, 852
Filling factor, 291, 328, 524, 544, 547–549, 586, 716
Film, thick, 815
Filter, 190, 192, 243, 451, 471, 505, 679
Filtering, time domain, 577
Five-spin system. 825
Flange, 253, 255
Flip coil, 368
Flow meter, 642
Fluorenone, 631
Fluorescent light, 750
Fluoroacetophenone, 632
Folding function, 412
Forepump. *See* Pump, mechanical.
Foster's theorem, 131
Fourier analysis, 469
Fourier series, 397
Fourier transform, 839
Franck-Condon principle, 676
Free radicals, 30, 327, 683
Freeze-pump-thaw, 629
Fremy's salt, 591
Frenkel defect, 690
Frequency
  conversion, 433, 443, 577

cutoff, 99, 102, 108, 116, 119, 120
deviation, 460
domain, 717
intermediate, 208, 443
meter, 208, 226, 242, 277, 278, 328, 497, 501
microwave, choice of, 851
multiplier, 439
standard, 208, 380, 497
Frölich-Kennelly relation, 354

G

Gadolinium, 719, 729
Gain-band-width product, 509
Gallium arsenide (GaAs), 440
Galvanometer, 486
Gamma function, 782
Gamma ray, 7, 602, 665, 666, 671ff, 831
  anisotropy, 742
Gap
  klystron interaction, 169
  magnet, 347, 364
Gas
  discharge, 488, 489, 679, 681
  paramagnetic, 602
Gas constant, 603
Gasket
  gold, 653
  lead, 641
Gaussian line-shape, *See* Line-shape, Gaussian.
Gauss' law, 58
Gaussmeter. *See* Magnetometer.
Gauss' theorem. *See* Divergence theorem.
Generator
  harmonic, 181, 185, 187
  microwave, 169
Germanium, 440
  ESR, 31
German silver, 500
Gettering, 629
g factor
  anisotropic, 16, 181, 589, 851
  determination, 319

EMIS